# Obesity Surgery

## Patient Safety and Best Practices

Stephanie B. Jones, MD
Daniel B. Jones, MD, MS

Distributed by: Ciné-Med, Inc.
127 Main Street North
Woodbury, CT 06798
(203) 263-0006



ISBN: 978-0-9788890-4-3

Notice: Our knowledge in clinical sciences is constantly changing. As new information becomes available, changes in treatment and in the use of drugs or medical devices become necessary. The authors and the publisher of this volume have taken care to make certain that the doses of drugs, uses of medical devices, and schedules of treatment are correct and compatible with the standards generally accepted at the time of publication.

**Acknowledgements**

Special thanks to Dr. Walter Pories for allowing us to showcase both his talents—surgeon and cartoonist.

Printed in Canada

# About the Editors

STEPHANIE B. JONES is the Residency Program Director, Department of Anesthesia, Critical Care and Pain Medicine, Beth Israel Deaconess Medical Center, Boston, Massachusetts, and Assistant Professor of Anaesthesia, Harvard Medical School. Her clinical focus is the anesthetic implications of obesity, bariatric surgery, and minimally invasive surgery, and she is frequently asked to lecture on these topics. She is an active member of the American Society of Anesthesiologists and the Society for Education in Anesthesia. Dr. Jones has recently co-edited an online educational program on bariatric surgery with CRICO/RMF.

DANIEL B. JONES is Chief of Minimally Invasive Surgical Services, Beth Israel Deaconess Medical Center (BIDMC), Boston, Massachusetts, and Associate Professor of Surgery, Harvard Medical School. Dr. Jones is the recipient of the SAGES Gold Laparoscope Award (2001) and of the James IV Association Travel Award (2005). He serves on the Society of American Gastrointestinal and Endoscopic Surgeons Board of Governors, and he is an active member of the the American Society for Metabolic and Bariatric Surgery, American College of Surgeons' Bariatric Network Advisory Committee, Blue Cross Blue Shield of Massachuseets Bariatric Advisory Committee, and Besty Lehman Center Expert Panel on Weight Loss Surgery. He received his medical degree from Cornell University Medical College and master's degree in medical management from the University of Texas at Dallas. An internationally recognized leader in the field, he is the author of more than 150 professional publications, including the *LAP-BAND Companion Handbook* and *Weight Loss Surgery: A Multidisciplinary Approach*.

# Obesity Surgery

## *Patient Safety and Best Practices*

Stephanie B. Jones, MD
Daniel B. Jones, MD, MS

# Foreword

Josef E. Fischer, MD

Unless you've been in a coma or on the moon, you must be aware that obesity in this country is an epidemic. Depending on how you look at the numbers, if the criterion is a BMI, or body mass index of greater than $40kg/m^2$, there are approximately 20 million potential patients for bariatric surgery if other nonoperative means of reducing weight are not effective. That number of patients is far beyond our capacity, which is in the range of 150,000 to 200,000 patients per year. However, quality and safety is the major issue concerning all of surgery, but certainly concerning bariatric surgery. I do not recall any other procedure whose outcomes have been scrutinized as closely and thoroughly as bariatric surgery. Although the claims are that the mortality for bariatric surgery is in the range of 1% and the leak rate is less than that, other data collected by third parties indicate that the mortality rate may be as high as 5%. This is as yet uncorroborated because it comes largely from insurance data, and particularly of that dataset in which 8 or 9 fields are available for ICD-9 diagnoses, because patients tend to be transferred when they do not do well following operations. And the initial surgeon or hospital may not even be aware of a poor outcome.

Nonetheless, safety in bariatric surgery has become a national issue with wide media coverage. It is highly appropriate that this institution is not only the site of the Patient Safety in Obesity Surgery (PSOS) postgraduate course, but the origin of the Betsy Lehman criteria for safety now generally adopted throughout the United States by institutions of all descriptions, as well as by the Bariatric Surgical Task Force of the Blue Cross Blue Shield Foundation, on which I serve. Thus, when I say that this book is a little different, it is because we are concentrating in this book on making this procedure, or these series of procedures, safe and available to a broad range of individuals who will benefit from such a weight reduction procedure(s). It is clear that following such a procedure, there are real benefits to this patient population, particularly in the area of reduction of adult-onset diabetes and, in some studies, hypertension. Therefore, we should concentrate on making these procedures safer and more available under excellent circumstances within the guise of accredited programs that not only do a total assessment of the patient preoperatively, but follow them at least 5 years in a multidisciplinary group—including internists, nutritionists, psychiatrists, social workers, and nurse clinicians, as well as other individuals, such as physical therapists, to deal with these patients' multiple needs.

These patients are quite ill, and they should be looked upon as, for example, transplant, cardiac, or neurosurgical patients, in whom the outcomes are very clearly dependent on a multidisciplinary approach, as well as, when needed, intensive care.

This textbook is authoritative as well as unusual because of the nature and diversity of the participants, including among others, the Surgeon General of the United States, attorneys, CEOs of large health insurance companies, the press, and students at Harvard Medical School. And I would be equally negligent if I did not mention the quality of the faculty and the multiple fields they are from.

I would be remiss if I failed to mention the excellent editors, who in addition to supervising the PSOS course are intimately involved in making a robust surgical obesity program at the Beth Israel Deaconess Hospital a model of attention to detail, quality, and safety, a program in which all members of the team, regardless of position, are empowered to deliver the best possible outcome for the patient.

# Preface

Problems surrounding the field of weight loss surgery and specifically issues of patient safety have led to increasing public scrutiny and to appeals for solutions. Healthcare providers are left to address a growing number of difficult questions regarding patient selection, risk reduction, and surgical outcomes. As a result, the Massachusetts Department of Public Health has identified the need to undertake a systemic review of the processes involved in weight loss surgery. The Betsy Lehman Center for Patient Safety and Medical Error Reduction assembled a panel of experts from throughout the state of Massachusetts to review the current evidence and recommend best practice solutions. The American College of Surgeons, American Society for Metabolic and Bariatric Surgery, and recent National Institutes of Health Consensus Conference have expanded on these recommendations and established accreditation criteria.

In 2005, Harvard Medical School and Beth Israel Deaconess Medical Center in Boston hosted "Patient Safety in Obesity Surgery: Defining Best Practices" as a forum to debate emerging regulations and issues related to obesity, bariatric surgery, access to care, insurance coverage, and escalating liability. This conference provided the caregiver with the most up-to-date consensus in an effort to promote the highest standards in patient outcomes and safety. Unlike other continuing medical education courses in which doctors train doctors, this symposium invited not just surgeons, but also scientists, lawyers, the media, journalists, insurance companies, and government to address issues affecting all aspects of society. The expert panel reconvened in 2007 to update their recommendations, and in 2008, Harvard Medical School sponsored "Patient Safety in Obesity Surgery: Implementing Accreditation Standards and Best Practices". This book updates the issues in a rapidly evolving and increasing regulated field by world experts across various disciplines and industries.

With one third of Americans overweight and one fifth of Americans with severe obesity, we need solutions to this epidemic. It is our hope to summarize the thought leaders and stimulate a lot of good ideas for how we might proceed with dealing with this national health problem.

Stephanie B. Jones, MD
Assistant Professor
Harvard Medical School
Program Director, Anesthesiology
Beth Israel Deaconess Medical Center
Boston, Massachusetts

Daniel B. Jones, MD, MS, FACS
Associate Professor
Harvard Medical School
Director, Bariatric Program
Beth Israel Deaconess Medical Center
Boston, Massachusetts

# Contributors

Ebaa Al-Ozairi, BMSc, MD, MRCP
Diabetes Consultant
Joslin Diabetes Center
Boston, Massachusetts

Jeffrey W. Allen, MD
Associate Professor of Surgery
Department of Surgery
University of Louisville School of Medicine
Louisville, Kentucky

Caroline Apovian, MD
Associate Professor of Medicine
Boston University School of Medicine
Director, Nutrition and Weight Management Center
Boston Medical Center
Boston, Massachusetts

Jerry Berger
Director of Media Relations
Beth Israel Deaconess Medical Center
Boston, Massachusetts

George L. Blackburn, MD, PhD
S. Daniel Abraham Chair in Nutrition Medicine
Associate Director, Nutrition
Division of Nutrition
Harvard Medical School
Beth Israel Deaconess Medical Center
Boston, Massachusetts

Loren J. Borud, MD
Instructor in Surgery
Harvard Medical School
Department of Surgery
Beth Israel Deaconess Medical Center
Boston, Massachusetts

George A. Bray, MD
Boyd Professor
Pennington Biomedical Research Center
Louisiana State University
Baton Rouge, Louisiana

Stacy A. Brethauer, MD
Fellow, Advanced Laparoscopic & Bariatric Surgery
Cleveland Clinic Health System
Cleveland, Ohio

Captain Patricia A. Buss, MC, VSN
Deputy Chief Medical Officer
TRICARE Management Activity
US Department of Defense
Military Health System
Falls Church, Virginia

Richard H. Carmona, MD, MPH
Distinguished Professor of Public Health
Mel and Enid Zuckerman College of Public Health
University of Arizona
17th Surgeon General of the United States
Vice Chairman, Canyon Ranch
Tucson, Arizona

Justine M. Carr, MD
Assistant Professor of Medicine
Harvard Medical School
Director, Clinical Resource Management
Beth Israel Deaconess Medical Center
Boston, Massachusetts

Ronna M. Casper, MEd, LCSW
Staff Psychotherapist
Bariatric Program
Beth Israel Deaconess Medical Center
Boston, Massachusetts

Jaime Wilson-Chiru
Medical Student
Class of 2008
Harvard Medical School
Boston, Massachusetts

Ram Chuttani, MD
Assistant Professor of Medicine
Harvard Medical School
Director of Endoscopy
Chief, Interventional Gastroenterology
Beth Israel Deaconess Medical Center
Boston, Massachusetts

Anita P. Courcoulas, MD, MPH
Assistant Professor of Surgery
University of Pittsburgh School of Medicine
Chief, Minimally Invasive, Bariatric Surgery
University of Pittsburgh Medical Center
Pittsburgh, Pennsylvania

Susan Cummings, MS, RD
Clinical Programs Coordinator
Massachusetts General Hospital Weight Center
Massachusetts General Hospital
Boston, Massachusetts

# Contributors

Kristina Day, RD, LD
Research Dietitian
Beth Israel Deaconess Medical Center
Boston, Massachusetts

Eric J. DeMaria, MD
Professor and Vice Chair, Surgery
Director, Bariatric Surgery
Duke University Medical Center
Durham, North Carolina

Karen A. Donato, SM, RD
Coordinator, NHLBI Obesity Education Initiative
Center for the Application of Research Discoveries
National Heart, Lung, and Blood Institute
Bethesda, Maryland

Diana Cullum-Dugan, RD, LD
Clinical Coordinator
Nutrition & Weight Management Center
Boston Medical Center
Boston, Massachusetts

James Ellsmere, MD
Therapeutic Endoscopy Fellow
Beth Israel Deaconess Medical Center
Harvard Medical School
Boston, Massachusetts

Jacob Enterkin, BS
Medical University of South Carolina
Charleston, South Carolina

John A. Fallon, MD, MBA
Chief Physician Executive
Senior Vice President
Blue Cross Blue Shield of Massachusetts
Boston, Massachusetts

Madelyn Fernstrom, PhD, CNS
Associate Professor and Director
Weight Management Center
University of Pittsburgh Medical Center
Pittsburgh, Pennsylvania

Josef E. Fischer, MD
McDermott Professor of Surgery
Chairman, Department of Surgery
Harvard Medical School
Surgeon-in-Chief
Beth Israel Deaconess Medical Center
Boston, Massachusetts

David R. Flum, MD, MPH
Associate Professor of Surgery
University of Washington School of Medicine
Director, Surgical Outcomes Research Center
University of Washington Medical Center
Seattle, Washington

Michel Gagner, MD
Chairman, Department of Surgery
Mount Sinai Medical Center
Miami Beach, Florida

Victor F. Garcia, MD
Professor
University of Cincinnati College of Medicine
Department of Pediatric and Thoracic Surgery
Cincinnati Children's Hospital Medical Center
Cincinnati, Ohio

James Garver
Director of Reimbursement
USGI Medical
San Clemente, California

Dean J. Geraci, MSc
Director, Global Market Development
Covidien Healthcare
North Haven, Connecticut

Judy Giusti, MS, RD, LDN, CDE
Research Dietitian
Joslin Diabetes Center
Boston, Massachusetts

Isaac Greenberg, PhD
Assistant Professor of Psychiatry
Department of Psychiatry
Tufts Medical School
Boston, Massachusetts

Jennifer L. Greenman
Medical Student
Class of 2008
Harvard Medical School
Boston, Massachusetts

Ronit Grinbaum, MD
S. Daniel Abraham Surgery Research Fellow
Beth Israel Deaconess Medical Center
Boston, Massachusetts

# Contributors

Giselle G. Hamad, MD
Assistant Professor of Surgery
University of Pittsburgh Medical Center
Magee-Womens Hospital of UPMC
Pittsburgh, Pennsylvania

Osama Hamdy, MD, PhD
Medical Director
Obesity Clinical Program
Joslin Diabetes Center
Boston, Massachusetts

Robert Hanscom, JD
Vice President, Loss Prevention and Patient Safety
Risk Management Foundation
Harvard Medical Institutions
Cambridge, Massachusetts

Alan M. Harvey, MD, MBA
Instructor in Anesthesiology
Harvard Medical School
Director of Quality Assurance, Quality Improvement and Patient Safety
Department of Anesthesiology, Perioperative and Pain Medicine
Brigham and Women's Hospital
Boston, Massachusetts

Edward A. Hatchigian, MD, MS
Medical Director, Bariatric Surgery Program
Beth Israel Deaconess Medical Center
Boston, Massachusetts

Marcelo W. Hinojosa, MD
Resident, University of California, Irvine School of Medicine
Department of Surgery
Irvine, California

Colleen M. Hutchinson, MA
Professor, Graduate Studies
Rosemount College
Managing Editor, Bariatric Times
Matrix Medical Communications
Edgemont, Pennsylvania

Matthew M. Hutter, MD, MPH
Instructor in Surgery
Harvard Medical School
Codman Center for Clinical Effectiveness in Surgery
Massachusetts General Hospital
Boston, Massachusetts

Thomas H. Inge, MD, PhD
Associate Professor of Surgery and Pediatrics
University of Cincinnati College of Medicine
Comprehensive Weight Management Center
Cincinnati Children's Hospital Medical Center
Cincinnati, Ohio

Thomas James III, MD
President
Edgewater Medical Consulting LLC
Louisville, Kentucky

Daniel B. Jones, MD, MS
Associate Professor of Surgery
Harvard Medical School
Chief, Minimally Invasive Surgical Services
Director, Bariatric Program
Beth Israel Deaconess Medical Center
Boston, Massachusetts

R. Scott Jones, MD
Department of Surgery
University of Virginia Health System
Director, Division of Research - Optimal Patient Care
American College of Surgeons
Charlottesville, Virginia

Stephanie B. Jones, MD
Assistant Professor of Anesthesia
Harvard Medical School
Department of Anesthesiology
Beth Israel Deaconess Medical Center
Boston, Massachusetts

Lee Kaplan, MD, PhD
Associate Professor of Medicine
Massachussetts General Hospital
Boston, Massachusetts

Farid J. Kehdy, MD
Fellow, Minimally Invasive Surgery
UT Southwestern Medical Center
Dallas, Texas

John J. Kelly, MD
Associate Professor of Surgery
University of Massachusetts Medical School
Chief of General and Bariatric Surgery
UMASS/Memorial Medical Center
Worcester, Massachusetts

# Contributors

Sang W. Kim
Medical Student
Class of 2008
Harvard Medical School
Boston, Massachusetts

Karen Miller-Kovach, MBA, MS, RD
Chief Scientific Officer
Weight Watchers International, Inc.
New York, New York

Kenneth A. Larsen, DMin, PhD
Director, Clinical Psychology
Department of Medicine
New England Baptist Hospital
Boston, Massachusetts

Meng-G Martin Lee, MD
Clinical Fellow in Surgery
Beth Israel Deaconess Medical Center
Boston, Massachusetts

Barbara Lightizer, MS, MA, CPHRM
Director of Risk Management
Beth Israel Deaconess Medical Center
Boston, Massachusetts

Kevin Lobo
President
Ethicon-Endosurgery, Inc.
Cincinnati, Ohio

John L. McCarthy, MBA
President
CRICO/Risk Management Foundation of
the Harvard Medical Institutions
Cambridge, Massachusetts

Michelle McCleerey, PhD, MA, MEd, RN
Director, Patient Flow Solutions
Hill-Rom IT Solutions
Cary, North Carolina

Kevin McGovern
President
Ciné-Med, Inc.
Woodbury, Connecticut

Joseph Nadglowski, Jr.
President & CEO
Obesity Action Coalition
Tampa, Florida

Ninh T. Nguyen, MD
Chief, Division of GI Surgery
University of California, Irvine Medical Center
Orange, California

Torsten Olbers, MD, PhD
Department of Surgery
Sahlgrenska University Hospital
Göteborg, Sweden

Robin F. Pearson
Senior Director, Project Management
SynerMed Communications
Califon, New Jersey

Tracy S. Pitt, DO
Clinical Fellow
Advanced Laparoscopic and Bariatric Surgery
Cleveland Clinic Health System
Cleveland, Ohio

Alfons Pomp, MD
Frank Glenn Faculty Scholar
Associate Professor of Surgery
Section of Laparoscopic Surgery
Weill Cornell Medical College
Mount Sinai Medical Center
New York, New York

Walter J. Pories, MD
Professor of Surgery, Biochemistry and Exercise and Sport Science
The Brody School of Medicine
East Carolina University
Greenville, North Carolina

Kinga A. Powers, MD, PhD
Minimally Invasive Surgery
Cambridge Hospital
Cambridge, Massachusetts

Gary M. Pratt, BS
Chief Executive Officer
Surgical Review Corporation
Raleigh, North Carolina

Janey S.A. Pratt, MD
Instructor in Surgery
Harvard Medical School
Assistant Surgeon
Massachusetts General Hospital
Boston, Massachusetts

# Contributors

Aurora D. Pryor, MD
Department of Surgery
Duke University Medical Center
Durham, North Carolina

Scott Rehrig, MD, LTCMC
Director
Bariatric Surgery
Walter Reed Hospital
Bethesda, Maryland

Christine Ren, MD
Associate Professor of Surgery
New York University School of Medicine
Department of Surgery
New York University Medical Center
New York, New York

Nancy Ridley, MS
Director
Betsy Lehman Center for Patient Safety and Medical Error Reduction
Boston, Massachusetts

Jo-Anne Rizzotto, MEd, RD, LDN, CDE
Joslin Hospital
Boston, Massachusetts

Malcolm K. Robinson, MD
Assistant Professor of Surgery
Harvard Medical School
Director, Program for Weight Management
Brigham and Women's Hospital
Boston, Massachusetts

Daniel S. Rooks, PhD
Assistant Professor of Medicine
Center for Nutrition Medicine
Harvard Medical School
Beth Israel Deaconess Medical Center
Boston, Massachusetts

James C. Rosser, Jr., MD
Chief, Minimally Invasive Surgery
Director, Advanced Medical Technology Institute
Beth Israel Medical Center
New York, New York

Thomas R. Russell, MD
Executive Director
American College of Surgeons
Chicago, Illinois

Donna H. Ryan, MD
Professor and Associate Executive Director
Pennington Biomedical Research Center
Louisiana State University
Baton Rouge, Louisiana

Kenneth Sands, MD, MPH
Assistant Professor of Medicine
Harvard Medical School
Vice President, Health Care Quality
Beth Israel Deaconess Medical Center
Boston, Massachusetts

Luke Sato, MD
Chief Medical Officer & Vice President
CRICO/Risk Management Foundation
Harvard Medical Institutions
Cambridge, Massachusetts

Philip R. Schauer, MD
Director, Bariatric Surgery Program
Cleveland Clinic Health System
Cleveland, Ohio

Benjamin E. Schneider, MD
Instructor in Surgery
Harvard Medical School
Department of Surgery
Beth Israel Deaconess Medical Center
Boston, Massachusetts

Robert S. Schneider, MSW
Vice President, Professional Relations
SynerMed Communications
Califon, New Jersey

Daniel J. Scott, MD
Associate Professor
Director, Southwestern Center for MIS
UT Southwestern Medical Center
Dallas, Texas

Scott A. Shikora, MD
Professor of Surgery
Tufts University School of Medicine
Tufts-New England Medical Center
Boston, Massachusetts

Peter H. Soderberg
President & CEO
Hill-Rom and Hillenbrand Industries
Batesville, Indiana

# Contributors

Jonathan Waks
Medical Student
Class of 2008
Harvard Medical School
Boston, Massachusetts

Angela Walsh, RN, MA, CNOR
MIS Nurse Educator
Lap-Band Program Coordinator
Beth Israel Deaconess Medical Center
Boston, Massachusetts

Katherine A. Wang
Research Assistant
Beth Israel Deaconess Medical Center
Boston, Massachusetts

Christina C. Wee, MD, MPH
Assistant Professor of Medicine
Harvard Medical School
Director of Health Services and Behavioral Research in Obesity
Division of General Medicine and Primary Care
Beth Israel Deaconess Medical Center
Boston, Massachusetts

Samuel E. Wilson, MD
Professor, Associate Dean, Affiliated Institutions
Department of Surgery
University of California, Irvine
School of Medicine
Irvine, California

Bruce M. Wolfe, MD
Professor of Surgery
Oregon Health and Science University
Portland, Oregon

James Zervios
Director of Communications
Obesity Action Coalition
Tampa, Florida

# Obesity: Public Enemy Number One

Richard H. Carmona, MD, MPH, FACS

The problem of obesity is a significant one. What is our country going to look like in 10, 15, 20, or 30 years? What will our society look like? Most likely, the economic burden will have doubled. The disease burden will be at least that much and, as such, will be unsustainable.

Add to these concerns the issue of what the workforce will be like in the future. Raising a generation that is not physically fit, presents the specter of higher rates of cardiovascular disease, cancer, and so many other comorbidities, leaving us to ask who will be the soldiers, sailors, firefighters, and police of tomorrow? Who will do the heavy work of construction, of building, when we're raising an infirm generation and doing nothing to break that cycle? And who is going to pay for all that health care? The fact is, we may be raising the first generation that will live fewer years than their parents.

Yes, we have an extraordinary challenge before us. But how did we get to this point? When I first came into office as Surgeon General, I was challenged with lawsuits. Everybody wanted me to file *amicus* briefs. "Go to court," they said. "Sue all the fast food places because they're why we have this obesity epidemic!"

That's not so. It's a multifaceted ideology. Lots of variables contribute to it and when you actually go back to the genesis, we see a society that changed over a period of decades.

In the past 20 years, the rates of overweight have doubled in children and tripled in adolescents. Today, nearly 2 out of every 3 American adults and 15% of American kids are overweight or obese. That's more than 9 million children—1 in every 7 kids—at increased risk of weight-related chronic diseases.

These facts are astounding, but they are just the beginning of a chain reaction of dangerous health problems, many of which were once associated only with adults. Today's pediatricians are diagnosing an increasing number of children with type 2 diabetes, which used to be known as adult-onset diabetes. Research indicates that one third of all children born in 2000 will develop type 2 diabetes during their lifetime. Tragically, people with type 2 diabetes are at increased risk of developing heart disease, stroke, kidney disease, and blindness. These complications are likely to appear much earlier in life for those who develop type 2 diabetes in childhood or adolescence.

Because of the increasing rates of obesity, unhealthy eating habits, and physical inactivity, we may well see the first generation that will be less healthy and have a shorter life expectancy than their parents. And the economic costs of obesity are staggering, second only to the cost of tobacco use.

The good news is that there is still time to reverse this dangerous trend in our children's lives. As US Surgeon General, I traveled the nation talking to students as part of my "50 Schools in 50 States" initiative. I've seen all kinds of kids—kids of different races, ethnicities, backgrounds, and upbringings. But one thing is constant: too many of them are living unhealthy lifestyles. You can tell this just by looking at them. I love seeing their bright smiling faces, full of hope and happiness. But what they don't know about excess weight could end up killing them in a few decades.

It is very important for parents to take responsibility. We must teach our children to enjoy healthy foods in healthy portions and encourage them to be physically active for at least 60 minutes per day. The average American child spends more than 4 hours per day looking at some kind of screen. "Parents," we must say, "make the healthy choices: turn off the TV and the video games. Go outside with your kids, play ball, go for a walk. Talk with your children. Spend quality time with them, and when you're together as a family, do something active."

Kids don't automatically know how important it is to be physically active for an hour a day. They don't all know that they need 5 to 9 servings of fruits and vegetables per day. That concept is part of what I'm talking about with Americans of all ages: increasing our "health literacy."

Health literacy is the ability to access, understand, and use health-related information and services to make appropriate decisions. We must close the gap between what health professionals know and what parents and children understand about physical activity and healthy eating. Every morning people wake up and, while they're sitting at the kitchen table, they read the newspaper and the cereal box. Throughout the day they read the nutritional information on their meals and on their snacks. But do they really understand the information they're reading? Can parents explain it to their children, who see tantalizing "kid food" products that they don't know are loaded with sugar and fat?

To make healthy choices, parents and children need easy-to-understand information that fits into their busy lifestyles. Many people, even educated Americans, don't know what a calorie is, or how to burn it. It's our job to make that kind of health information meaningful and helpful. We must promote healthy living, improve health literacy, and encourage healthier lifestyles so that we can end our nation's obesity problem before it has a chance to reach into another generation of Americans. Working together, industry, government, and individuals can achieve these goals.

*Richard H. Carmona, MD, MPH, FACS, is the 17th Surgeon General of the United States, vice chairman of Canyon Ranch, and distinguished professor of public health at the Mel and Enid Zuckerman College of Public Health at the University of Arizona. On October 12, 2006, Dr. Carmona addressed the 2006 Obesity Congress at Cleveland Clinic as a keynote speaker. The above remarks are excerpted from that address and are used with permission.*

# The Science of Weight Loss Surgery

Lee M. Kaplan, MD, PhD

This chapter provides a brief overview of the pathophysiology of obesity and the role of the gastrointestinal (GI) tract in body weight regulation. Recent studies suggest that many bariatric surgical procedures induce weight loss and improved metabolic function primarily by altering basic neuroendocrine physiology. Knowledge of these mechanisms is a necessary prerequisite to the most appropriate, effective, and safe use of these procedures. Moreover, this understanding will accelerate ongoing efforts to develop more effective surgical, endoscopic, and pharmacologic treatments of obesity and its complications, including type 2 diabetes and other metabolic disorders.

## A Balance of Energy

At the most basic level, body weight is simply a reflection of energy ingested vs. energy expended, with a modest adjustment to account for energy ingested and excreted in the stool unabsorbed. In most cases, less than 5% of ingested energy is excreted, so these losses have a minimal effect on total energy balance. By this analysis, obesity results from an excess of energy ingested compared with that expended. Although this approach is consistent with the laws of thermodynamics, it is insufficient to explain the physiologic mechanisms that govern weight and energy homeostasis in the human body. Superimposed on the laws of physics is a weight regulatory system in the brain that seeks to maintain an appropriate, usually stable, level of body energy reserves, nearly all of which are in the form of triglycerides stored in fat. This system is biologically determined (see "Genes and Environment" below) and varies widely from person to person. The net outcome of this physiological system is that the body defends its own "energy set point." Significant deviation—in either direction—from that set point results in the activation of a physiological response that tends to return the body to its chosen baseline. The effects of this powerful regulatory mechanism are felt over extended periods, with the body matching food intake and energy expenditure over days, weeks, and months. For most people, this homeostatic system is extremely accurate, matching energy intake and energy expenditure within a tolerance of less than 0.15% over one's adult life. Even in the setting of severe obesity, the long-term mismatch between energy intake and expenditure generally does not exceed a small percentage. The unanswered question is why some people defend an energy set point that puts them in the overweight or obesity category and why it is so difficult to return that set point toward normal. Achieving the latter goal is the "holy grail" of obesity therapy. Among currently available treatments for obesity, gastrointestinal weight loss surgery (GIWLS) may be the most effective. Unfortunately, highly effective GI surgical approaches also come with significant risks.

## Genes and Environment

A much debated subject is the role of genetic and environmental factors in the genesis of obesity. As with all biologic phenomena and diseases, both hereditary and environmental factors play an important role. Neither works in isolation, and obesity results from the unfortunate synergy between the two. Genes determine the basic design characteristics of the human body, the color of our eyes and hair, our height, and to a significant extent, our weight. But genes don't work in isolation. For both height and weight, our genes also determine how susceptible we are to the current environment. Since we have evolved as a species in an environment where food is occasionally scarce and where gathering or cultivation requires a great deal of physical effort, our genes have slowly adapted to this environmental reality. As a result, most of us have evolved genetically to protect us against starvation. While we have also evolved powerful protections against obesity as well, for many people, they are not powerful enough to protect against obesity *in the current environment.* The rapid rise in the rates and severity of obesity worldwide is a reflection of the changing environment. This fat-promoting, or *adipogenic*, environment causes susceptible individuals to generate weight gain and obesity, and each of us is variably influenced by these environmental factors, depending on our genetic makeup. Therefore, people whose ancestors may have experienced repeated famines may be particularly susceptible to the current adipogenic environment, and those whose ancestors never experienced food scarcity may be best protected against the current environment. Our current adipogenic environment results from a variety of changes in modern society, most notably the high abundance and accessibility of food and the dramatically diminished need for physical activity in order to live, succeed, and gain pleasure. Other aspects of the current environment that may play an equally important role include the *content* of highly processed food, irregular eating and meal patterns, increased stress, the rapid pace of life, chronic mild sleep deprivation, and lack of reward from our other activities and interactions. Indviduals react differently to these various environmental influences, and which of these factors is most important in promoting obesity likely varies from person to person. Therefore, rather than considering obesity as a single disorder, it may be better to consider it as a *symptom* of different disorders in different people. There may be several, or several dozen different *obesities*, each of which requires a somewhat different approach. We cannot identify each of them by name, but we recognize the differences among people with obesity by their size, body composition, distribution of body fat, age of obesity onset, pattern of comorbidities, resting and involuntary activity-associated energy expenditure, and eating behaviors, among others. There are at least several hundred different genes (some scientists estimate more than 1,000) that help determine body weight and metabolic activity, with countless minor variations or combinations that may predispose us to obesity and other metabolic diseases. Each of us has a unique genetic makeup, and thus each of us has a distinct *pattern* of susceptibility (or resistance) to the current adipogenic environment.

### Why Study Weight Loss Surgery?

Most importantly, weight loss surgery works. Gastrointestinal weight loss surgery works better than anything else that we currently have in our armamentarium, but we don't fully understand how. When gastric bypass was initially developed in the 1960s, it was thought to work primarily by simple mechanical restriction of food intake, augmented by malabsorption of ingested calories. More recent studies have dramatically altered our thinking about how this operation works, and we now know that durable weight loss and improvement in metabolic function result primarily from its ability to alter the basic physiology of body weight regulation. In effect, gastric bypass and other GIWLS procedures counteract the physiological response to the adipogenic environment. Even in operations that clearly cause malabsorption of ingested calories, such as the biliopancreatic diversion and the earlier jejunoileal bypass, weight loss mechanisms are more complex and physiologic. After these malabsorptive procedures, people eat *less* than they did before surgery, which would not be typical of a purely malabsorptive state. Other mechanisms must therefore be invoked to account for the observed clinical effects of these procedures, several of which are discussed below.

Clinical experience has shown that the effectiveness of each GIWLS procedure varies among individuals in ways that appear independent of variations in surgical technique, surgeon skill, and patient compliance. These variations suggest that these operations could be improved upon, perhaps by complementing them with other therapies. Understanding the physiological mechanisms by which these operations work and the basis for variation in clinical response will point the way toward improved surgical techniques, better procedure selection for individual patients, and development of appropriate combination therapies. In this way, the operations themselves can be made more effective for a greater number of patients without adding to their risk, thereby improving the overall benefit-risk ratio.

### The Pathophysiology of Obesity

At its core, obesity reflects excess body fat stores, which result from an imbalance between energy ingested and energy expended. However, this simple description does not reflect the body's normal—and powerful—homeostatic mechanisms, which are designed to maintain a very tight relationship between energy intake and expenditure. There is a very elaborate system to maintain energy balance within a very narrow range. Several feedback regulatory mechanisms, including proteins secreted from fat (e.g., leptin), signal body fat stores to the brain. The brain integrates these signals with information about recent food intake signaled by the GI tract, metabolic needs signaled by the liver, muscle, bone and fat itself, and the external environment signaled by sensory organs and the cerebral cortex, to make decisions about food intake, handling of ingested nutrients, and energy expenditure.

Communication between the GI tract and the central nervous system is mediated by endocrine and neuronal mechanisms. These signals have long been known to exert short- and long-term effects over food ingestion. The fact that they also have an important role in regulating body weight is evident from the effectiveness of GIWLS, which alters these signals in a manner that generates substantial and durable weight loss and improved metabolic function. The body, through all of these regulatory systems, defends a physiologically determined energy set point. If we arbitrarily move away from this set point by decreasing our food intake acutely, increased hunger is compensated for by conservation of energy expenditure so that a positive energy balance is maintained and that lost weight is regained. Acute overeating creates the opposite effect, with increased energy expenditure, decreased hunger, and fullness after smaller meals, all of which lead to negative energy balance and a return to the baseline weight.

Gastrointestinal weight loss surgery exploits these mechanisms to change the energy set point. Of the available options, Roux-en-Y gastric bypass (RYGB) is the most commonly used GIWLS procedure—exhibits the most favorable risk-benefit characteristics for most patients with severe or medically complicated obesity. As described by Pories and others more than a decade ago, RYGB is extremely effective, leading to excess body weight loss (EBWL) of approximately 70% within the first 1½ to 2 years and long-term average regain of 25% of the lost weight over the lifetime of the patient. Despite these excellent results overall, there is a substantial (>fourfold) variability in EBWL among individual patients. Interestingly, the EBWL is normally distributed, suggesting that biological variability among patients is responsible for the observed differences in outcome. Although many people have argued that the outcomes after surgery are largely dependent upon details of the surgical technique, surgeon ability, or patient compliance, none of these explanations is adequate to explain this highly normal and continuous distribution. This variation is most consistent with a *physiological* heterogeneity among patients in terms of their responsiveness to this operation. Moreover, it suggests that the response to surgery itself is physiological, that surgery somehow induces physiological changes to exert its weight loss and metabolic effects.

We and others have been trying to identify clinical predictors of weight loss after GIWLS. To date, the strongest independent predictors of limited EBWL have been restricted exercise or movement capacity, the presence of diabetes mellitus, higher initial BMI, increased age, and decreased participation in postoperative visits. None of these factors is strong enough, however, to determine the appropriate use of GIWLS. For example, even though patients with diabetes tend to lose less weight than those without diabetes, the improvement in the diabetes after surgery easily offsets the minor differences in weight loss. Similarly, none of the other predictors of diminished weight loss is sufficient to exclude patients from consideration of surgery. Together, these factors account for very little of the variation in outcome after GIWLS, suggesting that the variability may be due to as of yet undiscovered causes, which may serve as more useful guides for determining when obesity should be treated surgically and which operation is best for individual patients.

### Mechanisms of Action of GIWLS

Regardless of differences among procedures and among indvidual patients, the most important issue is why surgical weight loss therapy is so effective. Why is it so much better than behavior-based therapy, diet, exercise, or pharmacological interventions? Historically, surgery has been thought to work primarily by mechanical means—physical restriction of food intake and/or induction of malabsorption by bypassing digestive and absorptive GI mucosa. More recently, however, several lines of evidence have accumulated suggesting that these operations work by altering the physiology of body weight and metabolic control mechanisms. There are a number of clinical observations that support a physiological mechanism for the effects of weight loss surgery, particularly gastric and intestinal bypass operations. First, weight is remarkably stable late after surgery. After RYGB, weight regain over long periods of time (10 years and beyond) is about 25% of the weight lost initially. In the short term, however, most patients find that they regulate their body weight within a far more narrow range after the surgery than they did beforehand. Second, patients describe dramatic reduction in hunger, augmented and accelerated post-prandial satiety, and decreased reward-based, or emotional, eating after RYGB. As a result, they don't feel deprived after surgery as they typically do with restrictive dieting. Third, as noted above, there is a broad and normal distribution of weight loss after this procedure. Fourth, despite the fact that nearly all patients lose a substantial amount of weight, few (<5%) achieve a normal weight (BMI $\leq 25$ kg/m$^2$). More importantly, in the absence of surgical complications, virtually no patients become underweight. Fifth, patients who become pregnant after gastric bypass gain weight normally during the pregnancy, suggesting that there is a way for the body to temporarily override the effects of the operation. Moreover, in nearly all patients, food intake increased late after surgery, in most cases without an increase in weight. Although many surgical series have identified a correlation between a later increase in food intake and weight gain, patients in these series are generally identified by their increase in weight late after surgery. Most patients eat more late after surgery, and the vast majority of them don't regain a substantial amount of weight. Finally, using animal models, we have observed that RYGB *increases* total energy expenditure, which is the opposite of what one would expect if the surgery worked primarily by mechanical (restrictive or malabsorptive) mechanisms.

To examine the mechanisms of response to GIWLS, we and others have developed several rodent models of these operations. The effects are remarkably similar in rat and mouse models and in humans. We developed these rodent models because we thought that they could help characterize mechanisms of weight loss and improved metabolic function in more detail than can be done in humans. We have been particularly interested in determining the mechanisms of improvement in comorbidities, including whether improved insulin sensitivity results primarily from the associated weight loss, altered food intake, or other neuroendocrine mechanisms arising directly from the manipulation of the GI tract. These models also allow identification and examination of the parameters that are critical to the success of the surgery, including specific anatomic considerations (e.g., type of procedure, pouch size, anastomotic diameter, limb length) that have been suggested, but not proven to influence short- and long-term outcomes after these procedures. These models are also useful for identifying mechanisms and effective treatment of potential complications of surgery, most notably micronutrient deficiencies, metabolic bone disease, and alterations in other endocrine functions.

Of course, every model has its limitations. The anatomy of the GI tract and its innervation differs between rodents and humans. Patterns of food intake, sites and regulation of energy expenditure, and some aspects of the regulation of glucose homeostasis also differ among these species. However, the overall structure of these regulatory circuits and the major physiological, cellular, and molecular components are remarkably well conserved, making he animal models an important and very useful tool to further our understanding. Most importantly, the role of the hypothalamus, adipose tissue, and GI tracts in regulating weight appear highly similar across species, and we have obtained strong evidence for similar conservation of mechanisms of GIWLS.

What do the animal models of GIWLS reveal? In our earliest studies, we found that after RYGB, rats with diet-induced obesity lose approximately 25% of their total body weight compared with sham-operated control animals. Instead of continuing to gain weight over time as is typical for untouched or sham-operated rats, they stop accumulating body fat. Indeed, after RYGB, these rats initially lose some weight because of the overnight fasting and catabolic effects of the surgery, then their weights stabilize, and they maintain a stable weight for the rest of their lives. To determine mechanisms contributing to this profound weight loss, we examined food intake, nutrient absorption, and energy expenditure after RYGB. Not surprisingly, this operation leads to a 20% decrease in food intake across several months postoperatively. We found no evidence of macronutrient malabsorption or significant change in absorption after this procedure. We were surprised to find that RYGB causes a net *increase* in energy expenditure compared with animals that underwent a sham operation. Sham-operated animals, who were fed the same amount of food as was eaten spontaneously by RYGB-treated rats only lost half as much weight. Therefore, approximately half of the weight loss after RYGB in this model results from decreased food intake, and the other half from increased total energy expenditure. Further evidence that RYGB increases energy expenditure is that the animals that have undergone this procedure are warmer by about 0.4°C than their sham-operated counterparts. Therefore, GIWLS, particularly RYGB, has unique and remarkable effects that distinguish it from other forms of weight loss. After dieting, appetite increases as a result of increased hunger, decreased satiety after meals, and increased reward- or emotion-based desire to eat. Energy expenditure is conserved, and stress responses are enhanced. After RYGB, all of these effects go in the opposite direction. These effects of diet are consistent with the generation of a counter-regulatory response to reverse or limit the weight loss (i.e., to defend a set point for energy storage). In contrast, RYGB appears to alter the physiology of weight regulation to drive the animal or patient to a new, lower energy set point and stable weight. This effect likely results from altered neural and endocrine signaling from the manipulated GI tract to the rest of the body, including the brain, pancreas, and liver. The specific signals involved remain poorly understood, although there is accumulating evidence that diminished gastric secretion of ghrelin, and augmented postprandial secretion of peptide YY and glucagon-like peptide-1 contribute to the effects of several of these operations.

So which of the GI manipulations included in the RYGB are responsible for the effects of this operation? It is convenient to consider RYGB as 5 operations in one. These components include (1) isolation of the gastric cardia, the so-called "restrictive" component, (2) exclusion of the distal stomach from the nutrient flow, (3) exclusion of the duodenum and proximal jejunum, (4) exposure of the distal jejunum to undigested and unabsorbed nutrients, and (5) partial vagotomy necessitated by the division of the stomach. To sort out which parts of the RYGB are responsible for the physiological effects of this operation, we have developed several additional rodent surgical models, including a rat model of adjustable gastric banding (AGB). The structure of the adjustable band is similar to that used in humans, but adapted to accommodate the reduced size and altered gastric anatomy of the rat. In this model, after surgical placement, the band is adjusted every three days through the subcutaneous port rather than every 6 weeks (in humans) because of the accelerated metabolic activity and physiological processes in the rat. In diet-induced obese rats, AGB induces approximately half the weight loss of RYGB, similar to what is seen in humans. Band placement and adjustment is associated with significantly diminished food intake, although to a somewhat lesser degree than after RYGB in the same model. Most notably, there is no change in body temperature after AGB, suggesting that it does not cause the same stimulatory effect on energy expenditure as RYGB. Also, unlike RYGB, which induces decreased ghrelin levels in obese animals, AGB in rats causes an *increase* in plasma ghrelin levels. This is similar to the effect of AGB in humans and to the ghrelin changes after diet-induced weight loss in both humans and rodents. Therefore, there is a substantial difference in the mechanisms by which these 2 operations work, both in terms of their effects on energy expenditure and on circulating ghrelin levels.

Overall, these animal models appear to provide an accurate reflection of the human situation. Weight loss is substantial and durable in both species. The relative effects of RYGB and AGB are similar in both species, with AGB inducing one half to two thirds the weight loss associated with RYGB. The effects of the 2 operations on circulating ghrelin levels are similar in humans and rats, and the effects of these operations on food intake and nutrient absorption are similar. Rodent models can provide important information unavailable from human studies. There is broad variation in the human population that likely accounts for the observed variable response to surgery and can interfere with analyzing the mechanisms of these operations. Genetic, environmental, and behavioral variations are much easier to control in rodents, allowing for much more detailed and sensitive exploration of underlying mechanisms. Moreover, we can exploit the large variety of genetic models, particularly in the mouse, that can elucidate these mechanisms even more definitively.

In summary, GIWLS works by altering the physiology of body weight and metabolic regulation so as to move the patient to a new, lower energy storage set point. In the cases of AGB and RYGB at least, surgical therapy induces decreased food intake without nutrient malabsorption. Food intake also appears to decrease after biliopancreatic diversion and the duodenal switch operations, suggesting that even these malabsorptive procedures induce weight loss primarily by altering the basic physiology of body weight and metabolic regulation. The physiological changes induced by these surgical manipulations of the GI tract inhibit the adipogenic influences of diet and the environment. These operations defeat the powerful mechanisms for the defense against starvation that appears to be inappropriately overactive in obesity. The extraordinary effectiveness of GIWLS suggests that the search for new, effective therapies for obesity should aim to find those that share several critical features with the surgery. These critical features include promoting changes in the energy set point, influencing the weight regulatory system at multiple levels, and blunting the environmental influences on body weight and metabolic function that have caused the twin epidemics of obesity and diabetes in the first place. Surgery is a blunt tool that likely works by affecting several components of the weight regulatory system simultaneously. It is therefore likely that combination therapies will be the most effective approach, and that therapies targeted to individuals with different subtypes of obesity will provide the greatest benefit for the greatest number of patients. These considerations predict that single-drug therapies are not likely to be very effective in the majority of patients with obesity. However, combinations of drugs, or combinations of drugs and devices, in concert with behavior modification and dietary interventions, should one day be able to mimic the mechanisms and reproduce the benefits that, to date, have only been associated with GIWLS.

**Suggested Reading**

1. Badman MK, Flier JS. The gut and energy balance: visceral allies in the obesity wars. *Science*. 2005;307:1909-14.

2. Cummings DE, Overduin J, Foster-Schubert KE. Gastric bypass for obesity: mechanisms of weight loss and diabetes resolution. *J Clin Endocrinol Metab*. 2004;89(6):2608-15.

3. Kaplan LM. Body weight regulation and obesity. *J Gastrointest Surg*. 2003;7(4):443-51.

4. Morton GJ, Cummings DE, Baskin DG, Barsh GS, Schwartz MW. Central nervous system control of food intake and body weight. *Nature*. 2006;443:289-95.

5. Murphy KG, Bloom SR. Gut hormones and the regulation of energy homeostasis. *Nature*. 2006;444:854-9.

# NHLBI Clinical Guidelines on Overweight and Obesity in Adults

Karen A. Donato, SM, RD

The *Clinical Guidelines on the Identification, Evaluation, and Treatment of Overweight and Obesity in Adults: The Evidence Report,* released in 1998 by the National Heart, Lung, and Blood Institute (NHLBI) and the National Institute of Diabetes and Digestive and Kidney Diseases (NIDDK), presented the first federal, evidence-based guidelines developed for managing and assessing the overweight patient. The guidelines have been endorsed by the coordinating committees of the National Cholesterol Education Program and the National High Blood Pressure Education Program, the North American Association for the Study of Obesity, the NIDDK Clinical Obesity Research Panel, and the American Heart Association. These groups represent 54 professional societies, government agencies, and consumer organizations. This chapter includes information on the following topics: the development of the clinical guidelines, key recommendations from the guidelines, and examples of products and resources developed in order to put the guidelines into formats appropriate for practitioners and clinicians.

The creation of clinical guidelines depends on many things: the prevalence rates of obesity in the population, the existing science based on the health benefits from treatment, and the need for guidelines in primary care practice. For obesity, we examined the national data on adult overweight and obesity prevalence available from the National Health and Nutrition Examination Surveys (NHANES), as well as the Centers for Disease Control and Prevention (CDC) state-based maps. Regarding the issue of benefit from treatment, the panel examined the evidence on whether weight loss improves the health status for overweight or obese individuals. Lastly, an environmental scan was done to ascertain whether such a guideline was needed in primary care.

Getting clinical guidelines utilized in primary care is challenging. It is even more challenging when the issue is overweight and obesity. Primary care providers often don't feel comfortable addressing the issue, or knowledgeable enough to be successful in its treatment. Once the expert panel's clinical guidelines are final, NHLBI staff works to provide the information in a number of formats helpful to primary care. These include a variety of educational tools, continuing education modules, and patient materials based on the clinical guidelines for use in different settings.

### Development of Evidence-Based Clinical Guidelines

In 1995, prior to starting the clinical guidelines, the NHANES prevalence rate of overweight and obesity in adults was approximately 55% of the adult population, or 97 million Americans.

**Figure 1a**

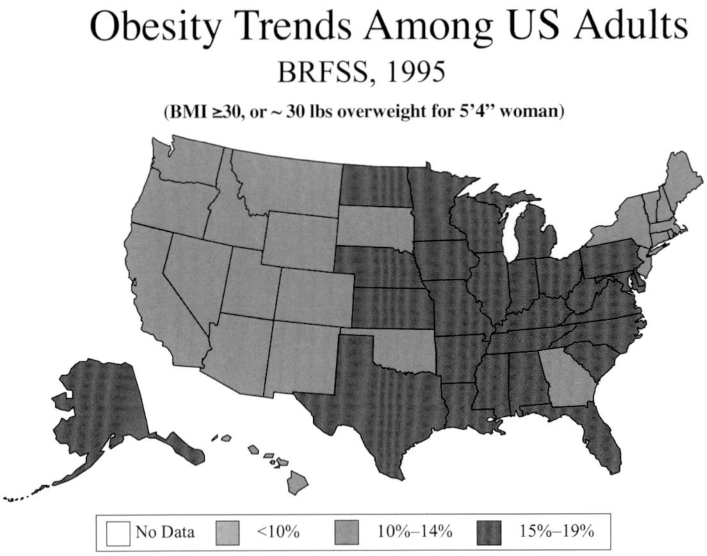


**Figure 1b**

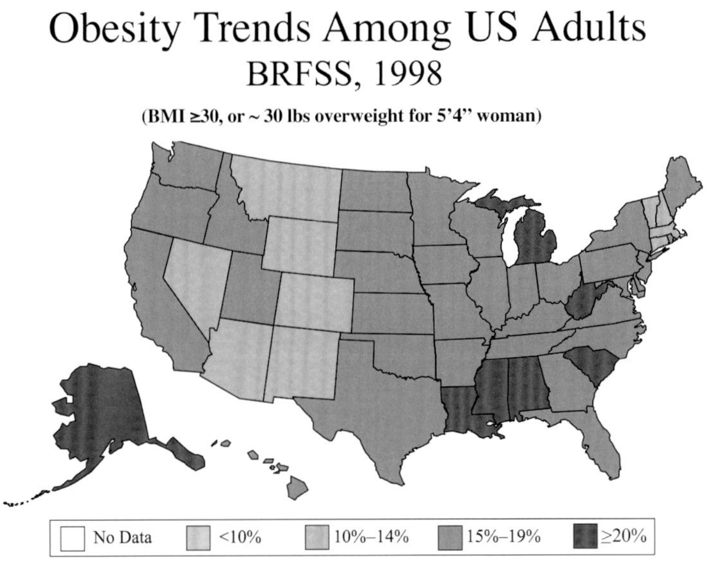


Looking at the CDC's state-based maps of the trends in obesity rates from the Behavioral Risk Factor Surveillance System (BRFSS) from 1995 (when we began the guidelines process) to 1998 (when we released the guidelines), it is clear that obesity was worsening (Figures 1a and 1b). The guidelines were needed more than ever. Even 5 years after we issued the guidelines, the maps continued to show even more states with high obesity rates in adults (Figure 1c).

Figure 1c

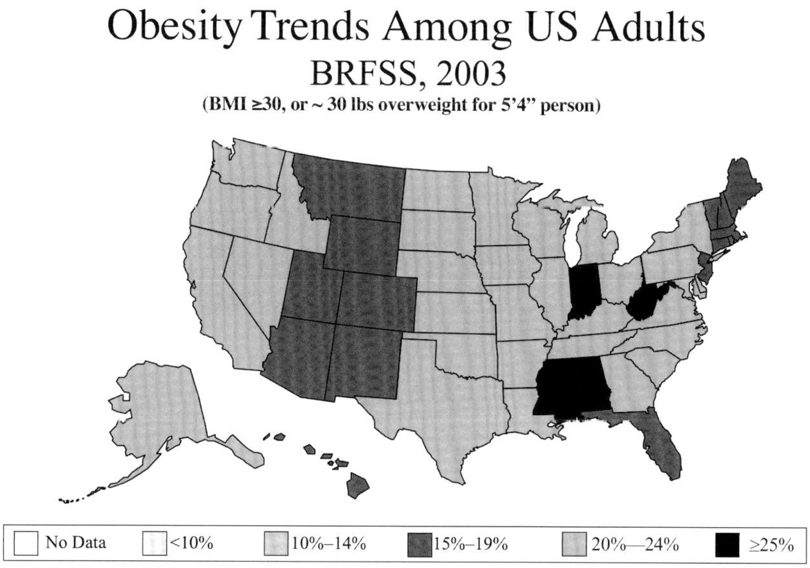


Creating evidence-based clinical guidelines requires that a methodology and a systematic review process be put into place. The following items were critical to the process: composition of the panel and its charge; creation of the evidence model; systematic review of the literature that involved inclusion and exclusion criteria, data abstraction, and development of evidence tables; and finally, development of criteria to rank the literature. The interdisciplinary expert panel consisted of 24 members, chaired by Dr. Xavier Pi-Sunyer from St. Luke's Roosevelt Hospital/Columbia University. The panel's charge was to examine the scientific evidence on overweight and obesity in adults as it pertains to: 1) other heart disease risk factors such as hypertension, blood lipid levels, and diabetes; 2) the distribution and amount of body fat as it influences risk; 3) the independent relationship of obesity to coronary heart disease (CHD); and 4) the relationship of obesity to sleep apnea. The panel also considered the evidence on

- Whether or not weight loss affects disease risk factors
- The impact of increased body fat on risk factors
- Options for treatment that can be performed in a clinical setting

In addition to the scientific review, the panel was charged to develop guidelines that would be appropriate for the practicing physician and other healthcare providers dealing with overweight patients, and to make the guidelines concise, comprehensive, and easy to use.

**Evidence Model**

In order to systematize the evidence review, the panel first had to develop an evidence model that outlined all of the topics for which the evidence had to be examined. The critical portion of the *evidence model* pertained to the evidence on the effects of treatment strategies on the overweight patient in terms of weight loss, and changes in fitness and abdominal fat, independent of weight loss. It also addressed various treatment strategies including diet, physical activity, behavior modification, combination therapy, pharmacotherapy, and surgery. The evidence examined pertained not only to the treatment options in terms of effects on weight loss, but also to whether or not the treatment options affected changes in abdominal fat or fitness. Ultimately, the main concern was cardiovascular (CVD) morbidity and mortality.

**Systematic Review of Literature**

The expert panel decided on the parameters and search terms for the literature review. The parameters included year of publication, country, language, and study design. The panel reviewed literature from January 1980 to September 1997. A priority was given to English-language randomized controlled trials (RCTs) and excluded editorials, letters, and case reports.

The evidence model comprised 39 questions requiring answers. A search of the literature revealed 43,000 records that had to be scanned to determine whether they were appropriate for this evidence-based review. After reviewing titles, approximately 25,000 of them needed additional review. The titles were screened again, and 8,000 abstracts were extracted for review. Of these, 2,400 abstracts appeared relevant and were sent to the San Antonio Cochrane Collaboration, which had been very involved in conducting systematic evidence-based reviews. The Cochrane Center staff abstracted 394 RCTs on the evidence related to obesity treatments. The staff also provided advice on multiple aspects of systematic review, including

- Searching and selecting materials
- Abstracting materials
- Organizing materials into evidence tables
- Conducting meta-analysis

The panel used the following criteria to determine whether a study should be accepted and included in the guideline:

- The timeframe for the intervention had to be at least 4 months (i.e., the minimum amount of time that must pass before the outcome measure is made)
- To consider long-term maintenance, studies had to include data collected after 1 or more years
- Studies were excluded if they used self-reported weights or patients that were not overweight, had dropout rates greater than 35%, or had no control group

The panel determined specific criteria to evaluate the evidence. These criteria ranged from level A to D, and were used to rank each evidence statement and recommendation provided in the guideline:

- A - Strong evidence: Evidence from well-designed, RCTs (or trials that depart only minimally from randomization) that provides a consistent pattern of findings. Level A therefore includes a substantial number of studies involving substantial numbers of participants
- B - Suggestive evidence: Some evidence from RCTs supports the recommendation, although the scientific support is not optimal. For example, either few randomized trials exist, they are small in size, the existing trials are somewhat inconsistent, or the trials were undertaken in a population that differs from the target population of the recommendation
- C - Suggestive evidence (from nonrandomized studies): Evidence resulting from the panel's interpretation of uncontrolled or observational studies
- D - Expert judgment: This is evidence gathered from clinical experience or experimental research derived from the consensus of panel members, based on knowledge that does not meet the other criteria. This level of criteria was used only in cases where the provision of some guidance was deemed necessary, but an adequately compelling empirical literature addressing the subject of the recommendation did not yet exist

**Assessment and Classification of the Patient**

The primary accomplishment of the clinical guidelines was the establishment of body mass index (BMI) ranges to define overweight and obesity in adults, as shown in the table below. Overweight was defined as a BMI of 25 to 29.9 kg/m$^2$, and obesity was defined as a BMI >30. Prior to these criteria, the measures determining weight status varied from study to study. Some used the definition for ideal weight derived from weight-for-height tables, others used skinfold measurements. Since the time the guidelines were released, most, if not all, scientific studies now use the same BMI criteria. Given the consistency in measurement across studies since the guidelines were released, evaluating the literature and updating the guidelines will be much easier.

| | Obesity Class | BMI (kg/m²) |
|---|---|---|
| Underweight | | <18.5 |
| Normal | | 18.5-24.9 |
| Overweight | | 25-29.9 |
| Obesity | I | 30.0-34.9 |
| | II | 35.0-39.9 |
| Extreme Obesity | III | ≥40.0 |

The panel reviewed the evidence on the relationship of BMI to disease risk and found that as BMI increases, disease risk increases across many diseases such as cancer, heart disease, and type 2 diabetes. They also acknowledged that there are limitations with the BMI measure since it varies across population groups and between individuals. The limits include possible overestimation of body fat in athletes and others who have a muscular build, and possible underestimation of body fat in older persons and others who have lost muscle mass. According to newer data available since the release of the guidelines, some experts suggest that the BMI cut-point for overweight in Asian population groups should be 23, while for African Americans, perhaps it should be higher than the current 25. The update of the clinical guidelines will consider this new evidence.

The panel also noted that BMI should be used as only one way of assessing the patient. The other measure requiring assessment is an individual's waist circumference as a measure of abdominal fat and disease risk. The presence of excess fat in the abdomen is an independent predictor of cardiovascular risk factors and morbidity. The panel defined high-risk waist circumference cut-points as follows: in men, it is defined as >102 cm (>40 in), and in women, it is >88 cm (>35 in). Since a larger waist circumference is associated with an increased risk for type 2 diabetes, dyslipidemia, hypertension, and CVD in overweight patients (BMI between 25 and 29.9), it serves as another measure of risk and ultimately signals the need for treatment for these individuals.

In addition to measuring BMI and waist circumference, assessment also includes considering the presence of CVD risk factors or comorbidities to determine absolute risk. Some diseases (e.g., CHD, type 2 diabetes, sleep apnea) place patients in a very high-risk category for subsequent mortality. These diseases require aggressive modification of risk factors, in addition to their own clinical management. Other obesity-associated diseases are less lethal, but still require appropriate clinical therapy (e.g., gynecological abnormalities, osteoarthritis). Overweight also aggravates several cardiovascular risk factors (e.g., hypertension, high blood cholesterol, low high-density lipoprotein [HDL], high serum triglycerides [>200 mg/dL], impaired glucose tolerance). Identifying these diseases or risk factors is required in order to serve as a guide in selecting the intensity of the clinical intervention used to treat the weight problem.

**Figure 2**

## Treatment Algorithm

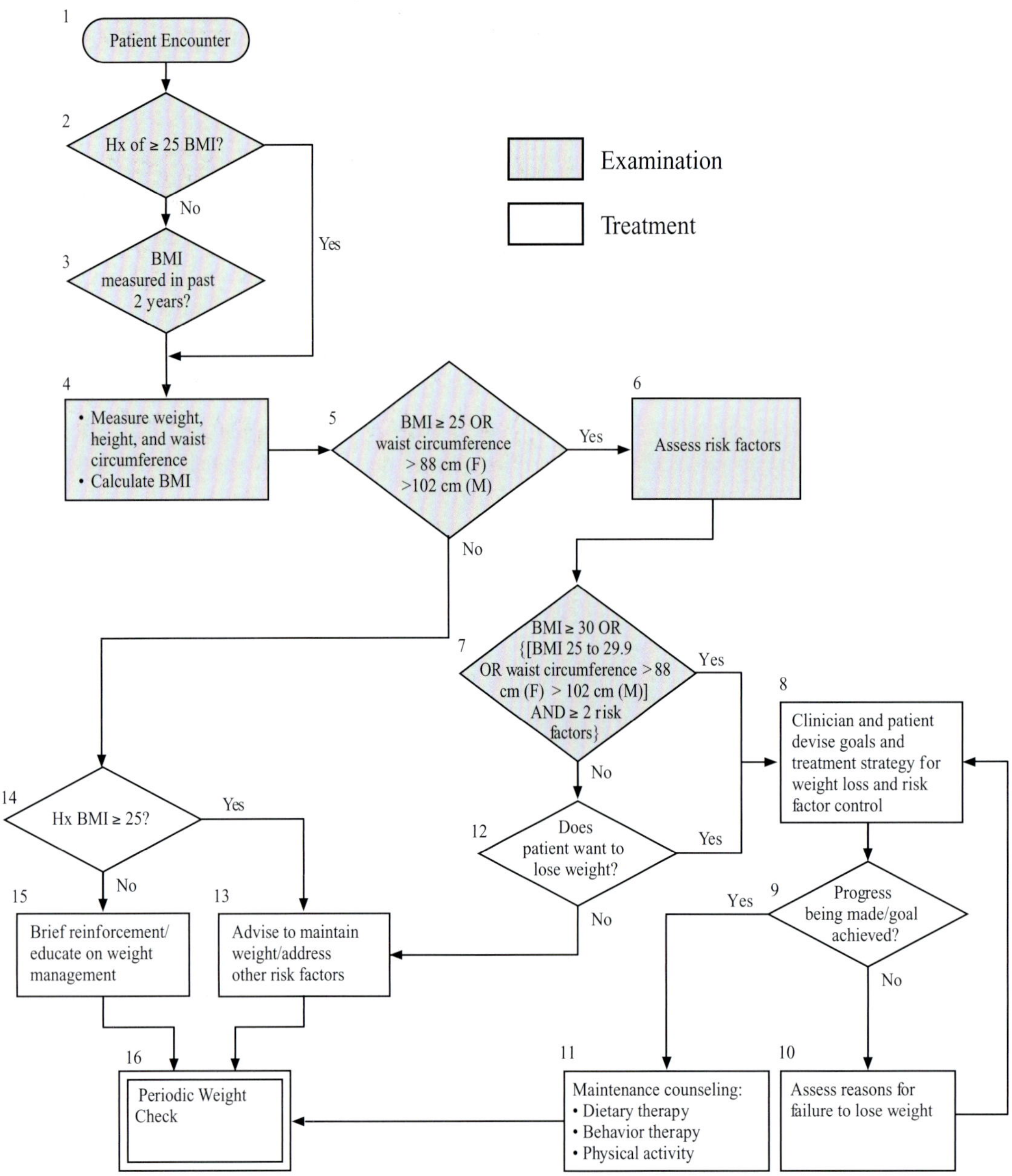


The treatment algorithm (Figure 2), developed by the panel and included in the guidelines, illustrates the various assessment and treatment steps. Some key features:

- In patients with a BMI >25 or with a large waist circumference, the presence of risk factors should be assessed
- Patients with a BMI ≥30, or BMI 25 to 29.9 or a large waist circumference AND 2 or more risk factors, need to work with their physicians to determine treatment goals and strategies
- The algorithm also points out the importance of determining the patient's desire to lose weight. Because of the cost implications for weight loss and follow-up, the patient's desire to lose weight is critical. If the patient does not want to lose weight, the emphasis is on the prevention of weight gain. The patient should maintain her/his current weight status,

not gain any more weight, and should be monitored periodically with a weight check every 5 years. For patients advised to lose weight, specific goals and treatment options should be discussed and their progress should be assessed periodically

- Any patient who achieves a 10% reduction in body weight in 6 months to 1 year, is making good progress. He/she can enter the weight-maintenance phase of counseling. If the patient does not lose sufficient weight, the provider needs to assess the reasons for the failure to lose the weight. These reasons should be used to develop new goals and treatment strategies

The initial goal for weight loss is to decrease body weight by 10%. Losing 10% of initial body weight has been shown to decrease severity of obesity-associated risk factors. This goal is achievable, realistic, and the weight loss can be maintained. A reasonable time frame is 6 months of lifestyle therapy. Once this target is achieved, further weight loss can be attempted if indicated.

Once weight loss goals have been achieved, maintaining a lower body weight becomes a major challenge. Weight maintenance efforts should begin after 6 months of weight loss, which is when it is difficult for most patients to continue to lose weight due to changes in resting metabolic rates and difficulty in adhering to treatment strategies. To achieve additional weight loss, the patient must further decrease calories and/or increase physical activity since energy requirements decrease as weight is decreased. If patients are unable to lose any weight, they should be encouraged to prevent further weight gain.

### Treatment Strategies

The guidelines include a thorough review of the evidence on 6 strategies for weight loss and maintenance: 1) dietary therapy, 2) physical activity, 3) behavior therapy, 4) combined therapy, 5) pharmacotherapy, and 6) weight loss surgery.

In terms of dietary therapy, the panel examined 86 RCTs that evaluated the effectiveness of different diets on weight loss. Thirty-four RCTs examined the impact of a low-calorie diet (LCD) (1,000 - 1,200 kcal/day). All of the studies showed that LCDs result in weight loss; those lasting ≥ 6 months brought about a mean loss of approximately 8% of body weight.

Three dietary recommendations supported by strong A-level evidence:

- Low-calorie diets for weight loss in overweight and obese persons. *Evidence Category A*
- Low-calorie diets (800-1,500 kcal/day) can reduce total body weight by an average of 8% and help reduce abdominal fat content over a period of 6 months. *Evidence Category A*
- Reducing fat as part of LCD is a practical way to reduce calories. Reducing fat without reducing calories would not be as beneficial. *Evidence Category A*

Very low-calorie diet (VLCD) is the other diet that was considered. Four RCTS compared VLCDs with LCDs (400-500 kcal/day vs. 1,000-1,500 kcal/day, respectively). There is strong A-level evidence to support the statement that VLCDs produce greater initial weight loss than LCDs. However, long-term weight loss is not different from that achieved through a LCD.

Physical activity is another important component of weight-loss treatment.

- There is strong A-level evidence that increased physical activity alone can create a caloric deficit and can modestly contribute to weight loss. Physical activity alone generally produces an average of a 2% to 3% decrease in body weight or BMI. *Evidence Category A*
- Physical activity may decrease abdominal fat. *Evidence Category B*
- There is strong evidence that increased physical activity increases cardiorespiratory fitness, with or without weight loss. *Evidence Category A*

In addition to playing a role in weight loss, physical activity is most important in helping to prevent weight regain. In addition, sustained physical activity has the benefit of reducing overall CHD risk beyond that produced by weight reduction alone. There were some studies that considered whether or not behavioral therapy was an important adjunct to diet and physical activity.

- The routine use of behavior therapy strategies to promote diet and physical activity is recommended. These strategies are helpful in achieving weight loss and weight maintenance. *Evidence Category B.*

Combined therapy, combining LCD, increased physical activity, and behavioral treatment, is the most successful strategy for weight loss and weight maintenance at A-level evidence. This kind of lifestyle intervention should be attempted with the patient for at least 6 months before considering any type of drug treatment or surgical treatment.

In terms of drug therapy, the evidence that drugs should be used after 6 months of lifestyle therapy was supported at Evidence Category B level, as shown below.

- Drugs approved for long-term use by the US Food and Drug Administration (FDA) may be used as part of a comprehensive weight loss program including diet and physical activity. *Evidence Category B.*
  - For patients with a BMI >30 with no concomitant risk factors or diseases.
  - For patients with a BMI >27 with concomitant risk factors or diseases (hypertension, dyslipidemia, CHD, type 2 diabetes, sleep apnea).

Only two drugs, sibutramine and orlistat, have been approved by the FDA for long-term weight loss. Sibutramine is contraindicated for those who have an increase in heart rate or blood pressure, and people taking orlistat have some problems with absorption of fat-soluble vitamins.

Weight loss surgery is also an option for patients with severe or resistant obesity.

- The guidelines state that surgery should be reserved for those patients who have failed in other attempts to lose weight and are suffering from the complications of obesity. *Evidence Category B.*
  - Patients who have a BMI ≥40 are potential candidates for surgery if they strongly desire substantial weight loss.
  - Less severely obese patients (BMIs between 35 and 39.9) also may be considered for surgery if they are at high risk and have other comorbid conditions (cardiovascular, sleep apnea, uncontrolled type 2 diabetes) or weight-induced physical problems interfering with performance of daily life activities.

The surgical procedures in current use (gastric restriction [vertical gastric banding] and gastric bypass [RYGB]) can induce substantial weight loss, and serve to reduce weight-associated risk factors and comorbidities. Compared with other available interventions, surgery produces the longest period of sustained weight loss. Assessing both perioperative risk and long-term complications is important and requires assessing the risk/benefit ratio in each case. An integrated program that provides guidance regarding diet, physical activity, and behavior therapy should be in place for all surgical patients.

Looking at the entire spectrum of the various treatment options, we see that lifestyle therapy begins at a BMI of 25 with comorbidities, drug therapy at a BMI of 27 with comorbidities, and surgery at a BMI of 35 with comorbidities.

One very important result from the release of these clinical guidelines was that health practitioners began to think differently about obesity. Obesity is now defined as a chronic metabolic disorder associated with significant morbidity and mortality. It is known to require long-term treatment and have a high incidence of relapse. The amount of weight that most people can lose and *maintain the loss of* is limited at 10%, but a modest weight loss confers significant health benefits.

### Outreach and Dissemination of the Clinical Guidelines

The ultimate package, the *Clinical Guidelines on the Identification, Evaluation, and Treatment of Overweight and Obesity in Adults: Evidence Report*, published by the NHLBI and NIDDK in June 1998, is more than 200 pages long. It includes all of the evidence reviewed and documented, hundreds of references, the treatment algorithm, and practical information, including menu plans for patients and even shopping tips. With the completion of any clinical guideline document, a new phase of work at the NHLBI begins. Getting the information into the hands of clinicians, providers, and the public in formats they can use and understand is the critical next step. The full report was first published as the September 1998 supplement in *Obesity Research*, and its Executive Summary was then published in the *Archives of Internal Medicine* and the *American Journal of Clinical Nutrition*.

Getting the guidelines read and utilized required many additional products. One important one was the *Practical Guide to the Identification, Evaluation, and Treatment of Overweight and Obesity in Adults* developed by NHLBI in partnership with the North American Association for the Study of Obesity. The guide is an abbreviated version of the full guideline, and includes many practical handouts for clinicians to use with patients. It has been marketed to many of the professional societies. The American Academy of Family Physicians provided 100,000 copies of the *Practical Guide* to its members.

Packaging also helps get information out to and utilized by the appropriate audiences. For obesity, this included the creation of the Primary Care Provider Education Kit, which contains the full guidelines, the *Practical Guide*, waist-measuring tape, tip sheets for use with patients, and a 3-step guide to start a conversation about weight management with patients.

Technology offers new opportunities to put the information in the palm of the hand using Palm OS and Pocket PC applications. The first Palm OS application that was developed was the BMI calculator, which has been received with overwhelming success. The second Palm OS application was the *Practical Guide,* which allows the provider to enter patient information to be directed to weight loss goals and treatment options. The software program will work on any device running the Palm OS or Pocket PC 2003, and it accepts English or metric-system input.

Other professional education efforts include a Clinical Guidelines slide show with 150 slides, as well as notes and two online CME modules—1) assessment of the overweight/obese patient and 2) management of the patient. Each module includes a free offer of 2 hours of Category 1 CME credits online at the NHLBI Web site.

All products related to the Clinical Guidelines for professionals, patients, and the public can be found at the Aim For A Healthy Weight Web site at http://healthyweight.nhlbi.nih.gov. The BMI calculator is the most popular item on the NHLBI site, receiving about 450,000 hits per month. A new Spanish-language version of the calculator has recently been added to the site.

One example of patient-education materials is tear sheets for providers to use with their patients. The *Your Weight and Health Profile* sheet allows providers to note BMI, waist circumference, and other risk factors, and to discuss a patient's overall risk. The other side of this sheet includes *Tips for Weight Loss Success,* which covers the importance of smart planning, keeping an eye on portion size, and balancing a "food checkbook." More recent items available to patients on the Web site are the interactive Portion Distortion Quiz and the *Aim for a Healthy Weight* booklet. "Portion distortion" shows how calories in very typical foods have increased over the past 20 years. In addition, it provides the amount of physical activity needed to burn up the "extra" calories associated with the larger portion. The site also includes PowerPoint slides.

**Other obesity-related activities**

Two more recent activities at the National Institutes of Health (NIH) include the Obesity Research Task Force and a new national education program on childhood overweight. This task force was created by the NIH director in April 2003, and it is chaired by the directors of two institutes, the NHLBI and NIDDK. The task force includes approximately 20 representatives from the various NIH institutes, offices, and centers, who meet periodically to discuss current research initiatives on obesity and to coordinate obesity research across the institutes. The charge of the task force is to:

- develop a strategic plan for NIH obesity research, based on identification of areas of greatest scientific opportunity and need;
- monitor implementation of the strategic plan;
- report to the NIH director and the Institute and Center (IC) directors, and
- serve as a point of contact for obesity-research–related issues between NIH and external agencies.

The *Strategic Plan for NIH Obesity Research* was published in August 2004 and is available on the NIH Obesity Research Web site (http://obesityresearch.nih.gov) along with a schedule of upcoming obesity-related meetings and links to request applications. The site can also be used to find program announcements or to review educational activities.

Another significant accomplishment of the NIH has been the efforts of 4 institutes coming together to promote *We Can!* (*Ways to Enhance Children's Activity & Nutrition*), a national education program to prevent overweight in children. *We Can!* is a collaboration of three institutes, namely the NIDDK, the National Institute of Child Health and Human Development (NICHD), and the National Cancer Institute (NCI), that have joined the NHLBI to promote a healthy weight among children between the ages of 8 to 13 years. These institutes are working together to bring the necessary resources to parents, practitioners, and community sites across the country. The NICHD also offers *Media Smart Youth*, a curriculum to use in after-school programs for children, and *Milk Matters*, another national educational resource. The NIDDK has materials for parents about helping the overweight child, and the NCI has Cancer Control Planet, which has catalogued evidence-based programs that can be used in communities.

*We Can!* was designed after a strategy development workshop, convened in February 2004, with leading researchers, public health experts, nutritionists and dieticians, youth marketing experts, and community center representatives from around the country. It also drew input from; a review of the science-based literature on obesity prevention; an environmental scan to review other agency work on overweight and obesity; and an assessment of the NHLBI Hearts N' Parks program. *We Can!* is unique among existing youth obesity-prevention initiatives in its focus on programs and activities for parents and families as a primary group for influencing youth audiences.

- *We Can!* offers a turnkey obesity prevention program that engages the entire community. *We Can!* uniquely offers a curriculum and materials focused on parents and primary caregivers, together with science-based curricula for youth and a community tool kit to help local organizations garner media attention and involve key partners in their efforts.
- *We Can!* is flexible. More than 86 community sites in 32 states around the country are implementing *We Can!* programs and curricula in a variety of settings, from community centers and parks to hospitals and schools.
- Finally, *We Can!* fosters collaboration by offering materials that draw community stakeholders together. Across the country, park and recreation departments, hospitals and healthcare professionals, schools, city government, and the private sector are all collaborating through *We Can!* to provide science-based information to families in their communities.

***We Can!* is being implemented through:**

➤ *Community Outreach: We Can!* is collaborating with 14 Intensive Community Sites around the country to take an active role in creating healthier hometown environments that promote a healthy weight. Sites comprise parks and recreation departments, state and county healthcare departments, healthcare systems, and local coalitions of medical practitioners and city planning groups. These sites are conducting parent and youth programs, as well as community events. In less than 1 year, 72 additional community sites committed to use and distribute *We Can!* program materials

➤ *National Media and Messages:* The national launch of *We Can!* involved Secretary Mike Leavitt and Surgeon General Richard Carmona at the National Institute of Environmental Health Sciences (NIEHS) conference on obesity in childhood, and Dr. Elias Zerhouni and Dr. Elizabeth Nabel in a radio and television satellite media tour. National promotion targets key constituencies with messages that introduce *We Can!* and motivate youth and their parents or primary caregivers to take individual and community action to maintain a healthy weight. Messages engage the public in recognizing both individual and environmental factors that influence their attempts to achieve and maintain a healthy weight, and ultimately reduce their risk of heart disease. Media outreach has occurred both at the national and at the local level, in television, radio, and print. As of this writing, approximately 403 stories have reached an estimated 206 million people

➤ *Partnership Development:* Providing an umbrella theme, materials, and support, *We Can!* has joined forces with approximately 18 other national organizations, including health-professional associations, federal agencies, corporations, and the media to provide parents and caregivers with the most up-to-date information on the prevention of overweight in children. Organizations collaborating with *We Can!* are tailoring their programs and promotions to include *We Can!* materials, messages, and activities

*We Can!* enables an unlimited number of community sites to receive free online access to many materials. *We Can!*

resources include: the parents' handbook—*Families Finding the Balance*, in both English and Spanish; a community toolkit for action that includes the parents' curriculum for a 6-week course; a *Who Can Make it Happen—We Can!* poster, and a trifold promotional brochure. Also available are *We Can!* wristbands for youth and adults. Three youth curricula (i.e., *CATCH Kids Club*, *Media Smart Youth*, and *S.M.A.R.T.*) are also available to the sites. Approximately 100,000 copies of *We Can!* materials have been put into circulation in less than a year. Two listservs have also been established: one for the intensive sites and one for the general sites. The first edition of the *We Can!* e-newsletter was launched in the winter of 2006; currently, more than 700 subscribers have signed up to receive the newsletter. Information on *We Can!* can be found on the *We Can!* Web site at http://wecan.nhlbi.nih.gov. A toll-free telephone number is available at 1-866-35-WECAN (866-359-3226), from which printed copies of *We Can!* resources can be requested.

**Suggested Reading**


1. National Institutes of Health, US Department of Health and Human Services. Clinical Guidelines on the Identification, Evaluation, and Treatment of Overweight and Obesity in Adults: The Evidence Report. Bethesda, Md: National Heart, Lung, and Blood Institute; 1998. NIH Publication 98-4083.

2. Flegal KM, Carroll MD, Kuczmarski RJ, Johnson CL. Overweight and obesity in the United States: prevalence and trends, 1960-1994. *Int J Obes Relat Metab Disord*. 1998;22(1):39-47.

3. National Institutes of Health, US Department of Health and Human Services. Clinical Guidelines on the Identification, Evaluation, and Treatment of Overweight and Obesity in Adults: The Evidence Report. Bethesda, Md: National Heart, Lung, and Blood Institute. *Obes Res*. 1998;6(suppl 2):51S-209S.

4. Executive summary of the clinical guidelines on the identification, evaluation, and treatment of overweight and obesity in adults. *Arch Intern Med*. 1998;158(17):1855-67.

5. Clinical guidelines on the identification, evaluation, and treatment of overweight and obesity in adults: executive summary. *Am J Clin Nutr*. 1998;68(4):899-917.

6. National Institutes of Health, US Department of Health and Human Services. The Practical Guide: Identification, Evaluation, and Treatment of Overweight and Obesity in Adults. Bethesda, Md: National Heart, Lung, and Blood Institute, National Institutes of Health and North American Association for the Study of Obesity (NAASO); 2000. NIH Publication 00–4084.

7. National Institutes of Health, US Department of Health and Human Services. Strategic Plan for NIH Obesity Research: A Report of the NIH Obesity Research Task Force. Bethesda, Md: National Institutes of Health; August 2004. NIH Publication 04-5493.

8. National Heart, Lung, and Blood Institute Healthy Weight Community Outreach Initiative, Strategy Development Workshop Report. Bethesda, Md: NHLBI Publication; January 2005. Administrative Use Only.

# Dietary Guidelines

George L. Blackburn, MD, PhD
Katherine A. Wang
Kristina Day, RD, LD

In January 2005, the US Department of Agriculture (USDA) and the US Department of Health and Human Services (HHS) released the sixth edition of the Dietary Guidelines for Americans.(1) The guidelines, published jointly by the USDA and HHS every 5 years, represent the federal government's most recent science-based advice for health promotion and for reducing chronic disease risk in people 2 years of age and older. In addition to promoting moderation, proportionality, and variety in food selection, they put a strong emphasis on reducing calorie consumption and increasing physical activity.(2)

These updated guidelines are particularly timely, given the recent rise in weight loss surgery.(3) Physicians advocate modest weight loss before undergoing bariatric surgery; patients with a body mass index (BMI) >50 kg/m$^2$ are advised to lose 5% to 10% of their initial weight.(4) Furthermore, the long-term success of bariatric surgery hinges on the patient's commitment to lifestyle changes of healthy eating habits and exercise.(5) It is, therefore, of prime importance to structure proper pre- and postoperative dietary practices that guide patients to restored health and long-term success. With the help of health practitioners, the new dietary guidelines will become a sound resource for patients attempting to lose weight and then maintain a healthy weight through prudent diet and exercise.

### Modest Weight Loss Benefits

For both pre- and postoperative weight loss and maintenance, the 2005 dietary guidelines offer sound strategies for a balanced diet that can be sustained for a lifetime. Modest weight loss can prevent or improve the dysmetabolism associated with obesity-related conditions such as hypertension, metabolic syndrome, type 2 diabetes, and insulin resistance by improving glycemic control, reducing blood pressure, and reducing cholesterol levels.(6-8)

Preoperative weight loss has been linked with improved sleep disordered breathing,(9) shorter operating times, and shorter lengths of stay,(10) indicating that modest preoperative weight loss may also improve the safety and efficacy of the surgery itself. After the surgery, the patient progresses through several stages of diet and eventually graduates from a liquid diet to normal healthy foods. By the time patients reach this final stage, they should be eating regular healthy foods within a reasonable portion size. The dietary guidelines can aid patients in this goal.

### Key Recommendations

Key recommendations in the dietary guidelines promote understanding of how energy balance can be achieved by consuming nutrient-dense foods, limiting non-nutritious foods and discretionary calories, and pursuing incremental physical activity that is both pleasurable and integrated into daily activities. Recommendations—including 9 servings of fruits and vegetables per day, a limit of 2300 mg of sodium per day, and 60 to 90 minutes of exercise on most days to lose weight—are grouped into 9 general topics:

- Adequate nutrients within calorie needs
- Weight management
- Physical activity
- Food groups
- Fats
- Carbohydrates
- Sodium and potassium
- Alcoholic beverages
- Food safety

Priority must be placed on the first three topics, as they lead patients directly to the essential skills of cutting calories, learning portion control, and promoting physical activity. Instilling these habits in patients is a top priority and can only promote the long-term success of weight loss surgery.

### Adequate Nutrients Within Caloric Needs; Avoidance of Nutrient Deficiencies

The 2005 Dietary Guidelines for Americans promotes intake of adequate nutrients within caloric needs. They recommend a balanced eating pattern that includes a variety of nutrient-dense foods and beverages within and among the basic food groups, while choosing foods that limit the intake of saturated and trans fats, cholesterol, added sugars, salt, and alcohol. This advice is invaluable to weight-loss–surgery patients, who must take care to avoid nutrient deficiencies as they reduce food intake.

Previous guidelines did not set specific limits or goals for most food categories, but offered vague statements such as "Aim for a healthy weight," and "Let the food pyramid guide food choices."(2,11) In addition to more specific recommendations, the new dietary guidelines tailor advice to special population groups and specify calorie requirements based on gender, age, and level of physical activity. They have been lauded by several health organizations for their specificity and emphasis on disease prevention. These organizations include the American Dietetic Association, American Heart Association, American Cancer Society, American Diabetes Association, and the Center for Science in the Public Interest, a public advocacy group.(12)

The "Estimated Calorie Requirements" table (categorized by age, gender, and activity level) and personalized recommendations from the USDA's MyPyramid(13) are tools individuals can now use to help them stay within daily energy requirements while meeting nutritional needs. Calories that remain after daily essential nutritional needs have been met and before daily energy requirements are exceeded have been coined "discretionary calories." Although these nonessential calories should comprise less than 15% of a person's daily caloric intake, data indicate that Americans obtain 25% to 30% of their daily calories from junk food.(14) For a balanced diet, specific recommendations from the Dietary Guidelines include

- 3 oz or more of whole-grain products per day
- 3 cups of fat-free or low-fat dairy products per day
- Total fat intake between 20% and 35% of calories
- Limited consumption of saturated fats and trans-fatty acids
- Foods and beverages with little added sugar or caloric sweeteners

**Figure 1**

# WAVE Pocket Card Tool

Weight Assessment Variety Excess

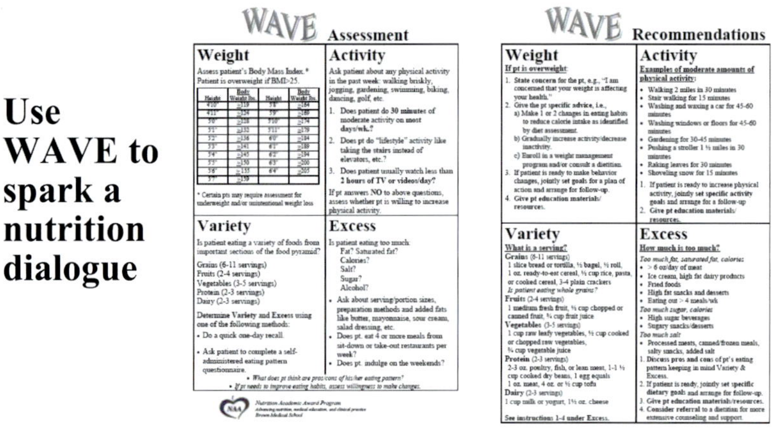


The WAVE (Weight, Activity, Variety and Excess) tool is a patient-assessment tool designed to spark a nutrition dialogue between patient and physician. Formatted as a pocket card, the WAVE features an Assessment side and a Recommendations side for the physician's reference.

**Figure 2**

# REAP Dietary Assessment Tool

Rapid Eating Assessment for Patients

Complete with patient
- or -
have patient complete
in waiting room

http://bms.brown.edu/nutrition/

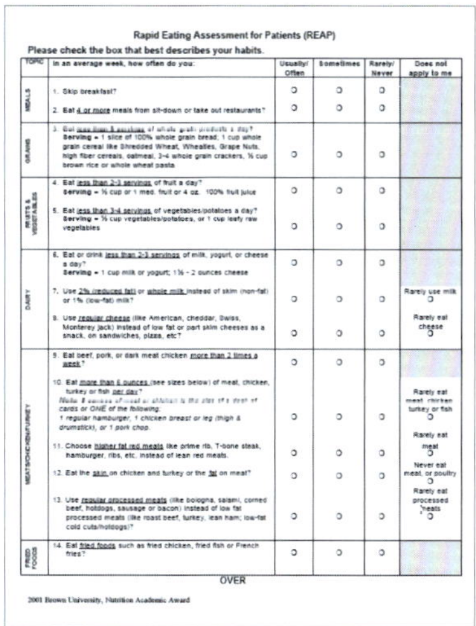

Rapid Eating Assessment for Patients (REAP)

Please check the box that best describes your habits.

| TOPIC | In an average week, how often do you: | Usually/ Often | Sometimes | Rarely/ Never | Does not apply to me |
|---|---|---|---|---|---|
| MEALS | 1. Skip breakfast? | ○ | ○ | ○ | |
| | 2. Eat 4 or more meals from sit-down or take out restaurants? | ○ | ○ | ○ | |
| GRAINS | 3. Eat less than 3 servings of whole grain products a day? **Serving** = 1 slice of 100% whole grain bread; 1 cup whole grain cereal like Shredded Wheat, Wheaties, Grape Nuts, high fiber cereals, oatmeal, 3-4 whole grain crackers, ½ cup brown rice or whole wheat pasta | ○ | ○ | ○ | |
| FRUITS & VEGETABLES | 4. Eat less than 2-3 servings of fruit a day? **Serving** = ½ cup or 1 med. fruit or 4 oz. 100% fruit juice | ○ | ○ | ○ | |
| | 5. Eat less than 3-4 servings of vegetables/potatoes a day? **Serving** = ½ cup vegetables/potatoes, or 1 cup leafy raw vegetables | ○ | ○ | ○ | |
| DAIRY | 6. Eat or drink less than 2-3 servings of milk, yogurt, or cheese a day? **Serving** = 1 cup milk or yogurt; 1½ - 2 ounces cheese | ○ | ○ | ○ | |
| | 7. Use 2% (reduced fat) or whole milk instead of skim (non-fat) or 1% (low-fat) milk? | ○ | ○ | ○ | Rarely use milk ○ |
| | 8. Use regular cheese (like American, cheddar, Swiss, Monterey jack) instead of low fat or part skim cheeses as a snack, on sandwiches, pizza, etc? | ○ | ○ | ○ | Rarely eat cheese ○ |
| MEATS/CHICKEN/TURKEY | 9. Eat beef, pork, or dark meat chicken more than 2 times a week? | ○ | ○ | ○ | |
| | 10. Eat more than 6 ounces (see sizes below) of meat, chicken, turkey or fish per day? *Note: 3 ounces of meat or chicken is the size of a deck of cards or ONE of the following: 1 regular hamburger, 1 chicken breast or leg (thigh & drumstick), or 1 pork chop.* | ○ | ○ | ○ | Rarely eat meat, chicken turkey or fish ○ |
| | 11. Choose higher fat red meats like prime rib, T-bone steak, hamburger, ribs, etc. instead of lean red meats. | ○ | ○ | ○ | Rarely eat meat ○ |
| | 12. Eat the skin on chicken and turkey or the fat on meat? | ○ | ○ | ○ | Never eat meat, or poultry ○ |
| | 13. Use regular processed meats (like bologna, salami, corned beef, hotdogs, sausage or bacon) instead of low fat processed meats (like roast beef, turkey, lean ham; low-fat cold cuts/hotdogs)? | ○ | ○ | ○ | Rarely eat processed meats ○ |
| FRIED FOODS | 14. Eat fried foods such as fried chicken, fried fish or French fries? | ○ | ○ | ○ | |

OVER

2001 Brown University, Nutrition Academic Award

The REAP (Rapid Eating and Activity Assessment for Patients) tool assesses dietary intake related to the USDA's 2005 Dietary Guidelines for Americans and the Food Guide Pyramid.

The WAVE (Weight, Activity, Variety and Excess) (Figure 1) and REAP (the Rapid Eating and Activity Assessment for Patients) (Figure 2) tools allow physicians to quickly assess a patient's dietary intake.(15-17) After actively listening to a patient about his/her habits and goals, a practitioner can help the patient set realistic expectations for nutrition that fit his/her particular medical needs.

### MyPyramid.gov and the DASH Diet

The 2005 guidelines suggest that individuals can follow either the USDA Food Guide Pyramid or the Dietary Approaches to Stop Hypertension (DASH) Eating Plan.(12)

MyPyramid,(13) an Internet-based interactive tool that offers information about the new USDA Food Guide Pyramid, provides personalized guidance for food selection from 5 food groups (grains, vegetables, fruit, milk, meat and beans) and features the key recommendations of the 6th edition of the Dietary Guidelines for Americans. Released in April 2005 by the Center for Nutrition Policy and Promotion (CNPP), an agency of USDA's Food, Nutrition, and Consumer Services, it replaces the 1992 USDA Food Guide Pyramid.(2,18)

The DASH diet,(13) which the guidelines conclude is applicable to the general public, emphasizes fruits, vegetables, and low-fat dairy foods and includes whole grains, poultry, fish, and nuts, and is reduced in fats, red meat, sweets, and sugar-containing beverages. Over the past decade, consumption and dietary patterns based on the DASH diet have emerged as effective strategies to reduce blood pressure,(19) maintain a healthy diet, lose weight, and address pre- and postoperative hypertension.

### Nutrient Density

Postbariatric surgery diet guidelines indicate that as patients progress from thin liquids to regular, healthy food, the food should be nutrient dense, with high-quality protein, carbohydrates, and essential fats. Consistent with this, the 2005 Dietary Guidelines for Americans also recommends nutrient-dense foods, or those foods that contain substantial amounts of key nutrients in relation to the dietary energy they provide.(20)

Low-energy, high-nutrient diets include a relatively high proportion of foods full of micronutrients and water, and low in fat such as fruits and vegetables. Those who rely on such diets consume fewer (nonwater) beverages (e.g., caloric carbonated beverages) and less fat. They also have higher intakes of several important micronutrients, including vitamins A, C, and $B_6$, as well as folate, iron, calcium, and potassium.(20) Data provide evidence of the importance of fruit and vegetable consumption for weight management.(21)

Adults on low-energy–dense diets are likely to eat more food (by weight) but have lower overall energy intake than individuals consuming a high-energy–dense diet. Data indicate that a relationship exists between the consumption of an energy-dense diet and obesity.(21) The energy density of a variety of dietary patterns, including higher-fat diets, can be lowered by adding fruit and vegetables. To achieve a low-energy–density diet, individuals should be encouraged to eat(21)

- A variety of fruits and vegetables
- Low-fat/reduced-fat, nutrient-dense, and/or water-rich grains
- Dairy products
- Meats/meat alternatives

**Weight Management**

To curb growth in the prevalence of overweight and obesity, the new dietary guidelines stress the need to maintain a healthy body weight through calorie control; patients must balance calories from foods and beverages with energy expended. To prevent gradual weight gain over time, they recommend small reductions in calorie intake and increased physical activity.

Body-weight control depends on calories rather than on relative amounts of fat, carbohydrates, and protein in the diet. Diets very low or high in specific macronutrient content, such as saturated and trans fats, are not advised for long-term use. Instead, the guidelines suggest that the healthiest way to cut calories is to eat less saturated fat, added sugars, and alcohol—all items that provide calories without essential nutrients.

**Figure 3**

# Understanding Portion Sizes

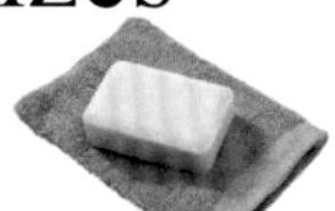

1 oz. meat: matchbox
3 oz. meat: deck of cards/ bar soap
8 oz. meat: thin paperback book
3 oz. fish: checkbook

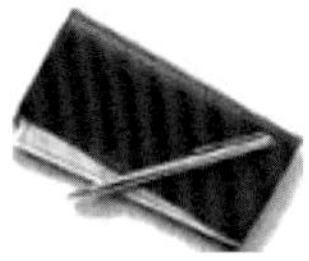

1 oz. cheese: domino

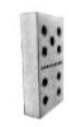

Medium potato: computer mouse
2 tbs. peanut butter: golf ball
½ cup pasta: ice cream scoop
1 oz. bagel: hockey puck

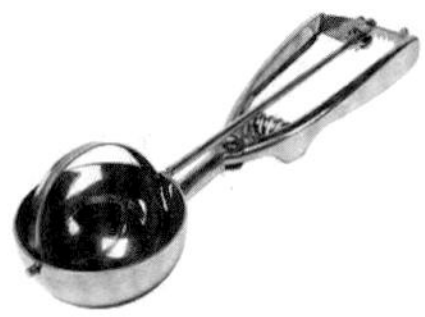

Understanding and controlling portion size are key factors in limiting caloric intake, especially when consuming energy-dense foods (i.e., those that are high in calories and low in nutrients).

Patients must also be counseled on the importance of portion sizes. Limiting portion sizes (Figure 3) is the key to regulating caloric intake, especially when consuming energy-dense foods.

Figure 4

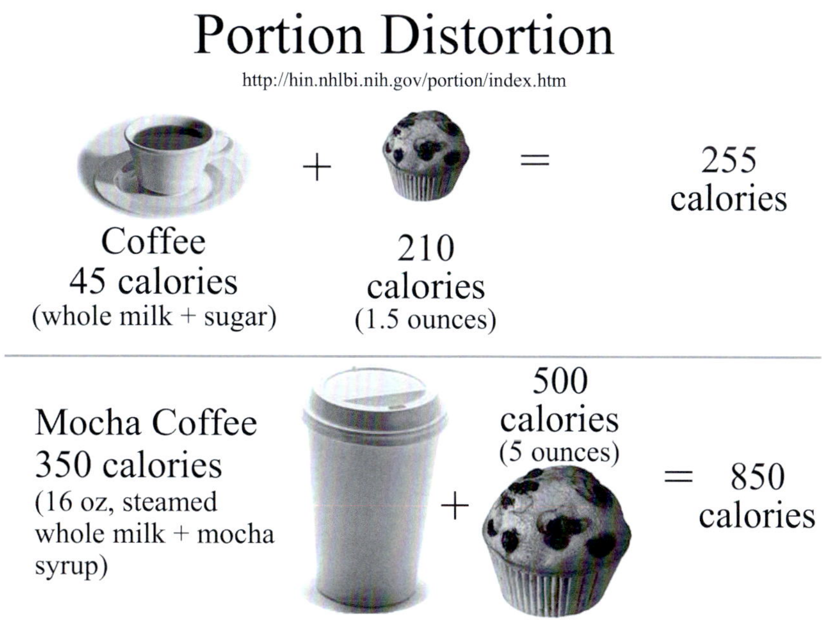


Portion sizes of foods and beverages served at restaurants and of foods packaged for single-serve sale have increased dramatically over the last 2 decades. The incidence of obesity has increased over the past 2 decades in parallel with growing portion sizes, and portion distortion may be a contributing factor.

Increased awareness of portion distortion(22) (Figure 4) can help individuals understand the impact of environment on food intake. However, because portion sizes are often difficult to imagine, patients must learn to recognize how portion size relates to the size of everyday items such as a deck of cards or a tennis ball.

### Physical Activity

Nearly 30% of American adults lead sedentary lifestyles. Even though small decreases in food and beverage calories and increased physical activity can help prevent gradual weight gain over time,(23) physical activity is a particularly important component of weight control for weight-loss–surgery patients.

New recommendations for adult physical activity are as follows:

- At least 30 minutes daily of moderate-intensity physical activity, beyond the usual activities at home and at work, to reduce chronic disease risk
- Sixty minutes of moderate- to vigorous-intensity activity on most days in order to lose weight and prevent gradual weight gain
- Sixty to 90 minutes of moderate-intensity activity to keep off lost weight.

For both pre- and postoperative weight-loss–surgery patients, practitioners must keep in mind the various barriers to physical activity. Practitioners can begin by encouraging patients to start small and gradually increase the number of steps they take each day. The National Heart, Lung, and Blood Institute's (NHLBI's) clinical guidelines on obesity suggest that patients start by walking 30 minutes a day, 3 days a week, increasing this until they include physical activity at least 5 days a week.(24) An overweight or obese person might have difficulty sustaining exercise for the recommended 30 minutes per day. Fortunately, short bouts of exercise are just as effective as—and sometimes more effective than—a longer sustained period of activity.(25) A pedometer is a simple tool that helps patients track their activity; eventually, patients should aim to be taking 10,000 steps per day.

### Changing Minds, Changing Behavior

A key tenet of the dietary guidelines is individual responsibility: helping patients make personal choices about physical activity and diet.(12) Healthcare providers can play an important role in helping patients achieve a healthy weight through diet and activity. Often, patients know what they "should" eat but have trouble incorporating that into daily living. Practitioners should focus on identifying and eliminating such barriers.(26)

Active listening is a key component of effective counseling. It might take only a few minutes for the practitioner to assess the patient's attitude, but even 3 to 5 minutes of active listening can establish a critical bond with the patient. Making suggestions based on what is heard will be much more effective than making blanket recommendations for health. It may be necessary to repeat recommendations over several visits, as people need to hear a message in a variety of ways before it sparks a change in behavior.(27-29)

Because patients benefit from concrete advice, a structured, practical plan is most likely to be successful. A treatment strategy based on the NHLBI's clinical guidelines on obesity(24) and the Surgeon General's reports on physical activity(30) and obesity(31) can be used as an easily adapted, evidence-based blueprint.

**Summary**

Modest weight loss through prudent diet and exercise is a very important component of successful weight loss surgery. The 2005 Dietary Guidelines for Americans offers recommendations for nutrition, weight management, and activity that can be tailored to be appropriate for pre- and postoperative weight loss.

As the prevalence of weight-loss–surgery increases, more specific guidelines on best practices for surgery are also being developed. For instance, an expert panel on weight-loss–surgery from the Betsy Lehman Center for Patient Safety and Medical Error Reduction published an executive report on patient safety in weight-loss–surgery.(32) The panel made evidence-based recommendations for weight-loss–surgery issues, including the necessity of modest weight loss both pre- and postoperatively.

The dietary guidelines recommend that individuals balance energy intake and expenditure by consuming nutrient-dense foods, limiting non-nutritious foods and discretionary calories, and adding pleasurable incremental physical activity that can be integrated into daily activities. Both the DASH diet and the USDA Food Guide Pyramid help patients achieve a balanced diet of fruits, vegetables, low-fat dairy, whole grains, lean meats, and other nutrient-dense foods.

Maintaining a healthy weight both pre- and postoperatively is critical to the success of weight-loss–surgery. Guided by the 2005 Dietary Guidelines for Americans, healthcare providers are uniquely equipped to influence patients' food and activity choices through effective counseling and the transfer of practical information.

**Acknowledgments**

The authors would like to acknowledge the support of the S. Daniel Abraham Chair in Nutrition Medicine at Harvard Medical School and the Harvard Center for Healthy Living. The authors thank Rita Buckley for assistance with medical writing.

## References


1. Dietary Guidelines for Americans. US Department of Health and Human Services and the US Department of Agriculture. 2005. Available at: http://www.healthierus.gov/dietaryguidelines. Accessed January 31, 2005.
2. Johnston CS. Uncle Sam's diet sensation: MyPyramid—an overview and commentary. *Med Gen Med*. 2005;7(3):78.
3. Smoot TM, Xu P, Hilsenrath P, Kuppersmith NC, Singh KP. Gastric bypass surgery in the United States, 1998-2002. *Am J Public Health*. 2006;96(7):1187-9.
4. Saltzman E, Anderson W, Apovian CM, et al. Criteria for patient selection and multidisciplinary evaluation and treatment of the weight loss surgery patient. *Obes Res*. 2005;13(2):234-43.
5. Lysen L. *Quick Reference to Clinical Dietetics*. Second ed. Boston: Jones and Bartlett Publishers; 2006.
6. Goldstein DJ. Beneficial health effects of modest weight loss. *Int J Obes Relat Metab Disord*. 1992;16(6):397-415.
7. Blackburn GL, Read JL. Benefits of reducing—revisited. *Postgrad Med J*. 1984;60(suppl 3):13-8.
8. Blackburn GL. Benefits of weight loss in the treatment of obesity. *Am J Clin Nutr*. 1999;69(3):347-9.
9. Peppard PE, Young T, Palta M, Dempsey J, Skatrud J. Longitudinal study of moderate weight change and sleep-disordered breathing. *JAMA*. 2000;284(23):3015-21.
10. Busetto L, Segato G, De Luca M, et al. Preoperative weight loss by intragastric balloon in super-obese patients treated with laparoscopic gastric banding: a case-control study. *Obes Surg*. 2004;14(5):671-6.
11. Nutrition and Your Health: Dietary Guidelines for Americans.US Department of Health and Human Services and the US Department of Agriculture. Available at: http://www.health.gov/DietaryGuidelines/dga2000/document/contents.htm. Accessed September 14, 2006.
12. Kuehn BM. Experts charge new US dietary guidelines pose daunting challenge for the public. *JAMA*. 2005;293(8):918-20.
13. US Department of Health and Human Services. Your Guide To Lowering Your Blood Pressure With DASH. Available at: http://www.nhlbi.nih.gov/health/public/heart/hbp/dash/. Accessed September 14, 2006.
14. Block G. Foods contributing to energy intake in the US: data from NHANES III and NHANES 1999–2000. *Journal of Food Composition and Analysis*. 2004;17:439-447.
15. Barner CW, Wylie-Rosett J, Gans K. WAVE: a pocket guide for a brief nutrition dialogue in primary care. *Diabetes Educ*. 2001;27(3):352-8.
16. Gans KM, Ross E, Barner CW, Wylie-Rosett J, McMurray J, Eaton C. REAP and WAVE: new tools to rapidly assess/discuss nutrition with patients. *J Nutr*. 2003;133(2):556S-62S.
17. Segal-Isaacson CJ, Wylie-Rosett J, Gans KM. Validation of a short dietary assessment questionnaire: the Rapid Eating and Activity Assessment for Participants short version (REAP-S). *Diabetes Educ*. 2004;30(5):774, 776, 778 passim.
18. The Food Guide Pyramid. US Department of Agriculture. Available at: http://www.usda.gov/cnpp/pyramid.html. Accessed September 14, 2006.
19. Appel LJ, Brands MW, Daniels SR, et al. Dietary approaches to prevent and treat hypertension: a scientific statement from the American Heart Association. *Hypertension*. 2006;47(2):296-308.
20. Darmon N, Darmon M, Maillot M, Drewnowski A. A nutrient density standard for vegetables and fruits: nutrients per calorie and nutrients per unit cost. *J Am Diet Assoc*. 2005;105(12):1881-7.
21. Ledikwe JH, Blanck HM, Kettel Khan L, et al. Dietary energy density is associated with energy intake and weight status in US adults. *Am J Clin Nutr*. 2006;83(6):1362-8.

22. Schwartz J, Byrd-Bredbenner C. Portion distortion: typical portion sizes selected by young adults. *J Am Diet Assoc.* 2006;106(9):1412-8.

23. Behavioral Risk Factor Surveillance System. National Center for Chronic Disease Prevention and Health Promotion. October 21, 2004. Available at: http://www.cdc.gov/brfss. Accessed October 27, 2004.

24. Clinical guidelines on the identification, evaluation, and treatment of overweight and obesity in adults. The Evidence Report. National Institutes of Health. National Heart, Lung, and Blood Institute. Available at: http://www.nhlbi.nih.gov/guidelines/obesity/ob_gdlns.htm. Accessed February 18, 2003.

25. Park S, Rink LD, Wallace JP. Accumulation of physical activity leads to a greater blood pressure reduction than a single continuous session, in prehypertension. *J Hypertens*. 2006;24(9):1761-70.

26. Foster GD, Makris AP, Bailer BA. Behavioral treatment of obesity. *Am J Clin Nutr*. 2005;82(1 suppl):230S-235S.

27. Blackburn GL, Waltman BA. Physician's guide to the new 2005 dietary guidelines: how best to counsel patients. *Cleve Clin J Med*. 2005;72(7):609-18.

28. Gardner H. Changing Minds. *The Art and Science of Changing Our Own and Other People's Minds*. Boston: Harvard Business School Press; 2004.

29. Blackburn GL. Teaching, learning, doing: best practices in education. *Am J Clin Nutr*. 2005;82(1 suppl):218S-221S.

30. US Department of Health and Human Services. Physical activity and health: a report of the Surgeon General. Washington, DC: US Government Printing Office; 1996.

31. The Surgeon General's Call to Action to Prevent and Decrease Overweight and Obesity. Available at: http://www.surgeongeneral.gov/topics/obesity/calltoaction/CalltoAction.pdf. Accessed August 4, 2004.

32. Lehman Center Weight Loss Surgery Expert Panel. Commonwealth of Massachusetts Betsy Lehman Center for Patient Safety and Medical Error Reduction Expert Panel on Weight Loss Surgery: Executive Report. 2005.

# Pharmacotherapy Pipeline

Donna H. Ryan, MD
George A. Bray, MD

Three medications approved by the US Food and Drug Administration (FDA) for long-term use in the treatment of obesity are currently available in the United States. Sibutramine (approved in 1997), orlistat (approved in 1999), and rimonabant (available in Europe and given FDA approvable status in 2006 for marketing in 2007) represent current approaches to medications used adjunctively for weight management.

The modern paradigm is that weight loss medications are used in clinical settings where health risk, rather than a cosmetic goal, drives prescribing. As demonstrated in large clinical trials of 2- to 4-year duration, these medications are associated with significant weight loss compared with placebo. Weight loss, when these medications are combined with an appropriate behavioral intervention, averages 8% to 10% from baseline; weight maintenance is demonstrated as long as adherence to medication continues. All medications have side effects that need to be considered. For sibutramine, there is a rise in blood pressure and heart rate that may require discontinuation of the drug in a small percentage of patients. For orlistat, gastrointestinal disturbances are the principal side effects. With rimonabant, nausea and other gastrointestinal symptoms are the chief tolerability issue; however, when compared with placebo, there are more reports of mood disturbance and anxiety with rimonabant. Once marketed, caution will be advised for those with depression when using this medication.

These three medications mark the first in a pipeline of drugs in development. There are medications for obesity in phase 2 trials that target the cannibinoid-1 (CB1) receptor, the 5-$HT_{2C}$ receptor, neuropeptide Y(NPY), peptide YY3-36(PYY), oxyntomodulin, and pancreatic lipase inhibition. Another trend is the investigation of combination therapy for weight management. Considering the epidemics of obesity and type 2 diabetes, pharmacologic approaches to obesity are likely to be the focus for discovery with the promise of yielding meaningful obesity treatment tools for the primary care physician.

At the time of this writing, there are some medications associated with weight loss that physicians sometimes prescribe off-label for obesity. We do not endorse off-label use and will focus on medications with a weight loss indication. Our focus will be on drugs approved for long-term use and those that are in development. For individuals desiring more detail or additional guidance in the use of currently approved medications to treat overweight, information can be found in a variety of sources. (1-4)

Our guidance on appropriate selection of patients for the use of weight-management medications is that health improvement be the goal of therapy. The prescribing guidelines for weight loss medications that have been approved for long-term use by the FDA indicate that the patient's body mass index (BMI) should be 30 kg/m$^2$ or greater or, if there are associated conditions such as hypertension, diabetes or hyperlipidemia, that the BMI be ≥27.

Our recommendation would also include two other conditions as comorbid conditions that would allow treatment of obesity with pharmacotherapy at BMI >27. First, we are supportive of the concept of using the diagnosis of the metabolic syndrome (modified criteria from the Adult Treament Panel III [ATP III] of the National Cholesteral Education Program [NCEP]) for determining eligibility for pharmacotherapy, because these criteria identify individuals who have a cluster of risk factors (lipids, blood pressure, and fasting glucose) at levels that, although not in the range that usually triggers intervention, when taken together identify increased risk for development of diabetes and cardiovascular disease. Second, the presence of a large waist circumference, specific to ethnic group, is an important criterion to consider when evaluating risk from overweight. The currently recommended upper limit for waist circumference in the NCEP ATP III definition of metabolic syndrome is 102 cm (40 in) for a man, and 88 cm (35 in) for a woman, but other cut-points have been recommended. The recent proposal from the International Diabetes Federation (IDF) for metabolic syndrome is useful, because it provides ethnicity-specific, waist-circumference definitions and also because it uses upper limits for waist circumference (>80 cm for females and >94 cm for males). (6) We would support the use of the IDF waist-circumference cut-points to identify candidates for pharmacotherapy.

Before initiating pharmacotherapy, an assessment of the patient's motivation must be made. Weight loss is hard work and patients must be highly motivated to be successful. The next step is to set a weight loss goal. Most patients have an unrealistic view of how much weight they can lose. For many, a weight loss of less than 15% would often be viewed as a failure. In contrast, weight loss using monotherapy with the drugs that are currently available is usually not more than 10%, even with a lifestyle intervention in addition to medication. Therefore, it is important for physician and patient alike to set a weight loss goal for initial therapy that is not more than 10% and to set a lower limit for weight loss of less than 5%, which would suggest the need for an alternative strategy.

The key to effective pharmacotherapy is to link the behavioral approach to the drug's mechanism of action. Patients must be fully informed of the drug's mechanism of action and side effects. The next step is to fully discuss the medication with the patient and then to ask him/her to sign a consent form indicating knowledge of the required behavioral approaches, potential side effects, and responsibility for follow-up.

We advise that physicians only prescribe medications approved by the FDA for long-term use. To our surprise, an algorithm sponsored by the American College of Physicians recommends 6 medications: orlistat, sibutramine, phentermine, diethylpropion, fluoxetine, and bupropion. (4) The first four have been approved by the FDA for treatment of overweight patients and may have some application, though phentermine and diethylpropion have approval for only short-term use. But fluoxetine, sertraline, and bupropion have not received approval for weight-loss indication and should not be used primarily for this purpose. In our view, fluoxetine and bupropion should not be used for weight loss, but may be appropriate choices for management of depression in overweight patients. Bupropion may also be helpful in reducing or preventing the weight gain when people try to stop smoking.

**Drugs Approved for Long-term Use**

There are only two medications currently available for long-term use in the United States—orlistat and sibutramine. We will not discuss these drugs in detail in this review, as there are others that review their efficacy and safety at length. (7-23) Instead, we will summarize the evidence-base supporting the use of these medications, as illustrated in Table 1.

**Table 1**

**Drugs Approved in the United States for Long-Term Weight Management**

| **Generic name** | Sibutramine | Orlistat |
|---|---|---|
| **Trade name** | Meridia | Xenical |
| **Date of FDA approval** | 1997 | 1999 |
| **Site of action** | Central | Peripheral |
| **Mechanism** | Serotonin and norepinephrine reuptake inhibitor | Pancreatic lipase inhibitor |
| **Weight-loss mechanism** | Induces satiety | Blocks absorption of 30% of fat in gut |
| **Dose** | 5-15 mg once daily | 120 mg tid before meals |
| **FDA approval** | Long-term use | Long-term use |
| **DEA class** | DEA Class IV | Not scheduled |
| **Weight-loss efficacy drug only (placebo subtracted)** | ~5% | ~3.5% |
| **Weight-loss efficacy drug + lifestyle (not placebo subtracted)** | 8-16% | 6-10% |
| **Advantages** | Once-daily dosing | Safety |
| **Disadvantages** | Cost and reimbursement, BP elevation | Cost and reimbursement, GI tolerability |
| **BP = blood pressure; GI = gastrointestinal** | | |

The two drugs have entirely different mechanisms of action. Orlistat is a lipase inhibitor and has a dose-dependent effect on fecal fat loss. When eating diets with 30% fat, about one third will not be absorbed. Thus, orlistat works to enforce a moderate fat-eating pattern, since indiscretion in high-fat meals and snacks will result in gastrointestinal consequences. Orlistat has little effect on subjects eating a low-fat diet. Sibutramine is a so-called selective serotonin and norepinephrine reuptake inhibitor. It reduces food intake in clinical studies. (24,25) If sibutramine increases energy expenditure, it is on the order of 100 kcal/day. (26)

The amount of weight loss that can be anticipated with sibutramine or orlistat is about the same. If one considers the effect of a drug alone on weight (i.e., placebo-subtracted weight loss), then the average weight loss at 12 months will be on the order of 2 to 3 kg for orlistat. For sibutramine, the placebo-subtracted weight loss would be 3.5 to 4.5 kg at 12 months. (20,21, 27,28) However, placebo-subtracted weight loss does not tell the whole story, as on average the placebo group lost approximately 5% of total weight due to behavioral approaches and the drug-treated patient gets the combined effect. What is critical to remember is that the goal of the modern weight-loss approach is a modest, sustainable weight loss. These medications assist patients in achieving that goal and enable more successes than would otherwise be possible in achieving the 5% to 10% weight loss goal. Because orlistat and sibutramine have different mechanisms of action, the behavioral approach that one would employ to maximize effects would differ for each drug.

Since sibutramine enhances satiety, a dietary program that takes advantage of this mechanism is likely to produce greater weight loss. Wadden and colleagues illustrated the advantage of a structured behavioral intervention in combination with sibutramine in a study where 224 subjects were randomly assigned to receive either sibutramine 15 mg daily delivered by a primary care provider in 8 visits of 10 to 15 minutes each, lifestyle counseling, alone delivered in 30 group sessions, sibutramine plus the 30 group sessions of lifestyle counseling, or sibutramine plus brief lifestyle-modification counseling delivered by the primary care physician in 8 visits of 10 to 15 minutes each. The weight loss at 12 months was -5.0±7.4 kg with sibutramine alone, and -6.7±7.9 kg when brief counseling was added. Lifestyle counseling alone had essentially the same effect as the drug + brief counseling, but when a 30-week behavioral plan was added to the medication group, the weight loss increased further to 12.1±9.8 kg (Figure 1). (29)

**Figure 1**

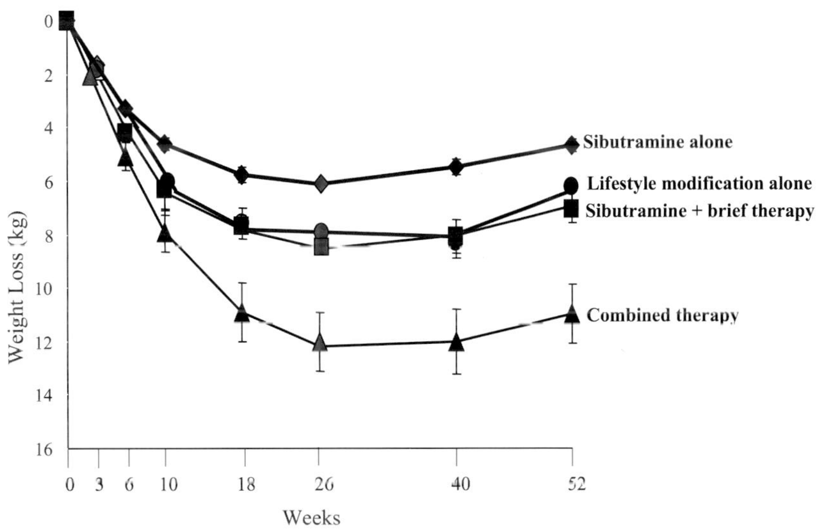


Effect on body weight loss of sibutramine alone or with additional supplementary behavior therapies
(Adapted from Wadden et al. *N Engl J Med.* 2005;35:2111-20.)

The efficacy of both orlistat and sibutramine are supported by multiple, large and well-designed clinical trials of up to 4 years duration, and both drugs have been used efffectively in special populations such as adolescents and persons with diabetes and hypertension.(7-16,18,19,29,39) Both drugs exhibit a dose-to-response relationship in terms of weight loss and, clearly, weight loss is maintained as long as medication is continued. For illustration, we will use the results of a 4-year, double-blind, randomized, placebo-controlled trial with orlistat, as illustrated in Figure 2.(11) A total of 3,304 overweight patients (21% of whom had impaired glucose tolerance) were included in this Swedish trial. The lowest body weight was achieved during the first year: more than 11% below baseline in the orlistat-treated group and 6% below baseline in the placebo-treated group. Over the remaining 3 years of the trial, there was a small regain in weight, such that by the end of 4 years, the orlistat-treated patients were 6.9% below baseline, compared with 4.1% below baseline for those receiving placebo. The trial also showed a 37% reduction in the conversion of patients from impaired glucose tolerance to diabetes, from 9% to 6%, for a relative risk reduction of 0.63 (95% CI 0.46 to 0.86). Essentially all of this benefit occurred in the patients who had impaired glucose tolerance at enrollment.(40)

**Figure 2**

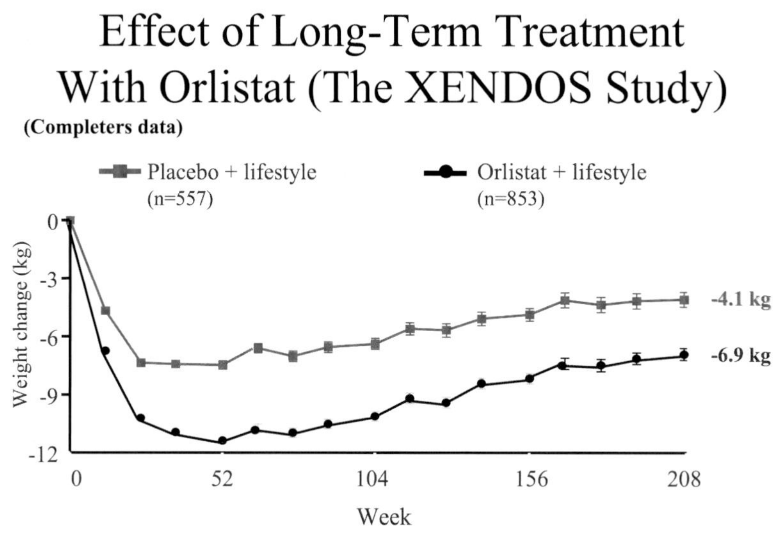


Torgerson et al. *Diabetes Care*. 2004;27:155-61. $P < .001$ vs placebo

The Xendos Study demonstrates efficacy of orlistat when used over 4 years (Sjostrom, ICO, 2002).

The weight loss observed with orlistat is associated with improvements in risk factors (lipids, glycemic control, and blood pressure), and the effect on LDL cholesterol reduction is actually greater than can be accounted for by weight loss alone. (3) Although weight loss with sibutramine produces improvements in lipids and glycemic control, sibutramine is not associated with the expected degree of improvement in blood pressure that one would expect with weight loss.

Safety is an important concern for medications used to treat obesity. The chief safety concern with sibutramine is the effect on blood pressure, which has been evaluated in a meta-analysis of 21 studies and in pooled data from placebo-controlled studies, with somewhat conflicting interpretations.(39,41) What is certain is that in clinical studies, mean data on blood-pressure change demonstrate a small increase in blood pressure, particularly diastolic blood pressure, when the drug is used. It also is evident that when weight loss is achieved with sibutramine, the decrease in blood pressure is less than expected with that degree of weight loss. The key points for practicing physicians to remember are that this drug can produce an increase in blood pressure in susceptible individuals and that patients who are taking the drug should have their blood pressure monitored. If sibutramine produces weight loss and the patient has an acceptable blood pressure, then the medication can be continued.

Orlistat is characterized by a remarkably positive safety profile. Fecal fat loss and related gastrointestinal symptoms are common initially, but they subside as patients learn to use the drug.(3) Orlistat can cause small and occasionally significant decreases in fat-soluble vitamin levels, but these usually remain within the normal range. A few patients may need vitamin supplementation. Because it is impossible to tell which patients need vitamins, it is wise to provide a multivitamin routinely with instructions to take it before bedtime. Orlistat does not seem to affect the absorption of other drugs, with the exception of cyclosporine; thus, the two medications should not be used concomitantly. It is anticipated that orlistat will be available over-the-counter in 2007 at a 60-mg dose. Physicians should be aware of the need for vitamin supplementation when this medication is used over the long-term, and should assess their patients for this use.

**Rimonabant**

The first in a new class was anticipated for release in the United States in 2007, but was withdrawn from consideration. The drug is marketed in Europe.

Rimonabant is the first in a new class of compounds that target the CB1 receptor. Marijuana and tetrahydrocannabinol stimulate the CB1 receptor and increase the intake of fat and sweets, and fasting increases the levels of endocannabinoids. Rimonabant is a specific antagonist of the CB1 receptor. It inhibits sweet food intake in marmosets, as well as high-fat food intake in rats but not in rats fed standard chow. Cannabinoid-1 receptor knockout mice are lean and resistant to diet-induced weight gain.(42-55)

The clinical evidence to support rimonabant's use is derived from four phase 3 trials of rimonabant for the treatment of overweight.(46-50) The Rimonabant in Obesity RIO-Europe trial, reported in 2005, enrolled 1,057 patients with a BMI >30 without comorbidities, or with a BMI >27 with hypertension or dyslipidemia.(46) Subjects were stratified based on whether they lost more or less than 2 kg during run-in and then randomized in a ratio of 1:2:2 to receive placebo, rimonabant 5 mg/d, or rimonabant 20 mg/d. The energy content of the diet was calculated by subtracting 600 kcal/d from the energy requirements estimated from the Harris-Benedict equation. The trial consisted of a 4-week run-in period followed by 52 weeks of treatment. Of those who started, 920 (61%) completed the first year. Weight loss was 2% in the placebo group and 8.5% in the 20 mg rimonabant group. Baseline weight was between 98.5 kg (placebo group) and 102.0 kg (for rimonabant 20 mg). During run-in, there was a mean 1.9 kg weight loss. From baseline to the end of run in, the placebo group that completed the trial lost an additional 2.3 kg, the low-dose rimonabant group lost 3.6 kg and the high-dose group lost 8.6 kg. On an intent-to-treat (ITT) basis, these numbers were a weight loss of 1.8 kg for the placebo group, 3.4 kg for the 5 mg/d group and 6.6 kg for the 20 mg/d group. Expressing the data as a responder analysis, the authors reported that 30.5% of the placebo group lost 5% or more, compared with 44.2% of the rimonabant 5 mg/d group, and 67.4% of the rimonabant 20 mg/d group. When a weight loss of 10% or more was considered, the numbers were 12.4% for the placebo group, 15.3% for the rimonabant 5 mg/d group, and 39% for the rimonabant 20 mg/d group. Waist circumference was also reduced by treatment. Triglycerides were reduced by 6.8% in the 20 mg/d group compared with a rise of 8.3% in the placebo group. High-density lipoprotein (HDL) cholesterol increased by 22.3% in the high-dose group compared with 13.4% in the placebo group. These changes in metabolic parameters were reflected in a change in the prevalence of the metabolic syndrome, which decreased by 33.9% in the placebo group compared with 34.8% in the rimonabant 5 mg/d dose group and 64.8% in the 20 mg/d group. In the 20 mg/d group, the low-density lipoprotein (LDL) particle size increased and adiponectin increased, while glucose, insulin, and C-reactive protein decreased and the metabolic syndrome prevalence was cut in half. There was no significant change in blood pressure or pulse between groups.

The second study was in dyslipidemic patients and is the Rimonabant in Obesity–Lipids (RIO-Lipids) study.(46) This was a 12-month, randomized, double-blind, placebo-controlled trial of rimonabant at 2 doses versus placebo in overweight subjects eating a hypocaloric (600 kcal/d) diet. The inclusion criteria were a BMI of 27 to 40, elevated fasting triglycerides (150 to 700 mg/dL), ratio of cholesterol to HDL cholesterol >5 in men and >4.5 in women, and no more than 5 kg variation in body weight in the previous 3 months. Subjects were stratified at run-in by triglycerides below or above 400 mg/dL and, at the end of run-in, by a weight loss of more or less than 2 kg.

Randomization was on a 1:1:1 basis of placebo: rimonabant 5 mg/d: rimonabant 20 mg/d. The drop-out rate was about 40% by the end of 12 months. Weight losses in this trial were almost identical to those in the RIO-Europe trial. After an approximate 2 kg weight loss during run-in, the placebo patients in the completers group lost an additional 2.3 kg, compared with 4.2 kg in the 5 mg/d dose group and 8.8 kg in the 20 mg/d dose group of rimonabant. Waist circumference also decreased in a dose-dependent way. Triglycerides, HDL cholesterol, the peak size of LDL cholesterol particles, adiponectin, fasting insulin, leptin, and C-reactive protein all improved with weight loss. Several liver enzymes fell with treatment, suggesting improvement in nonalcoholic steatosis. Blood pressure decreased significantly in RIO-Lipids in contrast with RIO-Europe. As might be expected from these metabolic changes, the prevalence of the metabolic syndrome in those who met the ATP III criteria fell from 54% at baseline to 25.8% in the rimonabant 20 mg group to 40.0% in the 5 mg/d group and to 41.0% in the placebo group.

The third randomized, double-blind, placebo-controlled study, RIO-North America, was also a 2-year study. It randomized 3,045 overweight subjects, each with a BMI >30 or with a BMI >27 with treated or untreated hypertension or dyslipidemia and without diabetes, to placebo, rimonabant 5 mg, or rimonabant 20 mg. Participants were instructed in a hypocaloric (600 kcal/d), diet. Randomization and baseline occurred after a 4-week, run-in period, when subjects had lost an average of 1.9 kg (Figure 3). The subjects were thus stratified by whether they lost more or less than 2 kg during run-in. At 1 year, half of the patients in each drug group were switched to placebo; completion rates were 51% to 55% for the three groups. During the first year, weight loss was 2.8 kg in the placebo group and 8.6 kg in the rimonabant 20 mg group. Weight loss declined steadily until week 36, after which it plateaued. For the second year, those individuals who were switched from rimonabant to placebo regained weight at almost the mirror image of the rate at which they had lost it during the first year. At the end of the study they were still slightly lighter, but no different from the group treated with placebo for the full 2 years. Waist circumference decreased, and the percentage of patients with the metabolic syndrome decreased from 34.8% to 21.2%, compared with a change from 31.7% to 29.2% in the placebo-treated group. HDL cholesterol and triglycerides improved on the higher dose of rimonabant.

**Figure 3**

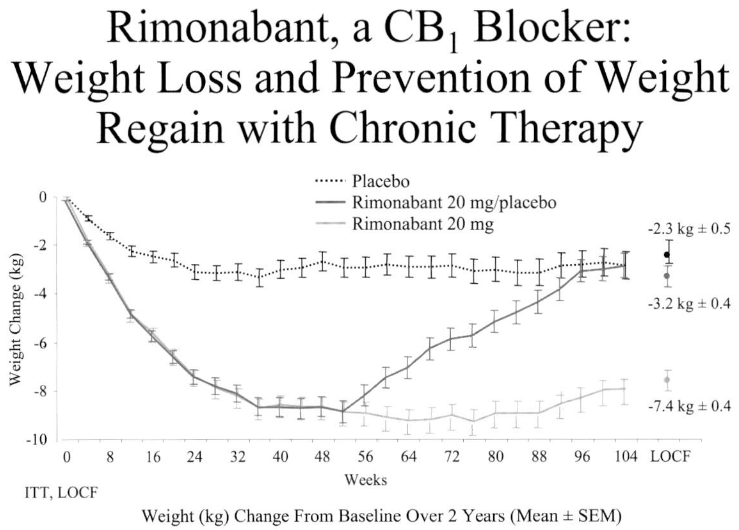


Effect on body weight of a rimonabant in a 2-year, randomized, placebo-controlled clinical trial.
(Adapted from Pi-Sunyer et al. *JAMA*. 2006;295:761-75.)

The fourth study, RIO-Diabetes, randomized 1,045 subjects in 151 centers in 11 countries to treatment. These subjects, who already had diabetes treated with diet, metformin or sulfonylurea drugs, received 1 year of treatment with rimonabant, 5 or 20 mg/d. Weight loss in the placebo group was 1.4 kg, compared with 2.3 kg in the rimonabant 5 mg group and 5.3 kg in the 20 mg group. Triglycerides and blood pressure declined more in the subjects treated with rimonabant 20 mg/d. Of completers, 55.9% lost >5% of body weight during treatment with rimonabant 20 mg/d, compared with 19.5% in the placebo-treated group.

The most frequent adverse events with rimonabant revealed by the four key trials outlined above were: nausea, dizziness, diarrhea, and insomnia. Each of these adverse events occurred at rates 1% to 9% greater than with placebo. However, the chief safety issue with rimonabant concerns potential effects on mood. Because rimonabant "dampens" the feedback systems for pleasurable responses, there is concern about its behavioral effects. In the studies outlined above, there was a dose-related and statistically greater increase in neuropsychiatric adverse events in rimonabant-treated patients. The rate of drug discontinuation for neuropsychiatric disorders (primarily depression and anxiety) was 2% to 5% higher in rimonabant-treated patients compared with placebo-treated subjects. It should be noted that in the RIO studies, patients with significant mental disorders were excluded, and thus, there is concern because of the high prevalence of depression in more extreme degrees of obesity. The drug was reviewed by an FDA Advisory Panel in 2007 and was withdrawn from consideration, based upon the panel's unanimous concern over the neuropsychiatric safety profile. Rimonabant is marketed in Europe, and ongoing surveillance of these aspects of its safety profile continue.

### Drugs on the Horizon

There are many pharmaceutical products targeting overweight, in various stages of development. Some notable investments have been made in evaluating leptin, topiramate, and, axokine (ciliary neurotrophic factor) pharmacotherapy for obesity. These products are no longer being pursued for the general obesity market, although there is interest in developing leptin for lipodystrophy.

The medications under development as of this writing have emerged from old clinical observations of potential targets (the 5-HT receptor) and, new clinical observations (the CB1 receptor), as well as from identification of new targets described in basic research experiments (the NPY and PYY receptors). The medications under investigation are shown in Table 2.

| | Site of Action | Mechanism of Action | Notes on Status |
|---|---|---|---|
| Rimonabant | Central | CB1 antagonist | Approved in Europe, FDA-approvable letter granted. |
| Lorcaserin | Central | 5-HT$^{2C}$ agonist | Successful phase 2 trial; phase 3 underway |
| MK 0557 | Central | NPY-5 antagonist | Phase 3 trial: weight loss not clinically significant; no studies underway |
| S 2367 | Central | NPY-5 antagonist | Phase 2 trial for weight-loss maintenance successful; phase 3 planned |
| PYY 3-36 | Central | GI peptide signal | Phase 1 trial completed |
| Oxyntomodulin | Central | GI peptide signal | Phase 1 trial completed |
| Cetilistat | Peripheral | Pancreatic lipase inhibitor | Phase 2 trial completed; phase 3 planned |
| AOD 9604 | Peripheral | Growth hormone fragment stimulates lipolysis | Phase 2 trial completed; phase 3 planned |

### Other CB1 Antagonists

There are a number of pharmaceutical companies that have agents in development targeting the CB1 receptor. We expect other agents to follow the rimonabant path to approval for indication in obesity.

### Serotonin 2C Receptor Agonist, Lorcaserin

Fenfluramine and dexfenfluramine are drugs that act on the serotonin system. (51-53) Although these were very popular weight loss medications, both were withdrawn from the market in 1997 due to cardiovascular side effects such as valvulopathy and primary pulmonary hypertension. Because of the robust effects of agonists toward the 5-HT$^{2C}$ receptors in suppressing food intake, and because this receptor is not associated with valvulopathy, a number of new agents are now under development. Only one of these, lorcaserin, has advanced to formal clinical trials as of this writing.

The results of a phase 2 dose-ranging study for APD356 (now named lorcaserin) were presented at the American Diabetes Association meetings in 2006.(54) A total of 459 male and female subjects with a BMI between 29 and 46 and with an average weight of 100 kg were enrolled in a randomized, double-blind, controlled trial comparing placebo with lorcaserin 10 mg/d, and lorcaserin 15 mg/d, each given once daily and lorcaserin 10 mg given twice daily, or 20 mg/d. Over the 12 weeks of the trial, the placebo group lost 0.32 kg (n=88 completers) compared with 1.8 kg in the lorcaserin 10 mg twice daily group (n=86 completers), 2.6 kg in the 15 mg/d dose group (n=82 completers) and 3.6 kg in the 10 mg twice daily, or 20 mg total group (n=77 completers). Side effects that were higher in the active treatment groups than in the placebo group were headache, nausea, dizziness, vomiting, and dry mouth. No cardiac valvular changes were noted. (54) A large (n=3,000) participant clinical trial of 6-months treatment is underway to assess the efficacy and safety of the lorcaserin. If no effects on heart valves are demonstrated, the drug has a promising future.

**Neuropeptide Y Receptor Antagonists**

Neuropeptide Y (NPY) is an attractive target for obesity drug development, since in animal studies it is an extremely powerful stimulant for food intake. It is widely distributed and has 5 receptors—Y-1, Y-2, Y-4, Y-5, and Y-6. Neuropeptide-Y stimulates food intake, inhibits energy expenditure, and increases body weight by activating Y-1 and Y-5 receptors in the hypothalamus. (55) Levels of NPY in the hypothalamus are temporally related to food intake and are elevated with energy depletion. Surprisingly, NPY-knockout mice do not exhibit an abnormal phenotype. NPY-5 receptor antagonists fall into two categories: those that reduce food intake and those that do not. Those that do reduce food intake seem to do so through a mechanism separate from Y-5. Therefore, Y-5 receptor antagonists may not be promising as anti-overweight agents. (56) Y-1 receptor antagonists may have greater potential as anti-overweight agents. A dihydropyridine neuropeptide Y-1 antagonist inhibited NPY-induced feeding in satiated rats. (57) Another Y-1 receptor antagonist, J-104870, suppressed food intake when given orally to Zucker rats. (58)

A study measuring serum NPY in obese humans casts doubt on the importance of the NPY antagonists in the treatment of overweight humans. Obese women had lower NPY levels than lean women and weight loss with a 400 kcal/d diet and adrenergic agonists (caffeine and ephedrine or caffeine, ephedrine and yohimbine) did not change NPY levels at rest or after exercise. (56)

Several clinical trials with a selective Y-5 receptor antagonist have been completed. After a 12-week proof-of-concept study demonstrated an optimal dose for MK-0557, a 52-week multicenter, randomized, double-blind, placebo-controlled trial involving 1661 overweight and obese volunteers was undertaken. There was a small but significantly greater response to the drug. The findings supported the hypothesis that NPY5R is a component of energy homeostatic pathways in human beings, although weight loss after pharmacological antagonism of the NPY-5R was not clinically meaningful in overweight and obese adults. (60)

A second NPY-5 antagonist has been studied and a clinical trial executed to test the effect of the antagonist on the prevention of weight gain induced by providing patients with a very low-calorie diet prior to randomization. The concept is that perhaps some stimulation of the NPY system is needed in order for the antagonist to be most effective. Those results have been reported in abstract format and show a small advantage to the NPY-5 antagonist.

**PYY 3-36**

PYY 3-36 is a hormone produced by the L-cells in the gastrointestinal tract and is secreted in proportion to the caloric content of a meal. PYY 3-36 levels are lower during fasting and after a meal in the overweight subjects compared to lean subjects. Development of a nasal-spray formulation for PYY 3-36 has undergone a phase 1 clinical trial. Based on the review of this trial, Merck and Company severed its commercial relationship with Nastech, the developer of the nasal formulation, in March of 2006. Nastech plans to continue developing this product.

Caloric intake at a lunch buffet was reduced by 30% in 12 obese subjects, and by 29% in 12 lean subjects after 2 hours, when PYY 3-36 was infused intravenously. (61) Thrice-daily nasal administration over 6 days was well-tolerated and reduced caloric intake by about 30% while giving 0.6 kg weight loss. (62)

**Oxyntomodulin**

Oxyntomodulin is a gastrointestinal peptide also produced in the L-cells of the intestine and is released in response to food. Animals injected with oxyntomodulin have a reduction in body fat and food intake.

In a short-term clinical study, oxyntomodulin reduced food intake by 19.3% compared to a placebo infusion. In a 4-week, randomized, double-blind, placebo-controlled trial, overweight volunteers injected oxyntomodulin subcutaneously three times a day, 30 minutes before meals. Body weight was reduced 2.3+0.4 kg in the group receiving oxyntomodulin compared with 0.5+0.5 kg in the placebo group. Serum leptin decreased and adiponectin increased in the group receiving oxyntomodulin. Energy intake in the treated group decreased by 170+37 kcal (25+5%) at the beginning study meal and by 250+63 kcal (35+9%) at the final meal.(63) Further studies on this intriguing peptide are awaited.

**Pancreatic Lipase Inhibitor**

Although orlistat, a lipase inhibitor, is already approved for the treatment of overweight, another lipase inhibitor, cetilistat, is under development. In a 5-day trial of cetilistat (ATL-962) in 90 normal volunteers housed at an inpatient unit, there was a three fold to seven fold increase in fecal fat that was dose-dependent. Only 11% of subjects had more than one oily stool, leading to the suggestion that this lipase inhibitor may have fewer gastrointestinal adverse events compared to orlistat. (64)

A 12-week clinical trial randomized 612 obese, diabetic subjects to cetilistat 40 mg, 80 mg, 120 mg, or orlistat 120 mg or placebo, given 3 times a day. Weight loss was 2.9 kg, 3.9 kg, 4.3 kg, 3.8 kg and 2.9 kg, respectively. The prevalence of gastrointestinal side effects was 11.6%, 1.7%, and 4% in the orlistat, cetilistat 120 mg, and placebo groups, respectively. (65)

**Growth-hormone Fragment**

A group working in Australia has identified a fragment of growth hormone that is lipolytic. This compound, called AOD9604, is a modified fragment of the amino acids in growth hormone from 177-191, and is orally active. It is said to bind to the fat cell, stimulating lipolysis and inhibiting re-esterification without stimulating growth. A 12-week, multicenter trial randomized 300 obese subjects to one of 5 daily doses (1, 5, 10, 20 and 30 mg) of AOD9604 or placebo. The 1-mg dose was the most effective for weight loss. Subjects on the 1-mg dose lost 2.6 kg compared to 0.8 kg in the placebo group, and the rate of weight loss was constant throughout the trial. (66) Phase 3 trials are evidently in the planning stages.

**Combinations**

Vivus, Inc. and Orexigen Theripeudics, Inc. are companies that have business plans for obesity treatment. These plans are based on the use of multiple medications in order to improve the amount of weight loss. The companies have identified medications approved by the FDA for other indications associated with weight loss, and are investigating, in clinical trials, the use of combinations of these medications. Three combinations have been patented and are under study: bupropion and naltrexone, bupropion and zonisamide, and topiramate and phentermine. The concept is to use medications with different mechanisms of action to maximize weight loss and, thus, be more appealing to the general public than the currently approved medications, which are associated with approximately 5% weight loss. The medications under study will have to be carefully evaluated for safety because of the long-term nature of medication use and the inherent risk-benefit issues when treating obesity. Tolerability will also be an issue to be carefully assessed in clinical studies.

While we believe that the future of obesity management holds promise for combination pharmacotherapy, we do not believe that combinations with topiramate and zonisamide are likely to be incorporated in primary care practices. If the management of other chronic diseases like hypertension and diabetes are guidance, then combination therapy is almost a certainty. A critical concern is safety, however, and although less critical, tolerability is also important. If we are to manage obesity as a chronic disease, then we need a pharmacopoeia of FDA-approved medications with good safety and tolerability profiles.

Although the drugs presently available for the treatment of overweight are few in number and limited in efficacy, the pipeline for development of drugs for overweight shows some promise. Since drug development is more sophisticated today than in the past, we anticipate that the development of safe and effective drugs for the treatment of overweight will proceed at a more rapid pace than was the case for other chronic diseases such as hypertension and diabetes, both of which presently have several classes of approved, safe and effective medications. Our view is that we are entering an era where obesity will be managed like type 2 diabetes. Multiple medications with different mechanisms of action will be FDA-approved for long-term management of obesity. Physicians of the future will be able to choose among many drugs, targeting multiple mechanisms of action, and combination pharmacotherapy will be common. The path to this future is paved with large clinical trials demonstrating efficacy, safety and tolerability. We also predict that advances in therapeutic approaches to lifestyle change will make the addition of medication to these programs routine, with the emphasis on prevention of obesity comorbidities. The medical management of obesity will be driven by health concerns rather than cosmetic priorities, and the approach will be long term.

**References**

1. The Practical Guide: Identification, Evaluation, and Treatment of Overweight and Obesity in Adults. National Institutes of Health. US Department of Health and Human Services. Bethesda, Md: National Institutes of Health; 2000. NIH Publication 00-4084.
2. Yanovski SZ, Yanovski JA. Obesity. *N Engl J Med*. 2002;346(8):591-602.
3. Bray GA, Greenway FL. Current and potential drugs for treatment of obesity. *Endocr Rev*. 1999;20(6):805-75.
4. Snow V, Barry P, Fitterman N, Qaseem A, Weiss K. Pharmacologic and surgical management of obesity in primary care: a clinical practice guideline from the American College of Physicians. *Ann Intern Med*. 2005;142(7):525-31.
5. Executive Summary of the Third Report of the National Cholesterol Education Program (NCEP) Expert Panel on Detection, Evaluation, And Treatment of High Blood Cholesterol In Adults (Adult Treatment Panel III). *JAMA*. 2001;285:2486-2497.
6. International Diabetes Federation. IDF Worldwide Definition of the Metabolic Syndrome. Volume 2006: International Diabetes Federation; 2006.
7. Sjöström L, Rissanen A, Andersen T, Boldrin M, Golay A, et al. Randomised placebo-controlled trial of orlistat for weight loss and prevention of weight regain in obese patients. European Multicentre Orlistat Study Group. *Lancet*. 1998;352(9123):167-72.
8. Davidson MH, Hauptman J, DiGirolamo M, Foreyt JP, Halsted CH, Heber D, et al.. Weight control and risk factor reduction in obese subjects treated for 2 years with orlistat: a randomized controlled trial. *JAMA*. 1999;281(3):235-42.
9. Rossner S, Sjöström L, Noack R, et al. Weight loss, weight maintenance, and improved cardiovascular risk factors after 2 years treatment with orlistat for obesity. European Orlistat Obesity Study Group. *Obes Res*. 2000;8:49-61.
10. Hauptman J. Orlistat: selective inhibition of caloric absorption can affect long-term body weight. *Endocrine*. 2000;13(2):201-6.
11. Torgerson JS, Hauptman J, Boldrin MN, et al. Xenical in the prevention of diabetes in obese subjects (XENDOS) study: a randomized study of orlistat as an ajunct to lifestyle changes for the prevention of type 2 diabetes in obese patients. *Diabetes Care*. 2004;27(1):155-61.
12. Hill JO, Hauptman J, Anderson JW, et al. Orlistat, a lipase inhibitor, for weight maintenance after conventional dieting: a 1-y study. *Am J Clin Nutr*. 1999;69(6):1108-16.
13. Hollander PA, Elbein SC, Hirsch IB, et al. Role of orlistat in the treatment of obese patients with type 2 diabetes. A 1-year randomized double-blind study. *Diabetes Care*. 1998;21(8):1288-94.
14. Kelley DE, Bray GA, Pi-Sunyer FX, et al. Clinical efficacy of orlistat therapy in overweight and obese patients with insulin-treated type 2 diabetes: A 1-year randomized controlled trial. *Diabetes Care*. 2002;25(6):1033-41.
15. Miles JM, Leiter L, Hollander P, et al. Effect of orlistat in overweight and obese patients with type 2 diabetes treated with metformin. *Diabetes Care*. 2002;25(7):1123-8.
16. Heymsfield SB, Segal KR, Hauptman J, et al. Effects of weight loss with orlistat on glucose tolerance and progression to type 2 diabetes in obese adults. *Arch Intern Med*. 2000;160(9):1321-6.
17. Mittendorfer B, Ostlund RE Jr, Patterson BW, et al. Orlistat inhibits dietary cholesterol absorption. *Obes Res*. 2001;9(10):599-604.

18. Chanoine JP, Hampl S, Jensen C, et al. Effect of orlistat on weight and body composition in obese adolescents: a randomized controlled trial. *JAMA*. 2005;293(23):2873-83.

19. Maahs D, de Serna DG, Kolotkin RL, et al. Randomized, double-blind, placebo-controlled trial of orlistat for weight loss in adolescents. *Endocr Pract*. 2006;12(1):18-28.

20. Avenell A, Broom J, Brown TJ, et al. Systematic review of the long-term effects and economic consequences of treatments for obesity and implications for health improvement. *Health Technol Assess*. 2004;8(21):iii-iv, 1-182.

21. Avenell A, Brown TJ, McGee MA, et al. What interventions should we add to weight reducing diets in adults with obesity? A systematic review of randomized controlled trials of adding drug therapy, exercise, behavior therapy or combinations of these interventions. *J Hum Nutr Diet*. 2004;17(4):293-316.

22. Norris SL, Zhang X, Avenell A, et al. Efficacy of pharmacotherapy for weight loss in adults with type 2 diabetes mellitus: a meta-analysis. *Arch Intern Med*. 2004;164(13):1395-404.

23. Zhi J, Mulligan TE, Hauptman JB. Long-term systemic exposure of orlistat, a lipase inhibitor, and its metabolites in obese patients. *J Clin Pharmacol*. 1999;39(1):41-6.

24. Rolls BJ, Shide DJ, Thorwart ML, et al. Sibutramine reduces food intake in non-dieting women with obesity. *Obes Res*. 1998;6(1):1-11.

25. Hansen DL, Toubro S, Stock MJ, et al. Thermogenic effects of sibutramine in humans. *Am J Clin Nutr*. 1998;68(6):1180-6.

26. Astrup A, Hansen DL, Lundsgaard C, et al. Sibutramine and energy balance. *Int J Obes Relat Metab Disord*. 1998;22 (suppl 1):S30-5; discussion S36-7, S42.

27. Haddock CK, Poston WS, Dill PL, et al. Pharmacotherapy for obesity: a quantitative analysis of four decades of published randomized clinical trials. *Int J Obes Relat Metab Disord*. 2002;26(2):262-73.

28. Li Z, Maglione M, Tu W, et al. Meta-analysis: pharmacologic treatment of obesity. *Ann Intern Med*. 2005;142(7):532-46.

29. Wadden TA, Berkowitz RI, Womble LG, et al. Randomized trial of lifestyle modification and pharmacotherapy for obesity. *N Engl J Med*. 2005;353(2):2111-20.

30. Bray GA, Blackburn GL, Ferguson JM, et al. Sibutramine produces dose-related weight loss. *Obes Res*. 1999;7(2):189-98.

31. Apfelbaum M, Vague P, Ziegler O, et al. Long-term maintenance of weight loss after a very-low-calorie diet: a randomized blinded trial of the efficacy and tolerability of sibutramine. *Am J Med*. 1999;106(2):179-84.

32. James WP, Astrup A, Finer N, et al. Effect of sibutramine on weight maintenance after weight loss: a randomised trial. STORM Study Group. Sibutramine Trial of Obesity Reduction and Maintenance. *Lancet*. 2000;356(9248):2119-25.

33. Mathus-Vliegen EM. Long-term maintenance of weight loss with sibutramine in a GP setting following a specialist guided very-low-calorie diet: a double-blind, placebo-controlled, parallel group study. *Eur J Clin Nutr*. 2005;59 (suppl 1):S31-8; discussion S39.

34. Wirth A, Krause J. Long-term weight loss with sibutramine: a randomized controlled trial. *JAMA*. 2001;286(11):1331-9.

35. Berkowitz RI, Wadden TA, Tershakovec AM, et al. Behavior therapy and sibutramine for the treatment of adolescent obesity: a randomized controlled trial. *JAMA*. 2003;289(14):1805-12.

36. Godoy-Matos A, Carraro L, Vieira A, et al. Treatment of obese adolescents with sibutramine: a randomized, double-blind, controlled study. *J Clin Endocrinol Metab*. 2005;90(3):1460-5.

37. Berkowitz RI, Fujioka K, Daniels SR, et al. Effects of sibutramine treatment in obese adolescents: a randomized trial. *Ann Intern Med.* 2006;145(2):81-90.

38. McMahon FG, Fujioka K, Singh BN, et al. Efficacy and safety of sibutramine in obese white and African-American patients with hypertension: a 1-year, double-blind, placebo-controlled, multicenter trial. *Arch Intern Med.* 2000;160(14):2185-91.

39. Jordan J, Scholze J, Matiba B, et al. Influence of Sibutramine on blood pressure: evidence from placebo-controlled trials. *Int J Obes* (Lond). 2005;29(5):509-16.

40. Padwal R, Majumdar SR, Johnson JA, et al. A systematic review of drug therapy to delay or prevent type 2 diabetes. *Diabetes Care*. 2005;28(3):736-44.

41. Kim SH, Lee YM, Jee SH, et al. Effect of sibutramine on weight loss and blood pressure: a meta-analysis of controlled trials. *Obes Res*. 2003;11(9):1116-23.

42. Bensaid M, Gary-Bobo M, Esclangon A, et al. The cannabinoid CB1 receptor antagonist SR141716 increases Acrp30 mRNA expression in adipose tissue of obese fa/fa rats and in cultured adipocyte cells. *Mol Pharmacol*. 2003;63(4):908-14.

43. Pagotto U, Marsicano G, Cota D, et al. The emerging role of the endocannabinoid system in endocrine regulation and energy balance. *Endocr Rev*. 2006;27(1):73-100.

44. Kirkham TC. Endocannabinoids in the regulation of appetite and body weight. *Behav Pharmacol*. 2005;16(5-6):297-313.

45. Juan-Picó P, Fuentes E, Bermúdez-Silva FJ, Javier Díaz-Molina, et al. Cannabinoid receptors regulate Ca(2+) signals and insulin secretion in pancreatic beta-cell. *Cell Calcium*. 2006;39(2):155-62.

46. Van Gaal LF, Rissanen AM, Scheen AJ, et al. Effects of the cannabinoid-1 receptor blocker rimonabant on weight reduction and cardiovascular risk factors in overweight patients: 1-year experience from the RIO-Europe study. *Lancet*. 2005;365(9468):1389-97.

47. Pi-Sunyer FX, Aronne LJ, Heshmati HM, et al. Effect of rimonabant, a cannabinoid-1 receptor blocker, on weight and cardiometabolic risk factors in overweight or obese patients: RIO-North America: a randomized controlled trial. *JAMA*. 2006;295(7):761-75.

48. Despres JP, Golay A, Sjöström L. Effects of rimonabant on metabolic risk factors in overweight patients with dyslipidemia. *N Engl J Med*. 2005;353(2):2121-34.

49. Munro J, MacCuish A, Wilson E, et al. Comparison of continuous and intermittent anorectic therapy in obesity. *Br Med J.* 1968;1(5588):352-4.

50. Scheen AJ, Finer N, Hollander P, et al. RIO-Diabetes Study Group. Efficacy and tolerability of rimonabant in overweight or obese patients with type 2 diabetes. *Lancet*. 2006;368(9548):1660-72.

51. Rogers PJ, Blundell JE. Effect of anorexic drugs on food intake and the micro-structure of eating in human subjects. *Psychopharmacology* (Berl). 1979;66(2):159-65.

52. Foltin RW, Haney M, Comer SD, et al. Effect of fenfluramine on food intake, mood, and performance of humans living in a residential laboratory. *Physiol Behav*. 1996;59(2):295-305.

53. Drent ML, Zelissen PM, Koppeschaar HP, et al. The effect of dexfenfluramine on eating habits in a Dutch ambulatory android overweight population with an over consumption of snacks. *Int J Obes Relat Metab Disord*. 1995;19(5):299-304.

54. Positive results from a phase 2b clinical trial of Lorcaserin demonstrated highly statistically significant weight loss. Available at: http://www.arenapharm.com/wt/page/lho. Accessed November 20, 2007.

55. Parker E, Van Heek M, Stamford A. Neuropeptide Y receptors as targets for anti-obesity drug development: perspective and current status. *Eur J Pharmacol*. 2002;440(2-3):173-87.

56. Levens NR, Della-Zuana O. Neuropeptide Y Y5 receptor antagonists as anti-obesity drugs. *Curr Opin Investig Drugs*. 2003;4(10):1198-204.

57. Poindexter GS, Bruce MA, LeBoulluec KL, et al. Dihydropyridine neuropeptide Y Y(1) receptor antagonists. *Bioorg Med Chem Lett*. 2002;12(3):379-82.

58. Kanatani A, Hata M, Mashiko S, et al. A typical Y1 receptor regulates feeding behaviors: effects of a potent and selective Y1 antagonist, J-115814. *Mol Pharmacol*. 2001;59(3):501-5.

59. Zahorska-Markiewicz B, Obuchowicz E, Waluga M, et al. Neuropeptide Y in obese women during treatment with adrenergic modulation drugs. *Med Sci Monit*. 2001;7(3):403-8.

60. Erondu N, Gantz I, Musser B, et al. Neuropeptide Y5 receptor antagonism does not induce clinically meaningful weight loss in overweight and obese adults. *Cell Metab*. 2006;4(4):275-82.

61. Batterham RL, Cohen MA, Ellis SM, et al. Inhibition of food intake in obese subjects by peptide YY3-36. *N Engl J Med*. 2003;349(10):941-8.

62. Brandt GAS, Quay S. Intranasal peptide YY 3-36: phase 1 dose ranging and dose sequencing studies. *Obes Res*. 2004;12 (suppl):A28.

63. Wynne K, Park AJ, Small CJ, et al. Subcutaneous oxyntomodulin reduces body weight in overweight and obese subjects: a double-blind, randomized, controlled trial. *Diabetes* 2005;54(8):2390-5.

64. Dunk C, Enunwa M, De La Monte S, et al. Increased fecal fat excretion in normal volunteers treated with lipase inhibitor ATL-962. *Int J Obes Relat Metab Disord*. 2002;26 (suppl):S135.

65. Kopelman P, DeGroot G, Rissanen A, et al. A randomised, placebo-controlled, trial of cetilistat (ATL-962), a novel lipase inhibitor and orlistat (Xenical®) for the management of obese type 2 diabetic patients. *Diabetes Metab*. 2006;55:A395.

66. AOD9604 Phase 2b Clinical Trial Successful. Available at: http://www.metabolic.com.au/files/T5SH4035T6/ASX_%20AOD9604_result%20announcement.pdf. Accessed November 20, 2007.

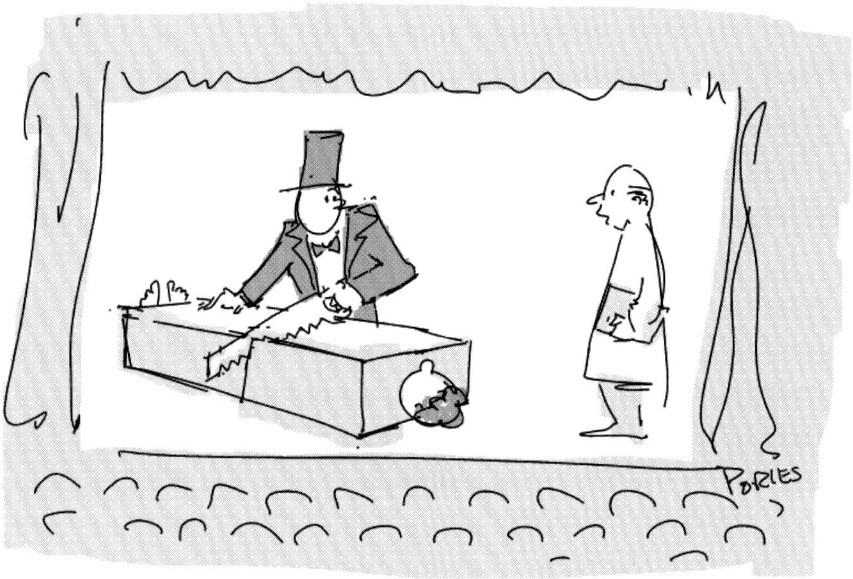


"Sorry for butting in but what happens to ghrelin, leptin, PYY, and GLP-1?"

# Meal Replacements

George L. Blackburn, MD, PhD
Katherine A. Wang
Kristina Day, RD, LD

## Introduction

Weight-loss surgery puts extremely obese patients at risk for complications and death from medical problems associated with obesity and from the surgery itself.(1) Weight loss prior to surgery has been used to reduce preoperative morbidity and reduce the risk of perioperative complications.(2) This approach is consistent with the current trend for initial weight loss prior to the completed bariatric procedure in high-risk, super-obese patients.(3,4)

Improved health status has been linked to preoperative weight loss. In a population-based, prospective cohort study, Peppard et al(5) found that modest weight loss improved sleep-disordered breathing, and data from van de Wiejgert(2) found that preoperative weight loss produced a major reduction in obesity-related morbidity (hypertension, impaired glucose tolerance, angina pectoris). Data suggest that preoperative weight reduction may also make bariatric procedures less technically challenging.(4) Fris (6) demonstrated that a 2-week preoperative low-calorie diet led to a significant reduction in liver size. Busetto et al(7) reported significantly shorter operating room times and length of stay after weight loss in patients with a BMI >50 kg/m$^2$.

Preoperative weight loss in high-risk patients with meal replacement is an established nutrition/medicine intervention. Several studies, reviews, and meta-analyses attest to the benefits of partial meal replacements (PMRs).(8) A systematic evaluation of randomized controlled trials (RCTs) using such plans for weight management suggests that these types of interventions can safely and effectively produce significant and sustainable weight loss(9,10) and improve weight-related risk factors of disease(10,11,12)(Figures 1 and 2). It is also thought that preoperative weight loss may optimize postoperative weight loss following bariatric surgery.(4)

**Figure 1**

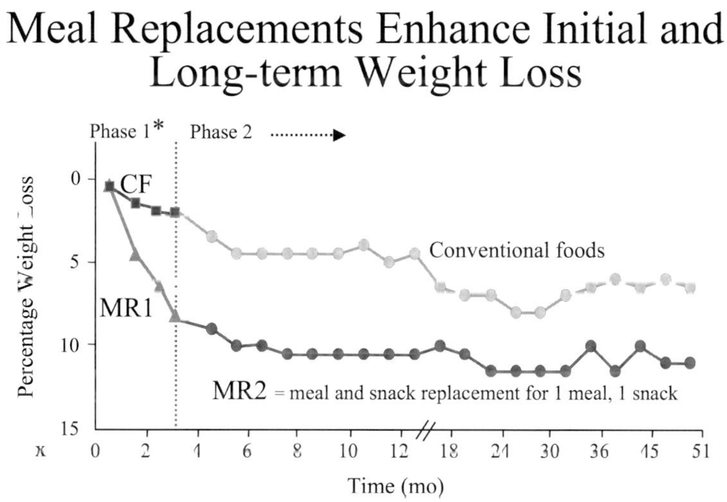


*1,200-1,500 kcal/d diet prescription
CF = conventional foods
MR1 = meal and snack replacement for 2 meals, 2 snacks

(Ditschuneit et al. *Am J Clin Nutr.* 1999;69:198; Fletchner-Mors et al. *Obes Res.* 2000;8:399.)

**Figure 2**
**Weight Reduction Maintained Long-term**

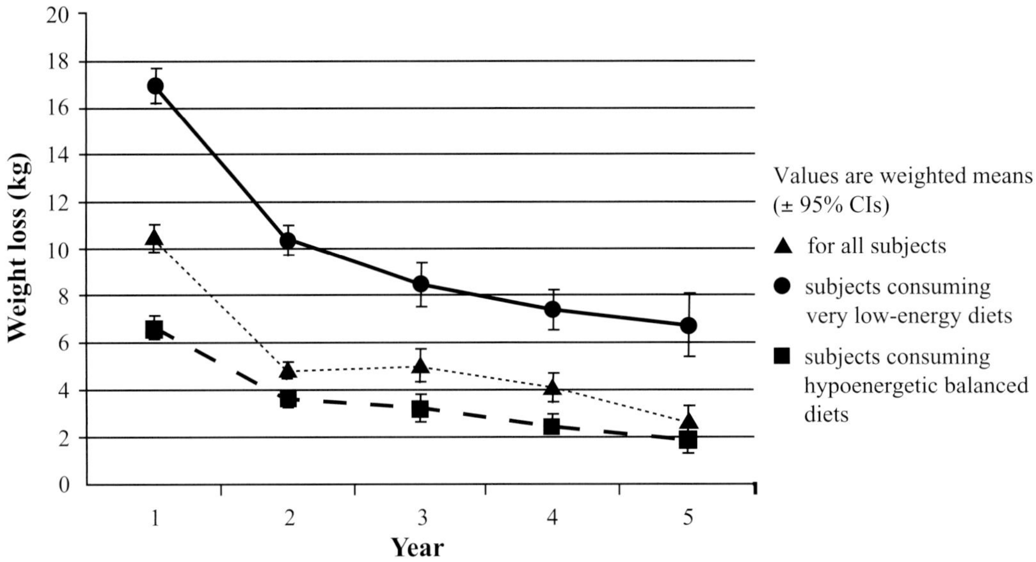


Anderson et al. *Am J Clin Nutr*. 2001;74:579-84.

Preoperative weight loss in high-risk patients can be achieved through short-term dietary means.(3) Reductions of 5% to 10% of initial weight are known to improve obesity-related hypertension,(13) lipid abnormalities, and glycemic control.(14) Pasulka et al(15) have shown that as little as a 10% weight loss may have dramatic effects on cardiopulmonary and metabolic function. Best practice in weight-loss surgery promotes preoperative weight loss in all bariatric surgery patients, and specifically a preoperative weight loss of 5% to 10% in patients with body mass index (BMI) >50 kg/m$^2$ or obesity-related comorbidities.(16)

**Meal Replacement Strategy**

Meal replacements are defined as "a single food or pre-packaged selection of foods that is sold as a replacement for one or more of the daily meals, but not as a total diet replacement."(8,17) These replacements, which provide a defined amount of energy, exert their effect through reduced portion size and, as a consequence, reduced energy intake.(18) A properly constituted, PMR exchanges a high-calorie, high-fat meal for a low-calorie, low-fat, good-tasting, nutrient-dense meal.(9,10)

It has been suggested that replacing two meals a day while maintaining one other main meal is effective for initial weight loss, while replacing 1 meal a day (preferably a meal high in energy such as lunch or dinner) sustains long-term weight loss maintenance.(19) In patients with morbid obesity (BMI >40, requiring large weight losses), specially formulated and medically supervised very-low-calorie diet (VLCD) forms of meal replacement have been used in place of all meals. However, the use of PMRs for one or two meals a day, with at least one usual meal consumed as part of an overall low-energy diet, is more common.(8)

**Principles of Meal Replacement for Weight Maintenance**

Food-based, meal replacement plans that emphasize the value of fruits, vegetables and portion control promote healthy eating patterns and produce safe, effective weight loss of 1 to 2 lbs per week.(20) Noakes et al(21) found the nutritional adequacy of a meal-replacement program equal and, in the case of some micronutrients, superior to a conventional diet with the exception of fiber requirement. Dietary calcium intake was increased in the meal replacement group, mostly as a consequence of the inclusion of milk-based shakes. In addition, the dietary structure (food choice and meal pattern) of both programs, meal replacement vs. conventional diet, resulted in similar energy distributions (i.e., moderate protein and carbohydrate intakes and relatively low fat intake) (Figure 3).(9,21,22)

**Figure 3**
**Meal Replacement Reduces Fat Intake to Recommended Level**

| | Group | Baseline | 3 mo |
|---|---|---|---|
| **Energy (kcal/d)** | A | 1797 ± 203 | 1663 ± 86* |
| | B | 1814 ± 84 | 1375 ± 43* |
| **Fat (kcal/d)** | A | 676 ± 79 | 547 ± 82* |
| | B | 655 ± 55 | 340 ± 43* |
| **Cholesterol (mg/d)** | A | 422 ± 57 | 244 ± 30* |
| | B | 378 ± 43 | 154 ± 14 |

Group A = conventional diet
Group B = meal replacement
$^*P \leq .05$

Ditschunheit et al. *Am J Clin Nutr*. 1999;69:198-204.
Ditschunheit et al. *Eur J Clin Nutr*. 2002;56:264-270.

**Structured Meal Plans vs. Traditional Dietary Options**

Various studies suggest that the structure of dietary interventions influences outcomes, but it is unclear whether meal replacements are superior to other structured weight loss approaches (e.g., those that provide menus, recipes, or financial compensation). Data indicate that most individuals in the United States who participate in structured weight loss programs do not regain all of their lost weight at 5 years, and that they maintain a long-term weight loss of approximately 3 kg.(11)

A meta-analysis by Heymsfield et al(11) found that individuals consuming meal replacements lost 7% to 8% body weight at 1 year compared with 3% to 7% body weight in those on a standard self-selected diet. These data are consistent with findings seen in other studies that compared meal replacements(9,19,23,24) or prepackaged entrees(25,26) with self-selected diets. Although some weight regain was observed over time, a greater reduction in weight was observed, even up to 4 years, in individuals who received meal replacements,(19) suggesting that replacing 2 of 3 meals with a liquid and/or solid meal replacement or at least two meals with a portion-controlled entrée resulted in greater weight loss than self-selected diets.

Wing and Jeffery(27) summarized a number of reasons why structured meal plans might improve weight loss and weight loss maintenance compared with traditional dietary options, including: increased attendance at treatment meetings, a positive impact on self-monitoring, more accurate assessments of portion size and calorie intake, improved meal-planning skills and reduced barriers to dietary adherence. They also found that structured meals helped instill regular eating patterns and promoted healthy modifications in the types of foods stored at home.

In a minimally controlled study in Australian adults, meal replacements were as effective a strategy for weight loss as a conventional diet when maintained over both a 3- and 6-month period. Participants found meal replacement easy to comply with and found it easier to dine out on this plan, facilitating longer-term compliance with a weight loss program and suggesting that meal-replacement programs are nutritionally sound if applied appropriately.

**Weight Loss With Meal Replacements**

Use of meal replacements once or twice daily in place of a usual meal can result in significant weight loss, but meal-replacement therapy must be continued if weight loss is to be maintained. A significant number of studies of this model used in behavioral programs that include emphasis on physical activity have been published.(23,26,28) Reports on these studies can be found in a supplement to *Obesity Research*.(29)

Meal replacements have been examined in a number of long-term studies. The results are positive and suggest that weight loss can be maintained by using this strategy.(9,10,19,23,28,30) In one such study, a 116-week follow-up study using meal replacements, weight loss was 6 kg overall.(31) After 1 year, 77% of subjects maintained >80% of the initial weight loss and

62% maintained >80% of the initial weight loss after 2 years, with only 7.4% of subjects above baseline weight. Flechtner-Mors et al(10) found that after 4 years in a single-arm intervention study using meal replacements, which had an initial 12-week, 2-arm meal-replacement and a conventional-diet intervention period, the original conventional-diet group had a 3.2% weight loss vs. 8.4% in the meal-replacement group. Ditschuneit et al(9) reported that weight loss after an initial 3-month phase (11.3% ± 6.8% in the meal-replacement group and 5.9% ± 5.0% in the conventional-diet group) was continued over 24 months.

While different forms of meal replacements have been used for weight loss over many years, controlled research on the effectiveness of PMRs is relatively recent. Several studies, reviews, and meta-analyses have reported benefits of PMRs, including usual weight loss of around 9% to 10% of total body weight in the short term (6-12 months), and 6% to 8% in the long term (e.g., 1-5 years), with no reported adverse effects when used as part of an overall low-energy diet plan.(18,19,32) Noakes et al(21) found similar decreases in weight in individuals using meal replacements (-9.0 kg or -9.4% body weight) and those following structured diets (-9.2 kg or -9.3% body weight) at 6 months. This compares with a 3%-7% loss on some other types of diet plans,(18,19,32) although at least one study showed similar short-term weight losses from meal replacements and a prescriptive, structured low-fat diet plan.(21) The benefits of PMRs are even more obvious when compared with no treatment. In a 5-year study, an average weight gain of over 1 kg per year occurred in control subjects, compared with a loss of 5.8 kg in men and 4.2 kg in women using PMRs.(28)

**Benefits for Practitioners**

Physicians often have the first opportunity to encourage weight control and primary prevention. Their clinical offices are the mainstay for treatment of obesity-related comorbid conditions.(33,34) Potential advantages of using meal replacements include wide availability to aid compliance, low cost, and minimal professional intervention.(31) Recent reports indicate that meal replacements coupled with a low-calorie diet can offer an effective option for long-term compliance or improvements in metabolic risk factors in clinic patients.(9,10,28,30,31) Compared with traditional diets, meal replacements have been shown to be an effective weight-management tool both in the medical-office practice and in traditional dietitian-led group settings.(30) For the physician, lifestyle counseling with meal replacement provides a useful tool that allows easy explanation and has demonstrated efficacy with patients.(24)

Anderson et al(35) report that meal replacements can be as effective as energy-restricted diets and low-energy diets with lower levels of intervention. Berkal et al(36) found that less traditional applications of behavior modification in the treatment of obesity (i.e., meal replacements, Internet interventions, telephone interventions) can be used effectively to apply the principles of behavior modification, specifically stimulus control and self-monitoring, to obese patients.

Meal replacements used in conjunction with practitioner intervention can be highly effective. A 1-year study using three lifestyle-based treatments showed that a meal-replacement intervention in a primary-care office setting was as effective at achieving weight loss (4%) as a dietitian-led, conventional dietary intervention (4% weight loss), whereas a meal-replacement combined with a dietitian intervention was more effective (9%) than either intervention alone.(24) A 2-intervention study (meal-replacement and restricted-calorie diet) achieved similar weight losses in both groups by using a pharmacy setting with structure built into visit times, incorporating the pharmacists as the focus for dietary advice and use of a 3-week visit program.(37)

**Benefits to Patients**

Partial meal replacements appear to have an effect across a range of ages and in both sexes (although men generally have better results than women).(28,38) Most studies show greater patient satisfaction and lower drop-out rates with PMRs than with other diets, possibly because meal replacements result in less hunger(39) and can be used with minimal supervision. Dietary compliance and convenience were also viewed more favorably by participants who consumed meal replacements than by those in a conventional weight loss program.(21)

Partial meal replacements also seem effective in people from low socioeconomic backgrounds,(40) who are currently more likely to be overweight and therefore in greater need of weight loss treatments.(8) Importantly, PMRs are generally cheaper than other diet plans, and certainly more so than nondiet meals. Meal replacements are not contraindicated in common weight-related diseases (e.g., diabetes and heart disease), but food sensitivities, such as lactose intolerance or food allergies, need to be taken into account when choosing specific products.(8)

Commercial meal replacements have become increasingly popular as a strategy among people trying to lose weight. Many American adults (15% of women and 13% of men) reportedly use meal replacements as their weight-loss strategy.(41) In one study, two thirds of 252 patients chose to use meal replacements at least once daily.(42) After 6 months, weight loss was 8.62 ± 1.81 kg for women and 7.03 ± 3.72 kg for men. According to Noakes et al,(21) participants found the meal replacement strategy convenient to use and provided manageable dining-out options. Management of, and compliance with, the diet, therefore, was good—supporting the notion that meal replacements offer an effective alternate strategy for long-term dieting.

**Meal Replacements and Type 2 Diabetes**

There is increasing scientific evidence to suggest that excess visceral fat in obese type 2 diabetes may play a key role in the evolution of the metabolic abnormalities manifested in this patient population. Several recent clinical trials have shown that weight loss in obese, type 2 diabetics can result in a favorable correction of several key metabolic disturbances.(43) Prospective, open-label, single-blind, RCTs have demonstrated that portion-controlled meal replacements are safe and effective and may prevent or treat such comorbidities of obesity as diabetes and cardiovascular disease.(9,10,19,43,44) Findings indicate that provision of a structured meal plan(45) or a liquid meal replacement(9,43) produces significantly increased short-term weight loss in obese diabetic patients(46,47) compared with the usual prescription of a low-calorie, nutrient-balanced diet of conventional foods. Yip et al(43) explored the effects of liquid meal replacements on immediate glucose response and 12-week glycemic control in obese patients with type 2 diabetes. Findings demonstrated that use of meal replacements in this population could help correct the metabolic abnormalities associated with excess body weight. During weight loss, there were associated reductions in glucose, insulin, and A1C levels (Figure 4). Furthermore, many participants were able to reduce use of oral hypoglycemic medications. In the 12-week study, weight reduction achieved through the use of liquid meal replacements resulted in improvements in glycemic control, insulin,(43) and lipid levels. Successful management of weight loss in obese patients with type 2 diabetes has been shown to be capable of correcting many of the metabolic abnormalities associated with the disease, such as hyperinsulinemia, hyperglycemia, and hypertriglyceridemia.(9,10,31)

**Figure 4**

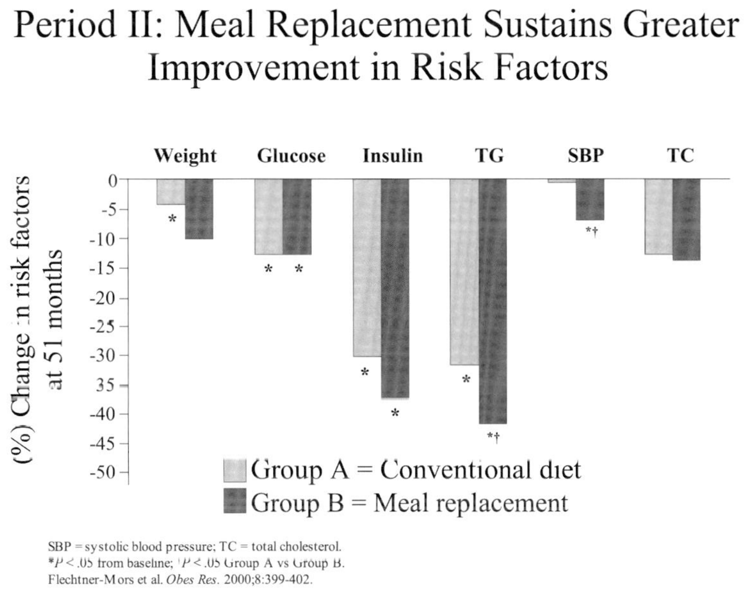


**Summary**

Best practice in weight-loss surgery encourages preoperative weight loss in all bariatric-surgery patients, and promotion of preoperative weight loss of 5% to 10% in patients with BMI >50 or obesity-related comorbidities.(16) Preoperative weight loss in high-risk patients with meal replacement is an established nutrition/medicine intervention(8); it has been used to reduce preoperative morbidity and risk of perioperative complications.(2) Data suggest that preoperative weight reduction may make bariatric procedures less technically challenging. It is also thought that preoperative weight loss may optimize postoperative weight loss following bariatric surgery.(4)

Compared with traditional diets, meal replacements have been shown to be an effective weight-management tool both in the medical-office practice and in traditional dietitian-led group settings.(30) A 1-year study using three lifestyle-based treatments showed that a meal-replacement intervention in a primary-care office setting was as effective at achieving weight loss as a dietitian-led conventional dietary intervention, whereas a meal replacement combined with a dietitian intervention was more effective than either intervention alone.(30) Data suggest that structured meal plans, which provide good nutrition and portion control for at least 1 or 2 meals a day, improve risk factors for the metabolic syndrome (e.g., blood lipids, glucose, insulin resistance, blood pressure) and help patients make healthy food choices, including increased consumption of fruits and vegetables.(27) Reduction of 5% to 10% of initial weight is known to improve obesity-related hypertension,(16) lipid abnormalities, and glycemic control.(14) Pasulka et al(15) have shown that a weight loss as small as 10% may have dramatic effects on cardiopulmonary and metabolic function.

Obese diabetic patients in a structured, skills-based behavioral approach for reducing caloric intake and increasing physical activity(46,47) have traditionally been prescribed a low-calorie, nutrient-balanced diet of conventional foods. Recent findings, however, suggest that provision of a structured meal plan(45) or liquid meal replacement(9,43) can significantly increase short-term weight loss and may play a positive role in facilitating weight maintenance.(9) Several recent clinical trials have suggested that weight loss in obese patients with type 2 diabetes can result in a favorable correction of several key metabolic disturbances.(43)

For many years, meal replacements have been promoted for weight loss and maintenance, but have only recently been subjected to rigorous scientific study. It is believed that these products offer numerous benefits to individuals who are seeking to control their weight.(10) In addition to the obvious benefits of convenience and relatively low cost,(9) meal replacements offer nutritionally balanced alternatives to the high-fat, high-calorie, fast-food meals that make up much of the American diet. The use of meal replacements also adds an element of structure to the patient's eating plan, reducing the number of food choices he/she must make each day, which may make it easier for patients to comply with dietary guidelines (e.g., increased consumption of fruits and vegetables) during "regular" meals. Use of meal replacements once or twice daily in place of a usual meal can result in significant weight loss, but meal-replacement therapy must be continued if weight loss is to be maintained.

**Acknowledgments**

The authors would like to acknowledge the support of the S. Daniel Abraham Chair in Nutrition Medicine at Harvard Medical School and the Harvard Center for Healthy Living. The authors thank Rita Buckley for assistance with medical writing.

**References**

1. Steinbrook R. Surgery for severe obesity. *N Engl J Med*. 2004;350(11):1075-9.
2. van de Weijgert EJ, Ruseler CH, Elte JW. Long-term follow-up after gastric surgery for morbid obesity: preoperative weight loss improves the long-term control of morbid obesity after vertical banded gastroplasty. *Obes Surg*. 1999;9(5):426-32.
3. Alfalah H, Philippe B, Ghazal F, et al. Intragastric balloon for preoperative weight reduction in candidates for laparoscopic gastric bypass with massive obesity. *Obes Surg*. 2006;16(2):147-50.
4. Alvarado R, Alami RS, Hsu G, et al. The impact of preoperative weight loss in patients undergoing laparoscopic Roux-en-Y gastric bypass. *Obes Surg*. 2005;15(9):1282-6.
5. Peppard PE, Young T, Palta M, Dempsey J, Skatrud J. Longitudinal study of moderate weight change and sleep-disordered breathing. *JAMA*. 2000;284(23):3015-21.
6. Fris RJ. Preoperative low energy diet diminishes liver size. *Obes Surg*. 2004;14(9):1165-70.
7. Busetto L, Segato G, De Luca M, et al. Preoperative weight loss by intragastric balloon in super-obese patients treated with laparoscopic gastric banding: a case-control study. *Obes Surg*. 2004;14(5):671-6.

8. Egger GJ. Are meal replacements an effective clinical tool for weight loss? *Med J Aust*. 2006;184(2):52-3.

9. Ditschuneit HH, Flechtner-Mors M, Johnson TD, Adler G. Metabolic and weight-loss effects of a long-term dietary intervention in obese patients. *Am J Clin Nutr*. 1999;69(2):198-204.

10. Flechtner-Mors M, Ditschuneit HH, Johnson TD, Suchard MA, Adler G. Metabolic and weight-loss effects of long-term dietary intervention in obese patients: four-year results. *Obes Res*. 2000;8(5):399-402.

11. Heymsfield SB, van Mierlo CA, van der Knaap HC, Heo M, Frier HI. Weight management using a meal replacement strategy: meta and pooling analysis from six studies. *Int J Obes Relat Metab Disord*. 2003;27(5):537-49.

12. Anderson JW, Konz EC, Frederich RC, Wood CL. Long-term weight-loss maintenance: a meta-analysis of US studies. *Am J Clin Nutr*. 2001;74(5):579-84.

13. Stevens VJ, Obarzanek E, Cook NR, et al. Long-term weight loss and changes in blood pressure: results of the Trials of Hypertension Prevention, phase II. *Ann Intern Med*. 2001;134(1):1-11.

14. Anderson JW, Kendall CW, Jenkins DJ. Importance of weight management in type 2 diabetes: review with meta-analysis of clinical studies. *J Am Coll Nutr*. 2003;22(5):331-9.

15. Pasulka PS, Bistrian BR, Benotti PN, Blackburn GL. The risks of surgery in obese patients. *Ann Intern Med*. 1986;104(4):540-6.

16. Saltzman E, Anderson W, Apovian C, et al. Criteria for patient selection and multidisciplinary evaluation and treatment of the weight loss surgery patient. *Obes Res*. 2005;13(2):234-43.

17. Food Standards Australia New Zealand. Australia New Zealand Food Standards Code. Available at: www.foodstandards.gov.au. Accessed September 7, 2006.

18. Keogh JB, Clifton PM. The role of meal replacements in obesity treatment. *Obes Rev*. 2005;6(3):229-34.

19. Ditschuneit HH, Flechtner-Mors M. Value of structured meals for weight management: risk factors and long-term weight maintenance. *Obes Res*. 2001;9 (suppl 4):284S-289S.

20. *Evidence-based Nutrition Principles and Recommendations for the Treatment and Prevention of Diabetes and Related Complications*. American Diabetes Association. *Diabetes Care*. 2002;25(suppl 1):S50-S60.

21. Noakes M, Foster PR, Keogh JB, Clifton PM. Meal replacements are as effective as structured weight-loss diets for treating obesity in adults with features of metabolic syndrome. *J Nutr*. 2004;134(8):1894-9.

22. Ditschuneit HH, Frier HI, Flechtner-Mors M. Lipoprotein responses to weight loss and weight maintenance in high-risk obese subjects. *Eur J Clin Nutr*. 2002;56(3):264-70.

23. Rothacker DQ, Staniszewski BA, Ellis PK. Liquid meal replacement vs traditional food: a potential model for women who cannot maintain eating habit change. *J Am Diet Assoc*. 2001;101(3):345-7.

24. Ashley JM, St Jeor ST, Perumean-Chaney S, Schrage J, Bovee V. Meal replacements in weight intervention. *Obes Res*. 2001;9 (suppl 4):312S-320S.

25. Hannum SM, Carson L, Evans EM, et al. Use of portion-controlled entrees enhances weight loss in women. *Obes Res*. 2004;12(3):538-46.

26. Metz JA, Stern JS, Kris-Etherton P, et al. A randomized trial of improved weight loss with a prepared meal plan in overweight and obese patients: impact on cardiovascular risk reduction. *Arch Intern Med*. 2000;160(14):2150-8.

27. Wing RR, Jeffery RW. Food provision as a strategy to promote weight loss. *Obes Res*. 2001;9 (suppl 4):S271-S275.

28. Rothacker D. Five-year self-management of weight using meal replacements: comparison with matched controls in rural Wisconsin. *Nutrition*. 2000;16:344-8.

29. Blackburn GL. Dietary patterns in weight management and health. *Obes Res*. 2001;9(suppl 4):S217-S218.

30. Ashley JM, St Jeor ST, Schrage JP, et al. Weight control in the physician's office. *Arch Intern Med.* 2001;161(13):1599-604.

31. Heber D, Ashley JM, Wang HJ, Elashoff RM. Clinical evaluation of a minimal intervention meal replacement regimen for weight reduction. *J Am Coll Nutr.* 1994;13(6):608-14.

32. Anderson JW, Hoie LH. Weight loss and lipid changes with low-energy diets: comparator study of milk-based versus soy-based liquid meal replacement interventions. *J Am Coll Nutr.* 2005;24(3):210-6.

33. Galuska DA, Will JC, Serdula MK, Ford ES. Are health care professionals advising obese patients to lose weight? *JAMA.* 1999;282(16):1576-8.

34. Kreuter MW, Chheda SG, Bull FC. How does physician advice influence patient behavior? Evidence for a priming effect. *Arch Fam Med.* 2000;9(5):426-33.

35. Anderson JW, Luan J, Hoie LH. Structured weight-loss programs: meta-analysis of weight loss at 24 weeks and assessment of effects of intervention intensity. *Adv Ther.* 2004;21(2):61-75.

36. Berkel LA, Poston WS, Reeves RS, Foreyt JP. Behavioral interventions for obesity. *J Am Diet Assoc.* 2005;105(5 suppl 1):S35-S43.

37. Ahrens RA, Hower M, Best AM. Effects of weight-reduction interventions by community pharmacists. *J Am Pharm Assoc.* 2003;43(5):583-9.

38. Winick C, Rothacker DQ, Norman RL. Four worksite weight-loss programs with high-stress occupations using a meal replacement product. *Occup Med* (Lond). 2002;52(1):25-30.

39. Rothacker DQ, Watemberg S. Short-term hunger intensity changes following ingestion of a meal-replacement bar for weight control. *Int J Food Sci Nutr.* 2004;55(3):223-6.

40. Huerta S, Li Z, Li HC, Hu MS, Yu CA, Heber D. Feasibility of a partial meal replacement plan for weight loss in low-income patients. *Int J Obes Relat Metab Disord.* 2004;28(12):1575-9.

41. Levy AS, Heaton AW. Weight control practices of US adults trying to lose weight. *Ann Intern Med.* 1993;119 (7 Pt 2):661-6.

42. Bowerman S, Bellman M, Saltsman P, et al. Implementation of a primary care physician network obesity management program. *Obes Res.* 2001;9 (suppl 4):S321-S325.

43. Yip I, Go VL, DeShields S, et al. Liquid meal replacements and glycemic control in obese type 2 diabetes patients. *Obes Res.* 2001;9 (suppl 4):S341-S347.

44. Franz MJ, Bantle JP, Beebe CA, et al. Evidence-based nutrition principles and recommendations for the treatment and prevention of diabetes and related complications. *Diabetes Care.* 2002;25:148-198.

45. Wing RR, Jeffery RW, Burton LR, Thorson C, Nissinoff KS, Baxter JE. Food provision vs structured meal plans in the behavioral treatment of obesity. *Int J Obes Relat Metab Disord.* 1996;20(1):56-62.

46. Pascale RW, Butler BA, Mullen M, Bononi P. Effects of a behavioral weight-loss program stressing calorie restriction versus calorie plus fat restriction in obese individuals with NIDDM or a family history of diabetes. *Diabetes Care.* 1995;18(9):1241-8.

47. Wing RR, Marcus MD, Epstein LH, Jawad A. A "family-based" approach to the treatment of obese type II diabetic patients. *J Consult Clin Psychol.* 1991;59(1):156-62.

# Weight Watchers®

Karen Miller-Kovach, MBA, MS, RD

Weight Watchers is a comprehensive weight-loss program that focuses on lifestyle modification. The efficacy of the program's approach has been demonstrated in randomized clinical trials and determined to be the only commercial program in the United States with convincing evidence to substantiate its weight-loss system.(1) It enjoys huge brand awareness, with approximately 98% of the American public (including healthcare practitioners) recognizing the Weight Watcher's name. Nevertheless, many people do not really know what goes on at a Weight Watchers meeting or what the program involves.

Founded in 1963, the Weight Watchers organization currently runs meetings in 30 countries around the world. There are 22,000 Weight Watchers meetings held each week in North America alone. Though a membership organization, its members are not required to sign a contract or pay a long-term membership fee at the time of joining. An initial registration fee of about $15 (waived during promotional periods or with a referral coupon from a physician) is collected and then a weekly membership fee—about $12 per week, although it varies around the country—is charged.

Many people are under the mistaken belief that the organization's food plan requires purchasing Weight Watchers brand-name foods. Because they see these foods in their grocery stores, they assume that these foods are a required part of the Weight Watchers program. This is not the case. In fact, members have a great deal of flexibility regarding their food choices and the Weight-Watchers–brand foods are in no way required in order to be successful in the program.

**Membership and leadership**

The Weight Watchers membership is about 90% female and 10% male, with the typical member being about 35 to 45 years of age with a body mass index (BMI) of about 32 kg/m$^2$ at time of joining. Membership policies require a BMI of approximately 21 to join, but the reality is that we have very few members join with a BMI of less than 25.

The typical meeting has about 35 people and is built around the concept of group support within a large group dynamic. There is no individual counseling, and weight loss recommendations are limited to strategies to assist in applying the defined Weight Watchers program to each individual's life. Based on public health guidelines, the program was created by credentialed healthcare professionals with expertise in weight management, but it is delivered by role models, meaning that each person who leads a Weight Watchers meeting has lost weight on the program, has achieved a BMI of 25 (or less), and is maintaining that weight loss on the program. All Weight Watchers staff members are extensively trained prior to leading meetings. Each must demonstrate proficiency in understanding and communicating the program as it is written. Deviation from the written program is not permitted, but leaders are able share their experiences and empathize with the weight issues that all members face.

This "developed by professionals and delivered by role models" approach is a key strength of the Weight Watchers method. Why? Healthcare professionals often face a significant barrier when working with overweight patients. If the professional is at a healthy weight, patients often assume that the person has never had a weight problem, and may discount the counseling being provided. On the other hand, if the professional is overweight or obese, the counseling is also discounted in the belief that, if the method were effective, the practitioner would not have weight to lose. One of the differentiating characteristics of Weight Watchers is that this "white coat resistance" simply does not exist. Every person who leads a Weight Watchers meeting has had weight issues, has lost weight, and is successfully maintaining a healthy weight. The result is an atmosphere conducive to bonding and empathy—one that encourages the kind of support that healthcare settings are sometimes handicapped to provide.

The Weight Watchers model works very well, but like all models, there are advantages and disadvantages. Among the advantages is the fact that there is a group meeting at a convenient location at virtually any time of the day or week. In the United States, meetings are conducted in places ranging from rural Nebraska to downtown Manhattan, at hours scheduled morning through evening, on weekdays and weekends. People demand convenience and having a wide choice of meeting options is a real plus. A potential disadvantage, however, is that Weight Watchers is not a medical organization and does not provide medical nutrition therapy. The staff is prohibited from modifying the program to meet a member's medical needs. Rather, the staff is trained (and audits are performed to make sure that policies are followed) to tell members with specific needs (e.g., those with diabetes, dumping syndrome, gluten sensitivity) to take the Weight Watchers program materials to a consultation with their dietitian or physician and follow whatever individual instruction they are given by the healthcare professional.

Weight Watchers has a rapid weight loss policy that is strictly enforced. During the first 3 weeks of a member's participation, there is a fair amount of water loss and close monitoring of the rate of weight loss is not done. After the third week, however, if a member is losing more than an average of 2 pounds per week, she or he is told that this is a more rapid weight loss than our program allows. The member is provided with two options: slow the rate of weight loss or obtain a physician's note approving a faster rate of weight loss, but with medical monitoring.

**Lifetime Membership**

Meetings are based on open enrollment. This means that when a person comes to Weight Watchers, he/she will be in a meeting with people who are at various stages of the weight loss journey, including some who have successfully lost weight and are lifetime members. A lifetime member is any member who reduces to either a BMI of 25 or provides physician advice specifying a weight goal deemed healthy for that individual; in either case, the member must successfully complete the 6-week maintenance plan. Lifetime members are encouraged to come back at least once a month for ongoing support and for the accountability of a weigh-in. All lifetime members who come in for monthly and are within 2 pounds of their weight goal attend for free.

Lifetime members are an integral part of the Weight Watchers meeting experience. In addition to the staff leading the meeting, these members provide motivation, encouragement, and support to the rest of the group. There is a lot of support and interaction between members during these meetings, where people are at all different parts of their weight loss process. At Weight Watchers, weekly meetings are an ongoing part of successful weight management.

**Weight Watchers: the 4 pillars**

Weight Watchers is committed to providing a science-based weight loss program that is continuously reviewed and periodically revised to reflect changes in members' lifestyles and the latest in scientific thinking. Despite the overwhelming awareness of the Weight Watchers brand, many people think of the program as essentially a diet and are often not aware of just how comprehensive the weight management program is. In fact, there are 4 pillars to the Weight Watchers program: food, activity, cognition (thinking skills), and support.

**The Flex Plan**

As of September 2004, Weight Watchers has offered two distinct food plans. The Flex Plan uses the patented *POINTS®* Food System and is a counting program not unlike counting calories, fat grams, or any other nutrient marker. Every food has a *POINTS®* value, usually a single digit like 1, 2, or 3. The small numbers make it easy to count. The *POINTS* value of a food is based on a formula that includes calories per serving, dietary fiber, and total fat. Members are provided with a paper calculator called the *POINTS®* tracker that enables them to calculate the value from the nutrition-facts panel of any packaged food. The number of *POINTS* values that a person gets in a day depends on his or her current weight and is called a daily *POINTS* target. By having a daily *POINTS* target and knowing how many *POINTS* values are consumed, a calorie deficit is created and weight is lost. The Flex Plan relies a great deal on portion control, but also provides a great amount of flexibility because every food has a *POINTS* value. As a weight loss plan, it is ideal for people who are numbers oriented and willing to keep track of their food consumption by counting. It is often the plan of choice for members who know that they need the structure and accountability that counting *POINTS* values demands. It is also very important for people who value the idea of being able to eat any food that appeals to them. These are the people who say, "I can't do without my wine with dinner," or "As soon as you start restricting me, I rebel and I fall off the wagon."

**The Core Plan®**

The Core Plan was introduced in September 2004 and is quite different than the Flex Plan. Many members refer to it as a "no counting" plan because it limits most food choices to a particular list, eliminating the need for counting. This plan focuses choices on wholesome, nutritious foods and is built on the foundation of limiting choices to foods low in energy density.

Low-energy–density foods tend to be high in water, rich in fiber, and less processed, so they tend to be filling. In addition, this plan also removes foods that people tend to overeat ("trigger" foods), and appeals to those who don't want to count. These are the individuals who say, "I can't be bothered with keeping track of all those POINTS." The Core Plan is also chosen by people who say, "Don't tell me I can eat everything. That isn't helpful. Telling me I can eat a little brownie that has a *POINTS* value of 2 doesn't help me. I do best when I structure my eating in a way that I can have it or I can't have it most of the time."

The Core Plan was thoroughly tested prior to its introduction. During its 18 months of development, approximately 10,000 Weight Watchers members across the United States followed the plan. The results demonstrated that those following the plan had nutritionally adequate diets and lost weight. The weight losses for both Flex Plan and the Core Plan are comparable.

**Self-Monitoring**

Self-monitoring is an integral part of the Weight Watchers program and that includes both food plans. Self-monitoring is inherent in the Flex Plan because *POINTS* values need to be tracked to ensure that the daily target is met. For the Core Plan, self-monitoring is achieved via a feature called the Comfort Zone. Members are taught how to assess their internal cues of hunger and satiety on a regular basis and to eat before getting too hungry and to stop eating when they begin to feel satisfied. Certainly there are people who say, "If I knew my Comfort Zone, I wouldn't have a weight problem!," and they have a good point. However, the Comfort Zone is something that can be learned. Members do have the ability to switch between the Flex Plan and the Core Plan on a week-to-week basis. However, most Weight Watchers members self-select into one plan or the other and then stay with it.

***POINTS* Allowance**

There are some elements of the Weight Watchers program that are common to both the Flex and the Core Plans. One is called the weekly *POINTS* allowance. All members get an "allowance" of 35 *POINTS* values per week. The weekly *POINTS* allowance is similar to the US Dietary Guidelines concept of the discretionary calories. One integral element of the Weight Watchers program is learning the skill of flexible restraint. Lasting weight loss demands some restraint in eating. However, many people with weight issues are black-and-white thinkers and they need to learn how to introduce some flexibility to their dietary restraint. The weekly *POINTS* allowance is a tool that helps people to learn this valuable skill. It can be used for indulgences, special occasions, or not used at all.

The weekly *POINTS* allowance is especially critical to those following the Core Plan, particularly people who chose it over the Flex Plan because they didn't want to count *POINTS* values. They would rather be told what they can and cannot eat. The reality is that following a limited food list can be done for a few weeks, but not for the long term. The weekly *POINTS* allowance provides a way to have foods that are not "on the list" and staying on the food plan for an extended period of time.

**Dietary Guidelines**

Another element shared by the two food plans is the 8 Good Health Guidelines. These guidelines shape food choices to resemble the DASH Diet and US Dietary Guidelines. Following these within the structure of the food plan ensures nutritional adequacy by prescribing amounts of fruits and vegetables, low-fat dairy, whole grains, and healthy oils. Weight Watchers also recommends taking a multiple-vitamin/mineral supplement that provides no more than 100% of the percent daily value (% DV) or recommended daily allowance (RDA).

**Activity**

Activity is the second pillar of the Weight Watchers program. In fact, the *POINTS* weight loss system includes both a *POINTS* food system and a *POINTS* activity system. The *POINTS* values for activity are based on a formula that considers exercise intensity (perceived exertion), the amount of time the activity is performed, and current body weight. People can do any activity, whether it is walking, gardening, going to the gym, and then calculate the activity *POINTS* values. The activity plan falls right in line with the American College of Sports Medicine and US Dietary Guidelines for weight management, progressing from health benefits to weight loss to maintaining weight loss. The program starts with a focus on reducing sedentary behavior and then doing enough activity to achieve health benefits (2 *POINTS* values per day). By the time a member reaches his or her weight goal and is ready to become a Lifetime Member, the emphasis on exercise is increased so that members are doing 60 to 90 minutes a day to help them keep the weight off.

### Thinking Skills

Thinking skills make up the third pillar in the Weight Watchers program. The most significant changes in behavior occur in the weekly meeting. The foundation of this aspect of the program is called Weight Watchers *Tools for Living*. *Tools for Living* is based on the tenets of neurolinguistic programming, or NL, and changes thinking patterns with 12 specific skills that are taught to members so they can enhance problem-solving, coping, and goal-setting skills as these relate to weight loss. While the *Tools for Living* are provided as part of the written program materials, their usefulness comes to life in the meeting. All Weight Watchers staff members have been trained on the use of the *Tools for Living* and how to facilitate their use during the course of the meeting. For example, one of the group members may raise a problem or a challenge or a concern and the meeting leader will say, "Well, let's do mental rehearsing for that. What are the steps for mental rehearsing? These are the steps that we take. Let's work with that." In this environment, members can really see how these step-wise skills, which are simple and easy to implement, can become part of their lives and help them manage their weight in a very proactive way.

### Additional Tools

An array of products exists to support the Weight Watchers program. For example, the Weight Watchers Web site provides a subscription service so that members, whether they choose to attend meetings or not, have access to all program information and tools in an interactive format. Weight Watchers foods, with *POINTS* values right on the package, are available at the grocery store and there is a Weight Watchers menu available at Applebee's. Books that contain the *POINTS* value and Core Plan status are available for generic and branded foods and for foods served at national restaurants. These small books can be kept easily in a purse or in the car so that food choices from fast-food restaurants can be assessed. And there are Weight Watchers pedometers and exercise videos. While not a part of the program per se, these tools can be used by members to enhance their compliance.

### Weight Watchers and the Bariatric Surgery Patient

Many health plans require 6 months of documented participation in a weight loss program to qualify for bariatric surgery. Weight Watchers has been the program chosen by many patients, often at the recommendation of their surgeons. This is not a practice that Weight Watchers recommends at this time. Why? The motivation to join Weight Watchers for these patients is different than the typical Weight Watchers members and these differing motivators can create discord in the group environment in which the meeting occurs. Certainly, the content of the Weight Watchers program can be very helpful for the bariatric patient who is preparing for surgery and will need to make significant lifestyle changes for lasting weight loss. The reality, however, is that the support that is so critical to the Weight Watchers experience can be lacking between those who are attending with an endpoint of surgery and those who are not. In summary, Weight Watchers does not prohibit people from using its method to qualify for surgery, but it does not market or recommend that Weight Watchers be a preferred weight loss program during the preoperative period.

As the number of bariatric surgeries is increasing, so is the number of postsurgical patients who are joining Weight Watchers. In general, these patients are not in their immediate postoperative period, but are 1 or 2 years out. They turn to Weight Watchers either because their weight has reached a plateau, or they want to lose that last 20 lbs or because they have started to regain weight. At this time, Weight Watchers can offer these patients a supportive environment with its weekly meetings and its proven weight management system. It does not provide any information or guidance that is unique to their postsurgical status, however. As with any member's medical condition, the Weight Watchers staff, if asked how to modify the program to meet that member's special needs, will refer the patient back to his or her physician or dietitian with encouragement to comply with any instructions that are given.

### References

1. Tsai AG, Wadden TA. Systematic review: an evaluation of major commercial weight loss programs in the United States. *Ann Intern Med.* 2005;142(1):56-66.

# Readiness to Change

Diana Cullum-Dugan, RD, LD

In weight management counseling, I hear hundreds of reasons why people can't change. I hear even more reasons why this or that diet doesn't work and excuses about why it's impossible to exercise. Hearing these "barriers to change" can lead to a high level of frustration, as a counselor and a provider. At some point, I began to feel there had to be something I could do differently that could make this dialogue a little easier, not only for me but for the patient as well. After being trained to use motivational interviewing (MI) as a style of counseling, I realized that MI was the tool that actually helped me best in this and I offer the following as an introduction to its use.

A surgeon in Rochester, New York, had a fairly extensive database with information regarding his own surgical patients over 8 years(1). This surgeon was keenly interested in figuring out what some of the behavioral factors were that led to success in some patients and not in others. The patients in his database were mostly women, all with gastric bypass or other types of weight loss surgery. He had asked them to complete lifestyle questionnaires before and 1 year following the surgery. Sixty percent achieved a 50% or greater weight loss, which left 40% who did not even achieve 50% weight loss.

As he was looking through this database, the surgeon came to the conclusion that those who had dieted previously had better success with weight loss after surgery. Most had dieted at least 7 times before they had surgery. Also, if they had greater weight loss success with these diets, they had better success after surgery. The greater their anticipated stress about the dietary changes that they had to make after surgery actually equaled greater success in weight loss. So the person who says, "Well, you know, my stomach's only this big (meaning 1 or 2 tablespoons), I'm sure I'll stop eating when I'm full and that should take care of it," doesn't succeed as well as the one who is a little more obsessive about what he/she needs to eat, how they're going to eat and how they will be able to make healthy and appropriate choices. Of interest: a prospective surgical patient with the greatest number of confidants had greater weight loss success. The surgeon concluded that the larger the social network, the better a patient would fare. The perceived level of stress experienced before surgery about impending dietary changes *after* surgery, along with a higher sense of coherence (in other words, a greater sense of confidence) led to less ambivalence. Less ambivalence meant that the patient was more intrinsically motivated to lose weight—and in this context, the less ambivalence a patient exhibits, the less MI you need to use.

Two providers in Boston realized that no standardized protocols existed for the interviewing process when it came to gastric bypass patients, so they put a protocol together.(2) The interview-style questionnaire they designed addresses 7 areas of interest, one being eating behaviors. The interviewers ask questions such as how fast the individual eats, what portion sizes he/she chooses and how many liquid calories are taken in. It also asks if the person eats when not hungry. They began addressing the patients' expectations regarding surgery and realized that some people have unrealistic expectations and goals. This gave the interviewers an opportunity to refer patients for further psychological counseling in an effort to assist them in developing more realistic ideas about what would happen after weight loss surgery. An example of an unrealistic expectation was belief that a bad marriage would be made good if the patient's body weight was less. Several people thought they were going to lose all of their excess body weight, which we know is not true as most surgical patients ultimately remain in the overweight category (body mass index [BMI] >25 and <30 kg/m$^2$). Also, looking at realistic motivations for surgery, it is critical to find out why a patient is going through this surgery: Is it for health reasons, or more of an appearance issue? Is it for increased mobility? Patients in these interviews perceived success in dietary compliance for multiple reasons. In other words, some felt they would be successful just by eating less food, even though this had not worked for them in the past. This line of questioning during the interview is directed more toward adherence to the tight and rigid structure of a postsurgery diet. If they were unable to do so before surgery for weight loss, how were they going to adhere to the rigid structure of a weight loss surgery diet? Another predictor of success is patients' ability to effectively solve problems, mostly life problems, such as how they handle the stress of marriage, divorce, or financial difficulties. Also, what relationships and support systems are in place? Again, individuals receiving strong support from friends or family have greater post surgery success. But, many of us do not realize that sometimes our greatest saboteurs are the people in our immediate family or close friend network who love us dearly.

Key to successful MI is the ability to recognize readiness to change, as well as ambivalence. What I'd like to share is that MI is a style of *talking*. It's not a rigid counseling technique that you must memorize and learn, or a strict algorithm of a step-by-step process. It is merely a style that is very empathetic and sensitive to your patient's needs and desires, a nonassuming, nonjudgmental *style* of talking. What you'll find, if you begin to use some of the skills and techniques of MI, is that they will enhance your patients' compliance and their commitment to change.

We all know about the stages of change, but what is important is being able to recognize that we don't always follow this continuum of change in the way the arrows on the figure suggest.

**Figure 1**

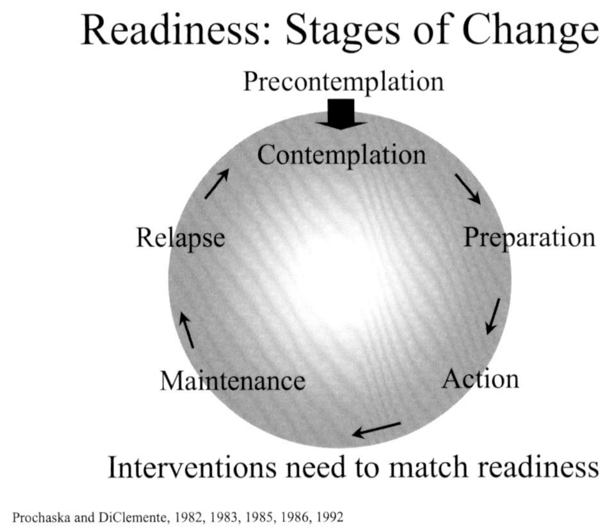


Often we bounce all over the place. We go from A to B to Z to K and we're all over the alphabet when we are looking at making behavioral change. Being able to understand two tools that I'll share with you about the importance and confidence level of your patient will help you identify where they are in their stage of readiness. Then the behavioral interventions have to match their readiness to change. If you have someone who doesn't feel it's important to make the changes, giving them a structured diet to follow is not going to be the appropriate intervention.

We argue for change (and I use that term loosely, theoretically) all the time. We persuade, advise, suggest, and make offerings of different ways that maybe someone can change; yet they dig their heels in ever more firmly and argue to stay the same. If a patient argues to stay the same, and we argue with them to stay the same, what's going to happen? You'll see that the opposite happens. The patient begins to argue for change. Ultimately the patient will always make the argument for change.

Rolling with resistance is a key term used in MI training. It simply means that if you're arguing with your patient and you're not getting anywhere, you are seeing no change, it's not your patient—it's you. That means you need to find a way to be a little bit different in reaching them, that you should consider evaluating your counseling technique and approach. I use "you" but include myself, because I was in the same situation. I was asking myself what can I do that will be more effective in reaching my patients? It turns out that, instead of being the expert and wagging our fingers at our patients and telling them what to do, we can be more effective by entering into a dual relationship with them. Stated another way, the dance of MI is just like a dance on a dance floor. And we serve as the lead dancer, the lead partner, as we safely guide our patient through the steps of behavioral change.

**Figure 2**

# Ambivalence is Normal!

| ⬇ ➡ | Eat What I Desire | S/P Surgery |
|---|---|---|
| Benefits of: | • I like the tastes<br>• Cheaper + more convenient<br>• Don't have time to shop<br>• Feel fine<br>• At least I don't smoke<br>• I'm not that bad a diabetic | • Improved health<br>• Decrease medications<br>• Less social distress<br>• Feel like I can make a difference<br>• *I don't want to die!* |
| Costs of: | • My doc lectures me<br>• I've gained another 20 lbs<br>• I can't control my sugars as well as I used to<br>• I don't like the meds | • Healthier food is expensive<br>• Too much measuring<br>• Hard to get protein<br>• Where will I dine out?<br>• My doc will still lecture |

Figure 2 shows my favorite tool in motivational interviewing. For practical purposes, however, it doesn't have to be this beautiful and well laid-out. You can rip a piece of paper in half when you're counseling, when you have a patient who is showing tremendous amounts of ambivalence about whatever change you're suggesting he/she consider making. Make a big plus sign on it. On the left, write "Benefits of" and "Costs of." On the top, write "Staying the same" or "Changing." Ask your patient what he/she feels are the benefits in life right now of staying the same, not making any changes. List these in the "Benefits of" square. Then ask the patient, "What are the costs to you of doing this?" You'll get a lot of different answers. But then ask what the patient perceives would be the benefits if they have surgery. Ask, "What are the benefits if you follow this dietary protocol? And what is it going to cost you?"

What you're going to find over time by using this tool is that there are a couple of squares or boxes that are going to be the "change talk," and two boxes that patients keep coming back to, which represent the status quo. The change-talk boxes are yours. Your power, your tool, is to know and understand the patient's perceived benefits of changing the behavior and why he/she wants to stay the same. This gives you greater power, because patients are going to come right back to the status quo. As long as you can stay dancing around the two boxes of "Benefits of changing" and "Costs of staying the same," they're going to start arguing for what you want. Remember, we always argue for change.

Motivational interviewing's strongest key feature is open-ended questions. By this, I mean a question that cannot be answered with a yes or no. It's very typical in counseling for us to ask questions that end in yes or no. In obtaining a 24-hour recall, for instance, I want to know everything the patient ate or drank the day before. I could start off by asking if he/she had breakfast yesterday, but there are two things wrong with that approach. I'm going to get a yes or no answer, and I am going to get a period and a stop sign. Then I'm stuck with no place else to go except to ask another closed-ended question. But, if I say, "Tell me what you had to eat or drink yesterday, starting from the time you woke up," I'm going to cast a really broad net—I am going to get more information than I really wanted. I am trying to get the patient to open up and share with me a wide variety of things, to share with me what it is like to be him/her. In addition, this approach is neither "assuming" nor "biased." I want to avoid casting assumptions when I'm speaking with a patient. The trick to open-ended questions is to ask no more than three questions. You may have an hour of counseling time, but try to limit your questions. Rely instead on reflective listening to get more information. As the patient talks, respond by offering statements rather than questions. If I'm asking what a patient had to eat yesterday and the explanation is, "Well, I didn't have anything to eat. I don't eat breakfast when I get up. I'm too busy, I've got to get the kids to school, etc., etc.," as I reflect back to them I can say, "So, it sounds like you don't have breakfast in the morning because you're too busy." Or I could say, "You don't eat breakfast?" The difference is that now I have turned it into a question. A downturn is when you take the rise, or upturn, out of your voice, eliminating the questioning tone. I can use that same sentence and say, "You don't have breakfast." I just made a statement out of a question. After that, allow for a pause. Someone has said this would be called a "pregnant pause." I really like that description so, I'm going to borrow it. Get comfortable with the silence that follows—that *pregnant pause*— when you reflect statements back to your patients. They may fidget a little but, I guarantee they'll start talking and tell you anything you want to know.

You can also use reflective listening as a way to test a hypothesis. A patient may not have said anything about feeling overwhelmed or lacking time-management skills, but you can interject that as you reflect back. Your reflective statements will validate everything your patients say, without judgment or bias, because what you are doing is simply confirming in their own words.

When speaking to your patients about their weight or the diet following surgery, or any special component that you know is going to be of a sensitive nature to them, ask their permission first. This will create a bond, because they're going to trust you whenever you ask to talk about something. Ask how they feel about what you shared with them so that you can freely go from there. "How do you feel about what we've talked about and what I said?," you may ask. "How do you feel about the diet after surgery?"

**Figure 3**

## Readiness/Importance

1. To assess *importance* of change:
   On a scale of 0 to 10, with 10 being 100% *ready* to take action, how ready are you to *(lose weight, eat less fat, stop smoking …)*?

0.........................................................10
*Not at all Ready* *Extremely Ready*

- Why are you at *x* and not at *0*?
- What would need to happen for you to raise your score a couple of points?

## Confidence/Ability

2. If you did decide to make a change, how *able* do you feel you are to do it? On a scale of 0 to 10, what number would you give yourself?

0.........................................................10
*Not at all Able/Confident* *Extremely Able/Confident*

- Why are you at *x* and not at *0*?
- What would need to happen for you to raise your score a couple of points?

When you're really stuck with ambivalence, you can use the importance/confidence scale. This is the first MI tool I used and it works quite well (Figure 3). Patients can be very ambivalent. On one hand, they know they need to follow through with these changes, but on the other, there are those 100 reasons why they can't. They vacillate back and forth as they have this tug of war inside. You can ask, "Well, if you were to decide to make any changes today, on a scale of 0 to 10, 0 being changes that are not at all important and 10 being extremely important, what number could you give yourself?" Let's say they reply that they are at an 8. Validate and affirm their answers: "Why are you at an 8 and not a 6 or a 7?" What you'll find as you validate their stated number by comparison to a smaller number, is the patient's perception of both readiness to change, and the importance of making that change. If their number is low, this will help you identify whether you need to share the benefits of change at this point. Remember, I mentioned earlier that if a patient is not ready to change, providing them a detailed and structured approach to dietary change is not effective. If the number chosen is high, you're good to go—there's no problem. If it is a lower number, offering all the benefits of change to get them to begin thinking about change would be appropriate. Validate again: "What would it take—what would have to happen—for you to change your 8 to a 9?" Here you'll identify barriers to change, the issues, excuses, reasons, and all the problems they feel they will experience. Problems you can now help them to solve.

When you get stuck on importance/confidence you can take a step back to what some call good/not so good, or good/bad, pros/cons, benefits of/costs of. You might ask, "What do you really like about your life without surgery? How does eating out help you? How does your life right now feel comfortable to you?" And then: "What's not so good about it?" Reflect back to them what they say. Hearing it back will trigger even more talking; then you can flip to confidence or ability—how able he/she thinks they will be if they follow through. I think this is critical, especially with regard to the postsurgery diet. "How able are you to follow this diet?" Again, on a 0 to 10 scale, let he/she give you the number. Validate that number, drop down below it so that you can identify any need to share "benefits of" and inquire again, "What would need to happen to get that number higher?"

The ambivalent patient may not make changes now. You may be counseling someone who thinks he/she wants surgery, and then realize that he really doesn't; or she may not be appropriate for surgery in your clinical opinion. Validate your patients' ambivalence, validate that they may not be ready to make these changes, but, they have control over the ultimate decision. "You may or may not be ready for changes," you might say. "Would you like a few options other than surgery to think about?"

Elicit, provide, elicit. Elicit their ideas. What do they know about the diet following surgery? Listen to what they say. Then provide information back to them. Fill in the gaps. You're exhausting their knowledge so that you don't have to give them everything. Give them what they don't know and then ask, "How does that sound to you? Is there anything else you need to know?"

In summary, using motivational interviewing is an extremely effective tool in many areas, especially in counseling for weight management or potential weight loss surgery intervention. You'll find that you do not have to work so hard. Put your patient in the driver's seat. When patients make the argument for change, they make the commitment to change; their compliance increases, their risks of surgery decrease and your visits are much more pleasant.

**References**

1. Ray EC, Nickels MW, Sayeed S, Sax HC. Predicting success after gastric bypass: the role of psychosocial and behavioral factors. *Surgery*. 2003; 134(4):555-63.

2. Sogg S, Mori DL. The Boston interview for gastric bypass: determining the psychological suitability of surgical candidates. *Obes Surg*. 2004; 14(3):370-80.

# Health Utility Assessment

Christina Wee, MD, MPH

Being overweight or obese is associated with serious health and social consequences. Not surprisingly, many populations place a high value on being thin. Describing one's health utility is a way of estimating the value one places on one's state of health and hence, measuring health utility may be a potentially important way of quantifying the value patients place on weight loss. It is important to understand how much a patient values weight loss. Knowing the different approaches that can be used to estimate that "value" allows us to assess health utility and adapt it as a measurement for use in helping obese patients.

**The Value of Bariatric Surgery**

Obesity is a major public health problem in this country.(1) Bariatric surgery is one of few effective weight loss treatments, but despite its overall effectiveness, it is associated with risks of mortality, complications, and side effects. Furthermore, this surgery is not universally effective.(2) Results from well-done, long-term, follow-up studies with low rates of attrition show a substantial variability in weight regain across individual patients.(3) The degree of sustained weight loss varies quite a bit, as well. For all these reasons, many in the medical community are ambivalent about whether bariatric surgery should be the treatment of choice for a large segment of patients with obesity.

When thinking about whether to pursue certain interventions, most clinicians tend to focus on health outcomes and the benefits of treatment. Health payers might also consider the economic consequences. Patients, on the other hand, often consider how their lives will change after treatment. This is especially true in the case of obesity treatment because, in addition to its adverse health effects, obesity can be very stigmatizing and can result in negative social and economic consequences.(4-7) These quality-of-life considerations are paramount in the minds of some patients when thinking about different treatments for obesity.(4)

In making decisions about whether to adopt a health intervention on a public health basis, policymakers should, and often do, consider all of these factors. This process can be achieved through decision analysis, a method of systematically considering the risks, benefits, and costs of a treatment.(8,9) In considering the benefits of an intervention, decision analysis usually accounts for patient preferences or the value that patients place on different health outcomes. Cost-effectiveness is one type of decision analysis familiar to many clinicians.(10) A cost-effective analysis considers treatment or intervention costs and treatment benefits usually in the context of a treatment prolonging a person's life. In assessing the number of life-years that an intervention might save on an individual patient level, cost-effectiveness analyses not only consider the actual number of years of life saved, but also the quality of that life, usually by assigning a weight to the life-year. For example, a patient who goes through treatment and has excellent health has a life year that is weighted more highly than a patient who suffered a stroke as a complication of the treatment and is now disabled. In this way, the years spent in the suboptimal state are discounted. In assessing the cost-effectiveness of different obesity treatments, quantifying the value of weight loss becomes particularly salient.

**Measuring Quality of Life**

One way of ascertaining the value of a particular health outcome from the patient's perspective is to measure the quality of life associated with that outcome.(10,11) Quality of life is the subjective value that an individual places on satisfaction with life.(10) Health related quality of life refers more specifically to the physical, psychological, and social domains of health.(12) Descriptive measures of quality of life provide a sense of patients' preferences and the value they attach to certain health outcomes. One can infer that a disease that produces a low quality of life would be valued much less than a disease or health outcome that leads to a high quality of life.(8)

There are many different health status questionnaire instruments that capture quality of life. Perhaps the most familiar instrument is the 36-Item Short Form Health Survey (SF-36),(13) a widely used generic health status measure. The SF-36 was initially developed and validated to capture quality of life in medically ill patients, but has been used for a wide variety of diseases, including obesity. The SF-36 captures 8 domains including: physical functioning; social functioning; role functioning;

general and mental health; pain; vitality; and health transition. While the SF-36 is a very good general health-status measure, it has several limitations when used to measure the quality-of-life impact of obesity because it does not capture many of the relevant domains that are affected by obesity. For example, the SF-36 does not capture self-esteem or self-image or the stigma associated with obesity.(7,14,15) Newer health-status measures have been developed in order to capture domains important in obesity. One of these measures is the Impact of Weight on Quality of Life (IWQOL),(14,16-18) a 74-item questionnaire that measures physical functioning, self-esteem, sexual life, public distress, and work life. It was developed specifically for obese patients and has been abbreviated to contain 31 items. Another measure is the Moorehead-Ardelt Quality of Life Questionnaire II used in the Bariatric Analysis and Reporting Outcomes System (BAROS).(19) The Moorehead-Ardelt questionnaire captures the same domains as the IWQOL, but consist of even fewer questions and its psychometric properties have not been as rigorously established.

While health-status measures elicit a lot of information and are easily accessible to most audiences, they have several limitations.(7,14,15,17) The first is that any health-status measure or questionnaire cannot capture all of the relevant domains or aspects of quality of life that are important to every patient. Second, the domains are often assigned scores or points by a researcher, and these often reflect their importance in studies on other patients or respondents. This scoring may not reflect priorities of an individual patient. For example, how does having a poor sex life because of one's weight compare with not being promoted in a job because of weight? How do researchers or clinicians assign values to these domains? When a patient responds to a questionnaire, the researcher or the person administering the questionnaire assigns a certain importance to each question item. Thirdly, health-status measures may not be able to capture how important the quality-of-life impact of being obese compares with having other diseases such as diabetes. Finally, while many of the generic health-status measures, such as the SF-36, are too generic, the specific measures, such as IWQOL and BAROS, are too specific and preclude interpretation in a broader context. If a patient is given the weight-specific questionnaires and scores poorly, how does one compare those results with those of another patient who has poor quality of life as a result of a disabling stroke? Is poor quality of life from obesity worse than having a stroke? Is it better than having a stroke? How do you compare the adverse quality of life associated with these different conditions?

**The Value of Weight Loss**

Different lines of evidence suggest that thinness is highly valued in our society and this value exceeds that which is attributable to the health benefits of being thin, meaning that there is inherent value to weight loss and thinness independent of their health effects.(4,5) In 2001, Foster and colleagues(20) surveyed several hundred moderately and severely obese patients who were seeking different medical, behavioral, and surgical weight treatments (Table 1). Both moderately and severely overweight patients desired "dream" weights that represented weight losses ranging from 38% to 49% of their current weight. They considered weight losses of 24% to 33% "acceptable," but up to 22% of severely obese patients would actually be disappointed if they lost less than 22% of their weight. This finding is striking since many patients sustain less than a 20% weight loss from bariatric surgery.(2,3,21)

**Table 1**

**Evaluations of weight loss among patients seeking weight treatment(20)**

| **Weight, kg<br>(% change from initial weight)** | **BMI 35-39<br>n=105** | **BMI ≥ 40<br>n=141** |
|---|---|---|
| Current | 105 | 135 |
| Dream | 65 (38%) | 67 (49%) |
| Happy | 73 (30%) | 79 (41%) |
| Acceptable | 80 (24%) | 88 (33%) |
| Disappointed | 90 (14%) | 104 (22%) |

Results from the Swedish obesity study,(3) which followed participants for 10 years after surgery, showed that only a minority of patients who had gastroplasty and gastric banding can sustain a weight loss of 20% or greater (Table 2). Even in patients with Roux-en-Y gastric bypass, which tends to produce higher weight loss, more than a quarter do not sustain 20% weight loss.

**Table 2**
**Percent weight loss 10 years after bariatric surgery: results from Swedish obese study(3)**

| | Type of surgery | | |
|---|---|---|---|
| **Weight loss** | **RYGB** | **Gastroplasty** | **Banding** |
| <5 % | 9% | 14% | 25% |
| >20 % | 74% | 35% | 28% |

Given these study findings, many patients may be disappointed with the results of bariatric surgery. However, being disappointed with an outcome does not necessarily mean that patients do not value that outcome at all.

### Measuring Health Utility

Health utility can be used to quantify how patients value a particular state of health.(10,11) It has been used very widely and for a very long time to capture patient preferences in a diverse number of conditions and, therefore, is the gold standard for obtaining quality-of-life weights used in decision analyses. Recently, our group adapted this methodology to quantify how much patients value weight loss.(8)

There are different ways of measuring health utility, the two most common methods being the standard gamble and time trade-off.(10) These methods use a universal metric in order to capture the value that a patient attaches to a health outcome. In the standard gamble, the individual is asked to express how much he/she values a certain outcome in terms of his/her willingness to risk death to achieve that outcome. In the time trade-off, the respondent is asked how much time alive they would give up to be in that better health state. Another well-known approach is to measure willingness to pay.(10) This method is straightforward and easily understandable for most patients—patients are asked how much they are willing to pay to achieve a certain outcome (i.e., a particular weight loss goal). However, a major problem with this method is that the value of a unit of money is not as universal as one might think. The value of any given amount is dependent not only on how desirable an outcome is to the individual, but also on the individual's wealth and how easy or difficult it is for them to acquire wealth. In measuring health utility the objective is to have people express what the value to them is for a certain outcome in terms of something that everyone values to a similar degree.

### Standard Gamble

The standard gamble is the gold standard for assessing health utility or health value.(10) Patients are given a hypothetical choice: 1) they can stay in their current health state for the rest of their life; or 2) they can take the gamble. The gamble typically involves a treatment, for example, a hypothetical treatment that will immediately give the patient perfect health since, in most diseases, the desired outcome is perfect health. The hypothetical treatment does not cause any side effects and is not inconvenient, but a number of the patients will die immediately from this treatment. In essence, patients are asked whether they are willing to take this gamble, the chance to get rid of all their health problems, but at a risk of dying. This process is not dissimilar to the one that clinicians and patients undergo when making medical decisions about potentially risky treatments such as surgeries usually associated with a risk of death.

The risk of death is then varied in the standard gamble scenario to see how high a risk the patient is willing to accept to achieve the desired outcome.(8) For example, patients might be asked if they are willing to take this treatment if the risk of death is 1%. If a patient says yes, then he/she is asked about a 2% risk of death. The risk is increased until the patient refuses to take the gamble. At that point, the patient's response is recorded as his/her value point. The rationale behind the standard gamble is that the worse a patient's health, the higher risk of death he/she is willing to take. For example, a patient with terminal cancer who has 6 months left to live might be willing to take an 80% risk of dying to achieve perfect health, whereas a patient with diabetes might only risk 10% to achieve perfect health. The patient's response, or value point, is converted to a utility. The patient with terminal cancer in this case would have a health utility of 0.2 and the patient with diabetes would have a health utility of 0.9. A utility of 0.9 can be translated to mean that life in that current state of having diabetes is worth 0.9 of life for someone who is in perfect health.

**Time Trade-off**

The standard gamble can be quite challenging and complex, however. Moreover, there are patients who are just not willing to gamble or not willing to take a risk of death no matter how much they value an outcome. To circumvent the problem of risk aversion in some respondents, a second approach called the time trade-off is used.(10) The time trade-off works on a similar premise of giving a patient a choice; but instead of asking them to risk dying, patients are asked to trade time. For example, a patient is given the choice of living in his or her current health for a certain number of years or living a shorter period of time, but in better health or perfect health. The important thing to consider when using the time trade-off approach is to pose the scenario in the context of a relatively short timeframe, (i.e., 10 years). Patients are asked to imagine that they only have 10 years left to live in their current health or they have a choice of living 9 years, but in better health. For the time trade-off to be valid, the patient needs to be in the mindset of trading current time, so that a younger patient should not be thinking, "I'm 20 now. It's not so bad to risk one year when I'm 80 so that I can be thin and healthy now and for the rest of my life," because just as with the value of a future unit of money, future life-years are worth less.

A few years ago, we adapted the standard gamble and time trade-off in a telephone survey of 365 primary care patients.(8) The study surveyed 121 overweight patients and 100 obese patients. Most patients had fairly optimistic "dream" weights (Table 3). On average, the obese patients wanted to lose 28% of their weight in order to achieve what they classified as their "dream" weight, and needed to lose 19% to get to their "satisfied" weight. Patients were also asked a series of hypothetical standard gamble scenarios. First, they were asked to consider a hypothetical treatment that would lower their weight permanently without any effort or side effects but could potentially result in death. The patients were then told that the treatment would guarantee them a 5% weight loss permanently. We then proposed other scenarios where the treatment guaranteed a 10%, a 20%, and a weight loss that would produce a body mass index (BMI) of 25 kg/m$^2$.

**Table 3**
**Body-weight preferences in primary care patients(8)**

| | **Equivalent weight loss as a percentage of initial weight** | |
|---|---|---|
| | Overweight n=121 | Obese n=100 |
| BMI of 25 kg/m$^2$ | 7% | 31% |
| "Dream" weight | 10% | 28% |
| "Satisfied" weight | 4% | 19% |
| Minimum weight loss to achieve any health benefits | 5% | 11% |

On average, overweight patients had a BMI of 27 and the obese patients had a BMI of 37. About one fifth of overweight patients and one third of obese patients were actually willing to risk death to sustain a 10% weight loss; 43% of obese patients were willing to risk death to sustain a 20% weight loss (Table 4).

**Table 4**
**Percent patients willing to risk death to lose weight(8)**

| | **Overweight** | **Obese** |
|---|---|---|
| **Initial weight (BMI)** | **177 lbs (27)** | **230 lbs (37)** |
| **Weight loss** | | |
| 5% | 13% | 25% |
| 10% | 19% | 33% |
| 20% | 16% | 43% |
| BMI, 25 kg/m$^2$ | 20% | 50% |

When we tried to calculate utilities from these data we encountered some challenges, because initially we had planned to use a BMI of 25 as the equivalent to perfect health, as that was the lowest weight of the scenarios posed. However, we found that 12% of obese patients actually preferred to be at a higher body weight than a BMI of 25. As a result, we recalibrated each person's reference state. For some patients the utility of 1.00 was assigned to a 20% weight loss. For other patients, the 1.00 was assigned to a 5% weight loss, depending on their most valued health state. Table 5 presents the utilities for the different weight loss states.

**Table 5**
**Utility or value for weight loss among primary care patients(8)**

| | **Overweight** | **Obese** |
|---|---|---|
| **Relative to most desired weight** | | |
| **Current weight** | 0.95 | 0.88 |
| 5% weight loss | 0.96 | 0.91 |
| 10% weight loss | 0.98 | 0.93 |
| 20% weight loss | 0.98 | 0.96 |
| BMI 25 kg/m2 | 0.98 | 0.98 |

Studies(11,22-25) suggest that utilities for patients with disabling strokes tend to be in the 0.6 range, slightly more than half the value of perfect health. Other studies suggest that patients with diabetes reported a utility of 0.88, whereas patients with clinical depression have a utility of 0.95.(24,25) Our study(8) suggested that, independent of the health consequences of obesity, being obese is similar to living with diabetes. For overweight patients, being overweight is similar to having clinical depression. Applying this finding to the average obese patient, you can calculate how much it is worth to each patient to lose 10% of his/her weight. To arrive at this value, you subtract the utility of the patient's current weight (0.88) from the utility he/she would have at a 10% lower weight (0.93); hence, losing 10% is valued at 0.05.

In conducting a pilot study of patients undergoing bariatric surgery at the Beth Israel Deaconess Medical Center, we followed patients to examine the changes in health utilities and quality of life before and after surgery.(26) Baseline results from our first 40 patients showed that the mean BMI was 47. Most study participants were white women. Most of them wanted to lose 43% of their weight permanently from bariatric surgery and would be very disappointed if they did not achieve at least a 23% weight loss from their surgery (Table 6).

**Table 6**
**Expectations for weight loss from bariatric surgery(26)**

| | n=40 |
|---|---|
| **Current weight (BMI)** | 284 lbs (47) |
| **Ideal/"dream" weight (% weight)** | 124 lbs (43%) |
| **Min. satisfactory weight loss (% weight)** | 67 lbs (23%) |

Patients were also presented with a series of standard gamble scenarios as in our early survey of primary care patients, with some additional health states such as their "dream" weights. Patients were asked if they would risk death for perfect health, so that our results could be compared with results of other studies that use perfect health as the reference state. Another scenario proposed a combination of both perfect health and "dream" weight as the desired state.

Most patients (95%) reported that they were willing to risk death to undergo bariatric surgery and they were willing to accept, on average, as high as a 5% risk of death. However, only 70% were willing to accept the treatment for a guaranteed 20% weight loss and these patients were only willing to take a 2% risk of death, on average. However, almost all patients were willing to risk death to undergo bariatric surgery, even though for many patients, surgery could produce less than a 20% weight loss. Our findings suggest that patients may have unrealistic expectations for this surgery.

**Table 7**
**Willingness to risk death to lose weight(26)**

| Health state | Willing to risk death, n (%) | Mean acceptable risk, % | Utility |
|---|---|---|---|
| **Current** | - | - | 0.92 |
| **10% weight loss** | 35 | 0.3 | 0.92 |
| **20% weight loss** | 70 | 2 | 0.93 |
| **BMI of 25 kg/m2** | 85 | 6 | 0.98 |
| **"Dream" weight** | 90 | 6 | 0.98 |
| **Perfect health** | 85 | 6 | 0.98 |
| **Perfect health + "dream" weight** | 98 | 7 | 0.99 |
| **Bariatric surgery** | 95 | 5 | - |

Not surprisingly, our results from the utility assessment showed that the most valued health state for these patients is being in both perfect health and at their "dream" weight. However, not all patients chose this scenario as their most desired health state. Some patients preferred perfect health alone or just their "dream" weight alone.

**Limitations of health utility assessment**

Health utility assessment is not without its challenges.(10) First, the methodology is cognitively complex—it may be difficult for some patients to understand and respond to these scenarios in a way that accurately reflects how much they truly value different health outcomes. Second, this method is very labor-intensive from the assessment standpoint, because the questions need to be administered by an interviewer either by telephone or in-person. Another challenge is deciding on the appropriate reference state. In the literature,(10) the gold standard is perfect health, but that may not be the most valuable health state for every patient. Finally, while health utility is arguably the most valid method of quantifying how much someone values a health outcome, it does not tell you why a patient values a particular outcome. However, using health utility in conjunction with a particular obesity-specific measure may provide important insights.

In summary, health utility is a method of quantifying the value of different health outcomes using a universal metric, and potentially can be used to measure the value of obesity and weight loss; however, there are many challenges to using this approach. Nonetheless, health utility does produce important information that is needed to facilitate policy formation. It may also give clinicians some insight into the patient decision-making process.

**References**


1. Ogden CL, Carroll MD, Curtin LR, McDowell MA, Tabak CJ, Flegal KM. Prevalence of overweight and obesity in the United States, 1999-2004. *JAMA*. 2006;295(13):1549-55.
2. Shekelle PG, Morton SC, Maglione MA, Suttorp M, Tu W, Li Z, et al. Pharmacological and surgical treatment of obesity. Evidence Report/Technology Assessment No. 103. Rockville, MD: Agency for Healthcare Research and Quality. July 2004.
3. Sjöström L, Lindroos AK, Peltonen M, Torgerson J, Bouchard C, Carlsson B, et al. Lifestyle, diabetes, and cardiovascular risk factors 10 years after bariatric surgery. *N Engl J Med*. 2004;351(26):2683-93.
4. Libeton M, Dixon JB, Laurie C, O'Brien PE. Patient motivation for bariatric surgery: characteristics and impact on outcomes. *Obes Surg*. 2004;14(3):392-8.
5. Rand CS, Macgregor AM. Successful weight loss following obesity surgery and the perceived liability of morbid obesity. *Int J Obes*. 1991;15(9):577-9.
6. Puhl R, Brownell KD. Bias, discrimination, and obesity. *Obes Res*. 2001;9(12):788-805.
7. White MA, O'Neil PM, Kolotkin RL, Byrne TK. Gender, race, and obesity-related quality of life at extreme levels of obesity. *Obes Res*. 2004;12(6):949-55.
8. Wee CC, Hamel MB, Davis RB, Phillips RS. Assessing the value of weight loss among primary care patients. *J Gen Intern Med*. 2004;19(12):1206-11.
9. Hakim Z, Wolf A, Garrison LP. Estimating the effect of changes in body mass index on health state preferences. *Pharmacoeconomics*. 2002;20(6):393-404.
10. Gold MR, Siegel JE, Russell LB, Weinstein MC. *Cost-effectiveness in Health and Medicine*. New York: Oxford University Press; 1996.
11. Tengs TO, Wallace A. One thousand health-related quality-of-life estimates. *Med Care*. 2000;38(6):583-637.
12. World Health Organization. Constitution of the World Health Organization: Chronicle of the World Health Organization 1. 2002. Geneva, Switzerland: World Health Organization; 1947.
13. Ware JE, Kosinski M, Dewey JE. *How to score v2 of the SF-36® Health Survey*. Lincoln (RI): QualityMetric Inc.; 2000.
14. Ballantyne GH. Measuring outcomes following bariatric surgery: weight loss parameters, improvement in co-morbid conditions, change in quality of life and patient satisfaction. *Obes Surg*. 2003;13(6):954-964.
15. Horchner R, Tuinebreijer MW, Kelder PH. Quality-of-life assessment of morbidly obese patients who have undergone a LAP-BAND operation: 2 year follow-up study. Is the MOS SF-36 a useful instrument to measure quality of life in morbidly obese patients? *Obes Surg*. 2001;11(2):212-8; discussion 219.
16. Herpertz S, Kielmann R, Wolf AM, Langkafel M, Senf W, Hebebrand J. Does obesity surgery improve psychosocial functioning? A systematic review. *Int J Obes Relat Metab Disord*. 2003;27(11):1300-14.
17. Dymek MP, Le Grange D, Neven K, Alverdy J. Quality of life after gastric-bypass surgery: a cross-sectional study. *Obes Res*. 2002;10(11):1135-42.
18. Wadden TA, Phelan S. Assessment of quality of life in obese individuals. *Obes Res*. 2002;10 (suppl 1):S50-S57.

19. Moorehead MK, Ardelt-Gattinger E, Lechner H, Oria HE. The validation of the Moorehead-Ardelt Quality of Life Questionnaire II. *Obes Surg*. 2003;13(5):684-92.

20. Foster GD, Wadden TA, Phelan S, Sarwer DB, Sanderson RS. Obese patients' perceptions of treatment outcomes and the factors that influence them. *Arch Intern Med*. 2001;161(17): 2133-9.

21. Buchwald H, Avidor Y, Braunwald E, Jensen MD, Pories W, Fahrbach K, et al. Bariatric surgery: a systematic review and meta-analysis. *JAMA*. 2004;292(14):1724-37.

22. Tsevat J, Weeks JC, Guadagnoli E, et al. Using health-related quality-of-life information: clinical encounters, clinical trials, and health policy. *J Gen Intern Med*. 1994;9(10):576–82.

23. Froberg DG, Kane RL. Methodology for measuring health-state preferences—II: Scaling methods. *J Clin Epidemiol*. 1989;42(5):459–71.

24. Brown GC, Brown MM, Sharma S, Brown H, Gozum M, Denton P. Quality of life associated with diabetes mellitusin an adult population. *J Diabetes Complications*. 2000;14(1):18–24.

25. Wells KB, Sherbourne CD. Functioning and utility for current health of patients with depression or chronic medical conditions in managed primary care practices. *Arch Gen Psychiatry*. 1999;56(10):897-904.

26. Wee CC, Jones DB, Davis RB, Bourland AC, Hamel MB. Understanding patients' value of weight loss and expectations for bariatric surgery. *Obes Surg*. 2006;16(4):496-500.

# Patients of Size (Culture of Sensitivity)

Janey Pratt, MD

Obesity is often described as the last acceptable form of discrimination based on physical appearance. How do we change this culture of prejudice? There are 6 things that need to happen before you can change it, and this chapter presents what we at Massachusetts General Hospital did to alter the culture of prejudice and bias against the obese when we initially started our bariatric program.

It is important to first recognize that prejudice and bias exist. We must also recognize that people who treat obesity, as well as those who suffer from the condition, are not immune to this bias. In addition, there must be acceptance that obesity is a disease with genetic roots and is not a character flaw. Finally, it must be understood that obesity is a painful and debilitating disease and that language can influence these biases and prejudices.

**Recognizing bias**

Both normal-weight and overweight children describe obese silhouettes as stupid, dirty, lazy, sloppy, mean, ugly, and sad, among other pejorative labels. When college students were questioned about marrying an obese person, the students preferred to marry an embezzler, a cocaine user, a shoplifter, or a blind person rather than someone that was obese. There is evidence that obese individuals are denied educational opportunities, jobs, promotion, and housing because of their weight. Clearly, bias exists.

During a conference of the American Society for Metabolic and Bariatric Surgery (ASMBS), a nurse practitioner got up and said, "A 40 BMI is not the same animal as an 80 BMI person." Clearly, there was bias reflected in the nurse practitioner's words. It was an unintentional bias, but it was there. And in a published study conducted at an open session of an international obesity conference, an implicit-associations test was given to the entire group. The results showed a significant pro-thin, anti-fat bias amongst the participants in this conference. Subjects endorsed stereotypes like "lazy," "stupid," and "worthless" when describing obese people. However, there were lower levels of bias associated with being male, older, weighing more, having a positive outlook on life, having obese friends, and understanding the experience of obesity.

At the same ASMBS meeting referred to above, an insurance CEO said this: "I have a colleague who had surgery. He's now eating through his surgery; it's his fault. I don't think he was a good candidate for surgery at all." This gentleman was stating this in front of a group of 2,000 surgeons.

I think that we surgeons have to stop blaming the patient when the procedure fails. We are disappointed. We want it to work for everybody. Is it possible that the patient this CEO was referring to was not really eating through the surgery, but that the surgery actually doesn't work for every single person who is obese? I believe it could be that we, as surgeons, have failed when a patient goes "bad." We have failed as healthcare providers to discover what it is that makes surgery work for some people and not for others, and to have this knowledge *before* we operate on an individual. Someday we'll be able to do that. For now, we can't—just like we cannot guarantee a cure for cancer with surgery. But we have to stop blaming the patients when it doesn't work.

We must remember that people who suffer from obesity are not immune to the same biases noted above. In another study, a group of severely obese patients who had lost weight from gastric surgery stated that they would prefer to be deaf, dyslexic, diabetic, or have serious heart disease or acne, rather than return to their previous state of overweight.

A study published in the October 2004 *International Journal of Obesity*, which also used the implicit-associations test, as well as explicit measures in one group, surveyed two groups—68 overweight individuals in one group, and 48 in the other. Again, a significant anti-fat bias was revealed in those taking the implicit-associations test. What this means is that people who are overweight themselves are also biased against being overweight or against others who are overweight. Those tested also endorsed explicit beliefs that fat people were lazier than thin people. Again, these overweight subjects were tested in the same way as the people who care for overweight people were, and they showed the same basic bias.

Next, we must accept that obesity is a disease with genetic roots and not a character flaw. Attitudes about obesity can be defined as prejudice when they exist in the face of mounting evidence that a person's weight is largely determined outside of volitional control. In twin studies, dizygotic twins (those who are not genetically identical), have a very strong difference in weight, whereas monozygotic twins have no weight difference. What this says is there has to be a strong genetic component to obesity.

Accept that obesity is painful and debilitating. Of all the conditions for which a person may be stigmatized in our culture, including race, ethnicity, religious affiliation, physical handicap, and sexual preference, the stigma of being overweight may be the most debilitating.

Dr. Deitel published a study in which he interviewed 1,549 patients and considered problems commonly overlooked in obese patients. Obese patients truly are debilitated: of the patients interviewed by Deitel, 73% could not cut their toenails, which means that they also couldn't put on their own socks or tie their shoes. There's a reason that many of our patients wear Velcro-fastened or slip-on shoes. And 85% of the interviewees couldn't cross their legs, nor could 27% of them buckle a seatbelt. Thirty-six percent couldn't fit into a theater, airplane, or bus seat, 21% could not even wipe themselves, and 52% of the men were unable to urinate accurately. In terms of relationships, 81% said they would not sleep in a room with—nor would 73% get undressed in front of—their significant other.

Finally, it is important to realize that language can influence bias and prejudice. There was a study done by Dr. Wadden published in *Obesity Research* in 2003 that interviewed 167 women and 52 men. The subjects were asked about the most- and least-desirable terms used in reference to them. The least desirable terms when discussing patients' obesity were "fatness," "excess fat," "obesity," and "large size." Far more favorably regarded were terms such as "weight," "BMI," "excess weight," "unhealthy body weight," "weight problems," "unhealthy BMI," and "heaviness." My own patients prefer the term "patients of size." It is a word that can describe either a very large or a very small patient. And "patient of size" is in fact a term that is now used fairly consistently at Massachusetts General.

A number of other terms are used commonly in bariatric surgery, such as "recidivism." This is one that should not be used because by definition, it means "one who shows tendency to return to a previous pattern of behavior, especially criminal behavior." Why do we talk about recidivism in our patients who are going back to eating more, who are regaining weight? Equating eating to criminal behavior reflects prejudice. Fat, defined as unnecessary excess or corpulence, is really not a very pleasant term. Finally, "morbid" is a term that we simply must take out of the realm of obesity. Morbid is "pathological or diseased." It can also be defined as "characterized by preoccupation with unwholesome thoughts or feelings." It's also "gruesome or grizzly." We should not be using this word with respect to our patients.

What is the better, alternative language we can use? Instead of surgical failure or recidivism, we could talk about weight regain. Instead of morbid obesity we could call it severe obesity. Instead of excess fat, we can talk about excess weight and instead of the obese patient we can talk about patients of size, patients with a weight problem or an unhealthy BMI.

In the first year of our bariatric program at Massachusetts General (1999), a very large number of complaints were received from patients regarding their experiences with the facilities. We had, for instance, been unable to establish a good place to see our patients and, therefore, we asked the directors of a geriatric group that had extra room in their practice if we might set up there. We were told, "Our building isn't able to handle the weight of your patients." Nevertheless we had to set up there, and then fights between patients broke out in the waiting room. An overweight individual sitting next to someone who was 85 and thin would find him/herself yelled at by the 85-year-old lady and being told to lose weight or stop being lazy. Our physical plant just wasn't ready, either. We had no large gowns available in the hospital. We'd give the gowns out to patients in the clinic and say, "Here, take this with you when you go into surgery." We broke wall-hung toilets, we broke beds, we broke CT scanners. We had a lot of difficulty starting out.

Because of these experiences, we started the weight-friendly hospital initiative. We developed seminars to help nursing staff by educating them on how to talk about obesity. Addressing the complaints we were hearing about nursing staff on the floor, we pointed out that one nurse had made the comment, "Look at this huge gown. Oh, my God!" Her careless words had severely upset our patients. We had role-playing meetings such as one where the nurses wore a "bari suit" to see what it was like to be overweight, and that was very well received. We also developed a bariatric-concerns group at the hospital to research bariatric equipment, procure it, and to train the staff to use it once it was in place. We requested that radiology order the largest possible equipment for all new purchases, and went on to get every department on board with that concept. The bariatric-concerns group has held more seminars for nurses and today we have bariatric equipment available throughout the hospital. There are large gowns available on every floor.

But we're still struggling to remove prejudice and bias from the hospital. We're still working at changing the language so that we speak of "severe obesity" instead of "morbid obesity." We're trying to consistently say, "patients of size." And we continue to push toward losing "recidivism" or "fat people" from our bariatric lexicon.

Even with this, at a tumor board not long ago, the discussion centered on the treatment of a severely overweight patient who had breast cancer, and it was clear there was a significant bias within the board. We need to continue to fight against this prejudice, because it's still there. While it is happily true that patients feel better about their experience at our hospital today than they did 5 years ago, we still have a long way to go.

What are the keys to establishing a successful practice or facility for bariatric patients? The keys are empowerment, education, and equipment. Empowerment means that you must take it upon yourself to change things, whether it's at your local hospital, in your office, or in your town. In terms of bariatric health care, as a professional you need to create a weight-friendly initiative in your own space. We can make a great difference if we all go out and do this even a little bit at a time. If everybody takes the initiative, feels empowered to do it, things will change.

The best way to change the culture is through education. We must educate everyone about obesity: all healthcare professionals; from the person who cleans the room to the nurses on the floor; from the psychologists and psychiatrists to the nutritionists, internists, primary care doctors, specialists, and surgeons—everyone. Once educated, healthcare personnel will accept the 6 realities about obesity noted at the beginning of the chapter, which are:

- bias against persons of size exists;
- people who treat obesity are not immune to this bias;
- people who suffer from the condition themselves are not immune to the bias;
- obesity is a disease with genetic roots and not a character flaw;
- obesity is a painful and debilitating disease;
- and language can influence the bias and prejudice that persons of size encounter.

Obesity is a disease that's treatable, a disease whose sufferers endure the double-punishment of cultural prejudice. To treat these individuals, your facility must have the equipment necessary to accommodate them. Patients feel good when they're treated to chairs and beds and clothing and toilets that fit them. So, quite simply, it comes down to empowerment, education, and equipment being all that you need to create a successful, weight-friendly hospital.

**Suggested Reading**


1. Deitel M, Shahi B, Deitel FH. Effect of Weight Loss in the Morbidly Obese Patient with Severe Disability. *Obes Surg*. 1991(4);1:419-421.
2. Wadden TA, Didie E. What's in a name? Patients' preferred terms for describing obesity. *Obes Res.* 2003;11(9):1140-6.
3. Wang SS, Brownell KD, Wadden TA. The influence of the stigma of obesity on overweight individuals. *Int J Obes Relat Metab Disord.* 2004; 28(10):1333-7.

# Web-Based Education

Caroline Apovian, MD

The literature on Web-based education is scarce. What is available is data that basically compare Web-based diet and exercise education versus the face-to-face-, typical physician or registered dietician interaction with the patient. In a study at Boston Medical Center, we used the Dietary Approaches to Stop Hypertension (DASH) diet, posting the information online to help people with their diet and health via the Web. The DASH diet is the only diet that has been very rigorously studied in a randomized, controlled trial and shown to reduce blood pressure, as compared with another healthy diet high in fruit and vegetables. One of the original primary investigators of the DASH diet at Boston Medical Center, Dr. Tom Moore, along with a team including this writer, decided to give the DASH diet information to millions of people by developing a Web-based educational tool called DASHFORHEALTH.com.

We asked, "How can we change the eating habits of millions? We have a diet that we know is healthy, but how can we disseminate that information and get people to use it? We have an obesity epidemic in this country and worldwide, but how can we get the message of healthy eating to millions of people beyond our own practices, or get healthcare providers to use this diet to teach their patients good eating habits?" We as individual doctors are not likely to be able to do that in our lifetimes and there are only about 30,000 nutritionists in this country, versus 50 million hypertensives and 60 million obese people. Not even a combination of doctors and nutritionists can do it—the task is too monumental!

However, there *is* the public health model and within the public health model there are mass-media and marketing and government agencies that have been effective at changing the health of Americans, at least to some degree. For instance, years ago the seat-belt initiative decreased deaths from car accidents. Tobacco cessation campaigns have reduced the numbers of smokers in this country. And, consider the success of the "back to sleep" campaign for reducing the incidents of sudden infant death syndrome (SIDS). These are good models to use.

But, how about using the Internet to get information about healthy eating habits to many people at once? Pro: it reaches many patients at one time, travel to appointments is not an obstacle. Con: it requires a computer-savvy audience.(1) It's less personal than a face-to-face discussion with your physician or nutritionist, but so is mass-marketing and government intervention.

So who has access? Seventy-five percent of Americans have access to the Internet from home, but in an indigent population (for instance, the population we see at Boston Medical Center), that's really not true. As a whole, however, it would seem that many Americans now have access to the Internet. You do have to have education about how to use a computer, of course, and so that could be influenced by your income, education, literacy, race, ethnicity, age, gender, geography, or disability. Just because you have access doesn't mean you actually can use the Internet effectively.

There are lots of criteria to help patients figure out what is reputable material on the Web. There are at least 22 sets of criteria, but the problem is that many are duplicative and only about 25% are intended for consumer use. So what are the preferred sources of health information? We have providers, medical universities, and the federal government with sites on the Web. Those are probably the preferred sites.

## Internet Usage by Individuals with a Chronic Disease

- 45.9% Use Internet to seek health info/advice (highest use 52% amongst those with depression or diabetes)
- 58% Internet improved understanding of disease and treatments
- 28.3% Internet improved their ability to manage their condition
- 17.9% Affected treatment choice
- 36.9 Affected the way I eat or exercise

*Preventing Chronic Disease* 2004;1(4).

What do people actually do? Of patients with a chronic disease, about 46% percent will use the Web to seek health information and advice. Approximately 58% will use it to improve understanding of their disease and treatments, 28% to improve their ability to manage their condition, and 18% permit it to affect their treatment choice.

People are using the Web quite a lot, in fact, so it isn't surprising to see that about 37% are using it for diet advice, or that it's affected the way they eat and/or exercise. Many feel that it doesn't take too long to find information on the Web, so they're using it effectively. They find the information trustworthy and easy to understand. They even use it to seek care from a different doctor, accessing the physician by e-mail. (Happily, only 6.6% use e-mail to communicate with a doctor; more, and there would be a problem of never being able to leave the office!)

But, how can we help patients find *reliable* Web resources? Search using Yahoo! for sites having to do with weight loss and you hit 69 million results! (Accessed October 2006.) How are patients going to cull through that many? Similarly, there are at least 18 million sites yielded on a Yahoo! search for weight loss surgery.

The fact is, the Web has reached a point of information overload. We must find a way to distinguish what is reputable and what's not and pass that on to patients. You can always find general information on the Internet that includes details on where to get more specific information, which you can then e-mail to patients or other healthcare providers. Group support, chat rooms, message boards—these are all available for your patient to use. And there are many tools offered that allow one to calculate BMI or target heart rate for exercise. You can use calculators to see how much exercise you're actually doing and how many calories you're burning and even to get your personal resting metabolic rate.

These are all tools that can help patients lose weight and then manage their weight. Downloads are available for food and activity records, recipes, diet assessments, food/nutrient analyzers, menu planners, diet plans, and treatment guidelines. Here are some tips for navigating the Web.

- .com - commercial; may have an agenda, such as selling a product.
- .net - can be excellent, but in many cases may be unreliable.
- .edu - university or school; usually reliable, or at least we think so.
- .gov - government; generally reliable.
- .org - nonprofit organization; very likely trustworthy.

Once a site is located, search for information about the site. Who created it? Get their credentials and find out when it was last updated. Is the information provided consistent with what you already know? Is the site hosted by a recognized company? Internet companies such as Yahoo! have too much at stake to publish inaccurate information. These are important things you can tell your patients to help them navigate the Internet.

**Figure 1**

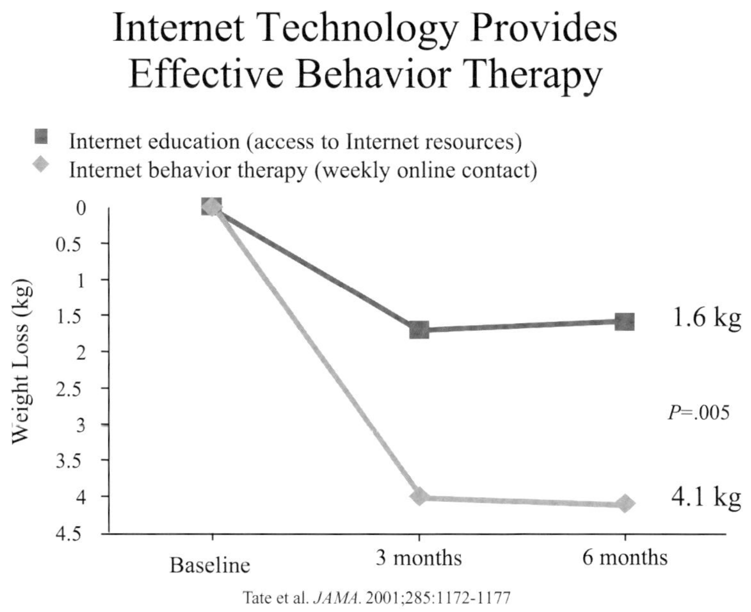


So what about the Internet as a medium not only for general information or support, but also for actual treatment? A study by Tate, et al looked at the difference between just having access to resources and providing, via the Internet, an adjunct to behavior therapy and a registered dietician. You might expect what they found at 3 months and then at 6 months—those who received the weekly interactive online content lost more weight than those who were just given access to information and support.

## Effects of Internet Behavioral Counseling on Weight Loss in Adults at Risk for Type 2 Diabetes

- 1 year, single center, randomized, controlled trial; 92 subjects, BMI 33.1, 48.5 yrs
- Internet program vs. Internet program with added behavioral "e-counseling"
- Both groups received one face-to-face counseling session and same core Internet programs; submitted weekly weights
- E-counseling group submitted calorie and exercise information and received weekly e-mail behavioral counseling and feedback from a counselor

Tate DF, et al. *JAMA*. 2003 Apr 9;289(14):1833-1836.

Another study, again from Tate et al, looked at patients who were obese and at risk for type 2 diabetes. This was a 1-year, single-center, and randomized trial, that looked at 92 subjects with a high body mass index (BMI). Again, the difference in treatment was between an Internet e-counseling treatment program and access to information only. The difference here was that both groups in this trial also received one in-person counseling session and both received the same core programs and submitted weekly weights. The e-counseling group also submitted calorie and exercise information and received weekly feedback from a counselor. This slightly altered study showed that the basic group lost weight; the group that received added e-counseling, however, lost about double that amount of weight, lowered their BMI points and lost waist circumference. Therefore, it appears that the Internet can provide a valuable opportunity for patients to receive intensive feedback.

## Positive Effect of Internet on Long-Term Weight Loss Maintenance

- 255 overweight and obese adults; 6-month behavioral weight control program conducted over interactive television
- Tx followed by a 12-mo weight maintenance program with either: internet support (IS), minimal in-person support (M-IPS) or frequent in-person support (F-IPS)
- RESULTS: no significant differences in weight loss (mean +/- SD) from baseline to 18 mos (IS 7.6 +/- 7.3 kg; M-IPS 5.5 +/- 8.9 kg; F-IPS 5.1 +/- 6.5 kg, *P*=.23)

Harvey-Berino et al. *Obes Res* 2004;12:320-329.

Another study, from a different group, looked at the effect of Internet programs on long-term weight maintenance. A cohort of 255 overweight and obese adults, were put on a 6-month weight control program, conducted over interactive television, with no in-person contact. This was followed by a 12-month weight maintenance program, with either Internet-program support only, or minimal in-person support versus frequent in-person support. Studying both the effect of using the Internet instead of face-to-face contact and the value of different degrees of face-to-face contact, the researchers found there was no difference in weight loss or maintenance of weight loss. They concluded that an interactive-television weight loss and support program can help people lose weight and maintain that loss as well as face-to-face interaction can.

The last study I want to mention was published by Leslie G. Womble, an expert in behavior modification. Womble looked at the difference between using a commercial Web-based program, eDiets.com, a good Internet program that has become very popular, and the LEARN weight loss manual (which we use in our clinic). Forty-seven women with high BMI were randomly assigned to either eDiets.com or the LEARN manual. At baseline, participants in both groups met with a psychologist and were instructed to follow as closely as possible whichever program they were randomized to. They also had brief visits with a psychologist at weeks 8, 16, 26, and 52. This was a 1-year program and the change in weight was the outcome measure. The study showed that the manual users did much better at losing weight, both at 16 weeks and at 52 weeks. These interesting results appear to demonstrate the exceptional effectiveness of the LEARN manual.

There is a review article, again by Tate, that looks at the use of the Internet for psychological treatment. The data strongly support using the Internet to submit behavioral assignments over the Web and to obtain social support from peers and other important information. It suggests that the Internet is excellent for receiving feedback and support from therapists, but obviously doesn't replace face-to-face psychological therapy. However, it can be used as an adjunct, with good results.

We can refer to these technologies as interactive behavioral change technology (IBCT), which has been known to be a partial solution to the competing demands of primary care practice. As primary care physicians, we're very busy, often only having 15 minutes per patient. We can't do everything. So the question becomes how do we use the Internet and other technologies to help us? There are CD-ROMs, interactive voice-response telephone calls, etc. A lot of research is being done at Boston University (BU) on using voice-response telephone calls, for instance, to help people lose weight and keep it off, and the results are pretty good. Although they're used as adjuncts and, again, are not going to really replace face-to-face contact, they can increase the effectiveness of what you're trying to do in your busy office practice.

At BU, we developed the DASH-based program, which has a Web site called dashforhealth.com (Figure 3). The DASH diet is rich in fruits and vegetables, but that's not the only difference between it and an American diet using the US Department of Agriculture (USDA) guidelines. It's also high in low-fat dairy and low in saturated fat, as well as in total fat and cholesterol, and it provides many more servings of fruits and vegetables than even the USDA guidelines do. The DASH diet provides a little more low-fat dairy than the guidelines do, and we add 4 to 5 servings of nuts per week. You may ask, "Why did you decide on this combination?" Simply, the decision was made to put in everything that was known in the literature to reduce blood pressure and see what the results would be when compared with those of a diet that is just high in fruits and vegetables. The DASH diet calls for several servings of low-fat meats or protein per day as well. Moderate in sodium to begin with, DASH's sodium content was decreased when the researchers did a lower-sodium trial that showed even larger decreases in blood pressure. In addition, the DASH diet limits sweets.

**Figure 2**

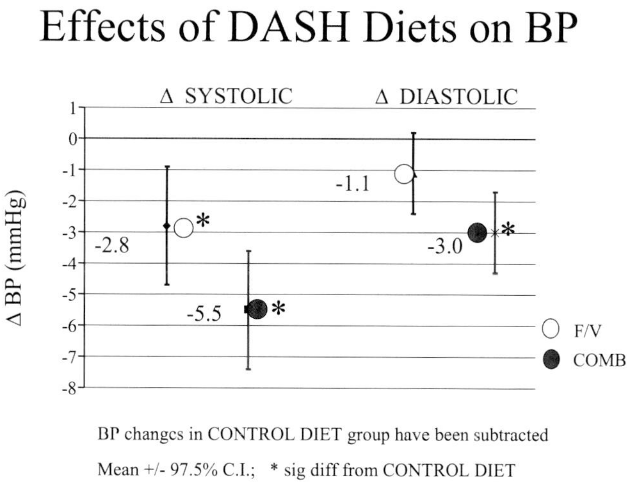


The effects of the DASH diet on blood pressure have been published in several papers, and this was one of the original studies that looked specifically at comparing DASH against another diet high in fruits and vegetables. While both reduced blood pressure in those patients with high blood pressure, the DASH diet did consistently better both in reducing systolic and diastolic readings.

We use the DASH diet on our Web site not only to help patients lower their blood pressure, but also to help them reduce their lipids and lose weight. On our commercial Web site (www.dashforhealth.com), we can help patients get to what their daily servings of DASH foods should be by putting in their height, weight, and age. We calculate their daily caloric requirements, showing they should have this many servings per day of fruits, vegetables, dairy, grain, meat, fish, poultry, nuts and beans, and fats and sweets. We also help them figure out how much a serving size is, because that's also key. They will have a folder called "YOUR STUFF" in which they can enter their weight, blood pressure, exercise, and steps each day, and they'll receive progress reports on how they are doing with each item they enter.

Figure 3

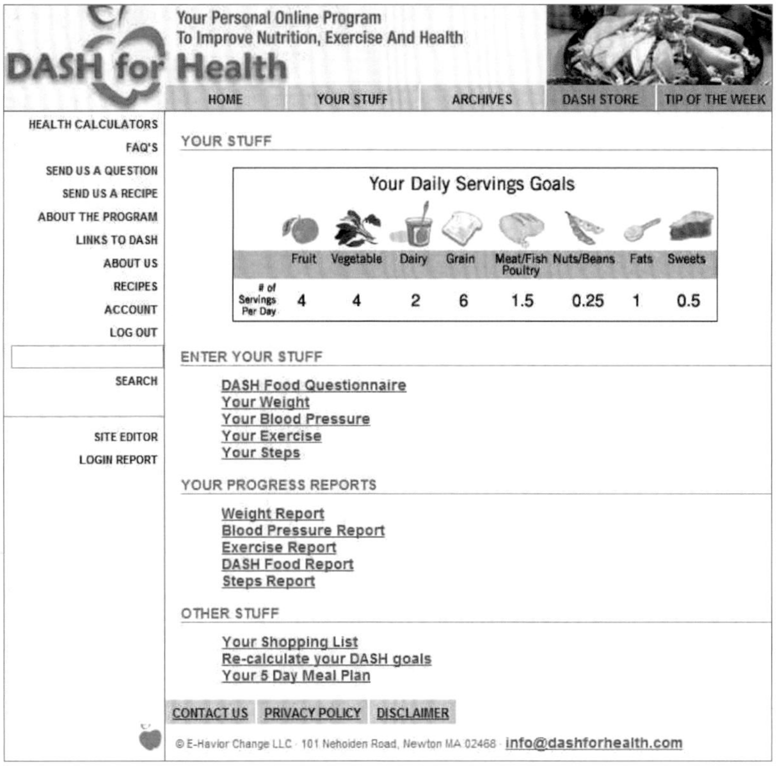


We also provide shopping lists, and offer 5-day meal plans as needed. So we try to be very interactive and multidisciplinary, with pop-ups for health calculators and "send us a question" tabs to click on to e-mail a question, to which we provide an answer within a reasonable amount of time. In addition, there are recipes and an invitation to send us recipes. Weekly messages are sent to the consumer, and a midweek tip goes out on things like how to use the diet when in a restaurant, how to exercise, or how to maintain DASH goals. A link is provided to archived messages so patients can look back on any they've received. We talk about whether or not they put cream versus milk in their coffee, for example. If they use light cream and have a cup of coffee every morning, they can expect to be consuming 7.6 sticks of butter every month—quite a shocking revelation to most people.

Our commercial Web site's information was initially developed from our 3-year pilot study. Boston Medical Center collaborated with $EMC^2$, a local software company and provider of information storage and management (there are also sites in North Carolina and California). We provided all the employees with access to this 3-year, Web-based nutrition and exercise education program, calling it "DASH for Health at $EMC^2$." The weight loss component was added due to demand; most people who joined wanted to lose weight. The program was offered as a no-cost benefit for the employees as part of their health-benefit package. They didn't have to join if they didn't want to, and how often they visited the site was totally discretionary. Just as the site does now, we provided nutrition advice based on the DASH diet, had a new topic every week, and offered a weight loss tip midweek. We reminded participants by e-mail to visit the site (they assured us that they didn't consider this harassment) and offered the options of recording their blood pressure, weight, and exercise. This is how we were able to glean information for our study. Again, participation was optional, and no one had to provide us with his/her information.

**Figure 4**

## DASH for Health at EMC$^2$:
## *Baseline Participant Data*

| | 2002 | 2003 | 2004 |
|---|---|---|---|
| **Number** | 3,997 | 710 | 455 |
| **M/F** | 2,207/1,790 | 443/267 | 248/207 |
| **Age** | 40.2 | 39.7 | 40.5 |
| **Weight (M)** | 204.0 | 202.0 | 196.1 |
| **Weight (F)** | 156.1 | 157.4 | 158.2 |

In order to keep interest in the site we held contests with prizes and people were excited about that. We gave away T-shirts and hats, free DASH healthy meals at their cafeteria and we also gave special discounts on healthy foods at Stop and Shop, one of our sponsors. We had several food-industry sponsors and lots of fruit and vegetable providers, like raisin companies. Even the dairy council was part of our sponsor list, so we were able to get a lot of funding for this site.

So—how to start and restart the DASH diet? Let's review. We were able to provide things like health calculators, a "send us-a-question" invitation, and recipes that were easy (because these were busy employees just like the rest of us).

**Figure 5**

***Sample Web Page: Serving Sizes***

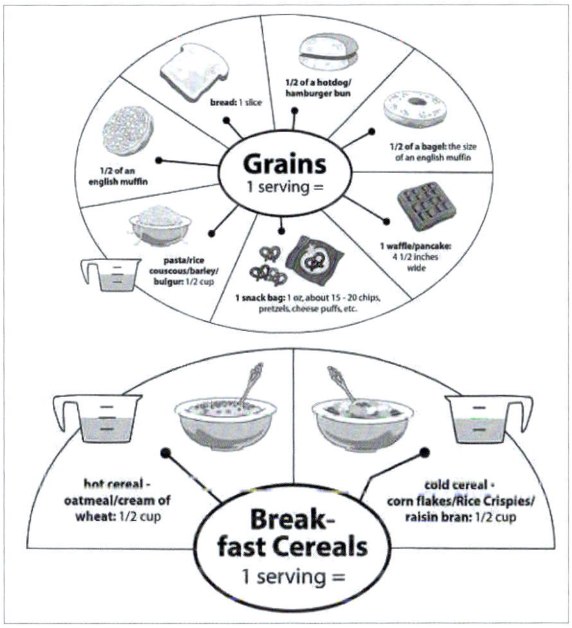


We were also able to teach serving size (serving sizes for the DASH diet are similar to USDA's, with slight differences) by developing a "wheel" that illustrated serving sizes of grains, for example, and of breakfast cereals. We had one for fruits and vegetables, one for meats, and another for sweets. We made sure progress reports were easy to read. Another valuable piece of information we gleaned from the response to the 24-hour food questionnaire we'd developed was how many servings of grains and fruits and vegetable patients were actually consuming.

## Summary

- Internet technology has been expanding rapidly and has had a dramatic impact on how people communicate, learn and share information
- The most reliable sources are by government, universities, and nonprofit organizations
- Data on Internet use for successful weight loss is convincing

The Web-based technology for Internet communication and education on diet and exercise has been expanding rapidly over the past few years. As noted, there are many Web sites available for anyone interested in learning about diet and exercise. As for data emerging on diet-effectiveness through studies specifically for postoperative bariatric patients, they are in the developing stage with more to come soon. In the meantime, healthcare providers should remember to stress to their patients that the most reliable Internet sources for information tend to be at sites run by government, universities, and/or nonprofit organizations. There are convincing data out there that you can use the Internet not only for communication, but also to help your patients lose weight and keep it off.

**References**

1. Tate DF, Wing RR, Winett RA. Using Internet technology to deliver a behavioral weight loss program. *JAMA*. 2001;285(9):1172-7.
2. Tate DF, Jackvony EH, Wing RR. Effects of Internet behavioral counseling on weight loss in adults at risk for type 2 diabetes: a randomized trial. *JAMA*. 2003;289(14):1833-6.
3. Harvey-Berino J, Pintauro S, Buzzell P, Gold EC. Effect of internet support on the long-term maintenance of weight loss. *Obes Res*. 2004;12(2):320-9.
4. Womble LG, Wadden TA, McGuckin BG, Sargent SL, Rothman RA, Krauthamer-Ewing ES. A randomized controlled trial of a commercial internet weight loss program. *Obes Res*. 2004;12(6):1011-8.
5. Tate DF, Zabinski MF. Computer and Internet applications for psychological treatment: update for clinicians. *J Clin Psychol*. 2004;60(2):209-20.
6. Glasgow RE, Bull SS, Piette JD, Steiner JF. Interactive behavior change technology. A partial solution to the competing demands of primary care. *Am J Prev Med*. 2004;27(2 suppl):80-7.
7. Sacks FM, Svetkey LP, Vollmer WM et al. Effects on blood pressure of reduced dietary sodium and the dietary approaches to stop hypertension (DASH) diet. *N Engl J Med*. 2001;344(1):3-10.

# Program Management

Madelyn Fernstrom, PhD

The key to a successful bariatric surgical program is having a comprehensive treatment program, as well as a strong support system for the patient. In addition to good patient education programs, successful outcomes are increased by providing resources for the patients' family members and physicians. Weight loss in general is a difficult endeavor and to have the additional requirements of managing patient information and medical evaluations certainly adds to the complexity of undergoing bariatric surgery. Thus, it is important to communicate not only to the patient, but also to their family and their primary care physician, that obesity treatment and surgery must utilize a continuity-of-care approach and work toward a chronic disease model of treatment. Lifestyle has to be the foundation of any obesity treatment. Medications can help and surgery is an option, but those are only tools to make the transition to a new lifestyle easier. In Pittsburgh, we have introductory workshops where patients come to get information. Initially, many patients think they have, and know, the correct information; but often they don't understand the complexity of the surgery or that changes in lifestyle truly are the key to weight loss and that surgery only helps to make those lifestyle changes more manageable. In order to accomplish these lifestyle changes, patients need constant support and education through daily or weekly access to programs, support networks, and even to other patients and potential patients.

Meeting surgical criteria is not the only preoperative issue of which patients need to be aware. They must fully understand the risk-to-benefit ratio. In our Pittsburgh clinic, we have a 6-month lifestyle preparation program. Our clinic strongly emphasizes that this program is not merely a hoop to jump through before surgery, but, instead, it is an introduction to the lifestyle that needs to be adopted. This presurgical program demonstrates to patients that they will have long-term follow-up, support, and help that will encourage their motivation by monitoring their progress. The most important part of the 6-month plan is not to lose 10 pounds, but to lose 10% of their weight. Thus, the 6-month presurgical lifestyle program teaches patients the discipline needed to monitor and understand the stress of long-term food restriction, and to be in touch with feelings and thoughts about what food does, and does not, do for them. It also shows them how to participate in programs in their community, in a medical clinic, or any kind of support program, whether it's one-on-one or through a Web site.

Successful programs must also address postoperative issues such as the immediate medical postoperative recovery, when to call the surgeon, and the different diet phases. Patients often think too far ahead and only focus on the phase when they can eat kid-size meals, while overlooking the very early phases of recovery, when they can only consume clear liquids. Again, the physical versus behavioral concerns influence the long-term follow-up and the barriers to long-term success. A successful surgical procedure can lead to a lot of positive outcomes; but identifying personal barriers early on, is equally important for the patient, rather than saying, after the procedure, "Well, I've had the surgery and now it's time to worry about other things." This can be addressed, in part through long-term participation in support groups or appropriate Internet sites.

**Figure 1**

## Fernstrom's Surgical Readiness Test

- Do you accept partial responsibility for your weight gain?
- Are you willing to work on regaining control?
- Are you willing to confront your eating sabotages?
- Are you comfortable managing the stress of long-term food restriction?
- Do you have realistic expectations of the surgery?
- Are you prepared for the regimentation of the postsurgical lifestyle?
- Are you willing to become more physically active every day?
- Are you willing to meet with someone/some group for ongoing support and connection?
- Are you willing to be in a follow up program for life?
- Are you willing to seek additional help if needed?

In the Pittsburgh clinic, I've developed a surgical readiness tool to help assess whether patients are prepared to do some things, but not necessarily everything, regarding their weight issues. For surgery, I developed a 10-point quiz (Figure 1). Responding affirmatively to every question often leads to a reasonable surgical outcome, or at least provides a fighting chance toward the direction of losing weight. One issue addressed in this readiness tool is whether the patient accepts partial responsibility for his or her weight gain. This is not to identify whether genetics or environment caused the obesity, or who is correct or incorrect, or if anyone was at fault for the obesity. These are moot points. In most cases, whether the cause stems from cognitive or biological reasons, a person eats too much food for their body's needs. If a patient can accept that there is too much food going in, then that's a good step toward progress.

Our tool will also evaluate the patient's willingness to work on regaining control. Body weight is really a barometer of control or a measure of being out of control. Eating disorders are similar, as patients frequently admit that they feel out of control. However, by agreeing to want to regain control, patients are neither expected to regain that control immediately, nor are they expected to achieve it easily. Instead, positive steps are simply to acknowledge that they've lost control and that they need help to regain it.

Assessing whether the patient will be comfortable managing the stress of long-term food restriction can also be achieved with the readiness tool. Understanding that he/she will not physically be able to handle larger amounts of food is essential in the patient's psychological assessments. Overeating during the preoperative stages results in mild malaise, but with time they will eventually feel better. Overeating during the postoperative stage has physical consequences that should be avoided. Does the patient have realistic expectations of the surgery? It cannot be emphasized enough that assessment must be made to determine whether the patient is prepared for the regimen and structure of the postsurgical lifestyle. Is the patient willing to become more physically active every day? Although this does not imply that he/she should go out and run a marathon or even exercise, he/she must be willing to find ways to increase their daily activity levels. The key here is "willingness." Surgery alone will not inspire patients to jump up and start to walk for 40 minutes if they were previously living a couch-potato lifestyle. However, as they become more able to engage in physical activity, patients must find the motivation to participate in increased activity and not focus only on issues of food intake.

Another key to success is whether the patient is willing to meet with an individual or group for ongoing support or connection. This person can be a spouse, a friend, a structured support group, or a Web site. Relying entirely on a Web site, however, can have a downside as interaction with a site is somewhat detached and isolates one from others, which is not always a positive experience. Often, it is good to be in a group so that feedback can be given and received. In the end, it is always important to be open to the fact that different strategies work for different people. Patients are encouraged to participate in follow-up programs to help maintain their new lifestyles for the rest of their lives. These individuals are not surgery patients forever, but instead are weight loss survivors whose work toward maintaining their healthier body weight does not end. Finally, we ask the patient whether he/she is willing to seek additional help if needed. Patients should be open to the idea that if they begin to struggle, they may need some additional help. This can come in the form of therapy, group counseling, or just a kind friend.

It is also important to identify the family's role in a successful weight loss program. Family support is critical and becomes important to help the patient identify family barriers to success. For example, family members can frequently be too "pro" surgery, perhaps because they have observed the success of a friend or a different family member's surgical procedure. Patients need to be certain that they are choosing bariatric surgery for the right reasons, meaning that they've chosen to do it for themselves. Therefore, because family support is so important, we have an extension of the patient program for the family members. Many times families want to help and ask whether they should avoid speaking about food, avoid offering desserts at a special occasion, or if they should police their family member's eating habits. These small gestures can often blow the situation out of proportion. Families want to help and do the right thing, but many members are uncertain about how to provide support. Family members often have concerns with the safety of the surgery itself. When time and effort are taken to discuss with them the risk-to-benefit ratio for the patient and the effects on the family, they often become wonderful advocates for the patient.

Equally important to the patient's education is the physician education component. Patients get a lot of mixed signals, which is why it is important that the patient and primary care doctor are on the same page. It is important to educate the primary care doctor about the care needed before and after surgery. In addition, the physician should know when he/she should provide a referral source when medical or lifestyle support is necessary. Further medical support may be needed, not because the physician is incompetent or uninterested in providing it, but because she or he may not have the time or resources to provide all the medical evaluations for patients who are at a higher medical risk for bariatric surgery or have other psychosocial issues.

A successful, comprehensive program should include an initial assessment to triage and identify patients at high medical risk, psychologically and nutritionally, so that the best program can be designed for varying individual needs. The program should have a referral service for specialists who will help the patient reach an optimal state before their surgery. This is not meant to exclude individuals, but it is important for patients to be in optimal health, and to have a positive psychological and nutritional status in order to have a successful surgical outcome. Clearly, nutritional education is important as patients must unlearn past eating behaviors and adopt a new bariatric diet and eating lifestyle, as well as understand the role of exercise or daily activity. Psychological evaluations help to identify issues surrounding the stress of food restriction or arising from intimacy problems that may not have surfaced before. Self-esteem issues may surface as the patient begins to be perceived differently by others—because now he/she is thinner. It is important to convey that these are all natural changes that may occur and support for these issues can come from the patient's primary care doctor, a structured program or the bariatric surgeon's office. Again, it is important to identify, both to the patient and the surgical team, what the primary care physician's role will be during this process, to avoid confusion about who conducts the follow-up of the patient. Many studies demonstrate that bariatric surgery patients are lost from follow-up protocols that are part of a structured program or are conducted from the surgeon's office—but not when the follow-up is done by their primary care doctor. In addition, involving the primary care physician as an active part of follow-up for the patient is important because, he/she can help identify community resources. Primary care doctors and structured regional programs like ours can't provide everything to every patient, so the issue of community resources becomes very important

The discussion up to this point has centered around external support resources, but we must also consider the patient's self-support. What can patients do for themselves? This becomes an empowerment issue for the patient, as he/she will spend more than 98% of the time outside of a doctor's office.

Patients need to have a toolbox of resources not just for weight management, but for other contingencies as well. Monthly meetings where people can meet each other through support groups and make in-person connections, or being able to count on telephone support are good resources to have. Even community support groups, church-based and/or YMCA groups, or exercise programs at different facilities can be helpful. Commercial programs that cost money, such as Weight Watchers, can be good for some, although we caution people who are participating in a commercial program to not advertise the fact that they've had bariatric surgery because so many people wrongly say, "You did it the easy way." That type of sabotage couldn't be further from the truth, as everyone in our program knows. Because the fact is, changing one's lifestyle after bariatric surgery is 10 times more difficult than anything that he/she has undergone before.

# Pushing the Envelope of Patient Education and Support With Technology-Enhanced Applications and Strategies

James C. Rosser, Jr., MD, FACS

Postoperative patient education and support has not been given enough attention with regard to bariatric surgery and long-term weight loss management. Many surgeons tend to have the mindset that surgery is the ultimate solution for the scourge of morbid obesity. Often they do not realize that the surgery is the first step, not the last step, of the weight loss journey. Patients must go "back to the future" in order to secure a future of freedom. They must go back to the same formula of establishing a balance of good nutrition choices, portion control, and physical activity that has been prescribed by the medical establishment for quite some time. The only difference is that the surgical procedure gives the patient a tool that can offset the tremendous obstacles to long-term success.

Weight loss surgery patients must adopt a "learning for life" philosophy because recovery is for life. Some may be offended by the term "recovery" in this context. Most frequently, the term is reserved for those who suffer from substance abuse. Contrary to public (and some professional) opinion, morbid obesity and substance abuse are not one and the same disease. But being committed to a long-term treatment effort is a broad proximity point of common ground. Patients recovering from weight loss surgery must be prepared to make this sacrifice every day in spite of challenges that go far beyond the physical.

To the general public, the choosing of a surgical treatment option may seem to be the easy way out of a problem that patients have created for themselves. This lack of knowledge and sensitivity by the public has lead to prejudice toward the ever-growing obesity community. It is well known that the human experience has always made room for the posture that "I will make myself feel better by highlighting the differences and deficiencies of others in order to assign inferiority." As I stated to Martin Luther King III, when I was presented the SCLC Charles Drew Award for Medicine, his father, Martin Luther King, Jr, was willing to die for 10% percent of this nation's population. His son's legacy could be defined by his willingness to fight for those of us who are "nutritionally challenged" and struggling under the yoke of this country's last bastion of bigotry, size discrimination. For those who are uninformed, this road to recovery is not easy and anyone who travels it is impeded by nonmedical factors that do nothing to help. At 5 o'clock in the morning when the patient is sweating from a 1-hour walk, and at night when he/she must decide to have fruit instead of cheesecake, it is not easy. It boils down to commitment to a never-ending struggle. The complexities and difficulty of treating morbid obesity dictate that we must identify, validate, and utilize technology and technology-enhanced applications and strategy methodologies to help make this lifelong effort easier to establish and maintain for all.

One of the keys to successful, lasting outcomes will be the adoption of a strategy traditionally employed in business, which is "if you cannot measure it, you cannot manage it." Our challenge as healers for the "nutritionally challenged" is the acquisition of data that can be used to guide postoperative treatment. Whether it is the amount of calories taken in by patients or how energy is utilized or expended, or where and how frequently patients go to eat out, data collection should inform not only physicians, but also their patients. In addition, new approaches to patient education and empowerment must be pursued. Patient support is sometimes an afterthought that offers more lip service than substance and its availability will vary widely according to race and socioeconomic lines. This disparity must be eradicated if our war on morbid obesity is to be successfully fought. Here, the use of technology and technology-enhanced strategies can help tremendously.

In 2005, more than 160,000 patients in the United States chose what is considered the ultimate weight loss weapon; for as it stands today, with surgery we have been granted an opportunity to impact a major healthcare menace. Unfortunately, in spite of tremendous success, a continuing problem has been the fact that more and more patients are becoming "weight loss surgery refugees." These are patients who have gone to programs that practice a "fire and forget" philosophy. Such programs concentrate on the surgery and not on the postoperative care. This is profoundly troubling. Some of those programs seem to say, "Well, we can't do any better. The demands on physicians and staff are just too great." Lack of patient focus and the fact that nobody wants to pay for aftercare may be valid obstacles, but they are not justification for this lack of effort in treatment continuity. If we are to move forward, the surgical and medical communities must honestly look at our shortcomings and admit that the responsibility for optimized success resides with us. We are the ones responsible for the proper preparation, education, and support of our patients. This is not to relieve patients of their responsibilities or to say that we, as physicians, have to do it all. But the shouldering of the responsibility and the taking of a leadership position is key to reform. Ultimately, we must strive to simultaneously promote measures that not only provide treatment to the stricken, but also prevent the disease from getting a foothold in the first place.

I have a unique vantage point on this subject as a weight loss surgery survivor. From this privileged eagle's-nest view of being surgeon, scientist, and patient, I would like to share some of the research and strategies that I feel will be key for my continued success and the successful treatment by the medical community as a whole of millions of other bariatric surgery patients.

**Support Groups**

Make no mistake about it, the ultimate victory resides in aftercare and traditionally the support group has been its pillar of presence. But what kind of presence has been truly established at this point? Dropout rates from support groups are significant. In one study of support groups conducted over 3 years, only 28% of patients actually consistently participated. Anyone unfamiliar with this arena may think that is a dismal failure, but considering that patients had to go to a remote location to participate, this data should not be judged too harshly. Still, these are not optimal outcomes and we must try to improve. The $300 million question is—how do we get this done?

A hint at one answer may reside in the blending of technology with "living lesson plans." Combining entertainment with education to increase knowledge and patient empowerment allows us to make use of popular culture icons for the greater good. This principle is basic to the world we live in, but our challenge is to tap into it when structuring patient education, aftercare programs, and support groups. Content, and the delivery of content, is king rather than the glitz of technology.

For the most part, traditional support groups have formats that are absolutely boring. Even patients who are faithful struggle with tolerating the focused onslaught of stimuli ineptness. Once again, looking at mass media and the data associated with mass-media marketing, we can employ an "edutainment" format similar to an Oprah Winfrey/Jay Leno talk show. This format captures the attention of the audience with a collage of stimuli. From opening monologues and expert guest interviews to multimedia presentations, a full-court press is aggressively pursued to keep observers engaged. The goal is not only to transfer information, but also to infect the viewer with an emotional connection to the subject matter. Imagine if we, as healers, could embrace the same strategies and methodologies in our weight loss surgery support groups! This could lead to a more effective experience that would have patients fighting to get a seat and maybe willing to pay. In addition, this type of support effort also taps into the emotional inspiration needed for successful recovery. When all is said and done, it must be remembered that great things are not accomplished solely with that which resides within the confines of the cranial vault, but rather with that which resides within the confines of the chest. Physicians who take up the cause of obesity treatment must never underestimate the potential impact of emotion and mass-media techniques that can provide new pathways to improve outcomes. So far, this has not been done and the situation must change.

In my practice, we have developed a prototype program that has the features previously mentioned. These programs occur every 2 months under my leadership. Monthly standard support groups supplement this effort. Anecdotally, the patients are much more engaged and attendance is better. In addition, the program expands the scope of content that goes beyond assistance to the patient. For instance, the plight of loved ones has been frequently overlooked. Support efforts must include spouses, family, and significant others, because they, along with the patients, also fight this battle—and more often than not, without any assistance. They can be the first line of defense against failure; thus, any program seeking to upgrade must involve them. We must not save our patients only to lose the ones who dare to love them. In my program, my wife has a recurrent session called Dana's Hymn to address these issues. There is also a Web site, www.DanasHymn.com, which acts as an expansion to scale technology-enhanced application of this important subject.

This strategy has another advantage that can help in bringing aftercare to the masses. The talk show is very conducive to being channeled into a broadband Internet format. Access to the Internet, especially with the proliferation of broadband, has increased at an exponential rate. The vast majority of American homes are now online and wireless broadband Internet is allowing access to take a voluminous leap forward. We now have the bandwidth to offer dynamic multimedia presentations on a scale similar to television. It only makes sense that the restructuring of the support-group format should follow closely that of proven television mass-media techniques. Imagine Oprah-like support group programs with dynamic interactivity universally available in the comfort of the patients' homes. In conjunction with Titus Duncan in Atlanta, we added this unique edutainment support format to his support group program and it was very successful. The program was interactive—people asked questions and were educated, empowered, and entertained. Patients all had pen and pencil at the ready and were busy writing, laughing, and crying. The patients attending via the Internet loaded the phones with questions. This exploratory effort was not conducted with broadband connectivity, but the possibilities for the future were clearly portrayed. We must prepare for the future by having physicians produce the scripts for these programs today.

**Pre- and Postoperative Evaluations**

As we survey the many problems that plague our efforts to address morbid obesity, it is imperative that I discuss access to bariatric procedures. When I started the process of qualifying for a weight loss procedure, the number of surgeons proficient at performing the procedure was very limited. When we look at outcomes even today, this still seems to be true. My schedule presented another obstacle to my efforts to address the disease. One of the areas I have always been involved in is telemedicine, the care of patients via telecommunication. My weight loss surgery journey presented an opportunity for me to not only "talk the talk," but also "walk the walk."

My initial preoperative evaluation was conducted with videoconferencing. I was at Yale University School of Medicine and my surgeon, Dr. Phil Schauer, was at the University of Pittsburgh. The videoconferences were done at 384 kb/s connectivity. It can be done at 128 kb/s, which broadband now features. All necessary data was gathered and everybody was comfortable with its precision and accuracy. Thus, telemedicine had allowed me to get the evaluation process moving forward. I then underwent the necessary preoperative tests. Telemedicine greatly condensed the number of visits that I would normally have and allowed the maturation of the necessary doctor-patient relationship that is so essential. Once the procedure was done and after staying onsite for 2 weeks to undergo postoperative evaluations, I was able to conduct more frequent postoperative exams utilizing telemedicine applications. For me this was pivotal to my successful surgical intervention. For many, access to care is still fraught with obstacles (i.e., the establishment of the "Center of Excellence" system and the limited expansion of the surgeon pool because of restricted payment based on rigid qualification criteria and our aggressive medical malpractice environment). The technology-enhanced techniques discussed above could prove beneficial in expanding treatment opportunities for the ever-increasing number of patients undergoing bariatric surgery.

**Fitness**

Fitness is another challenge for many patients and is a cornerstone of the triangle for successful long-term weight loss with or without surgical intervention. This triangle of success includes healthy dietary choices, establishment and maintenance of emotional well being, and commitment to a consistent exercise regimen. Unfortunately, maintaining a fitness regimen is an issue with which most people struggle. There are many reasons for this, not the least of which is the patient's unique height-to-weight ratio and other physical traits. Historically, up until this time, it has been difficult for most patients to establish a fitness program that works, without going through painful trial and error.

The popular television show, the "Biggest Loser," illustrates the core issue surrounding the treatment of obesity. One slogan, often repeated, is, "You're not going to have an easy way out, no liposuction, no stapling, no nothing, and you've got to puke in order to get better." Imagine what that does to someone who is 450 pounds and trying to duplicate the exercise regimen of a 110-pound, 24-year-old fitness instructor. Most people just give up.

The reality is that the workout regimen for one is not the one for all. Everyone is different. The problem is that data have not been readily available to delineate just how these programs should be structured. Parameters such as heart rate, maximum oxygen consumption ($VO_2$ max), blood pressure, oxygen saturation, speed, and distance can be used to help customize a fitness regimen that is effective and attainable for each individual. These data could also allow for the identification of nontraditional fitness programs that embrace everyday activities such as parking the car a little further away from work and taking the stairs.

The use of technology can be pivotal for customization of a fitness program because it can answer the question of, "How much should I do?" This is not something that won't be available until sometime in the future. It is available today. A Boston company named FitSense has both hardware and software solutions to help with the fitness dilemma. The hardware is a system of sensors on the foot, chest, and wrist that send data wirelessly to your computer whenever you get in range. All downloading of data is automatically done for you. This system has been battle tested throughout its development. In fact, it monitored sprinter Michael Johnson with real-time telemetry during the Olympics.

Data are sent to a Web site and archived using state-of-the-art encryption. It is then evaluated and a status report is generated with customized suggestions for your workout profile. Other parameters measured by FitSense products are blood pressure, GPS location and blood glucose. There is a scale that wirelessly captures accurate body weights. For bariatricians and surgeons, the acquisition and documentation of accurate body weights is a very important, but elusive, pillar of long-term obesity treatment.

Let's look at a real-world scenario that demonstrates the potential impact of this technology on the war against obesity. A 44 year-old male, 3-years post-op, originally weighed 460 pounds. He initially lost 180 pounds after laparoscopic Roux-en-Y gastric bypass. He reported that over the last 7 months, however, he had gained 40 pounds, but swears he has maintained his diet and workout routines. He was then outfitted with the FitSense system and the data obtained were very illuminating. It showed that the patient only completed 50% of the prescribed workouts. In addition, when he did work out, he only achieved the desired $VO_2$ max 50% of the time. When his daily weigh-ins were followed with the FitSense scale, the weight gain actually fluctuated between 40-47 pounds. Despite these data, the nutritionist and fitness expert could not totally explain such a significant weight gain. The GPS feature of the product was then engaged. As it turns out, the patient had made 8 trips to Pearl and Alexander Streets over 1 week. The address was investigated and found to be the location of a fried chicken restaurant.

Some would say that this level of data detail is obtrusive. But in another sense, being monitored in this way allows patients to be surrounded by a ring of accountability, which can inspire them to continue to fight the good fight. The power of data is that it can be not only inspirational, but also lifesaving. Again, as is said in business, "If you can't measure it, you can't manage it." This kind of technology adds a never-before-available weapon for physicians to treat patients who endure this sinister disease.

**Prevention: The Ultimate Solution**

In spite of the fresh-approach suggestions to treatment that I have mentioned here, the real prize in this fight is prevention of the disease in the first place. It is a lofty goal that seems unattainable, but it is within our reach. It will take many years and a blended approach involving societal changes, policy adjustments, and industry reform; but we have faced similar challenges in the history of this nation. Let's look back on the wearing of seatbelts while driving. Most drivers once thought that the level of compliance we enjoy today would be impossible. A key component of the decades-long seatbelt campaign's success was the targeting of children as the facilitators of long-range change. In relation to winning the war on obesity, we should go back to the future and empower our children to change the world again.

Contrary to popular belief, the children of today are not a collection of underachievers who are destined to squander all that mankind has accomplished on this planet. Nothing could be further from the truth. It is true that they are different in their interests and attention foci. But their potential to contribute dwarfs that of previous generations. As far as the war on obesity is concerned, I am depending on them to put the surgeon's scalpel out of business. The ultimate victory over obesity starts today, with the empowerment of our children. We as adults must begin this empowering, saving a future generation one child at a time. If we can establish an anti-obesity lifestyle posture for our children, it not only will help decrease the incidence of the disease in the future, but also will help us today. For the children, once educated, will be ever-present footnotes of awareness for the grown-ups. If a parent dares to drive a car without his or her seatbelt engaged, a child will quickly question this as unacceptable behavior. We need to harness that same powerful resource, and to accomplish the task we can use the pop culture icons that so capture their attention, imagination, and focus.

Over the past several years, I have attracted worldwide attention to my video game research, which demonstrated that those who are better at video games make excellent laparoscopic surgeons. This is one of the first examples of scientific research focusing on video games to identify skill acquisition that can be associated with real world applications. On average, children spend several hours playing video games (about 15 hours per week for boys, and 10 hours per week for girls). These games have unbelievable knowledge-transfer capability, powered by recognized education best-practice methodologies. The only problem is that they are not being employed for constructive objectives. This must change!

An Australian company by the name of Big Red Frog has targeted childhood obesity as its focus for its interactive video games, offering the resulting data as helpful to the war on obesity. The company has introduced body mechanics as super heroes for health and has produced a 3-D movie and an accompanying DVD interactive game. In these, good versus evil, heroes contend with bad guys, and all are dedicated to teaching children sophisticated physiological facts that will empower them to help themselves. Characters include "Dr. Bludd," the mission commander of the Worldwide Federation of Body Mechanics. There are heroes such as "Sue Lynn," who characterizes insulin, and "Gluc" for glucagon. This is an innovative way to tap into the power of gaming to inspire and empower children. It is also an example of technology and education being used to overcome a societal issue. The game is available in DVD format that plays on standard DVD players and some popular console platforms. This strategy enables children from underprivileged households, who may not have video game consoles, to have access. In addition, it takes the game into the family room and serves to bring the family together. The effort is part of a well thought-out AKA (Awareness-Knowledge-Action) intervention strategy to impart knowledge of the causes of obesity and offer routes of intervention. The Blue Earth Institute's physical activity program provides the "get up and move" energy-expenditure component. This approach showcases a change in strategy that is slowly taking hold. The Body Mechanics movie and game represent initial offerings resulting from a movement, where society is showing a willingness to use any and all resources without prejudice to promote an agenda for the greater good.

**Conclusion**

This chapter has focused on aspects of the care of the obese that desperately need more in-depth attention. This review goes "outside the box" of traditional healing methods, and some may say that it is inappropriate for physicians to play a role where there is so much foreign landscape. No one could blame an individual who believes that implementing these suggestions is beyond his or her skill set. But we must realize that to defeat this formidable enemy (obesity) it will take a heroic effort on the part of all of us—patients, physicians, and society. From my unique vantage point of being a patient, I continue to assure all that there are lives out there worth the sacrifices involved and worth saving.

# Longitudinal Bariatric Experience: Combined Reflections

Jennifer Greenman
Jonathan Waks
Sang W. Kim
Jaime Wilson-Chiru

Inherent discrepancies exist in all patient-doctor relationships. While institutionalized codes, laws, and regulations may guide a physician's actions, norms and values may guide his patient. Esoteric knowledge accumulated through years of training may influence a physician's recommendations, yet intimate stories and intensely personal concerns may color his patient's treatment expectations. Illness is understood as a routine part of a physician's workday but to his/her patient, illness may represent a unique, traumatic event of enduring impact. In an era when limited time often minimizes patient-doctor interactions, it is essential that despite these inherent patient-doctor relationship discrepancies, physicians remember that each patient is distinct. Physicians must address individual patient concerns thoughtfully. They must resist applying generic, reflex-driven templates to clinical problems. In short, physicians must always practice patient-tailored care.

Harvard medical students are keenly aware of this goal: development and practice of patient-centered care is a fundamental tenet of our curriculum. But as these students move into the clinical realm during their third-year clerkships, they face the risk of losing sight of this goal. As patient visits necessarily become shorter and more focused, we are prone to adopt template-guided, time-efficient medical practices that may threaten individualized care.

A new component of Harvard's medical education program, however, has been designed to address and minimize this potential hazard. Within the novel "longitudinal" curriculum, third-year medical students now follow one patient closely for 12 months in addition to completing all traditional clerkships. By forming a long-term relationship with at least one patient, students intimately appreciate that patient's perspective. Powerful memories from these experiences will hopefully help narrow the divide between patient and doctor, and encourage us to practice empathetic, individualized medicine. As medical students, we, the authors of this chapter, chose to work with weight loss surgery patients under the guidance of Dr. Daniel Jones.

**Jennifer Greenman, HMS III:** *Suzy*

Throughout adolescence, Suzy despised her annual family trips to the Cape. She had no model body; she never had, and those August excursions brutally underscored this. The moment the shore came into view, Suzy always immediately spotted the teens she envied most. Sporting the thriftiest bikinis, they pranced triumphantly along the water's edge, clearly confident of their bodies' pulling power. Her own elephantine Levis were no match for their denim minis, and she typically sank to the sidelines, rigid with mortification, hidden beneath an XXXL beach towel. Who were all these skinny teens, anyway, and how did they stay so impossibly thin?

By age 13, Suzy had grown to detest her thick figure, but early dieting proved enormously unsuccessful. Appetite suppressants, metabolism-enhancing supplements, weight loss shakes and fat-free foods only further ballooned her ever expanding abdomen. She surpassed the upper limit of heavy by age 17, sinking into the socially suicidal borderline-obese category as a high school senior. Although she pledged to "start over" in college and even fashioned a detailed weight loss plan before matriculation, comfort snacks were impossible to relinquish. After all, a pint of ice cream with a half box of coconut donuts would never disappoint, no matter how desperate her emotional crisis. A complementary exercise regimen constructed during this time proved equally ineffective. After being steered toward her first treadmill in the student gym one morning, Suzy stood paralyzed in self-conscious embarrassment. How could she even mount that machine in her mammoth tee and spandex leggings? How could she possibly compete with those flat-stomached sorority blondes running away from gravity on their

Stairmasters, modeling Lycra bottoms cut so high that the crotch material just had to be wedged somewhere in their livers?

Following graduation, Suzy again attempted to lose weight. The sudden diagnoses of obesity-driven medical conditions in immediate family members fueled her newfound inspiration. After her 52-year-old mother suffered a second myocardial infarction and her two younger sisters developed type 2 diabetes, Suzy forced herself to confront her own extra pounds. She wasn't going to become the next morbidly obese female in her family. She wasn't going to swell to jumbo 747 proportions after pregnancy, embrace her girth, and then claim that she had entered a more cerebral phase of her life where figure no longer mattered, as her mother and both of her sisters had done. The health consequences of excess weight were too grave.

Suzy aspired to kick those excess pounds, again persevering to restrict her food portions and increase her exercise by walking twice weekly. She enrolled in healthy-cooking classes, in self-help groups for horizontally challenged young women, and she even attended a fantastically pricey body cleansing retreat where organic, low-calorie diets were strictly enforced. Over the next several years, Suzy tried the Weight Watchers program at least 5 times, interspersing those attempts with sessions at Overeaters Anonymous. Occasionally she achieved success, losing 35 lbs during her greatest victory. But at other times, she caved. She understood that moments of imperfection would blemish any realistic weight loss course, but minor setbacks were often impossibly discouraging. Suzy would abandon her weight loss efforts, reinstating more familiar habits of "emotional" eating when things became too tough. Unfortunately, the lost pounds always reappeared.

Now, having just reached age 40, she weighs her record high of 330 lbs. Her back pain has worsened and she recently developed shortness of breath after climbing just the single flight of stairs to her apartment. In tears, Suzy laments her inability to play "chase" with her 4-year-old nephew, Connor, or to carry for any real distance her 11-month-old niece, Liza. She cherishes her role as "Auntie," desperately wishing to watch these children develop into adults. With a body mass index (BMI) of 44.8 kg/m$^2$, Suzy believes she has only one remaining option: bariatric surgery.

As a third-year medical student who volunteered to share Suzy's surgery experience with her, I heard her story and swallowed hard. This was my introduction to Suzy, a gastric bypass candidate. Typically, when I explore a patient's weight history in my weekly primary care clinic, I either receive vague complaints of failed weight loss efforts or, more often, listen while my patients skirt the issue entirely and focus on more immediate complaints. But removed from the compressed clinic setting, Suzy and I had chatted more casually and her intimate, colorful history had impressed me deeply. At the onset, I knew that future conversations would foster a reciprocal relationship in which we would learn from each other emotionally. This would be no traditional academic experience.

It is by no accident that recent titles such as "Fast Food Nation" or "Super-Size Me" have achieved enormous popularity. Indeed, overweight and obesity have reached epidemic proportions among adults and children in the United States. More than 65% of U.S. adults are classified as overweight or obese, while nearly 20% of children ages 6 to 20 are overweight.(1) These unacceptably high rates are serious public health concerns. In a 12-year follow-up of 336,442 men and 419,060 women, the mortality rates for those of either sex who were 50% above average weight were increased approximately twofold.(2) Moreover, obesity-related comorbidities, including hypertension, hypertrophic cardiomyopathy, hyperlipidemia, diabetes, obstructive sleep apnea, hypoventilation, degenerative joint disease, and psychosocial disorders have reached record highs in both adult and pediatric populations, while obesity-attributable medical expenditures increased from $39 billion in 1986 to $75 billion in 2003.(3, 4)

Such trends suggest a need to tackle the obesity epidemic from multiple fronts, including training of medical professionals in methods to identify, prevent, and treat obesity. Continuing research on the etiologies and factors related to obesity, as well as on interventional approaches to both prevent and reduce its occurrence, will generate improved recommendations that will require translation into practice. So, as a third-year medical student, what precise training on the medical care of overweight and obese patients have I received since entering medical school?

Harvard's curriculum devotes surprisingly few—though concentrated—hours to the topic of obesity. Students receive most obesity-related instruction during a preventative medicine course offered once weekly from January through March during year 2. Within that course, just one lecture, along with a 2-hour, case-based tutorial, a film documentary, and several suggested readings from leading academic journals are presented to formally address the topic. Specifically, we reviewed obesity prevalence, demographics, and cost-related trends. We also touched on obesity-related health consequences, including hypertension, dyslipidemia, coronary artery disease, stroke, type 2 diabetes, gallbladder disease, sleep apnea, osteoarthritis, and certain cancers, all of which were treated more comprehensively in systems-pathophysiology courses. We explored obesity as a result of an imbalance in energy homeostasis. Discussions reviewed appetite physiology, including the roles of the hypothalamus, stomach, and adipocytes in relation to obesity. Diagrams summarized that food intake is triggered by the release of the hormone ghrelin from gastric oxyntic cells, which subsequently stimulates the release of neuropeptides from the hypothalamus, increasing caloric consumption. To signal adequate caloric load, adipocytes release the hormone leptin, which activates the satiety center of the hypothalamus, thus decreasing food intake. Ultimately, students realized that defects within this intricate hormonal axis could lead to energy imbalance. Leptin-receptor deficiency, for example, might result in the loss of the satiety signal, thus promoting obesity, while ghrelin overproduction might stimulate hyperphagia leading to obesity, as seen in patients with Prader-Willi syndrome.

The remaining class discussion devoted to obesity centered on treatment options, including rectifying underlying drug and endocrine derangements, endorsing diet and exercise lifestyle modifications, administering pharmacotherapy, and offering the option of bariatric surgery to the morbidly obese. Before each of these were covered, however, students were reminded that health care for obese patients has been hindered by the traditional misconception that weight is not a physiologically regulated variable, but rather determined by gluttonous food habits and hedonistic desires. Indeed, much of our U.S. population considers morbidly obese individuals weak-willed, awkward, self-indulgent, and even immoral. This prejudice cuts across age, sex, religion, race, and socioeconomic status and often precipitates psychological distress in the obese. Of the weight loss treatment options presented, we learned that although behavior modifications may be effective for overweight patients, extensive research has shown that such options alone have not effectively achieved medically significant, sustained weight loss in morbidly obese patients.(5) Even combined with pharmacotherapy, results have been less than promising. In a nearly 4-year study utilizing a 2-drug regimen of phentermine and fenfluramine, coupled with behavior modification, diet and exercise, initial optimistic weight loss results were not sustained.(6) The study suffered a one-third patient dropout rate and in those who were followed for the entire study, the average final weight loss was just 3 lbs. Moreover, the drug combination used appeared to have an unacceptably high association with cardiac valvular disease and is no longer recommended.

In contrast to the disappointing results of nonoperative treatments for obesity, bariatric surgery was presented as a much more effective alternative. Five years following surgical intervention, one study revealed that 50% to 70% of obese patients had achieved weight loss, while programs of diet and exercise or pharmacotherapy achieved 5-year success rates of just 1% to 5% in similar patients.(7) Physical restriction and induced calorie malabsorption contributed to weight loss immediately post-op, but more of the surgery's success was attributed to its ability to modify physiology. Surgery effectively "reset" energy equilibrium and defeated the powerful mechanisms for defense against starvation that are inappropriately overactive in obesity. Patients experienced decreased appetite, increased energy expenditure, and a decreased stress response after undergoing surgical intervention, while patients on weight loss diets experienced just the opposite.

To treat morbidly obese individuals, bariatric surgery clearly seemed superior to alternatives. Scores of excited students were eager to suggest this option to patients they anticipated meeting during their third- and fourth-year rotations. It seemed like a "no-brainer." But what specifically would the suggestion of bariatric surgery mean to a patient? All too often physicians recommend treatments or tests to patients without really recognizing the potentially staggering significance of their impact. Bursting schedules and appointments often limited to 15 to 20 minutes, during which a whole host of problems must be addressed, often preclude thorough patient doctor discussions of any topic. Medical students, however, have the responsibility to explore, in greater depth, the implications of suggested treatment options. One facet of Harvard's new longitudinal curriculum allows us to accomplish precisely this.

As a medical student enrolled in the longitudinal curriculum, I had the opportunity to select a patient with whom I would be working for the duration of my third year. Suzy, the vibrant 40-year-old administrator who is my patient, has elected to undergo a Roux-en-Y bypass surgery to treat her obesity. Our relationship has not been restricted to a superficial greeting outside the operating room. Instead, after attending all of her preoperative informational and screening appointments, and after learning her hopes, successes, and fears during several evening telephone calls, I've grown to really know her. As she prepares for her surgery scheduled in several weeks, I feel much more equipped to offer her constructive emotional support and I am looking forward to following her closely after the operation.

Suzy has enlightened me immensely. Initially, I anticipated our meetings to be didactic. I envisioned explaining the multiple presurgery requirements, surgical contraindications, and even the anatomic differences between available surgical options. But Suzy quickly demonstrated her mastery of the presurgery syllabus. To review Netter drawings would have been embarrassingly inappropriate, given her knowledge of anatomic detail. Instead, our discussions have centered on her emotions. Take, for instance, her relationship with food. Admittedly, I originally assumed that mindless overeating had fueled Suzy's obesity. After all, she adored late night television, so it was plausible that she inadvertently inhaled extra bags of Doritos during midnight episodes of Family Guy. But Suzy firmly denied a habit of oblivious consumption, emphasizing that she's always been acutely aware of what passes her lips. She confessed to having a "food addiction," describing actions eerily similar to those of any narcotic addict. She fights them, yet food frequently commands the upper hand, reducing her to a state where she's totally out-of-control. Over the years, she's had no choice but to finish boxes and bags of food, often in tears, simply to satiate her intense cravings. To someone who rarely contemplates meals, realizing just how significantly Suzy's "food addiction" has impacted her psychologically was a slap in the face. But I would have never been able to look beyond my own perspective and understand her situation if we hadn't developed this trusting relationship.

Suzy has shared many more remarkable pieces of history. Recently, as I broached discussion on post-op concerns, our conversation almost immediately diverged from the path I had anticipated. Rather than reciting statistics on potential complications or accentuating the importance of post-op vitamin supplementation, the focus of our dialogue became social concerns. Since many of her closest friends share a similar body habitus, would they resent her leaner frame, ultimately forcing her to forge new social circles? And what about dating? Would this actually be a possibility, post-op? Or would it remain elusive, given her years of "inexperience?" Her condition had interfered with menstruation; if she regained menstruation, might she consider having her own children? And would having her own children jeopardize her cherished relationship with her niece and nephew?

Neither of us knew exactly how to address such concerns, but listening in spite of not knowing solutions to these types of uncertainties was unquestionably more meaningful than knowing statistical answers to more traditional post-op concerns on outcomes and complications. It wasn't important that I couldn't offer her rote answers; what was important was that we worked as a team, learning from and improving on each other's suggestions. Through rich, candid narrative, Suzy has taught me to relinquish assumptions, to empathize and—above all—to never forget to listen to my patients so that I can offer them what they really need.

**Jonathan Waks, HMS III:** *Mark*

I was standing outside a restaurant when a group of women—perhaps in their mid-20s—walked out commenting that they had over-indulged in dessert. One exclaimed her disgust and horror at having gained a few pounds over the past few weeks, presumably from other, similar indulgences. She asked her friends if she was becoming "too fat." One of them chuckled and commented that, if anything, she was "too thin." Silence. Then heads whipped around as the first woman responded, exclaiming, "You can't ever be too thin!"

There is nothing unique about this anecdote or the feelings it illustrates. A 2006 study of attitudes surrounding obesity found that people of all weights had a considerable "anti-fat bias" inversely related to each respondent's own weight. Forty-six percent of responders said that their negative feelings surrounding obesity were so strong, they would rather give up 1 year of life than be obese. Of this same group, 14% stated that alcoholism was preferable to obesity.(1) A similar study in 2005 showed that obesity carried a greater stigma than other physical disabilities, and that even people who were themselves overweight or obese attached a significant stigma to obesity.(2)

Just before my first meeting with my new patient, Mark, I thought about the anxiety that gaining "a few pounds" had produced in the woman outside the restaurant. Mark, a 26-year-old, 6'2" man who weighed 335-plus lbs, had concluded that obesity surgery was the only viable solution left for him to lose the more than 130 lbs of excess weight he had been carrying for years. I had imagined what a BMI of 43 would look like, but was immediately struck that he looked much smaller than I had anticipated. I had envisioned someone grotesquely larger.

That Mark looked no bigger than many of the people I see on a daily basis underscores the prevalence of obesity in society today. Although the idea of obesity surgery may still be somewhat of a novelty, obesity itself is not. The Centers for Disease Control (CDC) reported in 1991 that no states had obesity rates above 20%, yet by 2005 only 4 states had obesity rates below 20%.(3)

I have been following Mark's progress as part of the pilot program at Harvard Medical School and the Beth Israel Deaconess Medical Center since he formally began the screening process for surgery about 4 months ago. I had wanted to better understand the impact that obesity can have on a patient's life. Our medical education succeeds in conveying a great deal about the epidemiology and long-term health consequences of obesity. Lectures delve into the physiology of hypothalamic set points and the role of leptin in shaping people like Mark, and who can forget the pictures of the massive *ob/ob* (leptin-deficient) mice standing next to their wild-type brethren? The personal dimension, however, often falls by the wayside. In Mark, I saw a chance to better understand the physical and emotional struggle that comes with being obese and trying to fight it.

Is surgery the only option? Many doctors would agree that for people like Mark it can be. Mark would too. He views surgery as his last chance to lose weight after more than 2 years of unsuccessful diets, appetite suppressants, and exercise programs. His primary reason for wanting surgery is not cosmetic, which somewhat surprises me as he seems relatively secure about how he looks and readily admits, "I'm a big guy." He needs to lose weight because of chronic, severe back pain and to avoid heart disease and type 2 diabetes, which have claimed the lives of many similarly large family members. A few years ago, Mark went on a "starvation diet" in order to lose enough weight to qualify for surgery to repair a damaged spinal disc. At the time, he "never felt better," but the weight came back as soon as he resumed eating. Surgery offers him the chance to be healthy and pain free, and to enjoy a better quality of life. For him, the benefits clearly outweigh the risks.

Mark approaches his upcoming surgery with a zeal that would challenge anyone claiming that laziness or apathy were reasons for his heavy frame. He works two physical jobs in order to be able to have this surgery and remain financially secure. He loads packages overnight at the airport and hauls cargo in a truck in the early morning. Recently, he has been working double shifts so that he will be able to afford taking time off for his surgery without losing income or benefits. In the last year, he has researched the different types of surgeries and their respective trade-offs and benefits. In fact, Mark's knowledge of the subject, at times, rivals my own.

Now, after years of dieting, exercising, working, and researching, Mark will finally undergo a Roux-en-Y gastric bypass operation, during which his stomach and small intestine will be rearranged so that he is less able to tolerate large volumes of food and absorb calories and nutrients. To an outsider this may seem drastic, but to Mark and those who know his history, it's the next logical step. I have no doubt that he appreciates the magnitude of what he is about to undertake. It is a decision that he has not taken lightly. Mark is committing himself to a lifetime of watching his diet with intense scrutiny to avoid complications such as the dreaded "dumping syndrome" and to ensure that he maximizes his weight loss without compromising his overall health. Will it work? The chances are in his favor of shedding up to 70% of his excess weight in a relatively short period of time.

As I follow Mark's progress over the next 6 months, I expect to witness a physical and emotional transformation. He will likely not have to worry about being "too thin" any time soon, but I have faith that he will shortly be on his way to a life filled with less pain, as well as reduced risk of early morbidity and mortality. As he becomes smaller, I will surely "grow" in my own way, having been able to witness firsthand a physical and psychological transformation that few other medical students have been fortunate enough to observe on a personal level.

**Sang W. Kim, HMS III: Changing a paradigm**

Surgery is a very special discipline of medicine. A surgeon makes an incision on a patient's body and proceeds to alter the area in the most unnatural of ways. And over time, as the patient heals, his/her body becomes "new" and regains its functions.

This is why I am so fascinated with surgery—to me, it is the most intimate and direct mode of changing the course of disease and allowing the body to recover, returning back to its renewed homeostasis.

This is the second year that the Beth Israel Deaconess Medical Center of Harvard Medical School is running the longitudinal patient care program. This program affords participating medical students the opportunity to follow up on an assigned patient for 1 year. Interested students are given the choice of obstetric, oncologic, or surgical patients. I chose a surgical patient because this would provide an invaluable opportunity for me to experience, along with the patient, the journey through diagnosis, treatment, and recovery from a surgical disease.

However, on the day when I learned about my assigned patient, the case was something I had not expected; my patient would be an obese person planning to undergo an elective weight reduction surgery. I think that I did not expect a bariatric patient as my longitudinal surgical patient simply because I did not believe obesity was a medical condition that would warrant a surgical intervention.

Like most people, I remained within the paradigm of thinking of obesity as a lifestyle issue—a reflection of our society's preoccupation with consuming unhealthy food and our persistent lack of exercise. And also like most people, I feel uneasy about "fixing" obesity by reducing the size of the stomach to give the patient an artificial feeling of satiety, and/or to curb the caloric intake by shortening the length of the digested food's transit. Is this an appropriate and responsible medical approach? Is obesity a condition that should mandate a surgical procedure? What kind of people, I asked myself, would allow, or in fact *demand*, to have their bodies altered in such unnatural ways in order to escape their obesity?

Having spent almost a full year with my patient, I am beginning to realize some answers. Throughout this time, I have attended bariatric surgery information sessions with her, as well as numerous appointments with doctors, nutritionists, psychiatrists, and surgeons. We spent many hours talking while waiting for those appointments. The result was that I began to see through the eyes of this one individual—my patient, a 35-year-old mother of 2 who is a part-time nursing student with a degree in pharmacy and who has tried 6 different dietary programs over 10 years. She has at one time or another managed to lose 30 lbs or more, only to regain this weight back again and again.

My patient is an energetic, fun, ebullient person who is full of life. Despite having worked overnight on the day of our first meeting, I felt myself being energized after spending just a few minutes with her. From our conversation, I found that her overweight problem began during her pregnancy, after which she was never able to get back to her baseline weight. The body undergoes change during pregnancy and sometimes it may not return back to its previous state. That could happen to anyone. I learned that she enjoys outdoor activities with her family, and that she had recently picked up rowing. Listening to her, I thought to myself, this person does not fit with the stigma of obesity that I had in my mind. She tells me that often she feels her body becoming the limiting factor that prevents her from doing what she enjoys with her family and friends. She feels trapped in her body, despite being confident and independent. And after completing so many weight loss programs and always regaining the weight, she has accepted that in order to break from this wearisome, perpetual cycle of failures, she is going to need some help. Bariatric surgery will be the tool that she will use to break the cycle.

My patient has taught me that obesity is more than just lifestyle issues. I have read her dietary diary where she meticulously recorded all of her food intake for 3 days. From reading her diary, I realized that the quantity or the quality of food she ate was not very different from anyone I know or myself (I have never had overweight problems). She worked out an hour on her treadmill at least 4 times a week for the 2 months prior to her decision to undergo surgery (I felt very guilty reading this part as I have been trying and failing to manage any exercise during the weekday since starting my third-year clerkship). It is admirable how she has managed to regulate her diet and exercise, take care of 2 daughters ages 6 and 11 and a husband, and be a part-time nursing student as well. Now, 2 months after undergoing the procedure, my patient tells me that she has lost more than 35 lbs and has never felt better. She continues to attend Weight Watchers and maintain hour-long sessions on the treadmill 3 to 4 times per week.

I have learned that obesity can become a condition that goes beyond lifestyle issues. It is an altered physiological state that we still do not understand completely. Thus, we must strive to understand, treat, and educate people about it at the medical, as well as the social, level. Obesity is a condition that can limit a person's life and become extremely medically detrimental. Bariatric surgery will never be able to replace a healthy lifestyle and exercise; however, as a tool, it can help to dramatically improve the quality of life and overall health of persons who have been unable to find other ways out of the obesity dilemma.

**Jaime Wilson-Chiru, HMS III:** *Carrie*

Carrie Norton is an exceptional human being. She has a warm and open nature that allows her to befriend others with ease. She is a loving grandmother of 13 who exudes a young and vibrant personality. Carrie works hard to support her family, and manages to get to the gym at least 3 times a week. She even makes a special effort to participate in the Walk for Breast Cancer every year. Overall, she is a very active, happy individual. Yet she struggles with one thing—her weight. It is a problem she's been dealing with for more than 15 years.

As a teenager, Carrie weighed less than 100 lbs. Over the years, however, her girth has steadily increased. Today, at 5' tall and weighing 230 lbs, Carrie is not only overweight, she's morbidly obese. For the past decade and a half, she has been trying, unsuccessfully, to shed the pounds. She has gone through many different diets: Atkins, Weight Watchers, and Jenny Craig, to name a few. The dieting never lasted long. Even a special program with a personal trainer fell through. All of these attempts have seemingly backfired, and the whole time she has only gotten bigger.

To make matters worse, Carrie suffers from emphysema as a result of smoking for decades. She quit recently, but not early enough. Now she can barely make it up a flight of stairs without huffing and puffing at the top. Unfortunately, the treatment for her lung disease involves an ongoing course of steroids. One of the many side effects of this medication is weight gain and, in Carrie's case, an insatiable appetite.

Up until 6 months ago, Carrie would look at herself in the mirror and see the same young, skinny person that she was in her youth. She would compare herself to her relatives, who are even bigger, and dismiss her weight problem as trivial. Her self perception had been clouded for a long time. But she woke up one day and realized the skinny, youthful Carrie had vanished long ago. That Carrie had been completely absorbed into the folds of fat that had slowly and surreptitiously built up over time.

At that point, Carrie decided that she needed to do something drastic. Attempts at changing her lifestyle hadn't worked, so she turned to the only method that would guarantee weight loss: surgery. Several of her friends and family members had already gone through weight loss surgery with astounding results. A few had chosen the gastric bypass procedure, which involves the creation of a small (15 mL to 30 mL) pouch from the upper stomach. This is accompanied by bypass of the rest of the stomach and the beginning part of the intestine. As a result, the volume of food that can be eaten is greatly restricted, and the food that is eaten is not completely absorbed. This procedure is a major one that essentially rearranges the gastrointestinal tract. It is also a time-tested way to achieve rapid weight loss.

Other people Carrie knew had opted for adjustable gastric banding, which was a newer, simpler technique. This surgery, she understood, consisted of wrapping a hollow plastic band around the stomach. The band connected a small box implanted in the abdominal wall and could be constricted by filling the box with fluid, which had a restrictive effect on the stomach's capacity, forcing the patient to lower his or her food intake. The advantage of this procedure was that the restriction could be modulated by emptying or filling the box.

At first, Carrie wasn't sure which procedure to choose. She took time to weigh the options carefully, as this was no trivial decision. After much deliberation, she finally settled on the gastric banding. Frankly, she was intimidated by the invasiveness of the gastric bypass procedure. After all, she couldn't afford to miss much time at work, and recovery would certainly be quicker with the gastric banding. Once she had chosen the procedure she desired, it was time for the next step.

Now, in a tiny room in the bariatric surgery clinic, a half-dozen bulky men and women sit around a small table, their attention directed toward a thin, pretty woman as she demonstrates with empty cans of juice and protein drink. The woman, a nutritionist, is explaining the diet stages for someone who had just completed weight loss surgery.

Seated at the table, Carrie Norton listens attentively. She's dressed in pink sweatpants and a pink cotton T-shirt from a breast-cancer walk that reads, "Hope starts here." For someone who has tried to lose weight (and failed miserably) on every conceivable popular diet, the prospect of surgery has given Carrie hope once more. She is eager to get through the presurgery requirements, which include meetings with the nutritionist, exercise physiologist, psychologist, and other health professionals.

Carrie is so eager that she can't help but interject every so often as the nutritionist methodically gives her spiel. Carrie is very familiar with the multitude of sugar-free drinks and protein supplements on the market—she's already sampled them all. Once the group meeting ends, she finds herself having a one-on-one discussion with the nutritionist. But now that she's separated from the group, Carrie's jovial nature fades away and out comes a more serious attitude.

"I can't get rid of the hunger," she says in a heavy tone.

The nutritionist inquires about emotional eating. Carrie seems uncomfortable and skirts around the topic. "Oh...yeah, there's some history of that."

The nutritionist presses her for more. Reluctantly, Carrie divulges that food once gave her comfort, but for some reason she doesn't enjoy eating anymore. That's as much as she will say, for now.

The meetings are over and Carrie sets off for home, 45 minutes away by car. In the coming weeks, she will need to return several more times for further presurgery evaluation. Her journey toward weight loss is just beginning. But Carrie Norton isn't deterred by the burden of the commute, the testing, or the seemingly endless wait. For her, hope starts here. Hope, in the form of a shiny, silver scalpel.

**References (Greenman)**

1. Hedley AA, Ogden CL, Johnson CL, Carroll MD, Curtin LR, Flegal KM. Prevalence of overweight and obesity among US children, adolescents and adults, 1999-2002. *JAMA*. 2004;291(23):2847-50.
2. Lew EA, Garfinkel L. Variations in mortality by weight among 750,000 men and women. *J Chronic Dis*. 1979;32(8):563-76.
3. Daniels SR, Arnett DK, Eckel RH, et al. Overweight in children and adolescents: pathophysiology, consequences, prevention, and treatment. *Circulation*. 2005;111(15):1999-2012.
4. Finkelstein EA, Fiebelkorn IC, Wang G. State-level estimates of annual medical expenditures attributable to obesity. *Obes Res*. 2004;12(1):18-24.
5. Safer DJ. Diet, behavior modification and exercise: a review of obesity treatments from a long-term perspective. *South Med J*. 1991;84(12):1470-4.
6. Weintraub M, Sundaresan PR, Schuster B, et al. Long-term weight-control study. IV (weeks 156-190). The second double-blind phase. *Clin Pharmacol Ther*. 1992;51(5):608-14.
7. Flegal KM, Carroll MD, Kuczmarski RJ, Johnson CL. Overweight and obesity in the United States: prevalence and trends 1960-1994. *Int J Obes Relat Metab Disord*. 1998;22(1):39-47.

**References (Waks)**

1. Schwartz MB, Vartanian LR, Nosek BA, Brownell KD. The influence of one's own body weight on implicit and explicit anti-fat bias. *Obesity*. 2006;14(3):440-7.
2. Latner JD, Stunkard AJ, Wilson GT. Stigmatized students: age, sex, and ethnicity effects in the stigmatization of obesity. *Obes Res*. 2005;13(7):1226-31.
3. Overweight and Obesity: US Obesity Trends 1985–2006. Available at: http://www.cdc.gov/nccdphp/dnpa/obesity/trend/maps/. Accessed January 15, 2007.

# Health Economics

Daniel B. Jones, MD, MS

Morbid obesity is an epidemic in the United States and bariatric surgery is the only durable treatment likely to achieve sustained weight loss and health benefits. With growing demand for surgical services, will more third-party payers open access to care or will patients need to pay out-of-pocket for health services? To address whether surgical options are cost-effective, it is important to review the prevalence of morbid obesity, risks and benefits of surgery, and the costs of operative therapy, as well as to address recent changes regulating bariatric programs and how reimbursement programs may be tied to best practices and outcomes.

Nearly one third of Americans are overweight and one fifth are obese. Body mass index (BMI) defines obesity as a BMI greater than 30 kg/m$^2$. The most dramatic increase in obesity has been among the heaviest patients with a 2-fold increase among patients with a BMI greater than 30 kg/m$^2$ and a 4-fold increase among the population with a BMI greater than 40 kg/m$^2$ (Figure 1).(1)

**Figure 1**
**Prevalence of morbid obesity in the United States by BMI.**

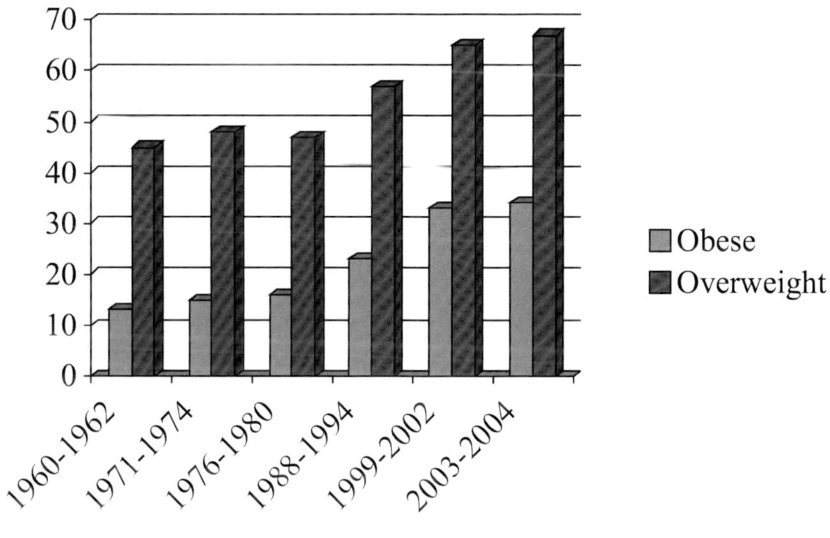


Sturm. *Arch Intern Med.* 2003;163:2146-2148.

Patient demand for surgical services has been exponential, but unable to keep pace with the epidemic of obesity. In 2007, more than 140,000 bariatric operations were performed in the United States.(2) With estimates of 11.5 million patients meeting medical necessity for weight loss surgery, millions of potential patients may not have access to care.(3)

Americans spend nearly 100 billion dollars annually combating obesity.(4) As insurance companies are facing rising healthcare costs and with policyholders increasingly unwilling to accept higher premiums, many insurance policies have excluded obesity coverage in the fine print. In Nebraska and Florida, the largest carrier (Blue Cross Blue Shield) discontinued health coverage for obesity surgery due to high demand and high costs.(5) Obesity surgery is often presented as an elective cosmetic option like plastic surgery, rather than treatment for a disease affecting all aspects of health and well-being. In these cases, patients are required to self-pay, often taking out loans. Other insurers have established rigorous approval processes, including monthly weight check-ins and psychological assessments. The private self-insured marketplace has similarly restricted healthcare coverage. For example, one of the nation's largest employers, like the majority of large employers, has recently discontinued bariatric coverage.(6,7) In Arkansas, bariatric coverage was eliminated from the state's self-funded employee benefit plan as its morbidly obese population increased from 5% to 25%.(6)

The Healthcare Cost and Utilization Project (HCUP) and the Agency for Healthcare Research and Quality track costs associated with obesity surgery.(8) In this database, inpatient costs for bariatric surgery were $16,541 in teaching hospitals, compared with $14,406 in nonteaching hospitals. Rural hospitals were slightly more costly at $16,741 compared with urban hospitals at $15,447. Comparisons of average costs per patient demonstrated no cost savings in high-volume centers compared with low-volume centers. Hospitals with low volume (<118 operations) had an average cost per patient of $16,402. High-volume hospitals (>387 operations) had an average cost per patient of $16,339. Inpatient mortality rates were low (teaching hospitals showed a rate of 0.21%; nonteaching hospitals, 0.18%; rural hospitals, 0.28%; and urban hospitals, 0.19%). Inpatient mortality rates were lower at high-volume centers compared with low-volume centers (0.12% versus 0.38%). Patients at teaching hospitals may be more seriously ill and high-volume centers may have better resources and processes to account for variations in outcomes.

The HCUP also reveals mean cost per operation by payers. In 2003, private insurance paid $12,822; self-pay, $12,822; Medicare, $19,030; and Medicaid, $17,844. Comparing 1998 with 2003, the HCUP demonstrated a 740% increase in the number of operations performed, from 13,386 to 112,435. Hospital inpatient costs to society increased from $173 million to $1.7 billion, and the mean cost per operation for all payers increased 21%, from $12,872 to $15,533.(8)

Bariatric operations reduce weight and improve health. A recent meta-analysis reported 62% excess weight loss for gastric bypass compared with 46% for gastric banding and 70% for biliopancreatic diversion/duodenal switch.(8) After weight loss, improvement of comorbid illnesses was dramatic, with resolution of diabetes in 77%, hyperlipidemia in 70%, and hypertension in 62% of patients.(9) With resolution of diabetes likely after weight loss and the annual costs of diabetes estimated at $10,683, gastric bypass appears very cost-effective.(10) Snow et al estimated the cost savings by eliminating medications. As comorbid conditions improved, medications decreased and gastric bypass paid for itself within 3 years (Figure 2).(11)

**Figure 2**
**Cost of gastric bypass versus savings in medication after gastric bypass.**

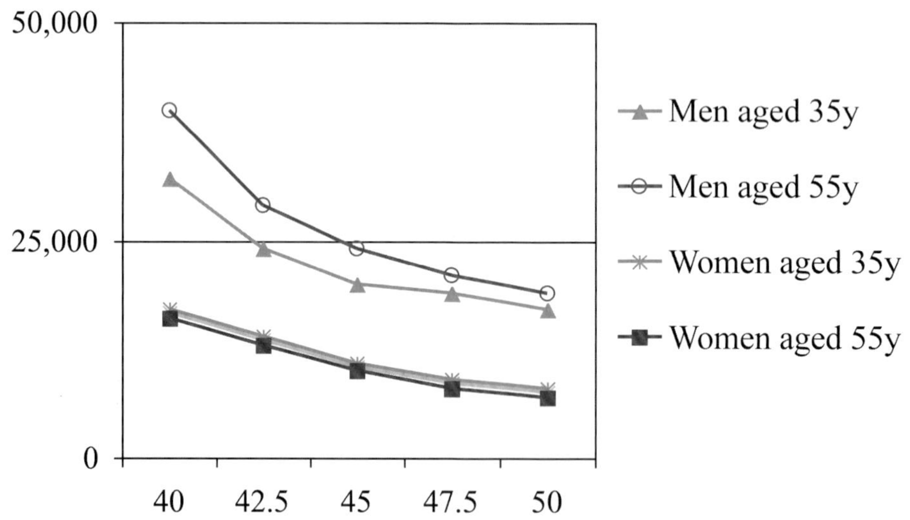


Snow, et al. The effect of Roux-en-Y gastric bypass on prescription drug costs. *Obes Surg*. 2005;14:1031-1035.

Cost-effectiveness is usually expressed as cost in dollars per quality-adjusted life years (QALY). The measure assesses quantity and quality of life generated by an intervention and is used by policy makers to prioritize resources. By convention, cost/QALY < $50,000 is cost-effective.(4) Craig et al demonstrated cost-effectiveness after open gastric bypass. Women were more cost-effective than men for BMIs greater than 40 (Figure 3).(12) Similarly, Clegg et al assessed weight change, quality of life, morbidity, mortality, revision rates, and obesity comorbidities, determining that surgery was cost-effective at $20,000 per QALY.(13)

**Figure 3**
**Cost-effectiveness after gastric bypass.**

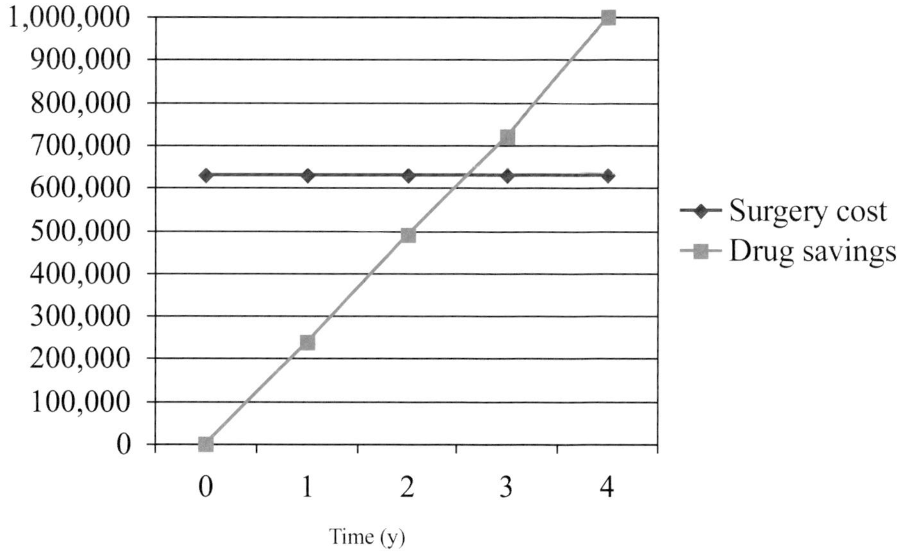


Craig. Cost-effectiveness of gastric bypass for severe obesity. *Am J Med.* 2002;113:491-498.

Laparoscopic gastric bypass achieves weight loss similar to open gastric bypass and costs less. Paxton et al demonstrated comparable excess weight loss between open and laparoscopic gastric bypass at 36 months.(14) This study compared hospital costs in open (n=6,425) and laparoscopic gastric bypass (n=5,867) and valued costs of the procedure, routine labs, x-rays, hospital room, complications, death, income lost, and risk of converting to an open procedure. Laparoscopic gastric bypass showed an average cost of $17,660 compared with the total costs of open gastric bypass, which was $20,443.(14) Likewise, Livingston et al compared charges and noted laparoscopic gastric bypass at $19,794, open gastric bypass at $22,313, and laparoscopic adjustable gastric band at $25,355.(15)

The decision to cover bariatric surgery should not skirt around the survival advantage after gastric bypass. For patients less than age 40 years, mortality over next 14 years is 3% after weight loss surgery compared with 13% without a bariatric operation.(16) In another study, gastric bypass reduced the relative risk of death by 89%.(17)

In response to the epidemic of obesity, many surgeons are adding weight loss surgery to their practice and bariatric centers are emerging to meet long waiting lists for surgery. Societies, licensing boards, and governmental agencies have published guidelines to standardize care and encourage hospital investment in its infrastructure for patients of size. In 2005, the Betsy Lehman Center for Patient Safety and Medical Error Reduction convened an expert panel in Massachusetts to establish best practices for weight loss surgery (www.mass.gov/dph/betsylehman/panel_summary.htm).(2) The American College of Surgeons has established the Bariatric Network to accredit hospitals based on Betsy Lehman Center guidelines and benchmarked outcomes. Similarly, the American Society for Metabolic and Bariatric Surgery and Surgical Review Corporation (SRC) have established an accreditation of surgeons and facilities based on volumes, personnel, and infrastructure. In 2006, Blue Cross Blue Shield announced its intent to tie payment for bariatric surgery to Betsy Lehman Center guidelines, and the media began to profile hospitals that fall short of volume recommendations for Centers of Excellence. In 2007, the Betsy Lehman Expert Panel reconvened and updated the recommendations.

Obesity is a major health problem and according to the National Institutes of Health weight loss surgery remains the best option for sustained and significant weight loss.(2) Strategies for prevention must be emphasized. However, after diet and exercise fail for the morbidly obese patient developing comorbid illnesses, bariatric surgery makes good sense and yields dividends worth society's investment.

**References**


1. Sturm R. Increases in clinically severe obesity in the United States, 1986-2000. *Arch Intern Med.* 2003;163(18):2146-8.
2. Kelly J, Tarnoff M, Shikora S, et al. Best practice recommendations for surgical care in weight loss surgery. *Obes Res*. 2005;13(2):227-33.
3. Encinosa W, Bernard D, Steiner C, Chen C. Use and costs of bariatric surgery and prescription weight loss medications. *Health Aff.* 2005;24(4):1039-46.
4. Salem L, Jensen C, Flum DR. Are bariatric surgical outcomes worth their cost? A systematic review. *J Am Coll Surg.* 2005;200(2):270-278.
5. Stein R. As obesity surgeries soar, so do safety, cost concerns. *Washington Post.* April 2, 2004:A01.
6. Alt S. Bariatric surgery may become a self-pay service. *Health Care Strateg Manage*. 2003;21(12):1, 12-9.
7. Haberkorn J. Obesity's new status will not affect insurers; but employers may pay more. *The Washington Times*. July 16, 2004.
8. Agency for Healthcare Research and Quality. Healthcare cost and utilization project (HCUP). HCUP NIS Database Documentation 2005. Agency for Healthcare Research and Quality. Available at: http//www.hcup.us.ahrq.gov. Accessed August 21, 2007.
9. Buchwald H, Avidor Y, Braunwald E, et al. Bariatric Surgey: a systematic review and meta-analysis. *JAMA*. 2004;292(14):1724-37.
10. American Diabetes Association. Direct and Indirect Costs of Diabetes in the United States: The per capita annual costs of health care for people with diabetes was $13,243 in 2002, compared to $2,560 for people without diabetes. American Diabetes Association. Available at: http://www.diabetes.org/diabetes-statistics/cost-of-diabetes-in-us.jsp. Accessed August 21, 2007.
11. Snow LL, Weinstein LS, Hannon JK, et al. The effect of Roux-en-Y gastric bypass on prescription drug costs. *Obes Surg*. 2004;14(8):1031-5.
12. Craig BM, Tseng DS. Cost-effectiveness of gastric bypass for severe obesity. *Am J Med*. 2002;113(6):491-8.
13. Clegg A, Colquitt J, Sidhum M, Royle P, Walker A. Clinical and cost-effectiveness of surgery for morbid obesity: a ,. review and economic evaluation. *Int J Obes Relat Metab Disord*. 2003;27(10):1167-77.
14. Paxton JH, Matthews JB. The cost effectiveness of laparoscopic versus open gastric bypass surgery. *Obes Surg*. 2005;15(1):24-34.
15. Livingston EH. Hospital costs associated with bariatric procedures in the United States. *Am J Surg*. 2005;190:816-20.
16. Flum D, Dellinger E. Impact of gastric bypass operation on survival: a population-based analysis. *J Am Coll Surg*. 2004;199(4):543-51.
17. Christou N, Sampalis J, Liberman M, Look D, Auger S, et al. Surgery decreases long-term mortality, morbidity, and health care use in morbidly obese patients. *Ann Surg*. 2004;240(3):416-24.

# Ensuring Access to Bariatric Surgery

Walter J. Pories, MD, FACS
Jacob Enterkin, BS
Gary M. Pratt, BS

Imagine, for a minute, that a pill had been invented that produced durable weight loss, usually more than a hundred pounds per patient. Then imagine that this is not the only effect. The pill also reverses diabetes, high blood pressure, sleep apnea … and this is only a partial list.

Would such a pill sell? You bet! Sales would very likely rapidly outstrip even the common antidepressants and antacids.

Well, there isn't such a pill, but there are several surgical procedures that produce these miraculous results. However, they have not been widely accepted and in fact, only about 1% of the patients who could benefit from bariatric surgery have access to the therapy. Of the 23 million Americans who have body mass indices (BMIs) greater than 35 kg/m$^2$ (the measure for obesity), only 180,000 (or 0.78%) undergo bariatric surgery each year.(1)

What are the reasons for this low rate of utilization? Is the surgery not always effective? Not safe? No, as a matter of fact, the operations are effective and have remarkably predictable positive results, as documented in numerous publications and in a meta-analysis (Table 1).(2) They are also safe, with national 90-day mortality rates of 0.34%,(3) about the same as hip replacements and cholecystectomies. That's approximately one tenth of most major abdominal operations, even though these morbidly obese patients carry significant increases in risk.

Table 1

**Comparison Of Bariatric Operations**
n = 22,094 patients; 2738 citations 1990 – 2002 (Buchwald)(2)

| | Adjustable gastric banding | Roux-en-Y gastric bypass | Duodenal switch |
|---|---|---|---|
| **Excess weight loss** | 47.5% | 61.6% | 70.1% |
| **Operative mortality (30 days)** | 0.1% | 0.5% | 1.1% |
| **Resolution of type 2 diabetes** | 47.8% | 83.6% | 97.9% |

Is it because the public is not informed? Again, no. Actually, we have the most informed public in history. There are few obese people who have not heard of "stomach stapling," or who do not have acquaintances who have had such operations. Many have even seen the numerous television programs that show each part of the operation in lengthy detail.

A more likely reason for the slow acceptance is that the public is well informed. Though there certainly have been many articles and broadcasts about the miracles of bariatric surgery, many obese persons were also familiar with a horror story of a friend with complications, or a patient in the intensive care unit, or a major lawsuit after an operation. The more sophisticated consumers i.e., employers, insurers, attorneys, and, indeed, our own colleagues—have become increasingly familiar with the 50-year history of failures, multiple operations, high complication rates, numerous law suits, prohibitive malpractice rates, and, finally, the refusal of carriers to pay for the procedures.

**2003: The Year of the Crisis**

By the fall of 2003, it was evident that the situation was unacceptable. We found ourselves confronted with the fact that obesity and diabetes had become the two most serious epidemics in history and that surgery was the only effective treatment. Yet the delivery system was seriously flawed. While some medical centers delivered effective and safe care, others were experiencing unacceptable morbidity and mortality rates. The initial response was an increase in malpractice litigation, soon followed by unaffordable malpractice rates. This, in turn, was followed by patients being denied the procedures by third-party payers, including Medicare and Medicaid. Some carriers developed innovative approaches to ensure denial: impossible measures such as requiring documentation of 5 years of physician-supervised diets. Others dealt with the problem by excluding bariatric surgery from their health plans, or by making it available only through expensive riders. Blue Cross Blue Shield of Florida(4) simply announced that they would no longer cover the surgery at all.

**The Carriers' Response: Centers of Excellence**

The draconian measure of cutting off access to bariatric surgery was not acceptable in the face of continuing evidence that, in the right hands, the results were remarkable. Durable remission of obesity, diabetes, sleep apnea, hypertension, stress incontinence, asthma, infertility, pseudotumor cerebri—even evidence of sharply improved arthritis—combined with reductions in mortality(5,6) and healthcare costs(7) prompted carriers to recognize that across-the-board denials were not acceptable strategies. They settled on a reasonable response: bariatric surgery would be covered, but only if the procedures were done by surgeons in hospitals with good outcomes—i.e., "centers of excellence."

By 2003, most major carriers had bariatric surgery Centers of Excellence programs. In general, the conditions under which the surgery would be reimbursed were sensible, usually based in part on the guidelines of the 1991 National Institutes of Health (NIH) Consensus Conference on the Surgery of Obesity,(8) which included a BMI ≥40 or a BMI ≥35 with comorbidities; a patient-age requirement of 18 to 55; full understanding of the potential outcomes of the procedures; evidence of control of previous emotional disorders; and, where alcohol and/or drug abuse was involved, treatment with agreement to long-term follow-up. In addition, there were requirements regarding the training of the surgeons and maintenance of data.

Unfortunately, each carrier also added its own individual requirements, usually not supported by evidence, such as documented attempts at dieting; evidence of weight loss; records of obesity dating back at least 5 years; and qualifications of surgeons in terms of training and experience. These variations led to unmanageable hurdles for surgeons and patients in the form of multiple applications for membership in panels and repeated denials because a particular condition, often not revealed, had not been met by the patient.

Most serious, however, was the failure of the carriers to share data either with each other or with the surgeons and hospitals. Each series was too limited and the data definitions too different to allow statistical interpretation. In spite of all effort and expense, the information was without value. Access to the surgery was still limited by bureaucracy and arbitrary decisions.

**Another Response: The American Society for Metabolic and Bariatric Surgery**

The leadership of the American Society for Metabolic and Bariatric Surgery (ASMBS) recognized that the situation was untenable. In spite of all efforts, patients were still denied access. The ASMBS also understood that the answer, the quality control of surgery, was a complex challenge that had been an objective of organized medicine, private carriers, and governmental agencies for over a century. Accordingly, the first steps were cautious—first, to determine the state-of-the-art as reflected by a meta-analysis of peer-reviewed articles and second, to hold a consensus conference with the format usually used by the NIH. The independent review of the bariatric surgical literature in the English language(2) and the consensus conference at Georgetown University(9) reflected the same conclusions: that bariatric surgery performed in "centers" (i.e., by experienced surgeons under appropriate conditions) was safe and effective. Based on this information, and with the support of the membership of the ASMBS, the Society explored the development of an ASMBS Centers of Excellence program that would address the two problems raised by the carriers' programs: developing evidence-based, uniform, nationwide requirements and ensuring the sharing of data.

This was not a simple challenge. The first hurdle was the warning that the ASMBS, as a professional society, should not undertake the initiative for two reasons: credibility and legal vulnerability. Consultants, carriers, and malpractice providers agreed that a "guild" would not have the credibility of an independent organization. Most convincing, however, was the advice of counsel that the Society was not in a position to respond to legal challenges by surgeons or hospitals who might sue following a denial of certification.

**An Independent, Nonprofit Organization**

In order to manage the program, three leaders of the ASMBS founded the Surgical Review Corporation (SRC) in November 2003 as an independent, nonprofit organization. Governance was split into two levels:

1. For policy, a board of directors was formed with a broad representation of shareholders (surgeons, nurses, a consumer, representatives from a health insurance carrier and a physician-owned professional liability company). Initially, one third of the seats were assigned to senior leaders in the American College of Surgeons (ACS), but the relationship ended when the ACS decided to start a competitive initiative in December 2004.
2. For professional decisions, a bariatric surgery review committee was set up, comprised of highly respected bariatric surgical leaders.

**Developing the Concept of Quality Control of Surgical Procedures**

Most challenging was the methodology for quality control of bariatric surgery. Although surgical outcomes data were collected even in antiquity, they were still generally limited to measures of operative morbidity, mortality, and long-term survival. Risk stratification was minimal, generally based on age, gender, and, for some cancers, the stages of the disease. With the exception of a few studies such as those of the National Cancer Institute, the series were usually limited and there was little standardization of procedures.

Consultation with engineers familiar with quality-control measures in the pharmaceutical industry emphasized the importance of the following criteria: standardization of procedures; uniform definition of data elements; inclusion of all outcomes data; identification of critical data indices (data vs. information); site inspections; and verification of the submitted information. Based on these guidelines, the review committee arrived at the requirements for certification as an ASMBS Center of Excellence. The requirements were derived from a review of the literature, multiple consultations among surgeons, and consultation with representatives from industry. In brief, these included:

- experienced bariatric surgeons with a major administrative role;
- an appropriately equipped hospital with a full complement of specialists;
- an adequate volume of cases for both hospital and surgeons;
- standardization of procedures and care paths;
- full reporting of outcomes; and
- follow-up of 75% of patients over 5 years.

To ensure support by the membership of the ASMBS, the requirements were widely published for public comment prior to adoption. Detailed descriptions of the current versions, somewhat changed from the originals, are available at www.surgicalreview.org.

The application process was divided into two levels, provisional and full approval. Provisional status was granted after the candidate surgeons and their center declared that they had the resources to provide bariatric surgery effectively and safely. Full approval required, in addition, submission of 1 year's bariatric surgical outcomes confirmed by a site inspection. To help ensure internal validity of the data, surgeons and hospitals are required to submit their data independently.

In December 2004, the ACS announced its own approach to certification of centers, based on requirements similar to those of the ASMBS. As of January 1, 2007, there are 210 ASMBS approved centers and 25 Level-1 centers approved by the ACS. In February 2006, based on the data presented at the Medicare Advisory Committee, the Center for Medicare and Medicaid Services (CMS) approved reimbursement for bariatric surgery, but only if the services were rendered in centers certified by the ASMBS or ACS.

**Current status of Centers of Excellence**

As of January 1, 2007, 210 ASMBS Centers of Excellence had been granted full approval. Based on application data for the previous 12 months, representing the experience involving 61,545 patients (11,017 males, mean age 42.98 [10-81], Medicaid 3,051, Medicare 4,216), bariatric surgery had been provided with an in-hospital mortality of 0.13%; a 30-day mortality of

0.29%; a 90-day mortality of 0.37%; a readmission rate of 4.9%; and a reoperation rate of 2.15%. These outcomes compare favorably with those of other common major operations (Table 2).(10) Bariatric surgery, when performed in Centers of Excellence, is now significantly safer than most common operations at the level of hip replacements and cholecystectomies—a remarkable accomplishment in view of the surgical risks posed by the severely obese.

**Table 2**

**Mortality Rates Following Common Operations In US Hospitals**
(Dimick)(10)

| | Aortic aneurysm | CABG | Craniotomy | Esophageal resection | Hip replacement | Pancreatectomy |
|---|---|---|---|---|---|---|
| **Number of hospitals performing operation** | 2485 | 1036 | 1600 | 1717 | 3445 | 1302 |
| **National average mortality rate (%)** | 3.9 | 3.5 | 10.7 | 9.1 | 0.3 | 8.3 |
| **Average hospital caseloads (median)** | 30 | 491 | 12 | 5 | 24 | 8 |

**Challenges**

The designation of ASMBS Centers of Excellence is an excellent start, but only a start. True quality control can only begin when the outcomes data lead to evidence-based improvements in care paths, operations, and long-term care.

To progress toward these goals, the SRC focused first on the data-collection process with the development of the Bariatric Outcomes Longitudinal Database™ (BOLD™), a surgical-outcomes software program solely based on defined choices rather than traditional free-text methods. For example, rather than allowing the provider to state whether the patient did or did not have diabetes, the program offers 5 choices:

- No diabetes
- Diabetes controlled by diet
- Diabetes controlled by oral medications
- Diabetes controlled with insulin
- Diabetes that is out of control

The approach forces objective, graduated entries that are fully retrievable in real time, essential for prompt recognition of problems and to achieve continued and current access to the clinical data. To ensure accuracy in communicating with other databases, SRC continues to pursue clearly defined common definitions for the data elements with other professional organizations.

BOLD™ is now available as a version called CORE™, which means it is limited to collecting only those data required for designation and maintenance of that designation. In the near future, BOLD™ will also be available as a COMPLETE™ version that will include more detailed descriptions of the medical history, physical examination, laboratory data, imaging results, and details of the surgery, as well as adverse events. The programs and definitions will also be available for adaptation by software vendors for surgeons who are already using such programs.

The second focus will be the "drilling down" on the deaths (0.34%) that occur within ninety days after the primary bariatric surgery. Each of the mortalities will be investigated anonymously in a "no-blame" manner similar to the investigation of aircraft accidents. The 90-day period offers fruitful opportunities for reducing mortalities because more deaths occur after discharge than during hospitalization. The nature of these deaths often remain unexplained; many may be preventable.

The third focus will be the conduct of prospective clinical trials conducted with a consortia of participating centers. The annual access to more than 100,000 new patients per year with real-time data in a central repository can provide a new and promising platform for clinical studies. Most importantly, the system will return the data to those who can improve care to our patients.

## Conclusion

Bariatric surgery is the only effective treatment for severe obesity and its comorbidities. The American Society for Metabolic and Bariatric Surgery Centers of Excellence now deliver this care with remarkable efficacy and safety. Future efforts include the maturation of the database, "no-blame" review of adverse events, and clinical trials for the benefit of our patients.

## References


1. American Society for Bariatric Surgery estimates. 2006.
2. Buchwald H, Avidor Y, Braunwald E, et al. Bariatric surgery: a systematic review and meta-analysis. *JAMA*. 2004;292(14):1724-37. Review. Erratum in: *JAMA*. 2005;293(14):1728.
3. Pories WJ. Yes, Virginia, bariatric surgery works, and it is safe. *NC Med J*. 2006;67(4):296-300.
4. Murr MM, Zeringue V. The ASBS "Florida Coalition." *Surg Obes Relat Dis*. 2006;2(4):493-4.
5. MacDonald KG Jr, Long SD, Swanson MS, et al. The gastric bypass operation reduces the progression and mortality of non-insulin-dependent diabetes mellitus. *J Gastrointest Surg*. 1997;1(3):213-20; discussion 220.
6. Christou NV, MacLean LD. Effect of bariatric surgery on long-term mortality. *Adv Surg*. 2005;39:165-79.
7. Christou NV, Sampalis JS, Liberman M, et al. Surgery decreases long-term mortality, morbidity, and health care use in morbidly obese patients. *Ann Surg*. 2004;240(3):416-23; discussion 423-424.
8. Gastrointestinal surgery for severe obesity. NIH Consensus Development Conference, March 25-27,1991. *Nutrition*. 1996;12(6):397-404.
9. Buchwald H; Consensus Conference Panel. Bariatric surgery for morbid obesity: health implications for patients, health professionals, and third-party payers. *J Am Coll Surg*. 2005;200(4):593-604.
10. Dimick JB, Welch HG, Birkmeyer JD. Surgical mortality as an indicator of hospital quality: the problem with small sample size. *JAMA*. 2004;292(7):847-51.

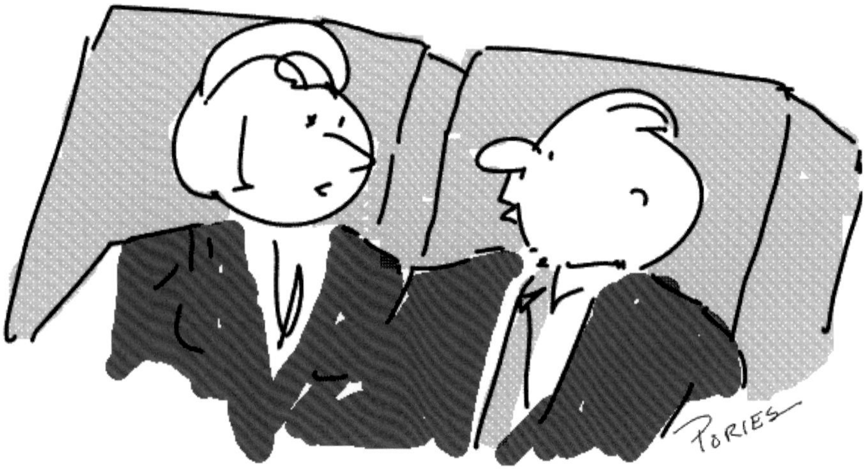


"What do you do?"

"I'm a bariatric surgeon."

"Oh, you make people thin?"

"No, I make people well."

# Access to Care

Joseph Nadglowski, Jr.
James Zervios

Today, the obesity and overweight epidemic impacts nearly 2 out of 3 Americans. It is estimated that more than 32% of Americans are obese.(1) Within the U.S. population, it is estimated that nearly 5% of Americans are considered morbidly obese, meaning 100 lbs or more over ideal body weight.(2) With numbers such as these, the obese population has needed representation throughout the United States.

In early 2005, during a meeting of legislators, a representative stood and said, "I could eliminate all access to obesity management services in my state today and nobody would say anything to stop me." This was a true and frightening statement. How could a population made up of more than 93 million people lack representation? Again, this was a frightening question. The appropriate response to the situation became clear: the obese population needed to form a coalition to represent them on a national level.

With the support of industry funding, and a great desire and determination on the part of the obese population, the Obesity Action Coalition (OAC) was formed. The OAC is a 501(c)(3) nonprofit, patient-based organization with a mission to elevate and empower—through education, advocacy, and support—those affected by obesity. The OAC aims to educate patients, family members, and the public on obesity, morbid obesity, and childhood obesity. In addition, the OAC increases obesity education, works to improve access to medical treatments for obese patients, advocates for safe and effective treatments, and strives to eliminate the negative stigma associated with all types of obesity.

By building a coalition of members ranging from patients and their family members to healthcare professionals, the OAC and its members focus national attention on obesity. They organize concerned individuals as advocates for action, advances, and change, and they visibly affect and impact the healthcare community and the public at large.

### The Current State of Access to Care

Over the past few years, access to obesity management services has become more and more difficult. The trend of "shortsightedness" on the part of the payers in regard to return on investment has led many insurance providers to downgrade or completely eliminate access to obesity management services in their policies.

This short-sighted decision is a very dangerous one. The rising rates of obesity, morbid obesity, and childhood obesity mean that more and more individuals are being affected by the many comorbid conditions associated with this disease as well. In fiscal terms, the management of these comorbidities over the course of an extended period far outweighs the cost of a patient's chosen obesity management service.

It is the OAC's goal to display to insurance payers that by allowing an individual access to care, they are helping the individual to take a proactive approach to pursuing an overall better quality of life, thus achieving a better quality of health. In addition, we would like to encourage these payers to develop a long-term mindset when calculating the cost of leaving this disease unchecked versus allowing the patient to pursue his or her chosen treatment option.

There is some hope in sight. Currently, there are four states (Georgia, Indiana, Maryland, and Virginia) with mandated coverage for weight loss surgery. Of these four, Indiana and Maryland have true mandated coverage. The other two states offer the access to care as an add-on feature with an extremely high premium. Mandates, however, only impact fully insured policies, which are regulated at the state level. Mandates do not impact self-insured policies, which are regulated at the federal level.

### Fully Insured vs. Self-insured

If the employer plan is **fully insured**, the insurance company is ultimately responsible for the healthcare costs, and the employer typically purchases a standardized package of coverage.

If the plan is **self-insured**, the employer is ultimately responsible for the healthcare costs, and therefore can customize the plan to include and exclude specific coverage, such as bariatric surgery coverage.(3)

Overall, many patients find it difficult to access care for obesity management services. Most of the time, working with the insurance provider can be a daunting task and often leads the patient to give up. To combat this, the OAC developed an insurance guide, "Working with Your Insurance Provider: A Guide to Seeking Weight Loss Surgery."(3) This guide provides patients with an overall assessment of the insurance process and offers helpful tips and information on how to successfully work with their providers.

**Advocating for Access to Care**

As any obese patient knows, obesity is a complex, chronic disease. It is not simply a condition caused by overeating. The obese often experience a wide variety of other health conditions (comorbid conditions), including diabetes, high cholesterol, high blood pressure, heart disease, sleep apnea, and cancer—all of which are serious medical risks. Adding to the challenge is the fact that patients are often denied access to needed treatment (medical weight management and/or weight loss surgery) as some payers (insurance companies, etc.) and employers do not recognize obesity as a disease.

**Why is it Important to Advocate?**

The obese population is often the target of discrimination. In fact, obesity discrimination is one of the last forms of acceptable discrimination in the country. Quite often obese individuals find themselves the target of discrimination in a variety of settings such as employment, health care, education, and much more.

**Consequences of Weight Bias**

Taken together, the consequences of being denied jobs, rejected by peers or treated inappropriately by healthcare professionals because of one's weight can have a seriously negative impact on quality of life. Obese individuals suffer terribly, both from direct discrimination and from more subtle forms of bias and stigma that are frequently encountered.(4)

Weight bias can have psychological, social, and physical health consequences for those affected by this disease. Psychological outcomes include, but are not limited to, depression, anxiety, low self-esteem, and poor body image.(4) The social effects can be rejection by peers, poor quality of interpersonal relationships, and compromised academic achievement. The physical health outcomes can include binge eating and unhealthy weight control practices.

**Reducing the Weight Bias**

Given how pervasive and acceptable weight stigma is in our society, transforming attitudes and enacting laws that prohibit discrimination based on weight are actions that can and must be undertaken. This requires enormous efforts in general, but there are important steps that also can be taken by both patients and their healthcare providers to help improve the daily functioning and well-being of obese individuals.(4) Patients who struggle with weight stigma can begin to approach this problem by becoming advocates for themselves. This includes identifying incidents in which they have been stigmatized because of their weight and deciding how best to handle such situations to achieve positive emotional health and help prevent similar incidents from occurring.

Obesity stigma is a crucial part of the access-to-care issue. In order to have adequate access to care, obesity must be recognized as a disease and the often and common negative stigma associated with it must be eliminated so that fair and safe obesity management services can be developed, supported, and made available to anyone requiring them.

**How Do I Begin Advocating?**

There are many avenues a patient can take to becoming an advocate for access to care. But first, the individual must understand the disease and understand what he/she is advocating toward. This is a quality-of-life issue. Weight loss surgery is not a cosmetic surgery. The OAC provides many resources for patients to draw on when educating themselves and others about this disease. From a weight loss fact sheet to an overview of obesity that promotes basic understanding of the disease, the OAC can provide the advocate with all the necessary tools to make a difference.

**Whom Do I Advocate Toward?**

It is important to educate our legislators. Elected US officials at the local, state, and federal levels play a significant role in our society and health care. Often, the laws they create directly influence our day to day lives or regulate the medical treatments we receive. However, the majority of legislators know little about obesity, its effects, and treatments.

As Americans, it is our right to build a relationship with our elected officials and to advocate for positive change. It is through the voice of patients, family members, and medical professionals that legislators learn how current, pending, and future laws impact Americans. The OAC encourages all to reach out to legislators.

There are a variety of ways to do this outreach, including communicating by mail, e-mail, phone; attending town hall meetings; or connecting in-person with legislators or other key individuals. Share your personal story with your elected official and encourage your family and friends to do the same. Keep in mind that you elect your lawmakers. They serve you and need to know the issues that are important to you.

Learn which individuals are key in the government regulating agencies—in particular, the healthcare regulating agencies. These include the Centers for Medicare and Medicaid Services (CMS), US Food and Drug Administration (FDA), National Institutes of Health (NIH), and Centers for Disease Control and Prevention (CDC), as well as many others. Regulatory agencies often welcome patient participation through public comment periods on proposed policies. Public comments are a great way to share views on a proposed regulation.

The media is one of the most influential groups in today's society. Educating the media is essential. Encourage local media productions of accurate stories about obesity. Do not hesitate to contact local newspaper reporters and/or television health reporters and share your story. Try to build a good relationship with the local media by providing accurate information and timely responses. If you see, read, or hear a story or article and believe it was inaccurate, one-sided and/or that it added to the negative stigma of obesity, write or call the media outlet and register your concerns.

The general public is bombarded on a daily basis by images, stories, and broadcast opinions of all kinds. Much of the content is one-sided or inaccurate. Reach out to your local media and encourage those in control to portray obesity accurately.

**The Importance of Educating Insurers and Employers**

Does your health insurance company offer coverage for obesity treatment? If you have been seeking treatment, you may already know. If you do not know, find out by calling the member services number on your insurance card. If coverage is not offered or you believe the procedures to access care are too complicated, do not hesitate to write the medical director of the insurance company and ask for an explanation.

Often, your human resources department or benefits manager at work plays a major role in deciding which health conditions are covered by your health insurance (and which insurance policies are offered). Share the seriousness of obesity and the importance of obesity coverage with them and encourage them to seek out policies that offer obesity coverage as a benefit.

**The Importance of Educating the General Public**

We have already discussed the influence the media has on the general public, but each individual can have an influence as well. It is important that the public receive accurate information on the risks and treatments of obesity, as well as about the numerous conditions (diabetes, heart disease, sleep apnea, etc.) related to the disease. You can be the source of such information by volunteering to speak on obesity at your place of worship, service club (Rotary Club, etc.) and/or your place of employment. Share your personal story; it will be tremendously influential.

Whichever route is chosen first, it is important for all advocates to remain positive and motivated. Changing access-to-care parameters takes time and dedication, but the results will benefit the millions of Americans affected by this disease.

**Examples of Access-to-care Issues**

Advocating for access to care for those affected by obesity is not a quick process. Often, when obstacles appear in the way of those seeking access to care, the true effectiveness of advocacy comes to light. In the examples that follow, advocacy played an integral role in changing the specific access-to-care issues.

- **Medicare National Coverage Decision**

  In February 2006, CMS released its new rules regarding access to weight loss surgery. The new rules allowed for Medicare to cover weight loss surgery as long as the procedure was performed under certain guidelines and criteria.(4)

  Prior to the decision, Medicare's policy only covered gastric bypass surgery if it was medically appropriate and if the surgery was used to correct an illness that caused the obesity or was aggravated by the obesity. In addition, coverage varied from region to region due to the absence of a national coverage decision.

  Medicare's endorsement of the safety and effectiveness of bariatric surgery provided the morbidly obese with increased opportunity to access care and decrease the many life-threatening, comorbid conditions associated with their disease. Although the decision was not without some controversy (mostly related to "Center of Excellence" requirements), it was a tremendous proactive step for the obesity community and was driven by the large numbers of patients and healthcare professionals who advocated for the change. It is the hope of the OAC that private insurers will follow suit in the future to also allow for coverage of weight loss surgery under the guidelines.

- **Blue Cross Blue Shield of Tennessee Requires IQ Testing**

  In 2006, the OAC learned of a new barrier to accessing care. Blue Cross Blue Shield (BC/BS) of Tennessee was requiring an IQ test as part of their psychological screening required prior to bariatric surgery.(4) Through research, the OAC learned that this was the first documented case of an insurance company requiring IQ testing on a patient wishing to access a medical procedure. From the OAC's perspective, requiring an IQ test to access any medical procedure is wrong and by implementing such a requirement, BC/BS of Tennessee set a dangerous precedent of denying health care based on intelligence. In addition, this decision further perpetuated the negative stigma often associated with obesity.

  The OAC immediately responded to this issue by sending multiple letters to BC/BS of Tennessee requesting that the company rescind its decision for IQ testing. Unfortunately, BC/BS of Tennessee did not respond. The OAC then issued a national news release asking BC/BS of Tennessee to rescind their decision to administer IQ testing to patients wishing to gain access to treatment for weight loss surgery. In addition, the OAC called on its constituents to take action and raise their voices by advocating for safe, fair, and effective access to care. Soon after the news release received national media attention, BC/BS of Tennessee decided to stop all IQ testing and removed the requirement from its coverage policy.(5) This decision was a tremendous example of how advocacy can make a difference in accessing care.(6)

The success of these two cases greatly increased access to weight loss surgery for all those affected by this disease. Medicare's decision allowed for a national basis of coverage under important and valuable guidelines and the decision to rescind the IQ testing advanced one of the OAC's important goals, which is to eliminate the negative stigma that is so often associated with obesity.

**Current Access-to-care Issues**

Although access to care in the United States is beginning to improve, there is still much work to be done. Each day, new issues arise where a patient is denied access based on various reasons. For instance, many patients are required, by their insurance contract, to participate in a medically managed weight loss program prior to weight loss surgery. Although some surgeons require medically managed weight loss as part of their programs, the OAC believes there is no evidence that suggests outcomes are better for patients who participate in such programs. One small study actually has shown the contrary.(7) The average length of time for this requirement is 3 months; however, many providers require 6 to 12 months of a medically managed weight loss program prior to surgery. It is the hope of the OAC to advocate for a 3-month length of time. Quite commonly, patients are in desperate need of care, have spent years struggling with numerous diet plans, and are debilitated by the many comorbid conditions often associated with this disease. It is our belief that insurance-required medically managed weight loss programs are simply a delay tactic and a significant barrier to care.

Another major issue on the horizon relates to insurers covering surgeries by type; that is, some insurers are considering, and at least one has implemented, rules that require specific surgeries for specific body mass index (BMI) ranges. For example, a patient with a BMI >50 kg/m² would only be permitted to be covered for gastric bypass, not laparoscopic adjustable gastric banding. The OAC strongly believes that patients, with input from their surgeons and healthcare team, should choose their surgery modality, and to this end it has begun efforts to discourage insurers from adopting protocols linking BMI to surgery type.

Thus, the OAC continues to advocate strongly for the rights of patients who wish to have access to bariatric surgical care. In 2002, the medical costs attributed to overweight and obesity reached an astonishing $92.6 billion in this country.(8) With the cost of care for comorbid conditions skyrocketing, treating obesity by improving access to care is an important national issue that must be addressed with open-mindedness, dedication, and compassion. Thanks to the many devoted individuals willing to advocate for their rights as Americans, it is our hope that access to the treatment of obesity in the United States will continue to improve for all those affected by obesity.

**References**


1. Centers for Disease Control and Prevention. Health, United States, 2003. Table 68: data according to the National Health and Nutrition Examination Survey (NHANES). Atlanta, GA: Centers for Disease Control and Prevention, US National Center on Vital Statistics; 2003.
2. Ogden CL, Carroll MD, Curtin LR, McDowell MA, Tabak CJ, Flegal KM. Prevalence of overweight and obesity in the United States, 1999-2004. *JAMA*. 2006;295(13):1549-55.
3. Working with Your Insurance Provider: A Guide to Seeking Weight Loss Surgery. Obesity Action Coalition. Available at: http://www.obesityaction.org/resources/insurance/oacinsuranceindex.php. Accessed February 7, 2007.
4. Puhl, R. Weight Bias. Presented at: Yale University Rudd Center for Food Policy and Obesity. September 29, 2006.
5. Centers for Medicare and Medicaid Services. Medicare expands national coverage for bariatric surgery procedures. Available at: http://www.cms.hhs.gov/apps/media/press/release.asp?Counter=1786. Accessed February 8, 2007.
6. Blue Cross Blue Shield of Tennessee. Bariatric surgery for morbid obesity. BlueCross BlueShield of Tennessee Medical Policy Manual. Available at: http://www.bcbst.com/MPManual/Bariatric_Surgery_for_Morbid_Obesity.htm. Accessed February 8, 2007.
7. Pinto, C. Insurer ends IQ test for obesity surgery—Blue Cross official: rule misunderstood. Available at: http://tennessean.com/apps/pbcs.dll/article?AID=/20070127/NEWS07/701270338/1024/NEWS. Accessed February 8, 2007.
8. Sentenac, H. Anger erupts over insurance company's IQ test for weight loss surgery. Available at: http://www.foxnews.com/story/0,2933,246519,00.html. Accessed February 8, 2007.


**Suggested Reading**


1. Jamal MK, DeMaria EJ, Johnson JM, et al. Insurance-mandated preoperative dietary counseling does not improve outcome and increases dropout rates in patients considering gastric bypass surgery for morbid obesity. *Surg Obes Relat Dis*. 2006;2(2):122-7.
2. Finkelstein EA, Fiebelkorn IC, Wang G, et al. National medical spending attributable to overweight and obesity: how much, and who's paying? *Health Aff.* 2003:w3: 219–26.

# Insurer Perspective: Massachusetts Blue Cross/Blue Shield

John A. Fallon, MD

I would like to give you an idea of the involvement that Blue Cross/Blue Shield (Massachusetts) has in the Betsy Lehman Center, but I will also look at bariatric surgery today and the whole issue of management of obesity. As an internist on the provider side my entire career, I joined Blue Cross in 2004. Blue Cross strived to focus strongly on quality, safety, and affordability and believed that these goals were all intimately tied together. Of course, we all know they are, but to have a health-insurance provider declare its intention to vigorously pursue these goals was really something quite unique. So, I decided to take Blue Cross up on its challenge. In this chapter, I'd like to share some of what I've seen happen since.

The Institute of Medicine (IOM) tells us we must be safe, effective, patient-centered, timely, and efficient healthcare professionals providing equitable care. However, whether we're treating obesity management or performing bariatric or cardiac surgery, we often come up short in this. We are also cautioned to pay attention to the value equation. We've all heard about affordability; you read about it every day in the paper. The problem of the uninsured continues to grow, as does that of the underinsured and those who are currently paying the bills, whether they are Medicare or Medicaid.

From the perspective of a company like Blue Cross, every day we encounter employers who ask, "What is the value I'm getting?," and for bariatric surgery they ask, "What is the value of that kind of procedure? I know the cost. I know the numbers are going up, but show me that it makes a difference. Show me the long-term outcomes, and where quality really takes place."

**Using Outcomes to Measure Quality Care**

There is a lot happening in the healthcare environment, in addition to the IOM and the value equation, which is very appropriate to note in a book about obesity management and bariatric surgery. We can't even consider a solution until we're aware of what's actually happening. You've heard about "pay for performance," a catch-phrase category that initially pertained to primary care physicians and Health Plan Employer Data and Information Set (HEDIS) measures. In our company, pay for performance has evolved into a system of rewarding clinical outcomes, as well as information technology (IT) investments and has now expanded from primary care physicians to specialists and hospitals. We have covered the entire spectrum, including bariatric surgery, because it involves specialty and hospital care. The Leapfrog Group keeps telling us that volume-counts and IT infrastructure are important—they're bridges of excellence as we look at meaningful outcomes and process redesign. It seems that the National Quality Forum comes up with an additional set of measures and evidence-based medicine guidelines every day that we must then follow.

The Centers for Medicare and Medicaid Services (CMS) has recently taken an enormous step regarding implantable defibrillators; we will see more of this happening in the future. They pay for procedures and for the implantable devices and in return, they expect outcomes data. These data are going to help further the guidelines development as the technology changes, and will be validating whether CMS's initial step in paying for implantable defibrillators was appropriate. We will be seeing a lot more of this, making this dialogue on outcomes measures in bariatric surgery a valuable "fit" with the Betsy Lehman Center report.

Other marked dynamics we're currently seeing is cost information and quality information coming forward in the tiering of providers. Again, you see Centers of Excellence in action across the country, but there are many other initiatives, which are not Centers of Excellence, starting to tier providers into 1, 2, and 3 segments, increasing co-pays, and with that, demanding quality outcomes in order to be in the appropriate tier. At the same time, high-cost radiology has been increasing its profile on the healthcare scene. Why is this important? It's important because employers are saying, "The costs are going up, there are too many tests being done! What is the value of my expenditure? Is the quality getting better or is it just that the cost is going up?" I hope you're starting to get the sense that in this country there is an enormous groundswell centered on health care, much of it focused on cost and quality regarding obesity management and bariatric surgery.

### Evidence-based Medicine

What works? What doesn't? What do we want to pay for? What do consumers want to pay for? You're paying your own bill as your own employer, but what is it that you think you get for your healthcare dollar? A lot of us in consumer-directed healthcare plans, including myself, have high deductibles. You may ask yourself, "What's the best company and plan? What kind of care am I getting? Is my doctor the best? How about my hospital? Is my healthcare program right for me?"

The US Food and Drug Administration (FDA) approval presents another interesting dynamic in the healthcare marketplace. However, FDA approval is often not based upon the criteria that we, as clinicians, would say is solid, evidence-based medicine. Sometimes lack of approval, quite frankly, is based on political or economic considerations. Unfortunately, the process of FDA approval is not always shaped by the rigor of evidence-based medicine.

In addition, we should understand that bariatric surgery is always subject to the continuum of care. The patient doesn't just enter the hospital, get the surgery, and go home, and it's done. The overarching question here is about *managing obesity* and you know that. As an insurer, those of us in the field are concerned about the long-term outcomes of bariatric surgery and how it fits in the long-term health of our members.

How do we help people who are overweight, who need to have some intervention, education, or access to support systems? What can we do to keep those individuals reasonably healthy so that the percentage of people who do require bariatric surgery remains as small as possible? And, for those requiring surgery, how can we make sure we use the appropriate selection criteria to facilitate that surgery?

I'd like to say evidence-based medicine is the be-all and end-all solution, but we know it only applies to a limited number of clinical situations. Even when we have these medicines or guidelines, disseminate them, and educate people—both providers and patients—about them, people often don't adhere to them. Studies are published regularly showing statistics, such as only 45% of people who need statins get them or only 28% of diabetics get the appropriate composite treatment, or 45% of people with hypertension receive the correct treatment. It would seem that we're not even able to provide the care we're supposed to. So what happens in bariatric surgery? Is it really any different?

Insurance companies are often asked, "We have this evidence-based medicine and it looks really good, so why don't you pay for it?" The answer is that there are criteria for deciding how claims get paid. The first is medical policy, which we would say is evidence-based. Next is coverage policy, meaning whether or not the treatment is actually covered by us. You might say, "Well, of course, it makes sense that if you agree it's evidence-based, you should cover it." What happens is that the benefit designs chosen by the employers may not have coverage for that evidence-based medicine. This does occur, especially with some of the national companies. There may be employers in Massachusetts, Texas, Florida, Indiana, and Seattle, Washington that do not want their benefit design to include reimbursement for bariatric surgery. Blue Cross as an insurance company may cover it, but if the employer's account does not include the procedure in its benefit design, Blue Cross is not going to cover it for policies under that employer. It is not just the involvement of those who initially pay the bill (the insurers), but those who ultimately pay the bill (the employers), who often make the determination of what will be included.

In some states, including Massachusetts, there are mandates for certain medicines and procedures to be covered. This doesn't apply to bariatric surgery, but good examples would be reproductive technology. These mandates do not exist for national accounts and certainly not for bariatric surgery.

Lastly, even if you've gone through the medical policy and the coverage policy, you're stuck with some methodology of payment. For the cases at Blue Cross Blue Shield, it's almost exclusively relative value units (RVUs); for others, it may be discounted charges. Therefore, you have to factor in a payment methodology as well. The world is not simple when it comes to those to whom we answer—not only our providers and our members, but also the accounts that pay the bill.

### What is Medical Policy?

There is a rigorous review to determine which services are really necessary—which are proven or unproven. It's ongoing and changes from month to month, supported not only by the medical literature, but also by the Blue Cross Association Technology Evaluation Center, which is composed of experts around the country who are not employed by Blue Cross/Blue

Shield Association or their other plans. This group regularly reviews the appropriateness of the evidence-based medicine criteria or any studies to improve certain procedures. For bariatric surgery, this is obviously one of the hurdles to get over, but that's true for many other procedures as well. This group determines the criteria, how often it is reviewed, and how the evidence looks. One study usually does not result in resounding changes; a collection of studies does. At Blue Cross we're not limited to that, however, because at times we will use local expert opinions. When making decisions we also have input from our providers. We bring in physicians to talk about the policy, whether it is the right thing to do, do we need to revisit any particular points. As you can see, this decision-making process is not run just by an internal group.

**Betsy Lehman Center Initiative**

It seems clear that although we're looking for evidence-based medicine we're really looking for outcomes, and we know these can take a long time to materialize. In the interim, we can look at processes. I had the honor and privilege of participating in the Betsy Lehman Center initiative and though I have been in medicine for a long time, I had never been part of something quite this remarkable. With the focus on the emerging field of bariatric surgery, this initiative amounted to someone saying, "I think we have a problem," and then proceeding to discover what might be the right thing to do. For instance, what standards could be set for the surgery? Shouldn't we, the stakeholders in Massachusetts, be able to come together to determine the right thing to do? Couldn't we determine what evidence-based medicine exists and adopt it for where it doesn't exist? How about the local experts? What do they think might be the best thing to do?

All the members involved in the initiative came representing their constituents. Soon after they became a team who understood that the focus was to improve the health care of the people in Massachusetts (and to show the country's healthcare community what cooperation and collaboration could produce).

Participation was not about my representing Blue Cross/Blue Shield or about others representing their institutions or programs. Rather, it was about coming together and defining what we could possibly do best. What type of cooperation and collaboration was required? We must be able to answer the tough questions, acknowledge when we don't have the answers, and determine ways that we can develop the answers. We must treat each other respectfully and honestly as we all try to get to a better place.

In terms of bariatric surgery, what does that better place look like? To begin with, it can be reached by professionals coming together at the Betsy Lehman Center and looking at the top 3 topics: medical policy, payment policy, and benefit design. True, benefit design may ultimately be in the hands of the employers—those who, at the end of the day, pay the bill. Other factors can be influenced directly with evidence-based information. Regarding medical policy, we can decide what is evidence-based or what we think is the best definition and make adjustments to the policy. As for payment policy, it will include everything that has been deemed appropriate per the Betsy Lehman Center report, with input from others who advocate solutions to bariatric surgery and obesity management.

It must be acknowledged that much of the current medical and payment policies are not up-to-date with regard to nutrition, behavioral health management, long-term follow-up, or even appropriate testing. We're not going to get where we have to go if payers and/or providers just keep banging their fists on the table and saying, "No!" or "You don't understand!" We have to be able to sit down and work together, to have a community definition of quality as it pertains to bariatric surgery. We must have measures and outcomes and we must have transparency. In addition, we have to make sure that we have the continuum of care before, during, and after any procedure. We have to have criteria for programs, not just surgery.

The Betsy Lehman Center has done all of that. It has put in front of us the opportunity to have a great group of professionals come together who are well-intentioned, and it has tasked that group to determine what it is that must be done, medically, in the obesity and bariatric surgery arena.

I have not personally seen this process occur around any other problem, any disease state, or any other program. Thus, the Betsy Lehman Center has set the stage for who should be at the table to make decisions about the right care by the right provider, done right the first time—with constant measurements—in a process that's supported by the right payment system that rewards quality. That may seem complicated, but the driving concept is simple: it is the right thing to do.

So we do the right thing. The providers set down the rules; which we will adopt though we will be tough, because not everybody is going to make the cut. If you want to reward quality and you want to set standards for process measurement, you're going to have to be transparent. Only with transparency are you going to be able to get the employer to say, "Okay, I will build this into my benefit design." Only with transparency are you going to get those who are in consumer-directed health plans to say, "There is a difference if you do 450 bariatric procedures versus 3. There is a difference if your program doesn't really have behavioral health or adequate nutrition or adequate follow-up built into it."

The question is very simple; Is bariatric surgery, in the context of obesity management, an opportunity to align and demonstrate value to all stakeholders, considering current local and national environments? The answer has to be yes. However, achieving that goal is not easy. The Betsy Lehman Center has provided an important start, but the dialogue must continue. Providers not only have to come together with patients but, in this case also with state and health insurers, and indeed with many other providers, including surgeons, nutritionists, anesthesiologists, and internists. We have a phenomenal opportunity with bariatric surgery—if we handle it correctly—to demonstrate how health care needs to change, how the value equation needs to be proved, and how at the end of the day we can see that quality has been improved. High quality will improve costs, whether by decreasing the amount of comorbid conditions that exist or by helping people live longer and healthier. That's our obligation. Not to decide whether we should pay 10 cents or 10 dollars more for something, but to define what it is we have to do and who the ultimate beneficiaries will be. It's *us—we're* all somebody's patient. It's the employers, who can't afford to pay another dime until we can prove we have outcomes.

It is a momentous and difficult challenge. At Blue Cross Blue Shield, we've been trying to figure out how we can blend quality and outcomes, manage our pay-for-performance initiatives, change our payment methodologies—and we are doing it so that we can truly reward quality. Not just quality in the bariatric sphere, but overall. I once asked a group of physicians, whom I use as a sounding board, if we should pay everybody the same. After careful consideration they said, "No." Then how should we pay people differently? Should we reward quality?

It sounds like a no-brainer. Of course we should reward quality. But changing a payment methodology to reward quality generally hurts somebody. The message is, "We're not going to pay you for this, but we are going to pay *them*." Or: "We're paying them more because they've shown they do better in this area." Over time, we're only going to pay the really good performers—only the professionals who can demonstrate outcomes, who really show that they can improve not only one individual patient's condition, but the condition of a population of patients. That's a far different message than just paying for performance, which we think of today as an incremental payment.

We're never going to change the healthcare system or bariatric surgery or obesity management until we get to the point of understanding what the goals must be, and what kind of reimbursement methodology we have to build to match them, and how we're going to hold each other accountable. There are metrics that providers must meet and ways in which payers must reward them. It is important to make this mind shift toward paying for quality, because it is going to make a difference. In encouraging this dialogue on bariatric surgery, the Betsy Lehman Center has enhanced the greater dialogue about what health care needs to be like in this country.

# Appealing Denials

Thomas James III, MD

Talking about appeals is like getting a child to eat spinach. This is not one of the things that people really relish. It's important to start by defining "health insurance"; and my own definition for it is "a system to serve for the fair, equitable distribution of limited financial resources so as to provide the policyholders with coverage or purchased benefits." Now, that's not what most people think they bought when they signed up with a company. Most people are under the impression that they have put down a certain amount of money per pay period so that they can get whatever kind of health coverage they want or need. The fact is, however, that there are limitations to resources and what we're really trying to accomplish, from a health insurance point of view, is to provide the coverage and administer the benefits the same way consistently. With that goal in mind, the various insurers around the country have purchased software packages that allow electronic or paper claims to be handled on a uniform basis. When you're dealing with something new or unusual, it tends to be handled on a manual basis by a claims processor, which presents the opportunity for inconsistencies. It's my experience that companies experience tremendous problems when things get handled by individuals.

The reasons why insurance companies will deny a claim fall into a number of categories. The person may not be a member or may be using an expired card, or he/she might have changed to another carrier. They may have two different insurance policies, and the one card they presented happens to be the secondary insurer. In the case of weight loss surgery (WLS), there may not be coverage provided. The denials that really "frost" most physicians, however, are based on judgment calls like the *surgery is not medically necessary* or that it is *cosmetic* or *investigational*. These become the basis for many appeals.

**Why Appeal a Denial?**

The reason why it's important to have a consistent process for reviewing appeals and handling them internal to the practice, is to correct errors. The benefit interpretation, especially when it is performed by an individual claims processor, may not be correct. The insurance company may have the wrong information on the person. When the appeal process is subject to physician input, it presents an opportunity to demonstrate medical necessity in individual cases and, on a broader level, gives the physician the opportunity to change medical policy. As an example, when Dr. Jeffrey Allen, who practices in Louisville, Kentucky, where I am located, came to me at Humana and said he would like to present a new technology for bariatric surgery, I was able to get him in front of Humana's medical policy board. As a result, he was able to help change the way that Humana reimbursed for a LAP-BAND. So it's a wonderful opportunity.

Dealing with the appeals process, however, is a truly daunting task. It takes a lot of energy and requires the same kind of discipline that surgeons must have when approaching the individual patient. Understanding the nature of each patient's individual policy is demanded. You have to understand the funding methodology, the time frames under which appeals have to be heard and what level of appeal a patient may have. This is almost Jeffersonian in the way that it's approached. On one hand, we have companies that are self-funded (increasingly, smaller companies are turning to a self-funded process so that they can control the benefits and not be subjected to state mandates; it also permits them to reduce the administrative overhead). On the other, we have those firms that want to be fully insured. These are firms that purchase a set of benefits from one insurer but will shop from year to year to find the insurance company that offers the lowest price for that set of benefits. Ultimately, these different funding mechanisms create different reasons or different methods for appeals

**Time Frames for Appeals**

The self-funded employer only has to deal with federal Employee Retirement Income Security Act (ERISA) laws. Those laws deal in terms of fairness and consistency of approach, but don't specify time frames or rules that must be followed with appeals. Firms that purchase individual insurance, on the other hand, have to follow the rules set by the insurance-regulating body in their state. If a company has employees in multiple states, the law dictates that the rules in the state in which the policy was sold are followed. These time frames for fully insured companies are usually well prescribed, meaning that an expedited appeal, where the member patient's health is in jeopardy and dependent on the decision, must be processed within 48 to 72 hours. In bariatric surgery, that would not be the case in most circumstances, so most are handled as routine appeals. Though some states require that they be handled in 15 days and others in 45 days, by and large, most require a 30-day turnaround. Do insurance companies follow that? Not often. But that's where a certain amount of clout comes in and I'll elaborate on that a bit later.

**Levels of Appeal**

There are different levels of appeals, the simplest being a "reconsideration." This is when, as the surgeon in a case that has lost an appeal, you get on the phone with the medical director and say, "Look, you didn't get all the right information. Let me talk to you about it." Together as professionals you and the director come to an understanding. When you get into the formal levels, however, there is the first-level appeal and the second-level appeal. The first is generally handled internally with the insurance company or a third-party administrator (TPA). It can be handled by any medical specialist unless the patient asks that it be done by somebody of similar specialty. I'm trained in internal medicine and in pediatrics, for instance, but as a first-level reviewer, I may be asked to review a bariatric surgery case, unless you as the patient or the surgeon say, "I want this reviewed by a surgeon, in particular somebody who does obesity surgery." However, when you get to the second level of appeals though (and this is for fully insured companies), it is sent out. The state takes over the appeal and rules that it will be reviewed by an external entity. There's greater opportunity to avoid the biases that may be internal to the insurance company involved.

Figure 1 shows my version of the appeals Krebs cycle, because it can get very complicated. The decision for surgery has always been a patient-doctor decision. It's fallen upon the physician to make the request to the health plan for having the surgery. Since this chapter is about appeals, we're going to ignore the portion of the flow chart on the left that says, "Health plan approved," with the patient having a successful surgery. Instead, we'll go down the other track that says that there's a denial. In most states, doctors are not given the right to ask for the appeal. It's the patient who has that right. So, the physician may have to help patients understand that this is something he/she needs to do. In general, most physicians will help the patient with that.

If a timely response is not obtained within 30 days (for a fully insured plan), it is advised to contact the insurer with a second letter. If there is a timely response, hopefully this is in the patient's best interest and he/she has a successful surgery. If, however, there is a denial and the denial persists, a more rigorous effort will be required to turn it around and charting the history of those efforts on a spreadsheet will help keep track of the progress.

**Second-level Appeal Process**

If the person is insured through a full insurance company, which cannot be known until contact is made with the health plan, then the second-level appeal request must come from the patient. When the request is submitted with physician-supported data and includes a request for a like-specialty reviewer, the state will ensure that gets sent out. If, on the other hand, the insurance is through a self-funded plan, the company may make the decision as to whether there will be a second-level appeal. I deal with a major Fortune 500 company that does not want any second-level appeals, that stops appeals at the first level. However, most employers do set up processes, which may include the use of committees where the patient can face a peer review to obtain a decision, or may go outside for further external review.

The point is that each plan has its own process. So, if you get a successful appeal through one insurance company, it becomes like case law helping any further cases that come through for that particular insurance company. It's only when surgeons keep track and follow through that they have more successful results, with a greater number of cases being covered. In this way, results may initiate changes in medical policy, with more patients likely to benefit from your skills in the future.

## Figure 1

## Appeals Process

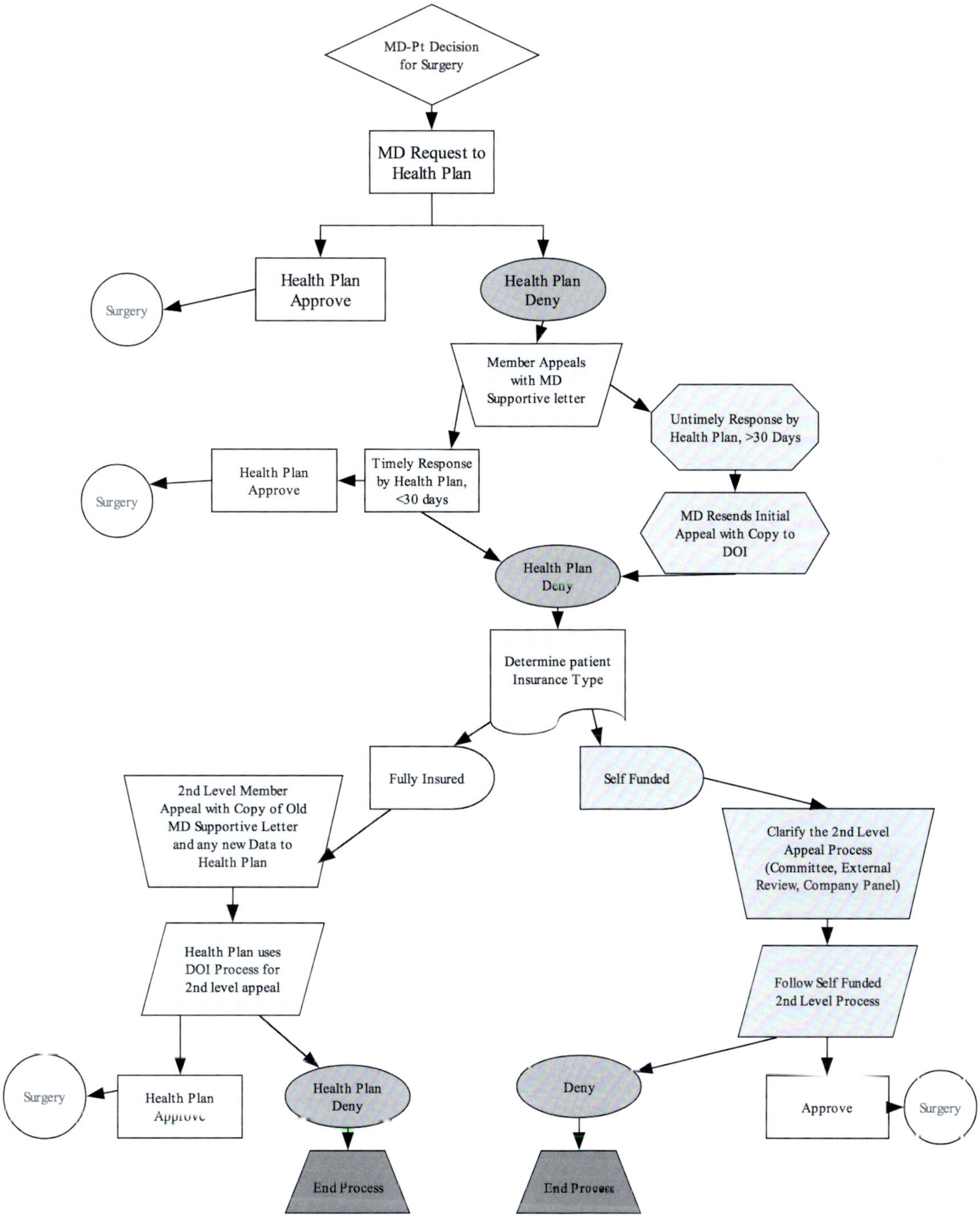

# Negotiating With Payers for New Technology and Procedures

Justine Carr, MD

Today's payment system is not where we want it to be. A major challenge is that care is paid for *a la carte*. We do not yet have an integrated medical system that recognizes episodes of care or a continuum of care related to a condition or disease.

## How Hospital Care is Paid:

### Inpatient Care

In 1983, Medicare (now Centers for Medicare and Medicaid Services, or CMS) introduced the compendium of diagnosis-related groups (DRGs). This now represents over 500 conditions that require inpatient care. Each DRG is assigned a case weight that parallels the resource intensity of the hospital (not the attending physician) care that is delivered to patients in that DRG. Hospitals are paid by an adjusted dollar multiplier for the relative case weight and this multiplier takes into account characteristics of the hospital's expenses, including academic teaching status, regional wages, and percent of underserved population. Many other payers have adopted the DRG system, although a parallel "All Payer" DRG system has emerged and is used by many managed care organizations. The All Payer DRG system has greater detail for conditions that are less common in the Medicare population. Non-DRG payers pay either a per-diem rate or, less commonly, a percent of hospital charges. Some payers will also provide a carve-out payment when a new expensive product/device is added to a procedure. Finally, Medicaid in Massachusetts pays a flat rate for each admission, based on admissions from earlier years.

### Outpatient Care

In 1997, Medicare/CMS developed a methodology for payment of outpatient care called Ambulatory Payment Classifications, or APCs. Similar to DRGs, APCs are groups of services that are clinically defined in terms of the resources they require. A payment rate is established for each APC. Unlike DRGs, hospitals may be paid for more than one APC for an encounter, depending on the services provided. Payment is made at a flat rate that is updated annually. Ambulatory Payment Classifications are not used by other payers. Many commercial payers pay a flat rate based on CPT codes, while others pay a percent of charges.

## How Payers Decide What to Cover:

### Government Payers (Medicare or Medicaid/CMS)

Government payers generally follow US Food and Drug Administration's (FDA's) approval in the decision to provide coverage. Local carriers for CMS can make a more restrictive policy and elect to consider something as a noncovered service. In addition, CMS may generate a national coverage determination, making payment contingent upon criteria related to the patient (e.g., comorbid conditions or degree of impairment from primary condition) and/or to the physician (e.g., volume of cases done) and/or to the hospital or facility (e.g., emergent or critical-care infrastructure). These decisions are arrived at through a process of review and public comment. Reviews are done by CMS research staff, at times supplemented by outside consultants. Medicaid is a state-run program and can have more restrictive coverage than Medicare.

### Private

With the proliferation of new technologies, a growing number of payers are developing formal technology evaluation programs. In 1985, Blue Cross and Blue Shield Association developed a national Technology Evaluation Center (TEC). Its mission is to provide healthcare decision makers with timely, objective and scientifically rigorous assessments that synthesize the available evidence on the diagnosis, treatment, management, and prevention of disease. In 1992, Harvard Pilgrim Health Care developed a medical director committee to make coverage decisions and then expanded in 2001 to include outside content experts and technology evaluation information programs. Appeals for special consideration for uncovered services may be considered on an individual basis. When payers do not have a formal technology evaluation process, coverage decisions are made in the context of the preapproval process.

### What Does "Coverage" Signify?

Covered services include those approved by the technology assessment and also included in a particular payer plan. Noncovered services are paid for out-of-pocket by the patient. The term "coverage," however, does not guarantee adequate payment, but only signifies that some payment will be made. In Massachusetts, the covered rate is the only amount paid. Billing for the balance between the cost and the amount paid is prohibited. Finally, coverage may be conditional, based on patient clinical criteria or the failure of past therapies.

### How Covered Service is Paid

#### Inpatient

Inpatient care can be paid for in a number of ways, including:

- Percent of hospital charges—This used to be the most common method, but was abandoned by many payers because it lacked incentive to manage costs.
- Case rate (DRG)—This approach continues to be used by CMS and many other payers. The rate is linked to the principle diagnosis and procedure. Except for extraordinary outliers, additional resource consumption or prolonged length-of-stay do not receive additional reimbursement, so there is an incentive to manage costs.
- Per-diem rate—Payment is dictated by length of stay, with longer stays receiving greater payment. This can result in an unintended incentive.
- Carve-out payment—This may be added to per-diem payments to ensure that high-cost technologies are adequately reimbursed. This may involve additional documentation/proof of utilization.
- SPAD (Standard Payment Amount per Discharge)—This is the flat fee that Medicaid pays to hospitals. There is an inpatient and an outpatient rate. It is the same fee regardless of the care that was delivered, although there is a review/reconciliation at the end of the year.

#### Outpatient

Medicare outpatient care is paid by Ambulatory Payment Classification (APC). Managed care is generally paid on a fee schedule based on CPT codes for procedure/billable services. Medicaid pays by SPAD-flat-outpatient rate, regardless of care that was delivered.

### Definition of Inpatient Versus Outpatient

The same procedure generally has a different hospital payment rate depending on whether it involves inpatient or outpatient care. The assumption is that a patient who is an inpatient for a procedure that could be performed on an outpatient basis has additional comorbidities or complications obligating additional care and resources. In recent years, payers have developed fiscal definitions of inpatient and outpatient and these definitions have diverged from the traditional clinical criteria.

| | **Inpatient** | **Outpatient** |
|---|---|---|
| **Clinical definition** | Patient sleeps in the hospital bed overnight after procedure | Patient goes home after procedure |
| **Fiscal definition** | Overnight patient whose care meets criteria for resource-intensity-of-care provision (e.g., complications or comorbidities that slow recovery) | Patient who goes home after procedure **OR**<br>Overnight patient whose care-resource intensity falls short of defined criteria |

Physician reimbursement differs from hospital reimbursement. Physicians are paid for skills and services. Hospitals are paid for resources consumed.

**Payment for Inpatient Care**

| | Physician | Hospital |
|---|---|---|
| **Reason to pay** | Based on physician time/skill expended | Based on institutional resources expended |
| **Unit of pay** | Payments for<br>Each operation<br>Each procedure | Single payment only—same rate for<br>1 operation<br>**OR**<br>10 operations |

**Diagnosis Related Groups (DRG)**

There are now more than 500 CMS DRGs. These are groupings that classify patients into clinically cohesive groups with comparable consumption of resources and length-of-stay (LOS) patterns. Patients are categorized by ICD-9 (International Classification of Diseases) diagnosis codes and procedure codes assigned on the basis of the documentation in the medical record. Each DRG has a weight. Reimbursement is based on weight times the individual hospital rate. Case weights may be adjusted annually based on national patterns. Academic medical centers get an additional supplemental education payment. Obesity surgery is paid for in DRG 288: OR Procedures for Obesity. This DRG includes ICD-9 procedure codes for open, laparoscopic and lap-band procedures. This DRG also includes plastic surgery procedures for adiposity. Below is listed the annual changes by CMS in case weight and length of stay. The changes in the LOS show the trend toward earlier discharge, and the increase in the cost weight between 1999 and 2003 suggests the recognition of the shift from open to laparoscopic procedure—shorter LOS, but increase in costs of operating room (OR) supplies.

| Fiscal Year | CMS DRG Case Weight | Average Length of Stay (in days) |
|---|---|---|
| 1999 | 2.02 | 5.9 |
| 2000 | 2.07 | 5.7 |
| 2001 | 2.16 | 5.7 |
| 2002 | 2.16 | 6.0 |
| 2003 | 2.22 | 5.4 |
| 2004 | 2.15 | 5.0 |
| 2005 | 2.13 | 4.5 |
| 2006 | 2.04 | 4.1 |

**Relationship of Cost and Payment Type**

Outlined below is the asymmetry of incentives implicit in various payment modalities.

| | Percent charges | Case rate (DRG) | Per diem | Carve-out |
|---|---|---|---|---|
| Supply cost | All ok | Low is favorable | Low is favorable | All ok |
| LOS | All ok | Low is favorable | High is favorable | N/A |
| OR time | All ok | Low is favorable | Low is favorable | N/A |
| Ancillaries | All ok | Low is favorable | Low is favorable | N/A |

## Negotiation

Negotiation with payers can take place at four levels.

1. Early: Recognition of a new technology or technique on the basis of published data and/or FDA approval is acknowledged by payers. Vendors often devote significant resources to recognition of the technology or technique. This involves working through ICD-9 and CPT committees to ensure there is a code that properly identifies the procedure. Once there is a specific code, payers can track the typical charges and LOS related to the procedure.
2. Adoption as a "covered" service: Payers decide whether to cover a service based on the findings of their technology evaluation committees. Some negotiation can be involved in the interpretation of the impact or importance of various outcome studies of short- and long–term-benefit superiority over existing modalities.
3. Individual patient eligibility: When a decision has been made not to cover a service, negotiation with payers on behalf of an individual patient may result in exception to the noncoverage rules. This may entail outlining the therapies that a patient has already failed.
4. Denials appeal: Similarly, if a payer has denied a claim, clinicians may challenge the denial, supplying additional information about the patient and/or from recently published literature supporting the benefit of the service for the patient.

## Negotiating Strategies: Understand Your Costs

In negotiations with payers, it is important to understand your costs. A key distinction is the difference between costs and charges. Charges are not the costs. They usually do not have a linear or uniform relationship to costs and may represent a legacy of pricing strategies that have been tweaked over years or even decades. To compare expense across institutions, it is possible to take the charges and apply the Medicare cost-to-charge ratio. This is a ratio that varies across institutions, but can somewhat normalize numbers on a large cohort of patients. It is much more accurate to work with costs, instead of charges. Costs are generally developed within a cost-accounting system with the total made up of the sum of the direct and the indirect costs. Direct costs are the resources used in the care of a patient (e.g., nursing care, drugs, supplies) Indirect costs are usually a fixed percentage of total costs and represent the cost of infrastructure (lights, heat, etc.) and administrative staff and other nonpatient expenses.

## Articulate the Benefits of the Procedure

Payers are interested in the cost/benefit analysis. It is useful to articulate both a short- and a long–term perspective. Information that is necessary to make the case include:

1. Target population with the greatest need and the greatest likelihood of benefit

2. Evidence of superiority of the new therapy as illustrated by immediate benefit (e.g., getting back to work quickly) and long-term care (e.g., preventing late complications of the condition).

**Understand Payer Constraints**

Government payers (e.g., CMS) often deal with major new expensive technologies through a national coverage decision. Prior to the decision, there is ample opportunity for input, but once published, it is not negotiable. Local Medicare carriers, however, can choose to be more restrictive than national, but may also be open to discussion. Managed care payers may vary in the sophistication of their electronic infrastructure. As a result, offering carve-out payments for select programs may be beyond the capabilities of their electronic programs and they may choose to negotiate with a hospital or network at the level of a "book of business" (total amount) rather than assessing the costs and payments of each individual program. Furthermore, payers may elect to cover a procedure, but the payment rate may not cover the full cost of the program.

**Negotiate Fair Payment**

Inpatient payments are generally more robust than outpatient because they take into account the resources required to care for a patient who needs additional monitoring, evaluation, and/or treatment. A flat-case rate (e.g., DRG 288) is preferable to a per-diem rate, particularly in treatment of conditions that have high technology and OR costs with short lengths of stay. When the payment is on a per-diem basis, additional carve-out payment should be sought.

**Payments: Importance of Complete Documentation**

Finally, once payment is negotiated, it is important to avoid denials or underpayments by providing complete documentation. This includes submitting a complete case history with enumeration of comorbid conditions. Timely notes should explain procedures done and devices utilized and the procedure notes should include indications for the procedure—in particular, failed previous therapies. Clinical pathways can be very useful in documenting variations and supporting indications for continued hospitalization

**Periodic Review of Payments**

It is useful to periodically review hospital costs and payment. This review benefits the hospital and clinician in understanding costs and payments. Denials or underpayments can be evaluated and addressed immediately and collaboratively by clinical and administrative staff.

**Conclusion**

Understanding how care is paid for is key to negotiating with payers, and building the clinical case for coverage is half of the battle. Helping a payer find a way to pay within the existing coding and payment structure is equally important. Partnering with administrative staff to build the case and suggest payer approaches and solutions can contribute to the success of the negotiation.

# Military Health System

Patricia A. Buss, MD, MBA

### The TRICARE Program

TRICARE, formerly known as the Civilian Health and Medical Program of the Uniformed Services, or CHAMPUS, is the Department of Defense's health program for active-duty and retired members of the 7 uniformed services, their families, and their survivors around the world. TRICARE serves more than 9 million beneficiaries (including approximately 1.4 million active-duty service members) through a worldwide network of 70 military inpatient facilities, more than 800 military medical and dental clinics, and the department's private-sector health-plan business partners. Our budget is about $25 billion a year and growing. TRICARE is not an insurance company; rather, it is an entitlement program, which means that the benefit flows directly to the beneficiary. The majority of our patients pay no premiums. We also don't have a payer dictating to us what the benefit ought to be, although benefits are constrained by Congress. As a general rule, medically necessary care that's proven and considered the standard of care in America will be a TRICARE benefit, unless it's expressly prohibited by law or regulation.

### Constraints on the TRICARE Obesity Benefit

We have constraints on our obesity benefit contained in both statute and regulation. Title 10 US Code [10 USC 1079(a)(11)] states: "Treatment of obesity may not be provided if obesity is the sole or the major condition treated." The Code of Federal Regulations [32 CFR 199.4(g)], which lists services excluded under the TRICARE program, specifically excludes "services and supplies related to obesity or weight reduction whether surgical or nonsurgical…except that benefits may be provided for gastric bypass, gastric stapling, or gastroplasty procedures in connection with morbid obesity as provided in paragraph (e)15 of this section." Paragraph (e)15 goes on to define the TRICARE morbid obesity benefit as limited to gastric bypass, gastric stapling or gastroplasty, and defines some eligibility criteria.

Additionally, we're constrained by the requirement [32 CFR 199.2(b) and 32 CFR 199.4(g)(15)] that TRICARE limit its coverage to treatments that have been proven safe and effective. The TRICARE hierarchy of reliable evidence is used to determine whether a drug, device, medical treatment, or procedure has moved from the status of unproven to the position of nationally accepted medical practice. Reliable evidence, as defined in 32 CFR 199.2(b), includes:

1. Well-controlled studies of clinically meaningful endpoints, published in refereed medical literature
2. Published formal technology assessments
3. Published reports of national professional medical associations
4. Published national medical policy organization positions
5. Published reports of national expert opinion organizations

Specifically not included in the meaning of reliable evidence are reports, articles, or statements by providers or groups of providers containing only abstracts, anecdotal evidence, or personal professional opinions. Also not included in the meaning of reliable evidence is the fact that a provider or number of providers have elected to adopt a drug, device, or medical treatment or procedures as their personal treatment or procedure of choice or standard of practice. Please note that in keeping with the requirement, we cost-share only appropriate medical care, which is defined, in part, in 32 CFR 199.2(b), as services that are in keeping with the generally accepted norms for medical practice in the United States. We may not consider foreign studies or medical literature, but only US studies published in US medical literature and other documents that relate to the standard of care in the United States.

We use a well-recognized process to search for and review reliable evidence, as well as policies of the Centers for Medicare and Medicaid Services (CMS) and other carriers to determine whether a procedure is safe, effective, comparable to conventional treatment, and the standard of care in the United States. The result is a balance between ensuring the safety and efficacy of the care our beneficiaries receive and access to better ways of practicing medicine.

**TRICARE Policy on Surgery for Morbid Obesity**

The TRICARE policy, then, is derived from the relevant law and regulation. The TRICARE benefit excludes nonsurgical treatment of obesity: weight loss medications, dietary control, weight loss counseling, wiring of the jaw, or any other similar procedure.

- Surgery for morbid obesity (gastric bypass, gastric stapling, or gastroplasty, to include vertical banded gastroplasty) is a TRICARE benefit when one of the following conditions is met:
  - The patient is 100 lbs over ideal weight for height and bone structure, according to the most current Metropolitan Life table, and has a comorbid condition as outlined in the TRICARE policy manual. Those comorbid conditions include diabetes, hypertension, narcolepsy, Pickwickian syndrome, severe osteoarthritis of the weightbearing joints, etc.
  - The patient is 200% or more of the ideal weight for height and bone structure.
  - The patient has had a gastric bypass or other surgery for obesity and, because of complications, requires a second operation.

At present, the TRICARE benefit for morbid obesity includes only the four CPT codes listed below:

| **Covered under TRICARE** | **Excluded under TRICARE** |
|---|---|
| Gastric bypass, gastric stapling, or gastroplasty, to include vertical banded gastroplasty:<br><br>• *Vertical banded gastroplasty (CPT 43842)*<br>• *Gastric restrictive procedure with short limb Roux-en-Y gastroenterostomy (CPT 43846)*<br>• *Laparoscopic gastric restrictive procedure with gastric bypass and Roux-en-Y gastroenterostomy (CPT 43644)*<br>• *Revision of gastric restrictive procedure for morbid obesity (CPT 43848)* | Unproven procedures:<br><br>• *Gastric restrictive procedure, without gastric bypass, other than vertical banded gastroplasty (CPT 43843)*<br>• *Biliopancreatic bypass procedure (Scopinaro) or distal gastric bypass (CPT 43847)*<br>• *Laparoscopic restrictive procedure with gastric bypass and small intestine reconstruction to limit absorption (CPT 43645)*<br>• *Biliopancreatic diversion with duodenal switch (CPT 43845 and 43633)*<br>• *Gastric bubble or balloon (CPT 43999)*<br>• *Mini gastric bypass*<br>• *Laparoscopic adjustable gastric banding [LAP-BAND® procedure] (CPT 43659)*<br>• *Bariatric surgery coded as unlisted laparoscopy procedure (CPT 49329)* |
| Nonsurgical treatment of obesity:<br>• *Patient- and parent-counseling on diet, nutrition, and physical activity (expected components of good medical practice) integrated into an appropriate office visit at no additional charge* | Nonsurgical treatment of obesity:<br>• *Diets*<br>• *Weight loss counseling*<br>• *Weight loss medications*<br>• *Wiring of the jaw or any similar procedure* |

Because of the lack of reliable evidence documenting their safety and efficacy, TRICARE considers as unproven the procedures listed on the right side of this table, including biliopancreatic bypass, biliopancreatic diversion with duodenal switch, mini-gastric bypass, and laparoscopic adjustable gastric banding (the LAP-BAND® procedure).

**Impact of Bariatric Surgery on Active Duty and Active Duty Family Members**

Separate from TRICARE policy, we have additional policies and considerations that pertain because of our uniquely military population. These affect both active-duty service members and their family members.

Because of the potentially adverse impact on medical readiness and worldwide deployability, bariatric surgery disqualifies an individual for service in any branch of the armed forces. In addition, service members already on active duty are not authorized to undergo bariatric surgery and are subject to administrative separation if they do so. There are additional service regulations that prohibit military surgeons from performing bariatric surgery on active duty service members.

There is no prohibition against active-duty family members (i.e., spouse, children, and any other immediate family members who live with an active-duty service member) undergoing surgery for morbid obesity. However, since follow-up care cannot be ensured in many overseas locations, a history of bariatric surgery may disqualify a family member from eligibility to accompany the sponsor on an overseas tour of duty. A family member already colocated with a sponsor overseas, who undergoes bariatric surgery may be subject to early and permanent return to the United States.

**The Road Ahead**

TRICARE recognizes that there have been many changes in the field of obesity surgery, and we are looking at this from several perspectives: conditions for coverage, procedures covered under the benefit, and outcomes.

TRICARE criteria for bariatric surgery, defined in the Code of Federal Regulations and the TRICARE policy manual more than 20 years ago, are at variance with current nationally recognized guidelines for bariatric surgery (for example, those published by the National Heart, Lung, and Blood Institute). TRICARE Management Activity (TMA) is considering revision of the relevant regulation and policy, consistent with statutory limitations on treatment of obesity, to align the TRICARE benefit more closely with current standards.

Review of procedures currently considered unproven continues on a regular basis.

Finally, as civilian activities proceed with certification of bariatric surgery centers, TMA will consider whether it may be possible to identify facilities with better outcomes. This information may then be used to direct patients to the appropriate center for their surgery. Finally, it may be of interest to note here that TRICARE uses a similar system for transplant surgery.

# The Cost of Setting Up a Bariatric Surgery Program

Malcolm K. Robinson, MD

Setting up a bariatric surgery program is quite complex and the cost can vary hugely depending on what resources are already available at the institution. For the purposes of this chapter, it is assumed that many of the physician resources are in place, including at least two bariatric surgeons, which obviates the need for surgeon-recruitment costs. It is also assumed that there are other physician resources—cardiologists, pulmonologists, intensive care specialists, emergency room physicians, etc., who otherwise would need to be recruited by an institution to make sure it has a high-quality program in place and can offer bariatric surgery that is appropriately and safely performed.

There are several unique features of bariatric surgical programs that directly affect setup costs

## Setup Costs: Unique Features of Bariatric Surgery Programs

- Obese patients require specialized equipment and facilities.
- Multidisciplinary professional staff is mandatory even though their services may not be covered by insurance.
- Lifetime patient follow-up necessary leading to long-term program growth.
- Quality assurance requires long-term (e.g., >5 years) data acquisition.

Obese patients require specialized equipment and facilities. Going through the exhaustive list of requirements is prohibitive for this chapter. However, things to think about include large-size wheelchairs, blood-pressure cuffs, gowns and beds. Many institutions already have acquired such things. However, many institutions do not have floor-mounted toilets in patient bathrooms, and these are preferred over the standard wall-mounted fixtures since the latter can be snapped off of the wall under excessive weight, which is an obvious safety hazard. Retrofitting bathrooms with floor-mounted toilets can be quite expensive, potentially running into tens of thousands of dollars. Alternatively, one may choose large-size bedside commodes with high-weight capacities. Although less expensive, patient privacy issues make this option less attractive.

Another important area for consideration is nonphysician professional staff. All comprehensive bariatric surgical programs require a multidisciplinary staff to provide excellent care. In addition, having such a staff is a requirement of the American Society for Metabolic and Bariatric Surgery and the American College of Surgeons for certification as a Center of Excellence. Many insurers also make this part of their program requirements. In the past, it may have been considered a "luxury," but now it is the standard of care. Unfortunately, although required, many insurance companies do not pay for such staff expenses. Hence, the cost is borne completely by the program and hospital. At a minimum, the program will require a dietitian trained in management of the bariatric surgical patient and a physician extender—nurse practitioner (NP), registered nurse (RN), or physician's assistant (PA)—to provide care. One of these individuals can serve as the program coordinator.

Lifetime patient follow-up is necessary. Thus, the number of program patients will continue to grow even if the same number of bariatric procedures is done annually. This translates into an ongoing need for increased staff expenditure to support the bariatric surgery program appropriately. And finally, there's a necessity for having an aggressive quality-assurance program, which will require longer than the standard 30-day, postoperative-course analysis. With bariatric surgery, postoperative analysis goes on indefinitely and some experts recommend that it continue for more than 5 years. This leads to certain issues regarding developing a bariatric database, which is absolutely necessary, as well as to concerns about monitoring the quality of data entry into the database and providing staff to assist with such efforts.

The specific costs of a bariatric surgery program can be considered by category. There are inpatient and outpatient care setup costs for a bariatric surgical program. In terms of inpatient costs, the standard now is that most programs will do minimally invasive or laparoscopic bariatric surgery. Most institutions that are going to consider doing this already have a minimally invasive or laparoscopic operating room (OR) suite, but if not, it will require a fairly large expenditure to obtain state-of-the-art OR equipment along with the appropriate bariatric surgical instruments. Laparoscopic bariatric surgical instruments, assuming there is already a minimally invasive OR suite in place, can be obtained for about $25,000. If a minimally invasive suite is not available (and depending on where the facility will be located), there may be very little construction renovation necessary or it may require large renovations that can cost upwards of $150,000 or more. Purchasing state-of-the-art equipment can range anywhere from $400,000 to over $1 million, depending on how fancy one wants to get with video conferencing, etc.

Many institutions are also moving toward specialized patient-care units, hiring trained inpatient staff, and building bathrooms that accommodate large individuals with fixtures such as floor-mounted toilets.

Ceiling-mounted, 1000 pound-capacity lifts alone are about a $10,000 investment. Obtaining the appropriate bariatric bed in the operating room will cost about $60,000. Finally, the most expensive single items are radiology equipment such as a large capacity CT scan or MRI, each of which cost more than $1 million.

These are just a few examples of the startup costs. Patient supplies are relatively inexpensive. Blood-pressure cuffs and wider wheelchairs may only cost $5000 to $10,000. Taken together, establishing the inpatient services for bariatric surgery can add up to as much, or more, than $2 million if an institution has minimal resources in place and is essentially starting from scratch.

Out-patient Care Setup Costs for a Bariatric Surgery Program

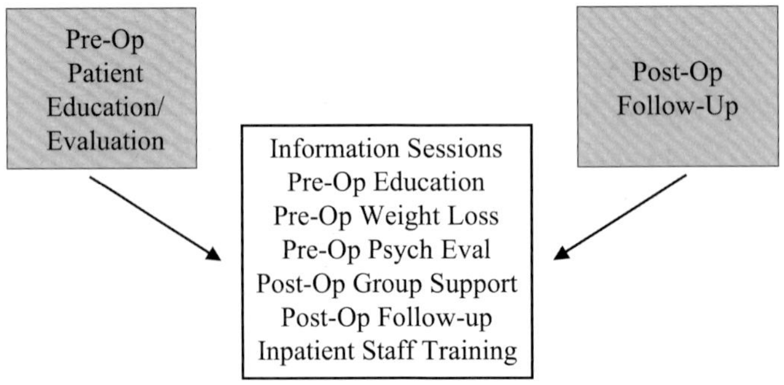


Minimum Staff Requirement:
RN/PA + RD

Outpatient-care setup costs for a program will include expenditures for preoperative patient education and evaluation, as well as for post-op follow-up. Most Center of Excellence programs offer information and preoperative education sessions for groups or on an individual basis, or both. For example, some insurance companies require preoperative weight loss, and so bariatric surgery centers are providing weight loss programs that are medically supervised. Even if the insurance companies don't require this, many surgeons feel that having their patients lose weight preoperatively is appropriate for optimizing outcome. In addition, there is also the need for preoperative psychiatric evaluation of patients who will be undergoing bariatric surgery.

Postoperatively, programs usually have support groups for their patients. Because there is an extensive post-op follow-up, surgeons need assistance to care for the high volume of patients. Again, this requirement usually translates into two individuals, a registered dietitian and a NP, RN, or PA. There are regional differences in pay for such individuals, but one can expect at least $150,000 per year or more to cover the salary and fringe benefits of two of these as full-time staff.

The final bariatric surgical program requirement is an active quality-assurance and data-monitoring program. This includes a comprehensive database, which can be purchased "off the shelf" for approximately $1,000 to $5,000, or custom designed (ensuring great flexibility and offering extensive features such as being able to pull laboratory values from other hospital databases) for $50,000 to well over $100,000.

Thus when setting up a program, one needs to think about inpatient care, preoperative patient education and evaluation, and postoperative follow-up with quality assurance in data monitoring. The idea behind this is to create a safety net for patients' success.

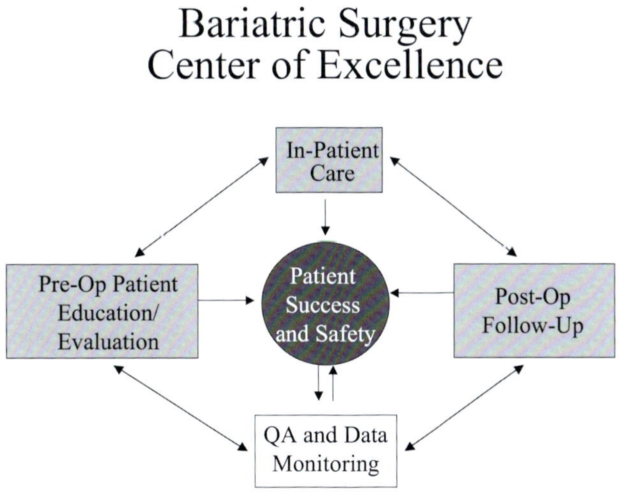


To not adequately address any one of these four areas is to leave a hole in the net that leads to a suboptimal outcome.

To fulfill the requirements for a bariatric center of excellence, a hospital/program can anticipate investing, at least initially, several hundred thousand dollars. Given such an investment, it must be carefully considered as to whether it is cost effective for hospitals and insurance companies to initiate or participate in such a program. In terms of physicians, bariatric surgery is generally covered by insurance; further, many patients are willing to pay out-of-pocket for surgeon services if insurance companies do not offer coverage.

Hospitals can benefit from offering this type of surgical program. Durham Regional Hospital was able to turn around a $26 million operating-income loss by initiating a bariatric surgical program. Within 1 year, doing approximately 310 bariatric surgery procedures, their operating income, which they attributed largely to bariatric surgery, went from -$26 million to $8.6 million in the succeeding fiscal year.

How do hospitals ensure profitability? The answer is that exquisite attention must be paid to four areas. First is high-quality clinical care. Whether the surgical program is referred to as a service line or a Center of Excellence, cutting corners in this area is not acceptable. Poor patient outcome can lead to complications, which are very costly from a financial, as well as human standpoint, and to patients avoiding the program. Second, the hospital itself needs to secure appropriate insurance reimbursement. This is a separate issue from surgeon fees as fees for hospitals are separately negotiated with insurance companies. If fees are not negotiated wisely by the hospital, significant revenue can be lost leading to low profit margin or net losses. Third, there needs to be efficient use of disposables. Surgical staplers are very expensive. The cost for using surgical disposables (e.g., surgical staplers, LAP-BAND) can vary from $2,000 to $8,000 per case. Unnecessary use or waste of surgical disposables can be quite costly and erode or completely eliminate hospital profit margins. Finally, the hospital (and surgeons) must compete successfully for adequate patient volume to make sure the program is financially profitable. The large setup and staff costs are "fixed" expenses. In a low patient volume setting the cost per patient may be prohibitively high. However, in a high-volume setting, the fixed costs per patient are relatively low and make financial success more feasible.

**Figure 1**

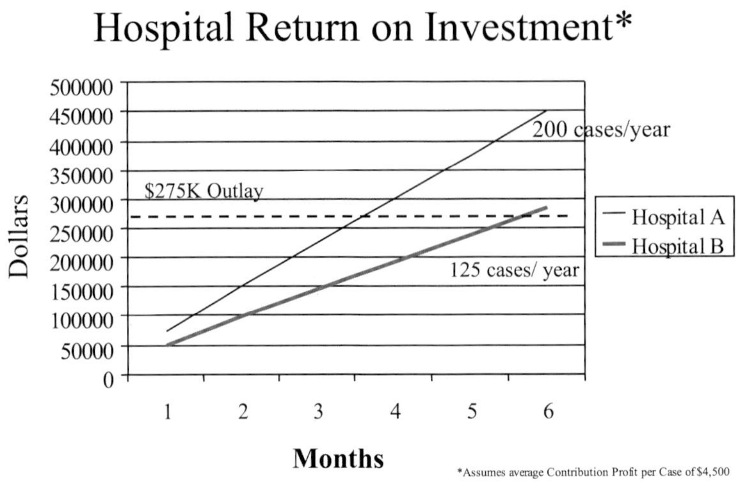


Finally, is bariatric surgery financially profitable for insurance companies? A study recently published in the online Web journal *Health Affairs* looked at the additional healthcare spending attributable to obese people, ages 18 to 64 that were covered by private insurers. The study found a tenfold increase in the amount of healthcare costs, from $3.6 billion to more than $36 billion over the past 25 years.

**Figure 2**

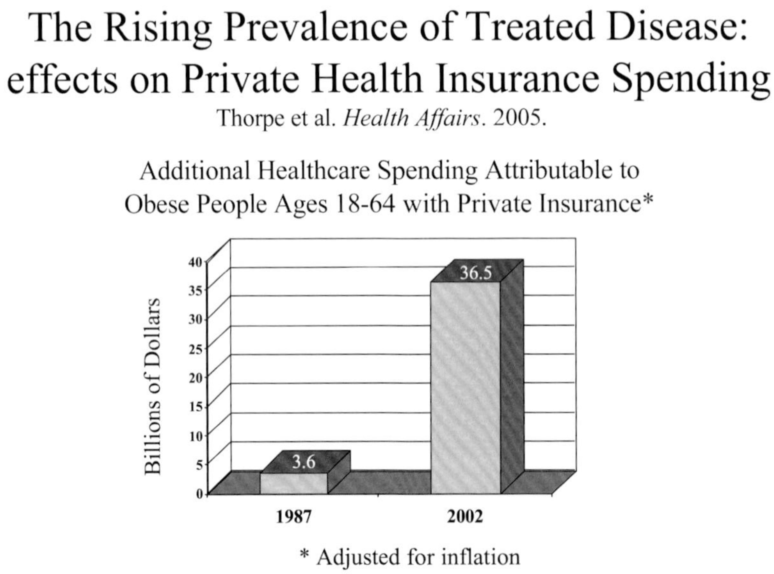


The question then becomes whether bariatric surgery decreases short- or long-term costs of obese patients, given the fact that obese patients are costly for insurance companies. Several studies indicate that despite the substantial initial outlay for insurers for surgical treatment of obese individuals, it is clear that there are long-term overall savings realized at about 3 years. This is related to decreased hospitalization, less use of medications, and fewer physician visits.

Figure 3

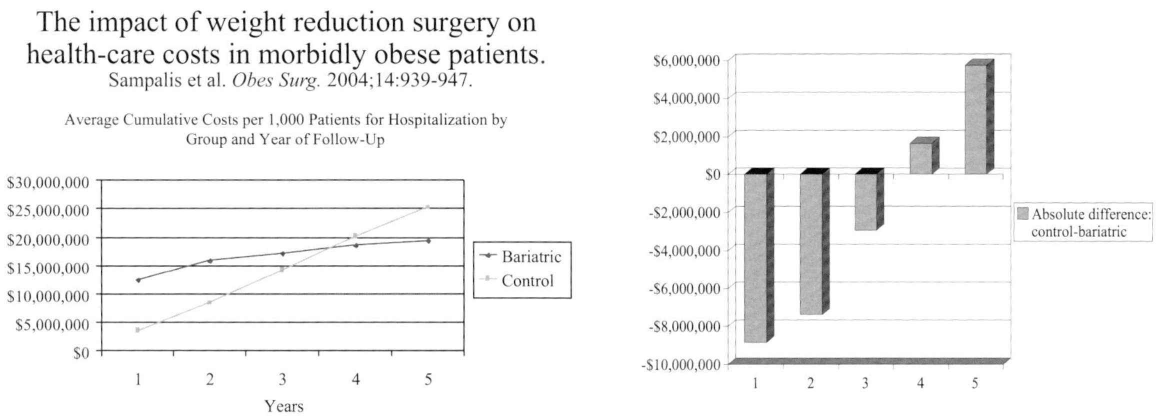


To summarize, bariatric surgery programs have several unique features that require significant hospital investment and expenditures. The investment must be in the areas of inpatient care, outpatient care, and quality assurance. Cutting corners or "doing the bare minimum" is not cost-effective in the long run, because of resulting expensive complications of poor patient outcomes. It is clear that these programs are profitable for hospitals where high-quality patient care is given, appropriate insurance reimbursement is secured, and there is adequate surgical case volume. Finally, it can be cost effective for insurance companies to support bariatric surgery programs due to reduced costs related to diminished outpatient visits, fewer hospitalizations and lower medication costs.

## Suggested Reading

1. Sampalis JS, Liberman M, Auger S, Christou NV. The impact of weight reduction surgery on health-care costs in morbidly obese patients. *Obes Surg.* 2004;14(7):939-47.

2. Thorpe KE, Florence CS, Howard DH, Joski P. The rising prevalence of treated disease: effects on private health insurance spending. *Health Aff* (Millwood). 2005;(suppl web exclusives):W5-317-25.

# Return on Investment

Anita Courcoulas, MD, MPH

I was asked to write about hospital decision making and, specifically, bariatric surgery and its return on investment. Is it a winner or is it a loser? I have to tell you from the outset that I'm not a hospital administrator. I'm a bariatric surgeon and my experience with hospital administration has been just my 10 years of working very closely with hospital administration at the University of Pittsburgh, in trying to grow a program. So, I hope that I'm going to reflect their perspective accurately.

Obviously, what's driving hospital leadership is the scope of the problem:

- According to the Centers for Disease Control and Preventions (CDC), nearly 12% of US medical spending today goes to treat direct and indirect costs of overweight and obesity;
- Health plans and employers are picking up more of these costs;
- Centers for Medicare and Medicaid Services (CMS) recently opened the way for coverage of obesity in the Medicare program;
- Some health insurers are launching disease management care programs aimed at reducing the incidence of obesity

None of these facts are new to anyone in the medical community.

From the hospital leaders' perspective, when they're either looking to grow their program, to start a program, or to expand to other centers within their program, they essentially address four different questions:

- What does it take to get a bariatric program started?
- What are the key factors that determine if a bariatric program will be feasible?
- How can a hospital increase its exposure to prospective patients?
- What makes a bariatric program or center pay off?

I'm going to spend most of my time on the last question, and will very briefly cover the other three.

**What Does it Take to Get a Program Started?**

I think there are three key components: planning, developing a multidisciplinary taskforce, and then identifying some key ingredients. I'll share my thoughts with you about all of those ingredients.

In terms of planning, the most important first step is general education of the management team that's going to be starting the program. This includes having a pretty detailed understanding of the surgical procedures themselves, both the pre- and postoperative components of surgical care, and all the elements of postoperative follow-up that patients need. We put together a very large group, a multidisciplinary bariatric taskforce that includes everyone from physicians and nursing staff to surgeons, nutritionists, pharmacists, facilities management, and others, in order to try and decide whether or not starting a program would be feasible to the institution.

Some of the key requirements we've discovered in our hospital over the years is to first and foremost identify skilled surgeons who've had appropriate training and significant experience, and have demonstrated quality outcomes. Availability of all related medical specialty services is necessary: cardiology, gastroenterology, pulmonary, anesthesia. Comprehensive weight management services are also key in the program development for presurgical education, medically supervised weight loss programs and many of the postoperative needs. This would include managing the support group, managing the patients who need extra attention, and providing help in guiding patients through the system.

Other key components are the clinical support services that can meet the needs of these patients. I'll talk more later about development of a bariatric surgery obesity service line, which is vital to the long-term success and return on investment from a hospital perspective. Clinical information systems and the database are important elements as well. And of course it is critical to understand and be able to analyze the financial issues related to bariatric surgical services, and to recognize how those financial issues are changing over time. Finally, and most importantly, the support and involvement of key senior leadership in the hospital is an absolute necessity.

**How Do You Conduct a Feasibility Assessment for a Bariatric Surgery Program?**

I can offer a few guidelines. One is to develop a relationship between hospital and physician that promotes excellence in bariatric surgery. You can't have an excellent bariatric surgeon who doesn't have a link with an administrator to make the program successful. Second is to integrate your services—weight management, minimally invasive surgery department that has the technical expertise, and your bariatric surgery program. If you can't integrate those programs, the long-term feasibility is probably not good. You need to be prepared to provide very extensive pre- and postsurgery services for reasons already discussed. Finally, you need to be prepared to track not only your clinical outcomes, but also your economic outcomes.

**Increasing Exposure to Prospective Patients**

Utilize the media and other methods to enhance public awareness. In doing this, clearly convey the benefits of bariatric surgery, and associate bariatric surgery not just with the treatment of obesity, but also with the treatment and prevention of comorbid conditions, most importantly diabetes and heart disease. Another way to increase exposure is to market your weight management services; market a global program, not just for surgical services, but also for behavioral and lifestyle intervention and pharmacological therapy. Lastly, by partnering with payers regionally and large employers, a hospital and its program can gain exposure to many more patients.

**What Makes a Bariatric Center Pay Off?**

What makes the return on investment a positive one and how is that assessed? Most institutions look at the obesity epidemic as both a challenge and an opportunity. I hope to convince you that, in order to overcome the challenges and meet this opportunity, you have to develop an obesity service line.

There is opportunity in the tremendous availability for bariatric surgical, and other weight and obesity services, because of the expanding problem in this country. There are, however, many resource and other challenges. I'm going to talk briefly about the different challenges from the hospital perspective. The first is equipment challenges. There are also many renovations involved; things that many don't even think of when they're first developing a program. Then there are the issues with staff training and injuries. Also to be considered are the very important payment and reimbursement issues, and the management and assessment of surgical risks.

**Specialty Equipment**

From the equipment perspective, we all know that patients who weigh over 400 lbs are going to need specialized equipment: gowns, blood-pressure cuffs, other routine supplies. This has now become a consumer-driven business and patients relate to one another. If you don't have appropriate equipment, your center will be assessed negatively among patients. The whole facility has to be right-sized. You have to examine the equipment from all aspects of bariatric surgery care: exam tables, wheelchairs, scales, blood-pressure cuffs, gowns, and all the other necessary equipment has to be acquired.

Equipment needed to move a patient to help avoid injuries can be rented or purchased. These are all decisions that have to be made in the context of program planning at each institution.

**Renovations**

This is a very costly component for hospitals. Wider doorways, larger rooms, potential ceiling railings, types of commodes and how they're mounted—all of these must be considered, not just for the bariatric unit, but throughout the hospital, as well. In addition, you have to right-size the entire facility looking beyond the bariatric inpatient unit. At our institution, when the task force meets, the members actually walk through the hospital and go to the different departments that a patient may visit, from the emergency room to the gastrointestinal (GI) lab, from radiology to the front entrance, side entrances, and admissions, carefully assessing the feasibility of the facility's size for these patients.

Facilities management is an area that is typically forgotten, but should be addressed throughout the hospital. Our hospital had significant problems early on because the types of tile used for flooring were not adequate for the beds for bariatric patients. The tiles had to be changed. So again, it is very important to assess all areas carefully.

### Staff Training

Staff training and injuries are very important from the hospital perspective. Sensitivity training for the physical and psychological needs of obese patients is significant. We all know that nurses and other patient-care staff are more likely to injure themselves attempting to mobilize severely obese patients. One back injury from a lifting incident can cost the hospital more than $500,000 in treatment costs and lost wages, so it's important that this be addressed on the front end.

Staff readiness is important and is mainly managed through education. It is imperative to train staff to know a good deal about the procedures and pre- and postoperative care that's required; the types of complications that might arise and how to recognize them early; follow-up care, both in the short and the long term; and how to provide the all-important training on the specialty equipment used in the care of these patients.

Sensitivity training for staff is also important. Patients do 1 to 2 years of research, on average, before choosing the facility where they're going to have their bariatric surgery. They're highly informed, particularly about things such as: "Is this a comfortable environment for me?"; "Were people nice to me?"; "Did I overhear someone in the operating room say something about how difficult it was to move me in the operating room?" Training caregivers about respect, teaching them to respect patients' diversity, and enhancing communication skills are key elements to providing the service well.

### Payment and Reimbursement Issues

This is one of the most important issues related to the hospital perspective. Actions to take when assessing or establishing a bariatric center:

- Stabilize program costs
- Contract for comprehensive services
- Obtain written preauthorization and perform procedure within timeline
- Attain coding expertise and ensure clear documentation of comorbidities
- Investigate state and local reimbursement levels

The business metrics on the hospital side, for either an established center or a hospital looking to establish a bariatric center, is to do the feasibility assessment, which was already discussed; perform a walkthrough with the taskforce and committee to determine what capital investment is needed; and then measure the financial incentives. This is one of the most interesting areas in the field because, as many of us know, this is what has been driving a lot of the growth in bariatric surgery and it's not always clear to the caregivers, surgeons, physicians, and nurses how the financial incentives are measured.

Hospitals, as you may or may not know, routinely perform profitability analyses. They are done at least on a quarterly basis, most certainly on an annual basis, and almost always when a change is going to be made in program structure or when there has been growth or expansion. These profitability analyses are broken down by individual surgeon, type of bariatric procedure, and by payer. There is tremendous variation across the country and from institution to institution, but in an established program providing comprehensive care, the direct contribution to margin of bariatric surgery procedures is approximately 40% to 60%. That is the highest of any other surgical procedure in the country. Traditionally, in an established comprehensive program, hospital administration will commit to reinvesting the majority, in the 70% to 90% range, of that contribution to margin back into the program in staff hirings, support services, and salaries to attract experienced staff.

Where the hospital really benefits, though, is from what's called the downstream revenue. This is composed of all the other services that patients will require, either before or after bariatric surgery. It's very much likened to a grocery store that sells milk at a good price to bring consumers into the grocery store to buy other products. The hospital never wants to negotiate with its downstream revenue. That is complete profit, and those numbers are fairly closely guarded. To compare in terms of medical services, for every dollar of internal medicine reimbursement, the hospital's downstream revenue is, on average, $8; for bariatric surgery services, for every dollar of reimbursement for bariatric surgery services, the downstream revenue varies from $20 to $35.

You can draw the conclusion that a financial pro forma to guarantee success on the hospital side for a bariatric program is to assess and understand your local reimbursement environment, because environments vary geographically, and to assess local coverage by commercial insurers and Medicaid. Know what your financial investment is going to be and be sure that you include both your capital and your staffing investment. Regularly ascertain your cost for surgery and try to keep those costs and complications limited as the program grows.

**Risks of Surgery**

This leads me to the final area of hospital assessment and that is the risks of surgery. Strategically, it is both a financial and clinical necessity to limit complications. We all know that complications are expensive. A single complication that requires a patient to stay in the hospital for 60, 90, or more days, could eliminate all profit on that surgeon's operations for that entire year. We all know from living in this geographic environment and others that both established and new programs can be closed down when a single high-profile death is brought to the attention of the media. Surgical risks have to be managed and assessed in the context of surgeon and hospital volume. Some studies have shown that 100 cases per surgeon and/or hospital per year, appears to be the threshold above which complications come down to an acceptable level.

Finally, the overall concept is to balance quality with the amount of volume. That is, limit readmissions to the emergency room, the number of complications, and reoperations. In our institution, all of those metrics are provided to us on a monthly basis so that we can track our quality along with our volume.

**A Service-line Approach: The Key to Success**

The key to success for a positive return on investment for the hospital, is to develop a service-line approach to obesity treatment. One of the most important factors is dedicated administrative support. We've been fortunate at the University of Pittsburgh, to have such dedicated administrative support that we've actually married our clinical data with our payment and claims data. We are doing some analyses to determine, based on body mass index and other demographic factors, which patients benefit the most from both a clinical and cost perspective. A service-line approach also requires that a full range of services be provided, before and after surgery and that specialized operating rooms and postrecovery units are staffed by trained personnel. It's very clear that a hospital's service-line approach to obesity treatment improves outcomes. It also attracts patients. There are significant financial benefits to the service-line approach for the hospital. It helps lower unit costs, as well as improving the collateral downstream revenues for all the other studies and procedures we do. At our institution, for every single bariatric patient on whom we operate, we make 14 internal referrals both before and after surgery.

Thus, a hospital service-line approach documents outcome so that your facility can establish itself as a regional Center of Excellence, and be able to negotiate preferential rates for preferred-provider status with payers. Specialized obesity treatment units can serve as a resource for improving care across the entire institution. We know that patients presenting for trauma or for oncologic surgery, for example, are all becoming increasingly obese and can benefit from some of this expertise and from a service-line approach.

**Future Trends**

So what are the future trends in bariatric surgery services from a hospital perspective? Clearly, the trend is that reimbursement is declining, and as that is happening we are going to be compelled to provide better service at lower cost. I predict that over time, by analyzing cost and clinical outcomes, the criteria for bariatric surgery will be subject to attempts at tightening up by insurance companies. I think that we, as providers and surgeons and physicians, have an opportunity to be involved in this analysis of the clinical and financial outcomes so that we can, in some way, help control and guide them. In addition, there are some strategic opportunities for surgeons to identify niche markets within bariatric surgery to provide new services.

In conclusion, "Can the return on investment in this area be a winner?" The answer is, yes. But, only if you can overcome the challenges and provide a service-line approach to meet the opportunity to provide cost-effective care, and do it with an excellent clinical outcome.

# Facilities Requirements

Barbara Lightizer, MS, MA

In 2004, the Beth Israel Deaconess Medical Center (BIDMC) in Boston formed a *Persons of Size* task force. The purpose was to improve the safety of care delivered to "persons of size" in medical facilities regardless of their point of entry or the particular service provided. The intention was to develop a risk-assessment and intervention strategy for patients at increased safety risk due to large body size. The rationale for focusing on this aspect of care was the growing area of literature suggesting that this was an imperative. An estimated 129.6 million Americans, or 64%, are overweight or obese. Obesity and overweight have been shown to increase the risk for developing type 2 diabetes, heart disease, some forms of cancer, and other disabling medical conditions. The total direct and indirect costs of obesity, including medical costs and lost productivity nationally, were estimated at $117 billion for the year 2000, according to the 2001 Surgeon General's Call to Action to Prevent and Decrease Overweight and Obesity. With 64% of the population overweight and many of them experiencing medical problems, it had become incumbent on hospitals to provide a safe environment for the delivery of healthcare services to this segment of the population.

The BIDMC *Person's of Size* task force, made up of representatives from the American College of Surgeons (ACS), American Society for Metabolic and Bariatric Surgery (ASMBS), National Heart, Lung and Blood Institute (NHLBI), and the Association of Perioperative Registered Nurses (AORN) began by defining the problem and population, drawing on input from these organizations.

Morbid obesity is generally defined as more than 100 lbs over normal body weight, or a body mass index (BMI) $\geq 40 kg/m^2$.

Any organization should be concerned with improving the services that are provided to persons of size. That means not just patients who come in for obesity surgery, but patients and their visitors who come into the organization for different reasons and through a variety of different portals.

**How do we Accomplish These Goals?**

It would be far more convenient, of course, if a facility were being built from the ground up, purchasing all new equipment and establishing accommodations "from scratch." But most organizations are not in that position and certainly that's not the typical situation.

It is important to start out by conducting an inventory and an assessment during which we focus on questions such as: "What are the priorities?"; "What can we do?"; and "What *must* we do?" Organizations should review each setting individually, even though many of the topics will apply to several or all of the settings.

**First Things First**

Conduct an assessment of what your facility already has. Chairs are a good example. These are present in meeting rooms, waiting rooms, and virtually every other area. The visitors' chairs in patient rooms, as well as the patient chairs themselves, should accommodate persons of various weights. It is often difficult to determine the maximum weight capacity for chairs purchased for common waiting areas or meeting areas since that information is not routinely provided with commonly purchased items. The challenge is to access that information, perhaps through the purchasing department or manufacturer.

It is also important to determine which population is being served. In facilities that offer bariatric programs, it is possible to establish limits for the size of patients the program can accommodate. But in terms of hospital emergency departments or other outpatient areas, these serve a public consisting of many sizes, weights, and shapes. Most hospitals, clinics, and emergency departments have no restrictions based on body habitus and find themselves having to deal with difficult circumstances in this regard.

**Wheelchairs**

Although it is likely that most organizations are not aware of the weight-bearing capacity of the basic chairs in their waiting rooms and other areas, it is more likely that the maximum capacity of their wheelchairs is known. As your assessment begins, this area of accommodation is critical. What do you have currently, in terms of wheelchairs? What are their maximum weight capacities? Most can certainly accommodate persons weighing 250 lbs, however, there are many people of far greater weight than that. And, in addition to weight capacity, wheelchairs must accommodate people of varying girths. It is important to know the needs of each individual patient and to have proper equipment to meet those needs. Your staff must know which piece of equipment to use for which patient, and be aware of how and when to access that equipment.

**Bathrooms**

Bathrooms are a big challenge. One of the things often observed in the literature is the problem of wall-mounted toilets that separate from the wall. It can be difficult to determine what, in fact, is the capacity of a wall-mounted toilet, but most are probably safe up to 300 lbs. Some national standards suggest a commode should be built to not break off at up to 350 pounds, but the hardware inside the wall may only be rated to 300 lbs. This must be considered when assessing accommodations. Take the number of toilets in your facilities—whether they be in public or patient areas or throughout—that may only be able to accommodate persons weighing up to 250 lbs or 300 lbs and calculate that against the percentage of the over 300-lb population your facility serves. That's an interesting challenge, again, when assessing your existing facilities. Consider what needs to be done about it. Is there a way to replace those accommodations, to retrofit? Research some of the products that are out there that may make retrofitting possible, providing safety and stabilization without total replacement costs. And for facilities that may be renovated, consideration should be given to replacing all wall-mounted commodes with floor-mounted fixtures.

**Exam Rooms**

Whether they are in inpatient, outpatient or physician-office settings, exam tables must be installed within all safety parameters. But, do those parameters include standards of width for persons of size? Are the tables bolted to the floor so that, with movement, they are not going to tip over? And what is the weight capacity? Do you know the answers to those questions for the exam tables in your facility? If not, how difficult is it to get the answers so you can gauge whether you will need to replace tables with equipment that will accommodate the populations being served? Again, organizations will always have to stop and think about who is being served in a particular setting and what will be needed to accommodate that population. The last thing any organization would want, obviously, is to have tables rated only up to 300 or 400 or 500 lbs and staff that are not informed of the weight ratings, and have someone of a larger size placed on that piece of equipment.

**Proper Supplies**

Does your facility maintain an inventory of the kind of supplies required to care for persons of size? Whether it is the right size blood-pressure cuff or scale, it is important for both patient and employee safety that proper supplies are readily available. Closely tied to this is the sensitivity issue. In order to responsibly serve people whose needs are not what perhaps in the past were considered typical or average, but whose dignity must be respected and who are entitled to the same care that all patients receive, your staff should be able to efficiently access appropriate equipment and supplies and do it with sensitivity and concern for the safety of all patients invited into your facilities.

**The Inpatient Setting**

For obesity surgery programs, consider maintaining a dedicated location. Ideally, this seems to be the most efficient and effective way to accommodate a specialized patient population; but of course in most organizations all comers are welcome and not everybody who is of size is coming for obesity surgery. Nevertheless, it may be possible to invest in creating an environment that anticipates a given time when bariatric surgery will be performed. It's really much more complicated than that, but where an organization's obesity surgery program is concerned, it may well be worth it. By having dedicated space, it is more viable to have staff with the sensitivity, safety, and equipment training required to meet the needs of that particular population.

For those organizations that do have the luxury of an available "dedicated" space that can be designed to accommodate the bariatric population, it is important to consider that it's not just having a particular floor where there are special beds and staff who know a little more than their coworkers about serving persons of size. The actual physical requirements are more complex than that. For example, take door widths. With larger equipment having to be brought into these rooms and the patient's visitors who might be persons of size themselves, it is recommended that the door widths be 60-inches wide. This includes the door to the bathroom. It is also recommended that there be 5 feet of space between the foot of the bed and the walls, and 5 feet between either sides of the bed and the walls. Again, the question that will arise as your assessment is being done may be, "Do we have that kind of space?" Because, once you start bringing in equipment that takes up more space, you are probably going to have more staff in the room too. And ideally, within a specialized bariatric unit, all patient rooms should be private to accommodate the previously stated needs. Can your facility accommodate those parameters?

**Bariatric Beds**

You have looked into what you currently have for beds, and you are questioning their capacity. Most beds accommodate up to 500 lbs. Will you have patients who exceed that weight? As a facility offering bariatric surgery, that would seem likely, but it may be that you can provide for those patients by using a rental service as needed.

Is your staff aware of the limits of existing beds and aware of options for patients whose needs exceed what is routinely available? Do staff members know how to get what they need for the particular patient in question? Again, if you have a dedicated floor or area for the bariatric patient population, maybe the rooms are all equipped for that population, but in terms of the kind of equipment that is rarely used and difficult to store, a rental agreement may make more fiscal sense when set up on an as-needed basis. For elective admissions like bariatric surgery, this works well as requirements are known in advance.

**Figure 1**

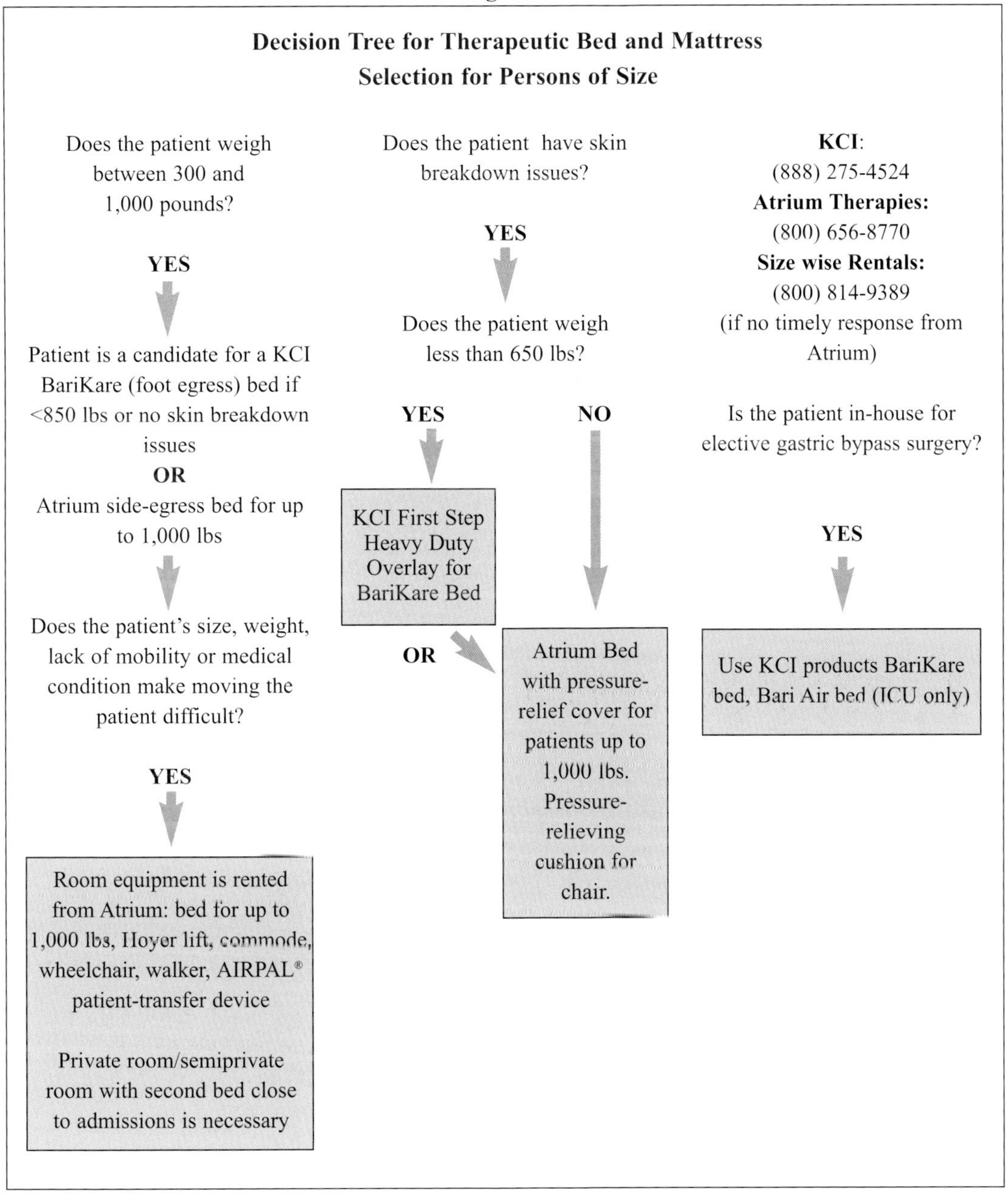

**Transfer-assist Devices**

Your staff is going to be moving patients from bed to stretcher, from bed to wheelchair, from bed to chair, etc. These moves must be performed in a manner safe for the patient and safe for the staff involved. Again, all staff should know what the capacity is of the equipment that they're using. Are they selecting the right equipment for the right patient, and is it available to them?

**Lifting Equipment, Walkers, and Effective Labeling**

If a patient falls to the floor, is your facility fitted with the right equipment that can safely raise that person? Do you have proper walkers? When it comes to wheelchairs, stretchers, gurneys, and other equipment used routinely for bariatric patients, this should be of great concern. It is important to consider the particular patient and the capacity of the piece of required equipment. Is all applicable equipment labeled with weight limits? In order to do that you must, of course, actually have that information. Once applied to the equipment, the labels should be able to resist cleaning and wear and tear. Staff should be aware of special cleaning instructions where required, and should be stringently trained to match patients who are persons of size to the equipment they know can accommodate them. Implementing a system that monitors these factors in a consistent manner should be part of the facility's overall patient/staff safety plan.

**Dimensions and Weight-bearing Safety**

As noted, most organizations have existing facilities that have been around for a long time. They are of certain dimensions. All redesign and retrofitting will have to take into consideration the square footage available for the change. In terms of bariatric patients, all doors will have to accommodate larger wheelchairs and wider walkers. Staff must be able to respond to an emergency situation that might occur in a bathroom and to be able to get potentially wider stretchers and more people into a room that's already crowded. In this regard, grab bars can be properly situated to help patients move, which means they must be capable of handling the kind of force that might be applied should a patient lose balance or slip to the floor. Improperly installed grab bars could be disastrous. And, what about existing shower stalls? Will those require expansion? Are the grab bars able to support weights up to and beyond 500 lbs?

**Procedural and Technical Equipment**

Bariatric patients who come in for surgery will have needs not limited to mobility and room accommodation. It is important to note whether the facility's CT scanning equipment can appropriately handle persons of size, for instance. Maximum capacity should be determined, and that applies, as well, to the space in which the scanner is located. Patients come into the hospital for a variety of reasons, not just for surgery. Any hospital would do well to be able to offer the various services they routinely offer patients outside the specialized area of bariatrics. Whether a patient, who happens to be a person of size, requires MRI, fluoroscopy, ultrasound, nuclear medicine, or interventional radiology, your facility should be evaluated for its ability to serve them.

**The Operating Room**

The operating room is probably a little bit easier to evaluate, simply because its equipment can be considered "fixed," and there are only a certain number of operating rooms. But it is important to check each piece of equipment for its capacity and efficiency in accommodating persons of size. Hydraulic lifts are generally labeled with their capacity, but it is crucial that staff know how to use them. This is true for operating tables as well. Although they are wide and have certain established maximum weight capacity, what happens when they are used at different angles? Does the weight limit change? Are personnel familiar with that and do they recognize under what circumstances they can and cannot change those angles? Is the proper perioperative instrument equipment available and readily prepared to be used in procedures on this population?

**Elevators**

Patients must be transported from the emergency department into the inpatient units, or from the inpatient units to radiology or to the operating room, or elsewhere. Most of the time, this transportation involves the use of an elevator. Do you know the weight capacity of your existing elevators? What about the width of their doors? Will the larger pieces of equipment you plan to have on hand fit, or will your staff have to wheel the patient a far distance to some special elevator that's really intended for freight? And if so, what does it say to your patients when they find themselves accommodated this way?

### Sensitivity Issues

Any discussion of "what it says to your patients" leads to the absolute need for hospitals to respond to sensitivity issues. Again it is necessary to compare what is being done currently with what needs to change in order to serve this population. Staff members must be educated, not only in the labeling, accessing, choosing, and handling of equipment, but also in the way in which they treat, communicate, and think about their patients. Providing training in this area, or periodic retraining to keep personnel aware of new methods or requirements, is essential to any facility wishing to best serve all of its patients.

Again, assessing these areas is critical whether a facility is concerned simply about being able to serve patients who are persons of size, or is considering offering a concentration in bariatric surgery services. It comes down to training, training, and more training; training on proper selection, proper use, proper body mechanics, and on sensitivity. The list goes on and on because in the arena of medical facilities and providing best care to patients, getting it absolutely right is always a work in progress.

### Suggested Reading

1. National Institutes of Health. The practical guide: identification, evaluation and treatment of overweight and obesity in adults. Available at: http://www.nhlbi.nih.gov/guidelines/obesity/prctgd_c.pdf. Accessed August 21, 2007.
2. Association of periOperative Registered Nurses. AORN bariatric surgery guideline. *AORN Journal.* 2004;79(5):1026-52.
3. Lehman Center Weight Loss Surgery Expert Panel. Commonwealth of Massachusetts Betsy Lehman Center for Patient Safety and Medical Error Reduction Expert Panel on Weight Loss Surgery: executive report. *Obes Res.* 2005;13:205-26.
4. Jones DB, Provost DA, DeMaria EJ, Smith CD, Morgenstern L, Schirmer B. Optimal management of the morbidly obese patient. SAGES appropriateness conference statement. *Surg Endosc.* 2004;18(7):1029-37.
5. Surgical Review Corporation. ASBS Bariatric Surgery Center of Excellence requirements. Available at: http://www.surgicalreview.org/pcoe/tertiary/tertiary.aspx. Accessed August 21, 2007.

# Equipment Considerations

Michelle McCleerey, PhD, MA, MEd, RN

As obesity rates have steadily climbed over the past 2 decades, hospitals have become sharply aware that the severely obese patient is no longer an anomaly.(1) Rather, the severely obese comprise a formidable patient population with myriad unique needs that many hospitals are ill-prepared to meet. The challenges of caring for this patient population have literally been revealed incrementally as new bariatric subpopulations have emerged. These include weight reduction surgical patients, chronically ill bariatric patients and geriatric, pediatric, and perinatal bariatric patients. In response, healthcare providers have scrambled to meet these challenges. Unfortunately, this often has meant attempting to bind together or reinforce existing equipment or utilizing a device or piece of equipment for purposes other than those for which it was specifically designed.(2) Many of these crude adaptations and improvisations placed both patients and caregivers in great peril.

In an attempt to meet the growing demand for bariatric equipment and devices, vendors first simply provided larger, more durable versions of standard models. Neither the great variability of weight, size, and shape of severely obese patients, nor the pronounced differences in their functional capacities were taken into consideration in the design of such equipment. Moreover, selection was markedly limited and quite often the equipment was industrial and darkly imposing in appearance. Thankfully, both the design and availability of bariatric equipment have greatly improved since then, enabling caregivers to more effectively meet the needs of this patient population.

One of the most significant obstacles to efficacious care of the severely obese has been the difficulty in providing optimal patient movement, both on a micro and macro level. Excellent healthcare delivery is dependent upon the ability to transition patients throughout the system of care: patients need to be seamlessly transferred from one location of the hospital or health system to the next. As well, patients must be mobilized while in their own bed or room. The ability to perform activities with ease and efficiency has traditionally been fleeting at best. Even prior to the great increase in the number of bariatric patients, caregivers suffered substantial pain and injury due to moving patients and managing their activities. In fact, according to the Occupational Safety and Health Association (OSHA), caregivers reported more work-related musculoskeletal disorders (MSDs) resulting in time away from work than did people in most other occupations, including truck drivers, construction workers, and maintenance personnel.(3)

The frequency of such debilitating injuries among caregivers is not surprising in light of the known biomechanical, work-related risk factors that contribute to the development of MSDs. They include forceful exertions such as grasping, pulling, pushing, and lifting; awkward postures or the need to engage in non-neutral positions such as bending while twisting; repetitious movements and activities; and prolonged duration, or the undue length of time, a task or movement is performed. Manual patient movement and handling, such as the lateral transfer of a patient from a bed to a stretcher or the transfer of a patient from a chair to a bed, incorporates all noted hazardous actions. Understandably, the movement and handling of severely obese patients increases the magnitude of risk-factor exposure. It has been well-documented that the cumulative effect of exposure to these risk factors places a worker at substantial risk for the development of MSDs.(4) Consequently, any technology able to reduce the degree of risk-factor exposure for caregivers will decrease the potential for injuries due to patient movement activities.

However, equipment designed to reduce biomechanical risk is essential but not sufficient to ensure consistent use by caregivers.(4) If not used, the ergonomic benefits of the equipment obviously cannot be derived. Therefore, equipment must also reduce nonvalue-adding activity. That is, it must eliminate those actions that consume time and resources but do not directly contribute to the health and healing of the patient. For example, if equipment is not immediately accessible and available, caregivers are less inclined to use it. The need to search and retrieve equipment or assemble components, all nonvalue-adding activities, dramatically reduces the likelihood of its use. Accordingly, equipment that can be operated by 1 or 2 caregivers eliminates the need to actively recruit the assistance of several coworkers. Another example of nonvalue-adding activity is the need for nontherapeutic patient transfers to other surfaces and the repetition of procedures that initially failed.

Another important characteristic of equipment designed for consistent use by this population's caregivers is that it should preserve the patient's dignity and comfort. Designs that resemble standard equipment, but can easily accommodate the patient's size and shape without requiring embarrassing positions or postures will gain much greater acceptance among both staff and patients. In this regard, there have been great advances in the design of bariatric equipment. The availability of flexible designs has eased the financial burden of capital purchases while reducing nonvalue-adding activities, by providing multiple features and functionality within a single piece of equipment.(2) For example, there are beds and stretchers that have telescoping features, expanding and retracting frames that ease transportation and can be adjusted to accommodate the patient's height and girth. Many bariatric beds have powered transport, so rather than requiring transfer to another piece of equipment, the patient is transported in bed by a single caregiver with minimal exertion and a neutral posture. In addition, beds capable of converting into chair positions allow a dependent bariatric patient to derive respiratory, cardiac and psychological benefits of an upright, seated position at the touch of a button. This is in stark contrast to the situation of caregivers who once had to recruit assistance to manually lift, twist, and transfer their patients to chairs. And bariatric beds are also designed to provide assistance with patient turning and repositioning, relieving the degree of force required to be applied by the caregiver and the awkward, unsafe posture he/she would have to assume. In addition, these beds assist caregivers with patient-egress and initial weight bearing by offering a foot-exit option.

Other flexible equipment designs include stretcher chairs (convertible equipment that can serve as wheel chairs, stretchers or exam tables) and surgical tables that provide lift and articulation, imaging capabilities, and interchangeable accessories for multiple surgeries. Built-in scales eliminate the need to transfer the patient to a sling scale, and integrated therapy surfaces eliminate the need to place the patient onto another surface. For hospitals and other care units, the incorporation of multiple ergonomic features into a single design also significantly reduces the need for storage space.

It is also imperative that bariatric-patient caregivers have appropriate lifts, lateral-transfer devices, stretchers, wheelchairs, and walkers at their disposal.(4,5) Powered air-transfer devices are commonly used to laterally transfer a patient from the bed onto a stretcher or between two flat surfaces. Again, such a device allows caregivers to perform this maneuver with less force exerted, no need for awkward posture, and requiring fewer assisting caregivers. In addition, bariatric stretchers and wheelchairs can be powered, decreasing the amount of physical exertion required to transport a patient.

Powered ceiling mounted lifts have become increasingly popular and offer the advantages of immediate accessibility and availability without the requirement of extra storage space.(6) However, floor-based models are necessary for moving patients who are located in areas where there are no ceiling lifts. Whether the lift is floor-based or ceiling-mounted, it is important that it has the capability to lift from the floor.

Lifts now have a variety of sling types and sizes. Slings are available for particular types of transfers (e.g., bed to chair or stretcher) and care activities (e.g., toileting and bathing), so choosing the correct sling is integral to patient safety and comfort. There are also types of slings available for use when repositioning the patient or for holding the patient in a particular position while care is being administered.(2)

When choosing the appropriate lift and sling, weight-bearing capacity is not the only consideration. The caregiver must also be aware of safety and comfort issues based upon the patient's body-weight distribution, level of dependency, and comorbidities. Patient factors to be addressed include biomechanical considerations (e.g., hip-angle tolerance, difficulty or inability to log-roll, limited trunk flexion); pressure points inadvertently created by an ill-fitting sling; susceptibility to respiratory distress (intolerance for the supine position or the inward rotation of shoulders); and balance and positioning challenges.

Several other factors must be taken into consideration to ensure that the proper equipment is available to enable efficacious care of the bariatric patient. One of the most apparent is that larger equipment consumes more space. Hence, having sufficiently large storage areas is a necessity. As noted previously, the closer this area is to where the equipment will be used, the better. In addition, any physical barrier, such as a locked room, or stacked or blocked equipment, will preclude use. Adequate storage space is only one environmental design recommendation. To properly accommodate the needs of the bariatric patient and larger equipment, as well as multiple caregivers, the design parameters of the room and the unit itself often must be modified.(6)

A popular inclination is to purchase the largest equipment available when first preparing for the bariatric patient population. However, it should be noted that the larger the equipment, the more likely it is that staff will have to reach and stretch and exert force to operate it when providing patient care. For example, bariatric beds can vary from 42 to 62 inches in width. Placing a patient in the widest bed made when a smaller bed would accommodate his/her size and shape will require caregivers to reach and strain in order to mobilize or care for the patient. Thus, it is recommended that a hospital provide a choice of equipment for caregivers.

Standard equipment usually has a weight-bearing capacity limit of 250 lbs to 300 lbs. The weight-bearing capacity limit of bariatric equipment can vary between 400 to 1,000 lbs. Thus, for safety purposes, it is useful to place a discreet label on each piece of equipment so caregivers do not exceed the limits.(7)

The investment in quality bariatric equipment does not automatically translate into derived benefits; the equipment must be used. However, there are many ways to promote consistent safe use of equipment by staff, beginning with the selection process. Staff members who will be using the equipment should be actively involved in the selection of these items. To be knowledgeable, they must be aware of the various types of equipment that are available. Such information can be obtained by reviewing catalogs, attending equipment fairs or exhibits, and exchanging information with other hospitals. Once staff members have identified potentially desirable equipment, following up with unit or department trials will provide further insight. All too often, though, equipment brought to a unit is virtually ignored by staff, leading to purchase decisions made without crucial information on the usefulness or implementation of the equipment being bought. Thus, a systematic process should be established to ensure that all staff members are knowledgeable on the use of the proposed equipment and that their feedback is solicited for purchase purposes.

Safe, consistent use of equipment requires more than just operational instruction for direct caregivers. The new technology must be integrated into the protocols of care for the bariatric patient. It is helpful for a multidisciplinary team to develop best practices that incorporate all of the care unit's available equipment.(5) The protocol then becomes the basis of all staff training. Direct caregivers will thus not be forced to learn equipment functionality in isolation; rather, they will understand the role and operation of the equipment within the context of care delivery.

Education and training should be directed at all levels of the hospital. Executive leaders must understand the importance of continued communication and demonstrated support of the bariatrics program. In addition, it is imperative that these leaders be aware of the need for continued investment in new care technology and the return to be gained from such investment. Further, education aimed at facility managers must inculcate the need for unit- department-level accountability concerning the consistent, safe use of equipment and compliance with care protocols.

Facilities are inevitably faced with the decision of whether to rent or buy bariatric equipment. Such decisions should be guided by capital and rental history, storage considerations, and accessibility needs.(14) Moreover, patient population mix, diagnoses and characteristics, as well as future demographic and reimbursement trends should provide direction in this regard. The recognition of obesity as a disease by Medicare has made it easier to collect reimbursement from insurance companies for specialized equipment.(15) The rental of bariatric equipment protects the facility from large cash outlays for seldom-used items, particularly if storage space is limited.

One of the greatest needs of the bariatric patient is mobilization. This includes biomechanical mobility and movement of the patient throughout the healthcare system. Both pose daunting challenges to healthcare providers and caregivers. New technology is enabling caregivers to more effectively address these needs as discussed in this chapter. Obviously, there are many other accessories and devices that are required in order to provide efficacious care to the bariatric patient population, and these would include appropriate blood-pressure cuffs, needles, gowns, bed pans, etc. The discussion of these items, however, falls outside the scope of this chapter.

**References**


1. Diconsiglio J. Hospitals equip to meet the bariatric challenge. Rising numbers of obese patients necessitates specific supplies. *Mater Manag Health Care*. 2006;15(4):36-9.
2. Harrell JW, Miller B. Big challenge. Designing for the needs of bariatric patients. *Health Facil Manage*. 2004;17(3):34-8.
3. Washington State Department of Labor and Industries. Concise explanatory statement. Ergonomics (RCW 34.05.325.6a) WAC 296-62-051; 2005.
4. VISN 8 Patient Safety Center of Inquiry (2001). Patient Care Ergonomics Resource Guide: safe patient handling and movement. Available at: http://www.visn8.med.va.gov/patientsafetycenter/safePatHandling. Accessed January 30, 2007.
5. Akridge J. Bariatric equipment puts ergonomics, safety to the test. *Healthcare Purchasing News*. 2006;30(2):24-29.
6. Akridge J. Weighty issues require careful planning. *Healthcare Purchasing News*. 2005;29(3):48-62.
7. Arzouman J, et al. Developing a comprehensive bariatric protocol: a template for improving patient care. *Medsurg Nursing*. 2006;15(1):21-26.

# Clinical Pathways in Weight Loss Surgery

Benjamin E. Schneider, MD

Clinical pathways, or integrated care pathways, define the care processes by which clinical interventions are outlined in the sequence of steps utilized for the treatment of a specific diagnosis or procedure. As a multidisciplinary algorithm, clinical pathways clearly delineate daily treatments of patients as they progress from the preoperative assessment through their surgical intervention, postoperative hospitalization, and ultimate follow-up. The aim of pathways is to enhance adoption of evidence-based treatment standards, or best practice guidelines, as well as to improve documentation and clinical data collection.(1) Successful care improvements may lead to standardization of care. They may improve the efficiency of resource utilization; reduce cost; shorten length of stay; improve patient compliance; improve implementation of research on evidence-based practices; encourage multidisciplinary communication; improve education of housestaff and new nursing staff; promote patient-centered care; and/or increase patient satisfaction. These improvements may ultimately result in more cost-effective and higher quality patient care.

### Clinical Pathways in Weight Loss Surgery

While it may seem intuitive that pathways result in healthcare improvements and cost savings, there is a paucity of supporting data on this. Despite somewhat conflicting evidence, the need for clinical standardization and economic force, has lead to the development and utilization of clinical pathways.(2,3) Weight loss surgery (WLS), with its high-acuity population and high costs, together with the rise in high-volume centers, lends itself well to attempts at reducing costs while maintaining quality care.(4)

The current literature evaluating WLS pathways is limited by a lack of randomization and is subject to uncontrolled analyses, which raises the possibility that improvement may be a result of secular trends rather than real changes in outcomes resulting from pathway implementation. Despite a lack of robust evidence to support WLS pathways effectiveness, there are limited data demonstrating some promise. Huerta et al retrospectively examined outcomes before and after implementation of a clinical pathway for open gastric bypass surgery.(5) A significant difference in hospital length of stay (4.05 days vs 3.17 days) and a reduction in length of stay in the intensive care unit (0.37 days vs 0.07 days) were noted between the pre- and postpathway groups. Also noted was a trend toward fewer complications in the postpathway group. This translated into a significant reduction in both readmission rate (4.2 vs 3.2%) and a 40% decrease in hospital cost per admission. Although prospective analysis is lacking at present, these reductions should not be discounted and the potential for clinical pathways to improve the quality of care necessitates rigorous, controlled investigation.

### Development of Clinical Pathways

The development of clinical pathways for both gastric bypass and laparoscopic adjustable gastric band at Beth Israel Deaconess Medical Center began as an initiative to streamline and improve levels of patient care. The strategic objectives of the pathways were developed based on national and regional recommendations as outlined by the American College of Surgeons Centers of Excellence and the Massachusetts Department of Public Health Betsy Lehman Center for Patient Safety and Medical Error Reduction Expert Panel on Weight Loss Surgery. Design and development were lead by the major stakeholders representing the core development team: surgeons, hospital administrators, nurses, dieticians, anesthesiologists, radiologists, pharmacists, and infectious disease and critical care professionals. The net result was the development of pathways formatted upon the patient's care progression from the pre- to postoperative periods (Table 1 & 2).(6) Computerized standardized order sets, based upon pathways for both gastric bypass and laparoscopic adjustable gastric band, are designed to improve adherence and reduce deviation from the intended plan of care. The pathway itself serves to simplify and streamline documentation. The construction of a dedicated bariatric wing of the hospital has had the desired effect of establishing a cohesive group of caregivers. Furthermore, by having an identified body of staff, ongoing educational sessions are focused specifically upon the nursing unit and rotating housestaff in an effort to familiarize all providers with the pathway.

**Table 1**

| | Before Your Surgery | Day of Surgery | Day After Surgery |
|---|---|---|---|
| **What to do today** | ☐ You may NOT eat after midnight before your surgery | ☐ You will not be able to eat<br>☐ You may walk short distances with assist at least once, more if tolerated<br>☐ You may perform breathing exercises 10 times/hour while awake<br>☐ Wear your compression boots when not ambulating to prevent blood clots in your legs | ☐ You will have a swallow study<br>☐ You may begin a Stage I diet and progress to Stage III diet if you pass your swallow study<br>☐ You may sit at edge of bed for all meals<br>☐ You may walk independently<br>☐ You may perform breathing exercises 10 times/hour while awake<br>☐ Wear your compression boots when not ambulating to prevent blood clots in your legs |
| **Activity** | • Continue with your normal daily exercise routine 30 minutes daily | • You may sit at edge of bed | • You should walk in the hall by yourself at least 3 times |
| **Education** | • Review the handout on pre-op dietary restrictions | • You will learn how to use the pain scale<br>• You will learn how to perform breathing exercises | • An inpatient nurse practitioner will review the patient education packet and support group information |
| **Tests/ Procedures** | • Your appointment with pre-admission test center is complete<br>• Please use your Hibiclens or pHisoHex® wash as per instructions from the nurse in the pre-admission test center | • The tube in your bladder may be removed<br>• Your incision dressing will stay on<br>• You may have your blood sugar checked | • Your incision dressing will be changed<br>• You may have your blood sugar checked<br>• You may have a blood test |
| **Medications** | • Please discontinue use of aspirin 10 days prior to surgery | • You may have IV pain medications | • You may have oral pain medications |

Table 2

**Your Name:** ______________________ **Date of Surgery:** ______________________

**Surgeon Name:** ______________________ **Case Manager:** ______________________

| Home Discharge Criteria | Patient Discharge Information |
|---|---|
| ☐ You can be discharged home when:<br>☐ Your vital signs (blood pressure, heart rate, etc.) are stable<br>☐ You can walk safely and at your activity level prior to surgery<br>☐ You are tolerating a Stage III diet<br>☐ You can urinate on your own<br>☐ Your pain scale is 1–4 on oral pain medication<br>☐ You and/or your family understand your medications<br>☐ Your wound care can be performed at home by you, your family, or a visiting nurse<br>☐ You and/or your family understand your diet instructions | ☐ You should understand the instructions for your discharge<br>☐ Prescriptions are given for medications to go home<br>Follow-up Bariatric appointment:<br>Place:__________ ______/______<br>Date Time<br>Next support group meeting:<br>Place:__________ ______/______<br>Date Time<br>When you are home, if you have any medical concerns, please call the Bariatric Clinic<br>If you have any nutrition questions, please call the Nutrition Clinic |

Although logistical challenges exist, randomized controlled trials are needed to assess the true impact of clinical pathways. Future areas of investigation may focus on not only the usual parameters (such as cost and length of stay), but also on variations of, or deviations from, the pathway.

## References


1. Campbell H, Hotchkiss R, Bradshaw N, Porteous M. Integrated care pathways. *BMJ.*1998;316:133-7.
2. Dy SM, Garg P, Puskal G, et al. Critical pathway effectiveness: assessing the impact of patient, hospital care, and pathway characteristics using qualitative comparative analysis. *Health Serv Res*. 2005;40(2):499-516.
3. Gadacz TR, Adkins RB, O'Leary JP. General surgical clinical pathways: an introduction. *Am Surg*. 1997;63(1)107-10.
4. Cooney RN, Bryant P, Haluck R, Rodgers M, Lowery M. The impact of clinical pathway for gastric bypass surgery on resource utilization. *J Surg Res*. 2001;98(2):97-101
5. Huerta S, Heber D, Sawicki MP, et al. Reduced length of stay by implementation of a clinical pathway for bariatric surgery in an academic health care center. *Am Surg*.2001;67(12):1128-35.
6. Beth Israel Deaconess Medical Center. Lap Band Clinical Pathway and Gastric Bypass Clinical Pathway: 2007. Boston, MA. With permission.

# Hospitals and The Joint Commission

Kenneth Sands, MD, MPH

As a general orientation to the Joint Commission (formerly known as the Joint Commission for Accreditation of Healthcare Organizations [JCAHO]), and in particular for those who interface with the organization only peripherally, it should be appreciated that the organization is increasingly shifting away from measures of structure. Past JCAHO surveys focused heavily on committee structure, documentation, and policy; but to its credit, the organization has made progress toward measures of assessing an organization's processes and maintaining a more limited focus on true outcomes. For example, the Joint Commission is less likely to have a standard mandating the presence of a specific committee such as infection control, but there will be standards regarding processes relating to infection control that must be demonstrable. Finally, it is clear that the Joint Commission has an increasing focus on patient safety. Other areas of particular focus include patients' rights, and standardization and coordination of care.

The Joint Commission has moved away from language that addresses specific programs, and toward a format requiring that a facility be set up with the right elements for the patient population being served. The survey is now largely focused on what is known as *tracer methodology*, which is an attempt to "walk the walk" of patients in the facility. This might involve the Joint Commission survey team requesting to be brought to a care unit for a patient with a certain condition or on a specific treatment plan. The survey will then "trace" the patient's episode of care in the hospital, either forward or backward in time, as the patient receives services in various parts of the facility. This may be a hypothetical exercise, or it may involve actual visits to the various areas where the patient has been seen or received care as part of his/her hospitalization. Patient tracers are chosen based on the ability to demonstrate the more challenging hospital standards, and therefore are likely to focus on patients with clinical, behavioral, or ethical complexities. The patient tracer is where bariatric care professionals are most likely to encounter a Joint Commission survey. In fact, there are no specific Joint Commission standards relating to persons of size; however, because these patients often demonstrate clinical, behavioral, or ethical complexities, they represent a good way to assess the degree to which an institution can meet standards when faced with challenges in providing patient care.

As already stated, Joint Commission standards in general do not contain parameters unique to bariatric surgery. Rather, the Joint Commission survey would be looking for evidence that the unique needs of this patient population were addressed as an illustration of a broader standard. However, there is a separate program within the Joint Commission known as "disease-specific care certification." Bariatric surgery is included among conditions and services for which an institution can seek specific certification. These programs are separate from the traditional Joint Commission survey process, and involve a separate fee.

Programs are evaluated on the basis of specific performance metrics and demonstration of a process for performance improvement, as well as a few additional elements. Based on information on the Joint Commission Web site as of this writing, there are three institutions that have received certification for bariatrics. This certification is clearly underutilized at present in relation to the number of bariatric programs in existence, for while there are no Joint Commission standards specific to obesity surgery or persons of size, there are many issues relevant to these patients within the standard survey process. Besides being interested in types of patients who allow assessment of how a particular institution manages their complex care, the organization will also focus on services that have been marketed in the community or have proven to be newsworthy. The Joint Commission actually monitors the media for events receiving coverage relevant to the hospitals it is surveying and will query those hospitals about such events or reports during its survey. So, if a bariatric program is being marketed, or has been in the news, this will very likely flag it for notice by the Joint Commission.

Clinicians will sometimes feel that an institution is taking action for no purpose other than to meet a Joint Commission standard. Personally, I do not believe there are many things in that domain at the interface with bariatric surgery. Issues that generally concern the Joint Commission are those that have already been addressed in this book and to which we, as providers, are already positively committed. For example, the Joint Commission requires that care meet the same standard for all patients across the hospital, that patient safety issues are addressed, and patients' rights are adequately addressed. In terms of the bariatric population, this may mean being able to demonstrate that patients have equivalent access to tests and procedures such as radiological services. There are likely to be special competencies relating to the care of bariatric patients, and the Joint Commission would be looking for the processes that ensure those are being maintained, such as credentialing and privileging or employee training and education. Does the environment meet the needs of patients and provide appropriate space and equipment? As we all know, bariatric patients need specialized equipment and spaces, and a facility is obligated to make sure that these are provided. Indeed, good bariatric programs can actually serve as role models for the caliber of processes that the Joint Commission requires institutions be able to demonstrate: attending to patients' rights, providing accurate patient education, displaying optimum hospital teamwork, and ensuring customization based on patients' needs.

# Betsy Lehman Center for Patient Safety

Nancy Ridley, MS

There is a unique and quite rewarding approach that government has taken in examining and addressing public policy aspects of bariatric surgery and its safety from a public health perspective. I have been fortunate, in my 25-year career at the department of public health to have had input in the regulation of health care and health policy; during those 25 years, I've learned that it doesn't always take regulations to solve a problem. There are alternative pathways and other approaches that one can take, as we see in the strategic approach that Massachusetts took when it established, as part of law, the entity called the Betsy Lehman Center for Patient Safety and Medical Error Reduction. I believe that most people in Massachusetts (and many from other areas) know that Betsy Lehman was a 39-year-old journalist for the *Boston Globe* who died in 1994 after a massive chemotherapy overdose. That event truly changed the culture of how we look at safety and medical errors here in Massachusetts. I think it was one of the seminal events that started the revolution that culminated in 1999 with the Institute of Medicine (IOM) report on patient safety and medical errors. I have always felt that the Massachusetts systems designers, from an academic, government and healthcare system perspective (as well as that of a medical practitioner), have been ahead of the curve in terms of how they have embraced challenges and moved forward, looking at things objectively as a "village" rather than as individual silos. Within a year or so of Betsy's death, Massachusetts had formed the Coalition for the Prevention of Medical Errors. It consisted of a voluntary group of individuals and organizations, including representatives from the Massaschusett Medical Society, the Hospital Association, the Massachusetts Department of Public Health, and the Joint Commission. The intention was to have these organizations and entities come together to formulate an agenda for patient safety, not as anything that had a statutory base, but really as a village of community practitioners, providers, and in some cases even payers, who had a vested interest in seeing what could be done to change the culture from one of blame to one of safety—in perception, as well as in reality—and to recognize what was good about what we were doing and to fix what was not.

The Betsy Lehman Center was actually codified in the statute several years ago; however, it wasn't officially launched immediately. By the time it was put into law, I had been able to secure a sizeable patient safety grant from the federal government's Agency for Healthcare Research and Quality (AHRQ). Using the grant to partner with a number of academic and medical institutions and the Coalition, we had a fairly secure source of funding to do patient safety work, as well as research. We also had access to the Health Care Quality Improvement Trust Fund, which came originally from user fees that were assessed in the long-term care area. We had money that some of our very forward-thinking legislators, like the Health Care Committee's Dick Moore, set aside for us to use—not for regulatory purposes, but for safety and quality projects. That funding was critical, as I was able to use some of it (about $90,000 in all) once the Lehman Center was launched to do the Patient Safety in Obesity Surgery project upon which this book is focused.

The US Department of Public Health and the federal government in general, has many different regulatory arms that are very familiar to anybody who practices medicine or works in a hospital. There is the Division of Healthcare Quality, for example, which licenses hospitals and clinics and any other service or system that's out there. Also found within the Department of Public Health are the boards of registration for all of the medical professions, from nursing and pharmacy to respiratory therapy and all other healthcare areas. Here we find the Board of Registration in Medicine, which differs a bit from the others with its own independent status. I should add here that the Lehman Center, which I direct in addition to my other roles within the Department of Public Health, also has independent status. The Center, while within our secretariat, is not under the Department of Public Health's supervision. There are a number of other entities, as we all know. For instance, the Attorney General's office on occasion gets actively involved in issues of consumer protection and the economics of health care.

The Board of Medicine Patient Care Assessment (PCA) program, which is separate from the Board's traditional role of licensing physicians, plays an important role as we look at the issue of bariatric surgery. Even before the Department of Public

Health and the Lehman Center began their combined approach to weight loss surgery, they had actually issued an advisory on the subject.

The question arises: why did the Department and the Lehman Center pick weight loss surgery as its first project? The Lehman Center was launched in January 2004 and in February of that year we were deciding what area would be first studied. Lehman is not a regulatory body itself. Rather, it focuses on best practices, on coordinating patient-safety initiatives and in developing or supporting research toward those goals. One of the things clearly on everybody's mind, as it had been front-page news almost everywhere, was bariatric surgery. We had, over an 18-month period, about 6 or 7 cases of morbidity or mortality that for one reason or another had triggered concerned reactions that made it into the media. Normally, 6 or 7 cases in an 18-month time period would not be that unexpected when the risk basis and complication rates of the surgery are considered. However, any event will get medical-sector attention when it causes concern with the public and media and begins to raise questions regarding economic impact and issues concerning patients, as well as third-party payers. Should the expense for these procedures be reimbursed?

**Figure 1**

Weight Loss Surgery in Massachusetts
(HCF&P)

FY 1996: 148 Gastric Bypass Discharges
FY 2004: 3,040 Gastric Bypass Discharges

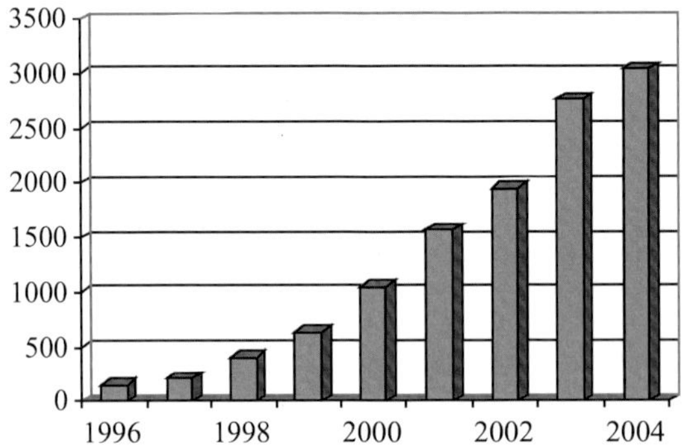


The numbers obviously prove the point. In Massachusetts, we have progressed from doing 148 bypass procedures a year in 1996 to more than 3,000 in 2004. That's a phenomenal increase. But numbers alone would not have justified our picking bariatric surgery as a project. One of the areas where I do regulatory oversight involves the external review process for individual patients who are denied third-party reimbursement for medical procedures theoretically covered under their plans. At the time of the news stories, I talked to one of my counterparts in California about the situation. In some parts of the country, it wasn't just an increase in the numbers of procedures, but also in the number of denials and external review of those denials. Gastric and bariatric surgery appeared at the top of the list in California, as well as other states. In Massachusetts, denials were practically nonexistent; however, we were starting to hear rumblings indicating they could potentially be on the horizon.

Another event—something a bit more personal—occurred. A leader within the Department of Public Health in Massachusetts at the time had bariatric surgery. We became pretty well versed on the risks and benefits of choosing bariatric surgery and what consumers were going through in the decision-making process. I would place calls to many of the experts (who are represented in this book) to inquire about the options. "What are the risks?," and, "What would be the benefits?" Through the research we learned a great deal about the risks and benefits and realized that one dilemma, from a public policy perspective, was that there was a perception out there that these surgical procedures were optional or cosmetic; or that they were being regarded as *elective* procedures. It became very clear that there were multiple comorbidities associated with obesity and that in the right circumstances these conditions rendered the surgery a necessary and viable option for individuals. And so, it must remain a necessary option for them.

The Lehman Center is an independent entity and, as such, it has many confidentiality protections that government regulatory agencies don't have. Those of us who have helped launch it were not going into it as regulators or with any intent to have regulations adopted as a result of what we did. The Commissioner of Public Health in Massachusetts made a request to the Lehman Center to form an expert panel to come up with recommendations for patient safety and guidelines for what would constitute best practice. In the course of naming the membership of the panel, I was very lucky to have as chair Dr. Alan Harvey, who was at the time the president-elect of the Massachusetts Medical Society, who had already adopted safety and quality as a key focus of his tenure, and I was also fortunate to have Dr. George Blackburn as vice chair.

My challenge was to put together a panel to address a high-profile, public policy issue. How would I approach it? One of the first things that George and Alan both advised was to make it multidisciplinary. The issue was not just an issue of surgery, they maintained, and not just one of physicians. It encompassed nursing care, nutrition, informed consent, consumers themselves, facilities, and certainly payers. So many things that go into making a safe, effective, and quality procedure aren't directly related to what the surgeons do, and so it really does take all of those components to have a safe program. Thus, developing recommendations for a panel that could address these several facets of bariatric surgery would take a multidisciplinary group.

The project itself could not have succeeded without the help of people like Frank Hu, our clinical epidemiologist, and Laurie Basinger who was our project manager. Others come to mind as key to the process: Elizabeth Fitzpayne, our medical librarian, and Rita Buckley, our medical editor for this particular project. It's also extremely important to note that the rigorous process Frank put us through in terms of classifying the medical literature was extraordinary. I think many of the medical scientists and physicians that were on the panel, and the nonepidemiologists, could barely believe what he made us do, but the objectivity and evidence base that resulted from such effort stands as proof. For within a very short timeframe for government—within 7 months, in fact— we were able to develop our 9 task forces, along with a comprehensive mission statement and an outline of objectives for the 9 areas we would study. These were fully representative of the multidisciplinary and multipronged approach we would take in looking at safety, quality, and recommendations for improvement in the arena of bariatrics. Each task force was chaired by an expert who kept members on target, communicating and doing what they needed to do. Rather than simply airing opinions as to what should be done, these groups presented clear evidence of what should be done. At the end of those 7 months, they had produced a very comprehensive executive summary, about 40 pages long. Included in those pages were 100 or more individual recommendations from 9 groups listed in Figure 2.

**Figure 2**

## Nine Task Groups

1. Surgical Care Group
2. Criteria for Patient Selection and Multidisciplinary (Psychological, Nutritional, Medical) Evaluation and Treatment
3. Patient Education/Informed Consent
4. Anesthetic Perioperative Care and Pain Management
5. Nursing Perioperative Care
6. Pediatric/Adolescent
7. Facility Resources
8. Coding and Reimbursement
9. Data Collection (Registries)/Future Considerations

The report was released in August 2004 along with a patient primer and FAQs. One asset I have within the Lehman Center is a patient safety ombudsman, a nurse, who was able to work with some of the consumers on the panel to develop a checklist and primer in consumer terminology that can be used when investigating surgical options. The report was sent to all

Massachusetts hospitals, as well as to all state health departments and commissioners throughout the country, along with recommendations that they use it internally within their departments. We were approached by the National Guidelines Clearinghouse of The Agency for Healthcare Research and Quality (AHRQ) as soon as they saw the rigor of our investigation and recommendations. We were able to translate the report into national guidelines, which are now available online through AHRQ. Everything culminated with the publication of the report's 10 articles in the journal *Obesity Research*.

We completed a survey of all Massachusetts facilities performing weight loss surgery, with an eye toward measuring the status of bariatric facilities since release of the guidelines. This was not done for regulatory purposes, but is a joint project between the Betsy Lehman Center and the PCA Committee of the Board of Registration in Medicine, which theoretically is not regulatory. We wanted to take an aggregate look and benchmark where we stood.

One of the things that George and I discussed was to reconvene the panel at intervals to take a look at the guidelines as time went on. Oftentimes, when research is completed it is put on the shelf. It takes vigilance to keep information fresh and relevant. You must make sure to remain aware of changes in technology, in the science, and in the work that's being done and to keep your recommendations as current and as informed by these changes as you can.

The model that was used to stay abreast of the evolving issues related to bariatric surgery is a model that we would like to see used to approach many other thorny issues in areas of medical care, such as patient safety and quality of care—issues that oftentimes end up in the legislature, being left to legislative solutions. We've seen it with cardiac surgery, transplants, and in many other aspects of health care. If you want the legislature to make laws prescribing or proscribing what medicine and health care should be doing, that's fine. If you don't, I think you must get on the bandwagon and become part of the village, adopting a proactive and prospective approach to how we as a field, an industry, and a group of individuals from many different backgrounds—government, private sector, academia—can develop evidence-based approaches that can be implemented to make health care safer for patients and for everyone else concerned.

# Betsy Lehman Center for Patient Safety and Reduction of Medical Errors

Alan Harvey, MD, MBA

Let me share my perspective—as a physician who was chair of the Betsy Lehman Center Weight Loss Surgery task-force project—on how we formed the team to accomplish this statewide, literature- and evidence-based process.

My own background includes an MBA with an additional concentration in health systems management. I had experience working on the first national practice parameters for the American Society of Anesthesiologists (ASA) with Dr. Stephen Woolf, methodologist for the US Preventative Health Service, and our ASA methodologists, Dr. Rick Connis and Dr. David Nickinovich. I could offer experience in leading physicians in both small and large committee processes as former Speaker of the Massachusetts Medical Society House of Delegates.

Let me review how the task group was formed, the process steps, and how we built a team to accomplish what none of us could do on our own. Take a look at our success as a template, which can be used for any other statewide, evidence- and literature-based, quality-improvement and patient-safety project. The "fun" part was that we had a blank slate. How do you create a state patient safety team to accomplish such a project? This process is applicable to any group of physicians and multidisciplinary team members working together with a patient focus. The first challenge was to create the core team. Nancy Ridley, with her extensive experience in government as Associate Commissioner of the Department of Public Health (DPH), set the tone of the deliberations by establishing the confidentiality of this new patient safety center. Her media savvy carried us through the initial flurry of the press wanting to be involved in every step of the process. The press, of course was interested, because there were 6 deaths in a 6-month period in Massachusetts, that had already received some media attention.

The Massachusetts Board of Registration in Medicine (BORM) has a confidential reporting system handled by the Patient Care Assessment (PCA) committee. This is an early-warning system for data coming into a state agency that monitors and identifies when something's going wrong in patient care and safety—something that needs to be analyzed. Through confidential reports from hospitals, the system identified weight loss surgery as an area of concern.

Once you have identified an area of concern, an independent task group must be formed because what follows will be an extensive effort. The BORM doesn't have the resources or expertise to do this properly, so we formed a team under the auspices of the Betsy Lehman Center for Patient Safety to take an in-depth look at the issues. In forming the team, a practicing physician was needed to lead the effort, but there was a lot of controversy involving who should be the chair. A surgeon, as head of the task force, could be seen as biased toward surgery. An internist could be seen as favoring noninterventional care and discouraging surgery. By having an anesthesiologist who is involved in the pre-op assessment of patients, as well as the risk assessment, perioperative period, and post-op care, we had somebody who could drive this process straight down the middle without bias and all points of view would be heard.

**Here are the Team Members:**

Dr. George Blackburn, MD, PhD, has spent his entire professional career in the area of surgical nutrition and obesity surgery, and has extensive national and international contacts. He really was the content expert for this process. Dr. Frank Hu, MD, MPH, PhD, is a world-class clinical epidemiologist at the Harvard School of Public Health. He instituted a rigorous literature search and evaluation of the literature process. We knew when we finished that this literature- and evidence-based task force report would be applicable to any group of patients in any state, as well as internationally.

Lori Bassinger, RPh, JD, was our project manager. Both a pharmacist and a lawyer, she had previous experience with the DPH in medication safety projects, so she knew the DPH process and was already part of a working team at DPH.

Elizabeth Fitzpayne, AB, DipLib, our librarian, was outstanding. She's the librarian with the Countway Library of Medicine at Harvard. She was able to offer her expertise in superb literature research and was involved in every step of the process. I've never seen a medical librarian contribute so much to such an important project.

Rita Buckley was the medical writer and editor of the final project, who managed to get uniformity across all the group reports.

As noted, the confidentiality of the task force was an extremely key issue, because we could not have functioned as a group if the media had been involved in every step of the process. This group was formed in response to patient deaths, thus, it is easy to imagine how intensely the media was interested in the project.

A conscious decision was made to only look forward. To look back at the cases that had already happened could mean compromising the court process in which many were still involved. Discussing the specifics of these cases, the group agreed, would have opened up our information for discovery, so we determined to just integrate what we knew had happened during those events into a forward-thinking, patient-safety–system improvement for the future. This emphasizes the advantage and importance of a statute-protected patient-safety center. Take a look at your protections for confidential, peer-reviewed, health-improvement systems in your own state. If your state doesn't have a statute-protected patient-safety center, it is important to have one established. It will enable your state's physicians and practitioners to work together, analyzing data and using a literature-based systems approach to improve patient safety.

Here at Betsy Lehman, we created a core panel of 24 members. We were trying to get our arms around all practitioners involved in the multidisciplinary care of weight loss surgery patients. We included the disciplines of surgery, internal medicine, anesthesiology, nursing, nutrition, psychiatric care, pediatricians, and educators. We also included hospital CEOs, which proved to be a wonderful step. Just as we've done in the patient safety movement, these represent the people who create the environment that will allow you the resources and the focus to improve patient safety and all systems of care. By involving the CEOs of Berkshire Medical Center, Bay State Medical Center, University of Massachusetts Medical Center, Newton-Wellesley Hospital, and Brigham and Women's Hospital, we gained important input and buy-in. Hospital risk managers and ethicists were also important members of the team. It was also critical to get health plans to buy-in, so we enlisted Dr. John Fallon, chief medical officer at Blue Cross Blue Shield, as well as key personnel from Harvard Pilgrim Health Care. We wanted the health insurance industry to see how we make critical decisions in medicine—not arbitrary coverage decisions that are pulled out of a black box, but evidence-based decisions that are applicable to all patients in all health plans.

We included the BORM Chair, Dr. Martin Crane and former members of BORM in our group. Because the PCA division of the BORM was the early warning system, we wanted the continuity of information—what they had discovered—and also their support throughout this process.

We also had a consumer representative to make sure we had the important perspective of the patient. The Coalition for the Prevention of Medical Errors is our statewide patient safety coalition. In Massachussets, we're fortunate to have some of the best working relationships in the healthcare sector combining to foster and ensure patient safety. The Coalition was our external group and reviewer, overseeing this process to make sure we were doing it right.

It was amazing in the first meeting that we were able to come up with a patient-focused mission statement using evidence-based recommendations for improving safety and well-being in weight loss surgery patients. Once everyone on the team had that focus, people who are usually economic competitors—you know, "My weight loss program is better than your weight loss program"—coalesced and worked together. It was important in the change-management process, with the pressure of media oversight, that everyone recognize something needed to be done. It drives change when you have great external urgency and need to work together.

What is the literature on patient safety for weight loss surgery? What are the real risks and how can we improve this care for patients? These were the questions we knew we must address in order to develop the system-based approach we wanted—one that would advance patient care based on the medical literature, reduce unnecessary variability, and improve surgical and patient outcomes. All healthcare centers across the Commonwealth, we were confident, would buy into and benefit from these literature-based recommendations, and they would be amplified to all 50 states and internationally. This wasn't just for academic programs. It was for everybody.

We had to get our arms around the scope of the project. Reviewing the weight loss surgical procedures to identify safety issues, we wanted to recommend specific concrete steps to improve patient safety and reduce medical errors. We would identify good existing studies, find literature with clinical guidelines and best practices, and be able to build on top of those. Identifying directions and areas for future research, we could direct research funding and investigative attention to where it would have the best effect. We left the most controversial issue—providing recommendations for credentialing and training providers—as the last topic, because we wanted people to first agree on the "easy" topics, the literature focus. Then, when the controversy came, you had already built a team with a shared perspective—you could tackle that difficult credentialing issue with confidence.

The 9 task groups were formed, and these followed pretty much the functional divisions in a hospital or an obesity surgery center. The groups were named as follows: surgical care, criteria for patient selection and multidisciplinary care, patient education/informed consent, anesthetic perioperative care and pain management, nursing perioperative care, pediatric/adolescent care, CEO/facility resources, coding and reimbursement, and data collection/registries and future considerations. The internal scaffolding was that each task group would analyze the literature according to 5 common criteria: patient safety recommendations, strategies for medical error reduction, strategies for system improvement implementation, needs for credentialing systems and practitioners, and research needed for the future.

For the task-group formation we took the data from the DPH database of hospitals doing the procedures and the volume at each center. Based on the Pareto principle (i.e., the 80-20 rule), we knew that we had to include 80% of the centers and people who use a system of care if we wanted change. We listed the highest- to lowest volume centers, and drew a line at the 80% inclusion level. In fact, there seemed to be a clear cutoff below this line: those centers below the line had only a handful of bariatric surgery cases each.

The 9 task groups included people selected from the centers in the 80% group, choosing from the different disciplines, as we wanted to create a social network across the state. By sharing information and working together in this process improvement, they would be more inclined to benchmark and keep in continued contact with this social network for their ongoing educational efforts. For example, the surgical care group could take the findings from the task group and present grand rounds at their own or other in-state institutions, or nationally. The message would be similarly amplified with each functional task group. The core group, leaders, and subgroup members totaled 94 statewide. We used electronic communications extensively, as well as coordinating face-to-face meetings for establishing the initial mission, organizing the groups, and analyzing the literature with the methodologists. We did the same with group presentations, using the other groups as a coordinating function and internal control, and using the Coalition for the Prevention of Medical Errors throughout as an external check on our process and recommendations.

Patient selection and multidisciplinary care was a large group. As we progressed, it became clear that we needed to split off to a separate report on the psychological evaluation and care of these patients. Patient education/informed consent was an amazing group, which, under the protections and with the confidence of the Betsy Lehman Center, was able to go to the centers doing bariatric surgery in Massachusetts and get them to share their pre-op patient education and their informed consent forms. We had samples from all across the state and we could see the variability. This group created one template for preoperative education and informed consent, in which key elements were identified, a template that will hopefully reduce medical liability risk in the state by providing an informed consent format all can follow.

The anesthetic perioperative care and pain management group pursued a key issue as many of the deaths that were reported occurred in the perioperative and post-op period. The nursing perioperative care group was challenged when, looking at the literature, it found very little to coordinate its effort. This was a significant group that approached all nursing organizations in Massachusetts and nationally to see what was being done, but not being published. They worked to amplify the best practices identified, to define what research is still needed and to develop ways to form the best nursing teams.

As for the pediatrics/adolescents group, we had phenomenal people at Boston Medical Center and Children's Hospital who were able to define the literature and make best-practice recommendations for pediatric and adolescent patients. The facility resources group where, as mentioned, the CEOs were in charge, made excellent best facility and hospital leadership recommendations. The coding and reimbursement group studied and recommended important measurement systems that we must have in the future. As we reviewed the existing coding, we found much that was not descriptive of current procedures. Descriptive, accurate coding is vital in order to identify data and best practices. This group came up with recommendations that were taken nationally to the American Medical Association, not only for the CPT coding process (the description of procedures performed), but also for the Relative Value Update Committee (RUC), which looks at the intensity of work, the valuation, and the reimbursement for physician services. The data collection and registries group tackled uniform data collection on the state and national level, as well as among the national specialty groups like American College of Surgeons (ACS), so that we are all measuring using the same standards.

Again, we had the 24 people in the original task group, which then amplified to 94 with all the subgroup members. Each subgroup had a coordinating person from the core group. Meetings were not only constructive, they were fun, with the "inner" table of the core group allowing participation and input to come from any of the other subgroup members at the "outer" table. This is very similar to the RUC process for national physician payment policy, a committee I served on for 5 years. The format works well, with the inner group recognized and working together almost as if in a fishbowl. The outer group sees everything that's going on in this transparent process and is able to comment. This style of interactive meeting allows for validation as you progress, and to check with your peers, asking, "Are we on track?"

Progress reports, as I mentioned, were made to the whole group tapping the subgroup members for feedback. The Coalition for the Prevention of Medical Errors was invaluable as an external advisory group. By statute, the Coalition is the group overseeing the Betsy Lehman Center itself; by attending the meetings, its members could validate that the process was open, transparent, data-driven, and that what would result from the process would be excellent recommendations to be implemented statewide.

We started the process in February 2004. The executive report with the task group recommendations was made available in August 2004, and it was immediately put online. Medical writer Rita Buckley, working with the subgroups, completed the editorial process and the executive report was published in February 2005. It includes an initial executive summary and the 10 subgroups' literature-based reports.(1)

Our goal was to have this amplified to all 50 states. In fact, it is being used by specialty societies such as the ACS, and the American Society for Metabolic and Bariatric Surgery in determining the criteria for their Centers of Excellence, and it is also being used internationally. We're trying to reduce the unnecessary variability in systems of care for weight loss surgery patients, involving a continuous improvement process on state and national levels, of measuring and benchmarking. The specific recommendations are as listed in the report. It is available electronically on the Web site *www.obesityresearch.org*. It's far easier to amplify and implement best practice recommendations in electronic form than in a paper-based format. Elizabeth Fitzpayne, our librarian, along with members of our task force, is continuously monitoring the medical literature for new information to be applied as updates to this evidence-based report. An update will soon be published.

In conclusion, this was an incredible process, performed in a short time frame. The groups came together initially in a sequential and then parallel process, where each group worked with the medical librarian, clinical epidemiologist, task group chair, and members—always using the 5 key questions as the internal framework. Developing the report was one of the most delightful and well-focused, professional efforts of which many of us had ever been a part.

If we can get measurement systems for weight loss surgical care, if we can measure its quality and effectiveness, we can improve upon it. This is why the data collection to standardize criteria and updating is so important within the social network formed as part of this project, working with colleagues across the state, we were able to benchmark against each other to determine what could be the best practices. By involving more than 80% of the centers in the state, it's possible to change a system of care for the better. We've developed some of the best patient-focused working relationships in Massachusetts simply by asking, "How can we improve systems of care for patients? How can we strengthen the doctor-patient relationship? What is the best education and best informed-consent procedure for patients?" We want patients and physicians to be informed, and to strengthen the key decision-making processes between them.

**References**

1. Blackburn GL, Hu FB, Harvey AM. Evidence-based recommendations for best practices in weight loss surgery. *Obes Res*. 2005;13(2):203-4.

# Ensuring the Safety of the Bariatric Surgery Patient

Thomas R. Russell, MD, FACS

In recent years, patient expectations that surgeons provide flawless care have greatly increased. At the same time, we as physicians have been presented with patients who tend more and more to be in poor health. This issue is especially common in bariatric surgery, where patients often have diabetes, high blood pressure, respiratory problems, and certain types of cancer.

As we head into the future, it is likely that ever-increasing numbers of operations will be required to prevent illnesses that genetics determine certain patients will be susceptible to developing. Similar procedures have been performed in the past, but again, the stakes are now higher as we're operating on more sickly patients.

There is no margin for error. Hence, we are being forced to more closely scrutinize what we do and ask why problems arise and how we can best ensure the well-being of our patients. Truth be told, there is nothing particularly revolutionary about this concept. It dates back to 1906, when Dr. Avery Codman postulated that all surgeons should look at how they perform procedures and analyze their outcomes. He called it the "end-results idea." Dr. Codman had the foresight to predict that this concept would not receive widespread acceptance and would not culminate in any plan of action for several generations. Well, here we are, 4 or 5 generations later, talking about the same notion albeit in different terms. Today we don't call it the "end-results idea." Instead we use terms like "outcomes analysis" and "quality assurance." Nevertheless, we are still seeking to answer the same question Dr. Codman posed, namely, *How do we reliably evaluate the safety and efficacy of what surgeons do?*

In another chapter of this book, Dr. David Flum has highlighted the difficulties of data collection and the potential for inaccuracies. This is the dilemma we are facing. Resolving these issues requires rigorous research and much review and discussion. There are no simple solutions.

### Why do Errors Occur?

Fueling public demand for improved patient safety was a published report entitled *To Err is Human: Building a Safer Health System*, put out several years ago by the Institute of Medicine. It noted that up to 98,000 deaths occurred annually in our hospitals due to medical errors. Whether that figure was correct or not, whether it was an over- or underestimation, remains debatable. But the intriguing concept this report introduced was that medical errors are caused by bad systems, not by fallible or "bad" people. This proposition is having a truly transforming effect on how we perceive and discuss patient safety. Five or 10 years ago, most of us were not thinking or talking about systems of care. We were blaming medical mistakes on the bad physicians, the inadequately trained surgeon, or the negligent anesthesiologist. We weren't looking at systemic problems.

This new way of thinking about medical errors is rooted in cognitive psychology, which shows that erring on occasion is normal human behavior and that the causes of errors are observable in the ways our hospitals function; that human error results from latent, environmental factors. Errors are the result of habits, interruptions, haste, fatigue, and stress—all the individual stressors that develop in response to our surrounding conditions. When these are allowed to fester, people experience anger, anxiety, boredom, or fear, which in turn increases their potential for making mistakes. Poor working conditions, long hours, overstaffing, inconsistent training, flaws in the design and maintenance of equipment—all of these factors create the right circumstances for the wrong action to occur.

The great British psychologist, James Reason, likens the situation to Swiss cheese—numerous potential problems in the system (latent errors) begin to align in a certain way so that "holes" develop in the mix, regardless of how many filters are in place. In surgery, these latent errors result in surgical teams operating on the wrong patient, or performing the wrong procedure on the right patient, or otherwise erring in some way during some stage of an operation.

### Changing Surgical Culture

Individual limitations such as poor communication or interpersonal skills, difficulty remembering, personal problems, etc, also lead to error. Maybe a patient gave contradictory information when describing the condition, or the physicians were confused and did the wrong type of operation. These are factors that can be counted as "human error," and are perhaps understandable, but surely avoidable if and when effective systems for catching them are in place.

Over the years, we've learned much from the aviation industry about how human factors affect outcomes. The American College of Surgeons (ACS) frequently invites airline pilots to speak at meetings about crew resource management and what pilots have learned through their experiences. Their observations and suggestions include the recommendation to avoid reliance on memory; to simplify and standardize procedures; to use restraint in forcing functions; to use protocols and checklists; and to avoid long hours and sleep deprivation, always matching workload to capacity.

Until only a few years ago, the concept of reducing work hours and workloads was unheard of in the medical arena, especially in residency training. Previously, it was considered that, as there were 168 hours in a week and the residents lived at or near the hospital, a 120-hour workweek was acceptable. In addition, residents and attending physicians were typically subject to an environment muddled with excessive workloads, double shifts, and high patient-staff ratios. Personnel functioned within an established hierarchy with autocratic leaders whose authority went unquestioned. This atmosphere led to a lack of teamwork, respect, and trust among health professionals and to "shaming and blaming" specific individuals when errors occurred. Now, however, our increased understanding of cognitive psychology has helped us to get our arms around some of the issues that we must address before we will be able to build safer healthcare systems.

**The ACS Response**

What we are witnessing is a sea change in the approach to safety and quality in patient care. Since its beginnings, the ACS has sought to ensure patient safety, hence the gracing of our seal with the phrase *omnibus per artem fedemque prodesse*—to serve all with skill and fidelity. This was our guiding principle in 1913 when the organization was established, and it remains that guiding principle today. Nonetheless, the renewed public focus on safety in the last few years has had a significant impact on everything we do at the College. From education to advocacy, from research to member services, we're involved at every level and as engaged as possible.

**Patient-safety Activities**

We are looking at the multiple factors affecting the healthcare environment and possibly impeding surgeons' ability to provide safe care. For example, because of the current liability climate, many healthcare professionals are afraid or reluctant to report near misses or mistakes, or they are actively resistant to reporting these. Their unwillingness to meet this responsibility acts as a deterrent to systems improvement. Such roadblocks to optimal patient care are discussed in a book that the ACS has published entitled, *Surgical Patient Safety: Essential Information for Surgeons in Today's Environment.*

In addition, the ASC has also worked with other groups, such as the Joint Commission (JCAHO), to develop protocols for ensuring that procedures are performed on the correct patient and the correct site, using the appropriate techniques. These guidelines are now being applied in hospitals across the nation. Needless to say, developing and implementing these standards has been a relatively simple and common sense process. The idea of taking time out before an operation to get the whole team together to make sure everybody understands the procedure and that we are operating on the right patient, on the correct side, in the right way, is a step in a positive direction. When we start developing guidelines for the more complicated aspects of surgical care in the future, the difficulty of reaching conclusions undoubtedly will increase proportionately.

**Trauma and Cancer Care**

The ACS also intends to enhance its reputation as a resource for the optimal care of trauma and cancer patients. Its Advanced Trauma Life Support® (ATLS®) program uses evidence-based medicine to teach healthcare professionals how to best care for the injured patient. Surgeons and allied health professionals around the world have undergone ATLS training and as a result, countless lives are saved every year. In addition, our committee on trauma verifies Level 1, 2, and 3 trauma centers and operates the National Trauma Data Bank®, a clearinghouse for causes of traumatic injury and the assignment of appropriate treatment.

Likewise, the ACS Commission on Cancer (CoC) started an approval program about 20 years ago that accredits cancer programs throughout the United States. More than 1,450 U.S. programs (which make up the majority of this country's cancer treatment programs) have received CoC accreditation. This total represents a small percentage of hospitals; however, those facilities add up to where about 80% of all major cancer surgeries are performed.

The ACS operates the National Cancer Data Base (NCDB), which tracks several million cases of cancer annually. Approximately 17 million patients are currently monitored through this repository. We believe the NCDB will prove a rich source of information that we will be able to mine in generating best practices and guidelines for application in a more systematic approach to cancer treatment.

**Quality Improvement Activities**

To further advance efforts to develop best practices for surgery, we borrow an approach from the Veterans Affairs (VA) healthcare system. The American College of Surgeons National Surgical Quality Improvement Program (ACS NSQIP) is aimed at promulgating risk-adjusted outcomes data on patients who have undergone major operations. The VA used this type of information to establish protocols in their hospitals, which resulted in significantly decreased mortality rates. The ACS is moving NSQIP into the private sector in anticipation of helping nonfederal hospitals analyze outcomes data and see how they compare with those of other medical centers. We believe NSQIP will ultimately be a powerful resource for improving surgical care.

At this time, NSQIP's risk adjustments are based on 52 preoperative, 15 intraoperative, and 33 postoperative variables. Hospital participation in NSQIP has involved substantial up-front costs (approximately $100,000 per year), but by helping to prevent major postoperative wound complications such as pneumonia or cardiac difficulty, the long-term savings will be well worth this initial investment.

The Centers for Medicare and Medicaid Services (CMS) is very interested in ACS NSQIP, and has indicated that it will incorporate it into the National Surgical Quality Improvement Program. This may influence physician reimbursement levels under Medicare as CMS moves ahead with plans to institute pay-for-participation and pay-for-performance policies.

For obvious reasons, the ACS considers NSQIP to be a long-term project. If it were possible to turn on a switch and suddenly improve patient care, we would have done so long ago. This project and the many other developing federal and organizational programs aimed at evaluating outcomes and improving quality of care demand a consistent and collaborative effort on the part of all stakeholders.

To further improve the quality of surgical care in this country, we need to start using the evidence gathered through clinical trials to produce best practices. Currently, the ACS conducts clinical trials in cancer care through the American College of Surgeons Oncology Group (ACOSOG). We must also manage clinical trials in hernia repair and foresee testing new technology and procedures for safety and effectiveness. Little research into the use of the laparoscope for gallbladder removal was done in the 1980s, although it was a defining moment in minimally invasive surgery. Laparoscopic cholecystectomy almost immediately became the standard of care, even though few clinical trials were conducted to determine its safety or efficacy. In the future, however, such innovations are likely to receive far more rigorous review and be promulgated through evidence-based education.

**The ACS Bariatric Surgery Program**

With respect to promoting safety for bariatric patients, the ACS has instituted a program for accrediting centers where these procedures are performed. To implement the program, we reviewed the literature, consulted with experts in bariatric surgery, developed standards, defined necessary resources, organized the means to collect data, and implemented guidelines for conducting site visits.

Bariatric centers that attain ACS approval must have certain resources in place. These include appropriate medical personnel, standards of practice, and means of documenting outcomes. High-volume institutions that have the physical resources and medical personnel necessary to safely and effectively manage the most complex and challenging cases are classified as Level 1a and 1b bariatric centers. Level 2a and 2b centers provide high-quality care to a lower volume of patients, who are less obese and have fewer comorbidities. In addition, the ACS recognizes outpatient bariatric centers that implement stipulated standards, maintain appropriate physical resources and medical personnel, and document their outcomes.

**Related Activities**

The ACS also is considering how it might evaluate overall systems of care. Currently, the Joint Commission rates institutional approaches to care, but doesn't definitively examine systems of care as they correspond to the overall treatment of surgical or medical patients. As a result, a real void exists in our ability to determine what approach, by which professionals, will yield the safest treatment in bariatric, breast, pediatric or geriatric surgery, or any other surgery.

Another important issue at this time is maintenance of certification and licensure for physicians. It has become apparent that successfully passing one's boards after completing surgical training does not guarantee a lifetime of competent performance. The primary emphasis of the ACS has been on surgical training—making certain that surgeons can meet the challenges of today and of the future. We recognize that surgical education is a lifelong commitment, and we are looking for ways to ensure that surgeons can remain competent throughout the 30- to 40-year career span of an active, busy professional. As the demand for physician accountability increases, surgery as a discipline must become involved in setting criteria for competent performance and ensuring that its practitioners recommit to continuing professional development. To satisfy such requirements, the ACS Program for Accreditation of Education Institutes was launched. This program certifies regional and local education institutes offering cutting-edge programs that address core competencies.

**The Surgeon's Role in Systems Safety**

Ultimately, it is the surgeon who is responsible for ensuring that the perioperative team delivers safe care. It is the surgeon who supervises and approves the series of events required and supervises the handing off of patients at various stages of major operations such as bariatric surgery. In the operating room, it is the surgeon who deals with anesthesia and with the fact that some anesthesiologists attend to the patient preoperatively, while others attend intraoperatively or postoperatively. Similarly, the nurses who care for patients before a procedure differ from those who do so inside the operating room. These constant hand offs create the right environment for something to go terribly wrong. Hence the surgeon must be involved and informed throughout each step of the process—from the time the patient is diagnosed with a surgical disease until the moment of that patient's hospital release.

Thus, we must standardize, simplify, and specialize our systems. Of course, the system of greatest importance to bariatric surgeons is the operating room, which is often misunderstood and highly complex. We, as part of the surgical team, are major stakeholders in the quality of the operating room function; therefore, we should have a major role in its design and management. In this way, we can ensure the safety of our patients, and offer the greatest chance for optimum surgical outcomes.

# ACS Bariatric Surgery Network

R. Scott Jones, MD

As the director of the American College of Surgeons (ACS) Division of Research and Optimal Patient Care, I would like to tell you a little about our work. This division of the College encompasses trauma programs, cancer programs, the Surgical Research and Perioperative Care Committees, and a large component called the Section of Continuous Quality Improvement. In that section we deal with evidence-based surgery, outcome studies and clinical trials, and quality improvement occupies a great deal of our time and energy. A few years ago, we developed an overall scheme that guides our approach, which I will review briefly.

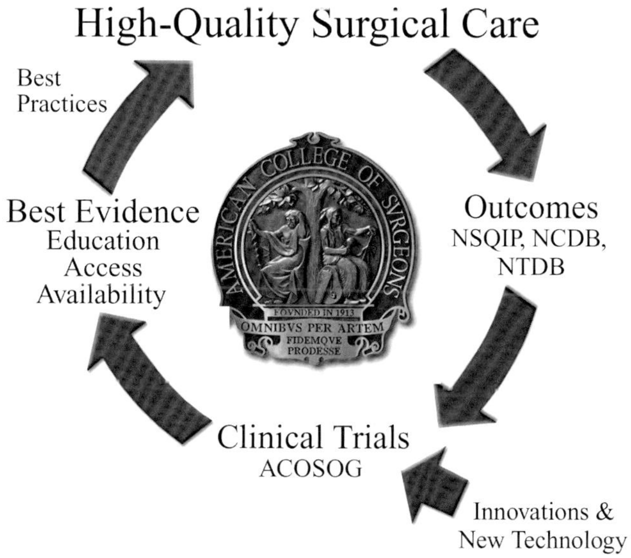


This overall approach to surgical quality improvement addresses the processes and outcomes of care and the introduction of new knowledge and technology. Our goal is to facilitate the application of best evidence into surgical practice. The first challenge was to identify best practices. We have identified more than 3,000 clinical guidelines and are editing those to find the ones with scientific validity and relevance to surgical practice. Then translating the best evidence into practice presents another challenge. Publishing guidelines in journals or putting them on the Internet is an ineffective way to get them into practice. The most effective way to get best evidence into practice is to develop disease-oriented specialty centers that incorporate guidelines into the structure of the center. Improving quality of care requires including evidence-based practices into the processes of care. In addition to application of best practices into these processes, surgical quality improvement requires documenting the outcomes of care. For that purpose, the ACS maintains three major databases, the newest of which is the American College of Surgeons National Surgical Quality Improvement Program (ACS NSQIP). This program has existed in the Veterans Administration (VA) for approximately 10 years and we had the opportunity to collaborate with the VA to move the program into the private sector using a 3-year grant from the Agency for Healthcare Research and Quality (AHRQ). We tested the NSQIP methodology in 18 hospitals and it worked operationally and methodologically. Over the 3-year study period, surgical morbidity fell by a statistically significant 10%. For that reason, the ACS offered this program to any interested private sector hospitals.

At the ACS, we operate the National Cancer Data Base (NCDB), which has records on more than 17 million cancer victims and dates back to 1986. We are working diligently to make the NCDB more relevant to quality improvement and to relate outcomes to episodes of care. We also manage the National Trauma Data Bank (NTDB), which is a little younger and has 1.5 million patient records. So we are very serious about applying outcomes, particularly risk-adjusted outcomes, to surgical care.

Much reference is made to the US Food and Drug Administration (FDA), whose main responsibility, of course, is drugs. The FDA also regulates devices, but it focuses more on safety than efficacy when evaluating devices. We have a professional responsibility to verify that new operations and new devices are both safe and effective before we put them into clinical practice. To do this, we need to develop a much more robust system of clinical trials for evaluating safety and efficacy of devices. The college has spun off a program called the American College of Surgeons Oncology Group (ACOSOG) funded by the National Cancer Institute (NCI). Our division works very closely in collaboration with ACOSOG to support clinical trials in surgical oncology. In addition, we are working to expand clinical trials for nononcologic, surgically treated diseases.

In brief, these matters comprise our mission: defining best practices, defining processes of care, measuring outcomes with scientific rigor, and introducing new technology into clinical practice. The things I have described briefly are in place in the ACS today. Obviously, some are rudimentary and some are fairly well developed; but our goal is to continue to develop these activities during the next several years.

The ACS has supervised, organized, and managed trauma centers for many years. There are more than 200 such centers in the United States operating under the aegis of the Committee on Trauma of the American College of Surgeons. The centers are stratified into Level 1, Level 2, and Level 3, according to the intensity of care provided. In addition, there are more than 1,400 cancer centers in the United States operating under the auspices of the Commission on Cancer, an organization in the ACS with more than 100 members representing more than 40 professional organizations, including the American Cancer Society. Thus, the trauma and cancer centers have been in place for many years, and we look at them as models for developing centers that require organization and leadership, as well as standards for equipment, buildings, and resources. Surgeons, anesthesiologists, nurses, and other trained personnel manage the care in the centers. Credentialing surgeons is an integral part of bariatric surgery centers and is another important function of ACS.

We also have center stipulations for processes of care, which, with suitable modification, will apply to bariatric surgery centers. Evidence-based guidelines and clinical pathways will direct the processes of care required for center certification. Outcome data will monitor the quality of care provided. Finally, all of the centers will undergo a verification process with a site visit every 3 years. This process has been effective for the cancer centers and trauma centers and in 2005, the Board of Regents of the ACS instructed the staff to develop additional specialty centers in addition to those in cancer and trauma, and to begin with bariatric surgery centers. Those instructions recognized the importance of the current epidemic of obesity in the United States. American Society for Metabolic and Bariatric Surgery (ASMBS) has provided great leadership in this endeavor and has led the way in developing bariatric surgery centers.

We recognize several additional opportunities for developing centers, including breast disease care centers. In addition, a committee of pediatric surgeons developed protocols to incorporate pediatric surgery into the ACS NSQIP. An ACS task force on geriatric surgery is working with the American Geriatrics Society to establish evidence-based processes of care and outcome measurements for standardizing and monitoring surgical care of the elderly.

We approached the development of bariatric surgery centers by reviewing the excellent material currently available from the Betsy Lehman report, the Surgical Review Corporation (SRC) of the ASMBS, the Society of American Gastrointestinal Endoscopic Surgeons (SAGES), and additional literature review of the subject. A group of 12 experts used this background information to establish the standards and operating procedures for ACS bariatric surgery centers. Several of them participated in the Patient Safety in Obesity Surgery program that produced this volume, and they should be thanked for their contributions. The ACS bariatric surgery center standards and operations manual is on the ACS Web site (www.facs.org) for review.

In closing, review of an outline of the ACS bariatric surgery center standards is in order. The committee recommended two levels of care. Level 1 includes larger or tertiary care hospitals with certain standards. The committee noted the problem of access to care for individuals who can benefit from bariatric surgery and that high-quality work can be done in hospitals other than tertiary care hospitals. Providing adequate access to bariatric surgery care will require inclusion of community hospitals as Level 2 centers. All ACS bariatric surgery centers must have approval from the Joint Commission or the American Osteopathic Association (AOA). A Level 1 center must perform 125 primary bariatric surgery operations annually in an organization with a program director, two or more bariatric surgeons, and a program coordinator. Level 1 certification requires at least two American Board of Surgery (ABS) certified surgeons performing 50 or more primary weight loss operations annually. Some centers will require additional ABS-certified surgeons to support the care of bariatric surgery patients. Those surgeons must have evidence that they can manage obesity surgery patients in the absence of a defined bariatric surgeon. Such surgeons and the bariatric surgeons will be responsible for the patients 24/7, 365 days per year.

The fundamental criteria of a Level 2 bariatric center are somewhat less stringent. We recommend that lower-risk patients, such as those with a body mass index <50 $kg/m^2$, may be operated on in approved community hospitals. The Level 2 centers should have performed bariatric surgery 24 months before seeking approval and should do no less than 25 weight loss operations annually.

**American College of Surgeons Bariatric Surgery Centers**

**Services**

- Multispecialty
- Anesthesia
- Recovery
- Critical care
- Operating room
- Emergency room
- Endoscopy
- Minimally invasive surgery
- Imaging services
- Postoperative rehabilitation
- Bariatric surgery for adolescence

The criteria stipulate the services necessary for a center, including certain equipment and facilities required. I emphasize the requirement for a multidisciplinary team to evaluate patients preoperatively to identify suitable candidates for operation.

The designation as a bariatric surgeon requires volume criteria and criteria for continuing medical education. New surgeons coming out of training must have performed 25 laparoscopic bariatric operations during residency or fellowship.

We expect the centers to employ quality improvement programs, a defined patient selection process, patient education with counseling, well-documented informed consent measures, and a standardized discharge process and follow-up plan. The future will bring a greater need for outpatient facilities for bariatric surgery, so we have developed stipulations for standards of care, approval, and evaluation of outpatient bariatric surgery centers.

In summary, the ACS looks at the matter of evidence-based surgery, outcomes, research, knowledge introduction and application, and overall quality improvement as a professional responsibility. The ACS will continue to direct its resources to ensure inclusion of quality and safety into surgical care of the future.

# Understanding Levels of Evidence

David Flum, MD, MPH

Based on the presumption that patient safety in bariatric surgery is a critical issue, two new initiatives were introduced in 2004 by the Surgical Review Corporation (SRC) and the American College of Surgeons (ACS), to establish standards in bariatric surgery. These initiatives include a Center of Excellence designation and an accreditation model approach. The motivation for these programs came from several sources of evidence, including case series, observational trials, reports in the press and medicolegal claims. Almost none of the motivation for these programs was the result of high-level evidence. Seeing that the SRC and ACS programs are linking certification to mandatory, contemporaneous, standardized data collection, these programs have the opportunity to change the paradigm for gathering evidence about bariatric surgical safety.

**Is There Currently a Problem With Safety?**

The title of this book presumes there is a safety problem with bariatric surgery. The problem of bariatric surgical safety needs to be viewed in a broader context of all surveillance for safety in surgical practice. In industries that rely on high-risk operations, such as the aviation and nuclear power industries and chemical plants, the risk of high-impact adverse outcomes needs to be mitigated. In most high-risk industries, complete surveillance of all procedures is at the heart of a system designed to identify all outcomes, understand the root cause of these events, and move through a cycle of understanding, minimizing, and tracking improvements in variability. These industries have recognized variability in adverse outcomes as a major threat to their success. While no such system exists in the surgical community, building one will help to understand if we have a safety issue. In the absence of such a system, we are left with inferior levels of evidence to make inferences.

This lack of a surgical surveillance system needs to be contrasted to other industries in order to really understand the impact of such a system. Since the early part of the 20th century, the aviation industry and federal government has initiated a series of regulations and policies that have proven their worth. When commercial aviation began in the United States, the public was appropriately fearful. In the early 1920s, when the precursor of the Federal Aviation Administration (FAA) began, 30 of the first 40 cross-country mail flight pilots died in flight-related events. When the Air Mail Act was enacted in 1925, the US Postal Service began contracting out its airmail services to various airlines, and a mandatory reporting system was initiated to track these events and learn from them. The level of evidence that the FAA currently uses to maintain air-flight safety is complete surveillance. Today, only one plane in 13 million flights per year will crash (www.transtats.bts.gov). This, in many ways is the product of a system-level approach to both tracking all flights and learning from those that can teach us something about safety. This is not a center of excellence approach, not "I'm a best airline—these are my great results," but a 100% surveillance approach. The public response to these programs has been increased consumer confidence over time.

**Evidence for Safety Issues in Bariatric Surgery**

The medical community suspects there is a problem with safety in bariatric surgery, but it may not be the same problem that the media has suggested. Most surgeons suspect that there is unnecessary variability in rates of adverse outcome between centers and surgeons, and that we don't know all the predictors of adverse outcomes (Figure 1). The medical community has based these opinions on two main assessments, scientific and pragmatic, that have been driving the debate. The pragmatic assessments come from media reports, medicolegal claims, and the court of public opinion. With respect to scientific assessments, there are levels of evidence that range from strongest to weakest.

**Figure 1**

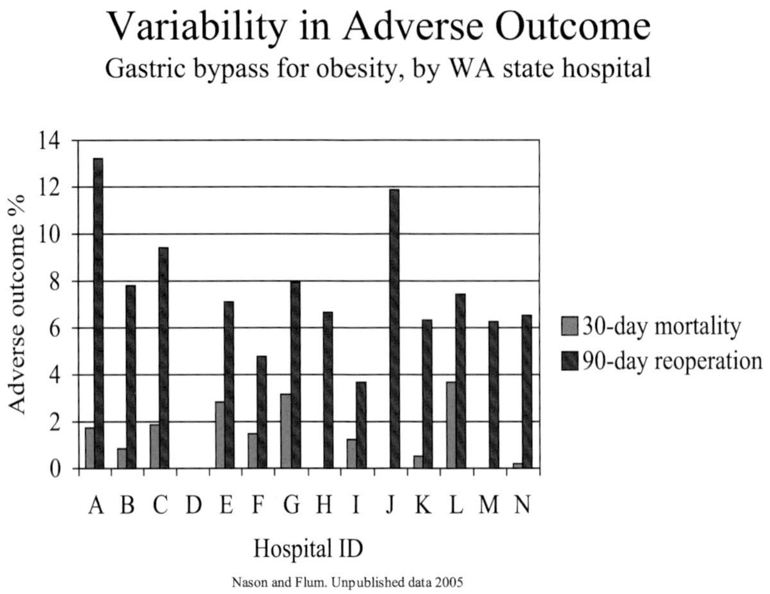


The best level of information about safety would be based on total surveillance of outcomes of all patients undergoing bariatric surgery in the nation. Such a national registry would be tremendously valuable, but does not currently exist and would require a national health service or organized-care–delivery system. Links to multiple Health Maintenance Organizations (HMOs) and Veterans Administration hospitals give a subset of this national surveillance, but represent only a fraction of the whole. Administrative data from large payers or purchasers of health care can also be used to evaluate national outcomes, but these are limited by their construction, the data they include, and the populations of patients they cover.

There is an established hierarchy of evidence for results of bariatric surgery reported by investigators in peer-reviewed journals. The highest level of evidence is repeatedly identified using the highest-level methodology (Figure 2).

**Figure 2**

## Levels of Evidence

- Category A: At least one well-controlled RCT
- Category B: At least one well-conducted prospective cohort study, registry or meta-analysis of cohort studies, or population-based case-control studies
- Catergory C: Uncontrolled/poorly controlled trials, case series, case reports
- Category D: Opinion

US Preventative Services Task Force

The highest level of study is the randomized controlled trial (RCT). If multiple RCTs demonstrate a significant finding, this represents the best level of evidence. Single reports using this best methodology would offer the second best level of evidence. Obtaining repeated findings with a suboptimal methodology is similar to what is available for most issues in bariatric surgery and specifically those related to bariatric surgical safety. The next level down includes single reports with a suboptimal methodology. The lowest level of evidence includes reports based on an individual's experience related through case series and expert opinion. The US Preventative Health Task Force has categorized these tiers of evidence into Category A and B, C, and D together. Category A has at least one well-controlled trial; Category D is opinion. Most often people prefer that scientific decisions be based on this level of evidence (Category A); however, in almost all issues related to bariatric surgery we are making inferences based on Category D evidence.

Since so much of the evidence in the field comes from expert opinion, it is worth considering some threats to validity of this common level of evidence. The strength of expert opinion is based on the strength of the experts selected, their experience and training that constitutes their expertise, and the extent to which that experience may be generalized. Ideally, panels of experts represent a broad group of clinicians from various communities of care: academic and private practice, large and small hospitals, older and younger, conventionally trained and fellowship trained. These panels work best when they utilize formal techniques for distillation of opinions and less well when they are single-setting "roundtables" aiming to garner consensus. One formal technique for data distillation and consensus-opinion generation is the Delphi method developed by the RAND Corporation. This technique involves a systematic approach to considering all available evidence including expert opinion. It is an iterative process of weighing evidence and distilling the strongest components. Since there are many issues in bariatric surgery that because of pragmatic or ethical restrictions will never be addressed using randomized trials, effectively distilling expert opinion is key to driving consensus. A good example of this process at work is the Betsy Lehman Center report on bariatric surgery (Appendix), which employed a Delphi-like method of data gathering, classification, and distillation. That group took advantage of many experts' opinions to help to generate their reports. They were able to evaluate the best levels of evidence including expert-opinion data from clinicians at more than 80% of the hospitals performing bariatric surgery in the Commonwealth of Massachusetts. It is telling that for so many of the domains and metrics of interest, most of the conclusions of the group were based on Category C and D data. Unfortunately, it is difficult to judge the quality of these conclusions, but they are enriched by the heterogeneous nature of the participants, the formalized approach used to distill evidence, and the group's willingness to re-evaluate when challenged by emerging data. Recently, the RAND group itself has applied the more formal Delphi method to the topic of quality indicators in bariatric surgery. As expected, there is overlap in the recommendations of these two groups as both reflect, in large part, expert opinions.

That there are similar conclusions between two groups of clinician experts who distill available evidence (including their own opinions) is both reassuring and a problem. Expert opinion usually reflects common practice and common experiences, but the old adage that common sense is rarely sensible should be considered. For one thing, boosterism (i.e., promoting one's own organization) is a common complaint about expert opinions derived from those who have most to gain from the conclusions they render. Do these panels adequately involve skeptics in the groups or does the definition of an expert include prominence in the field based on publishing or clinical excellence? Unless the group comprising a panel is heterogeneous enough to involve the full spectrum of opinion on a topic, its findings may not be as enriching as would be hoped. Then there is the component of expert opinion that speaks to the ability to be generalized. If a group of academic surgeons talks about academic medical centers, its members' various expert opinions will no doubt be portrayed, but where do those opinions come from and are they relevant in the nonacademic world? Furthermore, these opinions don't develop in a vacuum. They are the product of a training culture that thrives on "this is how I do it" approaches, which are then passed on to trainees. We surgeons train one another, so we should not be surprised to hear that we have similar opinions about things. There is also a group-think problem that people develop in expert-opinion groups, which stifles contrary opinions that may be as poorly supported by data as the conventional opinion but, as an "outlier," doesn't see the light of day in discussions among groups of experts. This is common when there are power differentials in these groups, where senior and junior experts are working together and the typical hierarchy of surgical training and practice invades the panel. Lastly, experts are human and like all of us surgeons, are particularly vulnerable to the "last case syndrome." In this scenario, expert opinion is weighted more heavily by anecdote than evidence. The last bad case is a very powerful influence on opinion and like all of these limitations, needs to be actively addressed by the moderator of these panels. As evidence is interpreted by clinicians and stakeholders, it is important to acknowledge the degree to which expert opinion has influenced the recommendations and the likelihood that the above limitations were addressed.

### Case Series

The next level up for evidence is that which is related to suboptimal methodology that is data (rather than opinion) based. The case series is the way surgeons have communicated experiences to one another for centuries. By convention, the more cases a surgeon reports the more credibility is given to the report. Case reports are not widely considered relevant for those who distill evidence, while the larger the case series and the better the results reported the more it seems the evidence is considered helpful. This concept of "strength in numbers" is not consistently valid. Case series, large or small, do not really help inform the important debate about bariatric surgery. While sometimes these are reported as "observational cohort studies," that term is typically applied when a cohort is followed over time. In higher quality observational studies, questions are usually decided ahead of time and data collected for the purpose of answering the question. In a case series, the temporal sequence is most often revered. The cohort exists, time has passed, questions are asked, and then data about the cohort (most often medical records) are evaluated to answer these questions. These studies are noted by lots of missing data, varying definitions over time, nonstandardized data-collection techniques, and changing patient characteristics in the cohort over time; and they include the biases that come from looking at a single surgeon or single clinical site. This issue of single surgeon/clinical site is relevant because, while that may show variability in the way a procedure is performed over time (i.e., one surgeon can discuss his specific technique for an operation), it can also be problematic. Based on the strength-in-numbers approach, case series are often pooled together to represent a broader experience. The meta-analysis of bariatric surgery published in *JAMA* in 2004 included 136 studies from 91 different populations. While these case series reported on more than 22,000 patients, these impressive numbers obscure the fact that these were essentially dozens and dozens of case series. While the numbers that can be generated with such reviews are influential in the debate, the validity of an aggregated study of case series is no worse—and many times may be worse—than the individual case series. For example, one of the important findings of this meta-analysis regarding surgical safety was that deaths from the most common bariatric surgery, Roux-en-Y gastric bypass (RYGB), occur in about 1 out of 200 procedures. There are several potential problems with this conclusion. The first has to do with sample-size bias in individual repots. For example, in a case series published by a surgeon who has operated on 100 patients without any death, the mortality rate appears to be 0%. A simple statistical rule of thumb is that the upper bound of the 95% confidence interval, when there are zero events in $n$ trials, is 3/n. In this case, the rate of mortality may very well be 0%, but after only 100 patients the upper bound may be closer to 3%—well above the aggregate estimate of 1 in 200. Aggregations of case series rarely consider this variability based on sample size. This is sometimes referred to as the "zero mortality paradox" which says that if a surgeon has never had a death in a series of patients—watch out, it's coming soon. Another way to think of this is that the data from case series are difficult to generalize to the population. If a surgeon has operated on 100 without a death, what does that mean for patient 101? There are also the twin issues of publication and selection bias. These are common in all forms of evidence, but the case series is particularly vulnerable to it. Publication bias is often considered "the best publishing their best." This phenomenon is challenging to evaluate and has many components. It is undoubtedly common in the bariatric surgical literature where there is little incentive and much disincentive to publish results with bad outcomes. When it comes to looking at safety in bariatric surgery, there is a genuine disincentive to publish results that are worse than those previously published. In a competitive commercial environment, this would not be self-serving. Since we still have a "captain of the ship" mentality in surgery, these results are potentially embarrassing and may even expose the center to medicolegal challenges. Generally, people do not make the effort to write up work that is going to put them out of the mainstream—some find it less interesting and it rarely captures the type of investigator interest needed to motivate a writer through the uphill process of creation, revision, submission, revision, and then publication. It can also be difficult to get a study with "out of mainstream" results published in a journal. Editors tend to be even more skeptical about results that deviate from the prior work. Skeptical editor and reviewers question the work, but studies with unexpected results necessarily receive even greater scrutiny. These fundamental limits are at the heart of case series and they get no better through aggregation. Meta-analysis is a technique that was designed for randomized trials to help pull together patients who had similar enrollment characteristics and for whom differences in confounding variables were limited by the randomization process. Conversely, when case series are aggregated using these techniques, the considerable heterogeneity in the populations, the high levels of confounding variables that are differentially found in the groups and the variation in techniques limit the conclusions of the aggregation.

**Observational Cohorts**

The next level of evidence also reflects a less-than-optimal methodology. If completed in a retrospective fashion, the observational cohort study shares many of the limits of the case series. When completed prospectively, the quality of the data gathered is often improved because it can be specified, rigorously defined, and collected in a systematic fashion. Large, prospective, multicenter observational cohorts are currently underway in the United States to understand the relationship between patient and provider characteristics and outcomes. These include both safety outcomes and those related to other domains such as weight loss, quality of life, and healthcare utilization. Data on safety from these multicenter trials will be critical in understanding the relationship of these factors to outcomes.

### Administrative Data

A variant of retrospective observational studies includes the use of administrative data. Administrative data are those gathered most often for billing purposes and, though used to represent clinical care, have a tenuous link at best to the clinical activity actually delivered. There is interest in using these data sets to address clinical questions because billing codes do reflect care received. Outcomes of care can also be evaluated using codes that reflect the discharge status of the patients (died in hospital, discharged to skilled nursing facility) and/or postdischarge status in the few data sets that allow linkage of patients over time (such as the Medicare data set). These outcomes can be evaluated in large populations of patients who live in different geographic regions, states, or the entire nation. Administrative data are also used for evaluating changes in these safety outcomes over time. These data are also used to examine the features associated with outcome such as the age or sex of the patient, surgeon features such as the number of cases performed, or hospital features such as for-profit status. Some administrative data sets can be used to evaluate the use of other associated procedures concurrent to the bariatric surgery admission such as blood transfusions. Unfortunately, most of the components that define the question of safety are not discrete, billable events. In Washington state we evaluated the longitudinal hospital discharge database and found that among 66,000 people who were hospitalized with obesity, nearly 3,000 had gastric bypass surgery between 1987 and 2001. In this series we identified a 2% mortality rate. Although this risk of death is higher than many case series identified during a similar time period (Buchwald, 2004), it corresponds to long-term series by other clinicians. This study also evaluated high rates of inter-hospital variability that seemed to be associated with the number of cases performed at that institution, but these associations are quite limited. Administrative databases do not include information on body mass index, a major determinant of patient outcome, undoubtedly a component of risk (and therefore safety) after surgery. Such limits in the data set undermine the relevance of these data sources in assessments of safety.

### Randomized Trials

The highest level of evidence is the RCT. Randomized controlled trials are the best way to distinguish the effect of the procedure from the confounding effects of patient, hospital, and surgeon features. Randomization is an effective way to distribute measurable and unmeasurable covariates equally between groups of subjects who then receive an intervention. There have been RCTs in bariatric surgery, such as those evaluating open versus laparoscopic surgery and long- versus short-limbed gastric bypass. These RCTs have all been technical studies of the components of the procedures, but none have used safety as an end point. Many have suggested that RCTs of bariatric surgery and nonsurgical interventions that aim to address safety and survival are not ethical. For example, there is little equipoise regarding the safety of surgical and nonsurgical techniques and, in the absence of equipoise, randomization may not be reasonable. Recent studies have even questioned whether or not randomized trials offer benefits compared with observational trials of effectiveness and whether they are adequate for infrequent events such as safety in bariatric surgery. Randomized controlled trials are also impractical for rare events like death after surgery—the ultimate safety issue. In addition, RCTs are not adequate because it may take thousands of patients to look at differences in safety between different interventions.

### Pragmatic Evidence of Safety - Lawsuits

From a medical-legal perspective, some may claim there is a problem with safety in bariatric surgery. Although there is a widespread perception that the number of medicolegal claims is increasing with the growth of bariatric surgery, the evidence behind this statement is limited. These data are not publicly available and there is up to a 5-year lag in claims and the cases they relate to. Many surgeons who have been asked to review medical-legal cases think that there is a growth of these claims, but it is hard to say that there is a problem unique to bariatric surgery. For example, bariatric surgery is not even on the top-10 list of most common procedures that move to litigation. Furthermore, medicolegal claims are not necessarily a marker of negligence related to safety. They often represent adverse outcomes, communication breakdown, or mismatched expectations of risk and benefit. Whether or not there truly is a problem with the safety of bariatric surgery, based on medicolegal claims in at least one state, it has been reported that insurance carriers are closing down coverage of bariatric surgeons. It has been reported that liability related to bariatric surgery or the perception of that liability exposes these companies to too much financial risk. These pragmatic assessments of safety need to be reconciled with scientific evidence if they are to be grounded in truth.

**Challenging Conventional Wisdom**

Even in the absence of high-level evidence to suggest there is a problem with surgical safety unique to bariatric surgery, regulatory and self-regulatory bodies have taken up the mission of making bariatric surgery safer. This includes the American Society for Metabolic and Bariatric Surgery and the American College of Surgeons creating accreditation programs and stakeholders like Medicare and private insurers embracing these programs. In many ways, bariatric surgery is being approached as the cardiac surgery of the new millennium. In the 1990s, cardiac bypass programs, widely perceived as having excessive variability in mortality rates, were given increased scrutiny, regulation, and reporting that ultimately restricted the number and type of centers delivering care. The data that drove this scrutiny was driven by public perception that too many people were dying, begging the question of just how many deaths are acceptable when considering high-risk procedures in sick patients. Regardless of the acceptability of the data that drove this scrutiny, there was a dramatic temporal reduction in the rates of adverse outcomes surrounding cardiac care despite a rising level of case complexity. That scrutiny improved the quality of care for cardiac surgery and it may do the same for bariatric care, but it's important to acknowledge that while the perception of a problem can be a powerful force for positive change, perception alone does not equate to truth. Bariatric surgeons should be aware of the parallel. For example, even if an "acceptable" rate of bariatric perioperative surgical mortality is 0.5%, if one considers all the bariatric surgery performed in the United States from 1990 to 2005 (15,000 to 150,000 per year), then thousands of deaths would be expected to have occurred. People are occasionally going to die after bariatric surgery because it is a high-risk operation in a high-risk population. This may not represent a safety issue as much as a recognized rate of occurrence that is inevitable. Recognizing that others may view this as a safety "problem" and use it as a driver of increased scrutiny of the field will be important in understanding the pragmatic evidence that informs the issue.

**Conclusion**

Over time, the field of bariatric surgery will undoubtedly reduce the associated risk of the procedures, both by selecting patients better, using safer techniques, and creating better systems to deliver care. Just because safety will improve over time does not mean that evidence exists to support a widespread problem in surgical safety today. There may be a problem with safety in surgery, but there is definitely a problem with the quality of evidence that is used to assess safety in surgery. Furthermore, surgeons cannot restore confidence in the system if they cannot assess its safety with confidence. A lack of a complete surveillance system in surgery allows weaker evidence, including media reports, medicolegal claims, and man-on-the-street evaluations, to drive the debate about surgical safety. Thus, implementation of a complete surveillance system will ultimately be the only way to solve the problem of evidence in bariatric surgical safety.

**Suggested Reading**

1. Buchwald H, Avidor Y, Braunwald E, et al. Bariatric surgery: a systematic review and meta-analysis. *JAMA*. 2004;292(14):1724-37.
2. Concato J, Shah N, Horwitz RI. Randomized, controlled trials, observational studies, and the hierarchy of research designs. *N Engl J Med*. 2000;342(25):1887-92.
3. Flum DR, Dellinger EP. Impact of gastric bypass operation on survival: a population-based analysis. *J Am Coll Surg*. 2004;199(4):543-51.
4. Lehman Center Weight Loss Surgery Expert Panel. Commonwealth of Massachusetts Betsy Lehman Center for Patient Safety and Medical Error Reduction Expert Panel on Weight Loss Surgery: executive report. *Obes Res*. 2005;13(2):205-26.
5. Maggard MA, O'Connell JB, Liu JH, Etzioni DA, Ko CY. Sample size calculations in surgery: are they done correctly? *Surgery*. 2003;134(2):275-9.

# Continuing Medical Education

Robin Pearson
Robert Schneider, MSW

With the rapidly evolving nature of the bariatric specialty, it is critical for surgeons and other bariatric specialists to keep current with the latest information about surgical devices, techniques, and pharmacologic agents that are becoming available to help patients cope with the dangerous and defiant disease process of obesity. In this field, as in all fields of medicine, continuing medical education (CME) plays an increasingly important role in helping clinicians not only stay up to date, but maintain their licensure. The EMBRACE™ (Exploring Multiple Bariatric Surgery Research Advances Through Continuing Education) CME initiative, designed to bring together the many disciplines involved in bariatric surgery, sought to do just this.

Currently, 60 state medical boards require an average of anywhere from 12 hours to 50 hours of CME per year for license re-registration.(1) This follows the American Medical Association (AMA) Principles of Medical Ethics, which states that "a physician shall continue to study, apply and advance scientific knowledge, maintain a commitment to medical education, make relevant information available to patients, colleagues, and the public, obtain consultation, and use the talents of other health professionals when indicated."(2)

The AMA has clearly defined CME that meets this commitment as: "...educational activities which serve to maintain, develop, or increase the knowledge, skills, and professional performance and relationships that a physician uses to provide services for patients, the public or the profession. The content of CME is the body of knowledge and skills generally recognized and accepted by the profession as within the basic medical sciences, the discipline of clinical medicine, and the provision of health care to the public."(3) In the field of bariatrics—where a great deal of misinformation and misperceptions surrounding bariatric surgery exists among both patients and physicians—the need for credible, fair balanced, scientifically rigorous educational activities that provide such knowledge is especially important. This is particularly true among primary care physicians, who are often the gatekeepers in the management of obese patients.

To address these issues, SynerMed® Communications, a third-party medical education organization founded in 1984, worked with NAASO, The Obesity Society (formerly the North American Association for the Study of Obesity) to develop an educational initiative—EMBRACE that would offer comprehensive education addressing the management of extreme obesity.

## The EMBRACE™ Educational Initiative: A Case Study

### Developing the Proposal

Following the Accreditation Council for Continuing Medical Education (ACCME) guidelines in developing EMBRACE™, we put together a strategic team that included a scientific director, professional relations specialist, and a project management team to develop a proposal that would address the needs of the larger clinician community, as well as potentially interested professional associations.

The first step in the process was to develop a needs assessment that would appeal to both these associations and a potential grantor (i.e., a commercial supporter who might be willing to fund such a program). This needs assessment document, fully researched and referenced, was based on ongoing discussions with experts in obesity management, along with a review of current literature. Much of what we uncovered and addressed has already been discussed in this book. However, our aim in developing the needs assessment was not just to review the current data, but also to identify unmet educational needs and how they might best be addressed. Our research revealed several treatment issues and specific educational needs:

- Management of severe obesity continues to challenge clinicians
- Diligent, long-term management of severe obesity is critical for successful patient outcomes, yet this is not the norm
- Clinicians continue to request information regarding the impact of pharmacologic therapies and newer surgical treatment modalities in the management of severe obesity

- There is a need to further evaluate current clinical data and explore treatment guidelines that facilitate safe and optimum use of these therapies in this patient population
- An overall misunderstanding of who to treat, when to treat, and the safety vs. therapeutic benefit of newer treatment strategies contributes to the need for education in this area

In addition, we determined that for an educational initiative such as the one we were proposing to achieve its goals and have an impact on the clinician audience, it was crucial to include major medical associations in the project. Their commitment would encourage the various professional specialties involved in patient management of severe obesity to address the challenges that were being discussed. This would necessitate the societies' direct participation in providing education that would be instrumental to both the advancement of innovative treatment strategies, as well as the reinforcement of conventional therapies that continue to improve patient outcomes.

**Offering a Unique Approach**

The involvement of such special-interest professional associations was key to the successful implementation of the EMBRACE™ program—especially for the sponsorship of the initiative. A myriad of universities and independent CME providers exist today who are available for sponsorship opportunities. In addition, a large number of professional organizations are accredited by the ACCME. After reviewing the many possibilities for a sponsor accredited by ACCME, we decided to approach NAASO, The Obesity Society. We thought that NAASO, a highly respected and visible organization with a multidisciplinary membership of individuals who have a clear interest in the topic, was the optimal choice for this initiative.

Our company has a more than 20-year history of working with both the federal government and professional associations in the presentation of educational activities. Our experience has included presenting programs with various National Institutes of Health (NIH) institutes and centers, including the National Eye Institute, National Institute of Allergy and Infectious Diseases, National Institute of Neurological Disorders and Stroke, etc. We have also worked with other federal organizations such as the Department of Health and Human Services Office on Women's Health, the Centers for Disease Control and Prevention, and the Department of Veteran's Affairs in the development of these types of programs. However, NAASO was new to us. Working with thought leaders in the bariatric field, we gained an introduction to the organization, its executive director, president, and educational committee chairman, and presented our proposal. We also provided this group with examples of educational initiatives we had successfully completed in other therapeutic areas with some of the organizations described above. A series of discussions took place, clearly defining our role, along with that of NAASO, and the EMBRACE™ initiative moved forward.

**Approaching Interested Participants**

In today's environment, funds for CME from universities, professional associations, governmental, and nongovernmental, bodies are increasingly limited. Our role as a third-party, medical education provider is often to bring together professional medical organizations with potential funding sources—that is, to demonstrate how the professional medical education needs of these groups may be similar and mutually inclusive. To this end, an unrestricted educational grant is obtained from one or more commercial supporters who may be interested in supporting a CME activity or initiative. SynerMed then works with an accredited CME provider to independently develop the initiative. For the EMBRACE™ project, we approached Allergan Medical (formerly Inamed), the manufacturer of an adjustable gastric band (LAP-BAND®) used in bariatric surgery.

Like many pharmaceutical companies, Allergan has long been a supporter of CME and recognizes that its funding of evidence-based, scientifically rigorous programs allows clinicians to better meet the healthcare needs of their patients. Allergan understood that ACCME guidelines allowed it no role whatsoever in the development of content for the initiative. However, the opportunity to advance the understanding of bariatric specialists and other interested clinicians regarding the continuing developments in bariatric surgery was appealing, and the company agreed to provide an educational grant for the program.

**Continuing Outreach**

With funding provided, and NAASO participating as the CME sponsor, we then implemented the second part of our proposal, which was to involve appropriate, interested cooperating organizations in the initiative. These organizations are professional associations whose membership has an inherent interest in the initiative topic. Research undertaken in the proposal stage identified a number of organizations with an interest in the EMBRACE™ learning objectives, and we approached their leadership via a concentrated campaign of teleconferencing and electronic communication. As we anticipated, the involvement of NAASO as CME sponsor was critical to our approach and was an important factor in helping us initiate discussions with these organizations.

Another key ingredient to involving cooperating organizations in the EMBRACE™ initiative was the quality of the agenda that was developed by the program co-chairs, as well as the potential faculty (Table 1). At this writing, the American Society for Metabolic and Bariatric Surgery (ASMBS), the American Society of Bariatric Physicians (ASBP), the Society for Laparoendoscopic Surgeons (SLS), the Society of American Gastrointestinal and Endoscopic Surgeons (SAGES), the American Association of Clinical Endocrinologists (AACE), the National Association of Bariatric Nurses (NABN), and the American Association of Nurse Practitioners (AANP) have agreed to participate. We are still pursuing the participation of other cooperating organizations, including the American College of Physicians (ACP) and the American College of Surgeons (ACS).

The role of cooperating organizations in an initiative of this kind is a study in contrasts. There can be only one sponsoring organization providing input into the development of the educational activities and its content—in this case NAASO. However, cooperating organizations—in offering educational elements of the initiative to their members—are invited to participate in live events and study enduring materials as both discussants and final reviewers. Their input and final approval is required before any materials with their names and logos can be published.

**The EMBRACE™ Educational Initiative: Program Elements**

The strategy underlying the EMBRACE™ proposal was a comprehensive, credible, scientifically rigorous and evidence-based initiative that would offer multiple activities over several months—and potentially years—to the many clinicians involved in the treatment of severe obesity. These clinicians include not just bariatric surgeons, but also primary care physicians (family practitioners and internists), psychologists, nutritionists and dieticians, nurse practitioners, physician assistants, registered nurses, and program coordinators. Thus, the program needed to be multidisciplinary in scope, encompassing the specific needs of varying specialties. In addition, the activities had to incorporate multiple media and formats in order to address the varied educational learning styles of the proposed audience.

Consequently, along with the initial needs assessment, we developed a series of educational goals and objectives that would appeal to these clinician audiences. These global objectives included

- Encouraging dialogue among multidisciplinary specialists, via evidence-based studies, that explored the efficacy, safety, and therapeutic benefits of both pharmacologic and surgical intervention techniques in the management of severe obesity
- Engaging and expanding the national core of leading experts (including teaching institutions, fellows, and residents) as advocates to identify and address issues relevant to the optimum prevention and management of severe obesity
- Educating bariatric specialists, surgeons, and other healthcare professionals in order to advance the issues on evidence-based decision making and implementation of therapeutic strategies, including bariatric surgery for severely obese patients
- Building advocacy among bariatric surgeons, and obesity specialists in order to facilitate the development of bariatric surgery Centers of Excellence
- Facilitating ongoing scientific endeavors that allow for the optimizing of severe-obesity treatment strategies that maximize short- and long-term outcomes

The EMBRACE™ initiative began in December 2006 with a multidisciplinary scientific roundtable held at the Emory University Conference Center in Atlanta, Georgia. Ten expert faculty members participated under the co-chairmanship of

Marc Bessler, MD, assistant professor of surgery and director of the Center for Obesity Surgery at Columbia University College of Physicians and Surgeons, and Patrick M. O'Neil, PhD, chairman of the education committee for NAASO, The Obesity Society, and professor and director of the weight management center at the Medical University of South Carolina Department of Psychiatry and Behavioral Sciences. Representatives from several of the cooperating organizations, including ASMBS, ASBP, and SAGES, were also in attendance.

The agenda, developed by the co-chairs, covered an 8-hour program that included identifying and defining extremely obese patients and discussing options for treatment, including behavioral and pharmacologic management, as well as bariatric surgery options (Table 2). Critical discussions included risk vs. benefit of the most commonly performed surgeries (adjustable gastric banding [LAGB], Roux-en-Y gastric bypass [RYGB], and biliopancreatic diversion [BPD]); defining successful outcomes; and the resolution of comorbidities via successful bariatric surgery. Aftercare of bariatric surgical patients, including nutrition, band adjustment, and the collaboration of the bariatric surgical team, were also discussed. The purpose of the scientific roundtable was twofold:

- to define the extremely obese patient and ways in which bariatric surgery could best optimize patient outcomes,
- and to generate content for ongoing enduring materials to be included as part of the EMBRACE™ initiative.

A multidisciplinary scientific roundtable such as this provides an opportunity for expert faculty and thought leaders to meet in an educational environment and offer often divergent points of view on the topic at hand. While prepared lectures are key elements of the live event, even more important are the discussion periods, when all faculty members have the opportunity to participate in lively dialogue on the subjects under discussion. This type of "live" event provides a forum for discussion that peer-reviewed articles and enduring materials cannot replicate, and can also introduce both established national experts and up-and-coming faculty to one another in a collegial environment.

In addition, this kind of scientific roundtable offers thought leaders the opportunity to debate ongoing issues in their field. While the goal of this activity is not usually to provide a consensus document, it can bring new thinking to the table and pave the way for the consideration of new clinical trials. In the case of the EMBRACE™ scientific roundtable, the faculty members were treated to hot-off-the-press publications by several fellow participants and were able to discuss ongoing, and as yet unpublished, investigations that were underway.

The EMBRACE™ scientific roundtable also offered the faculty a unique opportunity to discuss a number of issues related to bariatric surgery that will continue to have an impact on patient outcomes. For instance, long-term studies on the outcomes of LAGB have not yet been completed, as this device was only approved by the US Food and Drug Administration (FDA) in 2001 for use in the United States. Hence, there is currently no definitive, long-term comparison between LAGB and RYGB in the United States. However, members of the faculty were able to discuss their clinical experience, available international studies, and their thoughts for the future regarding this issue—which will certainly impact patient outcomes in the long term.

Also, because this meeting occurred under CME auspices, the faculty members were able to discuss off-label uses for the various forms of bariatric surgery. These discussions included bariatric surgery for adolescents (currently, bariatric surgery is approved by the FDA for patients 18 years of age or older) and surgery for patients with a lower body mass index (BMI) (currently bariatric surgery is approved for patients with a BMI $\geq$40 kg/m$^2$, or BMI $\geq$35 kg/m$^2$ with comorbidities). While no recommendations regarding these off-label uses will be made in subsequent enduring materials, the scientific roundtable afforded participants the opportunity to discuss both their clinical experience and future portents.

Among the key discussions were those that addressed potential enduring materials that might be included in the EMBRACE™ initiative, as well as the audience for these materials. Our original proposal to NAASO and Allergan Medical included a wide variety of materials and potential audiences, dependent on faculty input and available funding. However, the expert faculty members of this roundtable and panel were keenly interested in further defining content, potential activities, and potential audiences. Within this context, critical points were raised, including the following:

- Nomenclature. Both patients and physicians often react negatively to the term "morbid" obesity used to define these patients (BMI $\geq$ 40 kg/m$^2$, or BMI $\geq$ 35 kg/m$^2$ with comorbidities). A discussion of other common terminology, including "severe" and "extreme" obesity, was raised.

- Defining outcomes. Published studies look at two different outcomes: percentage of excess weight loss (%EWL) and total weight loss. In measuring outcomes and comparing studies, it is important to determine which outcome is being used and which might be more meaningful to both patient and clinician
- Counteracting negative conceptions regarding bariatric surgery. The popular media, patients, and even primary care physicians may look negatively on bariatric surgery. It is important to continue to define extreme obesity as a dangerous and defiant disease, as much in need of medical/surgical treatment as other disease states

Independent, evidence-based, scientifically rigorous CME is increasingly important for physicians, and especially for bariatric specialists who perform in an often controversial field. It is vital that these specialists—and potentially referring physicians as well—are offered accredited enduring materials and opportunities to attend live events at which discussions of the ongoing issues associated with bariatric surgery are included. Ensuring that they are has the potential to positively impact patient outcomes by providing clinicians with resources that address the multifaceted options available to them.

**EMBRACE™ Scientific Roundtable**

**Robin Pearson**
Senior Director, Project Management
SynerMed® Communications

**Robert Schneider, MSW**
Vice President, Professional Relations
SynerMed® Communications

**PROGRAM CO-CHAIRS**

**Marc Bessler, MD, FACS**
Assistant Professor of Surgery
Director, Center for Obesity Surgery
Columbia University College of Physicians and Surgeons
New York-Presbyterian Hospital
New York, New York

**Patrick M. O'Neil, PhD**
NAASO, The Obesity Society
Chairman of the Education Committee
Director, Weight Management Center
Professor of Psychiatry
Department of Psychiatry and Behavioral Sciences
Medical University of South Carolina
Charleston, South Carolina

**FACULTY**

**Susan M. Cummings, MS, RD, LDN**
Clinical Programs Coordinator, MGH Weight Center
Massachusetts General Hospital
Boston, Massachusetts

**Thomas H. Inge, MD, PhD, FACS, FAAP**
Associate Professor of Pediatric Surgery Cincinnati Children's Hospital Medical Center
Surgical Director of the Comprehensive Weight Management Center
Cincinnati, Ohio

**Daniel B. Jones, MD, MS**
Associate Professor of Surgery
Harvard Medical School
Chief, Minimally Invasive Surgery
Director, Bariatric Program
Beth Israel Deaconess Medical Center
Boston, Massachusetts

**Robert F. Kushner, MD, MS**
Professor of Medicine
Northwestern University Feinberg School of Medicine
Academic Medical Director
Wellness Institute
Chicago, Illinois

**Chris Nelson, MN, RN, FNP-C**
Nurse Practitioner
Surgical Specialists of Louisiana
Covington, Louisiana

**David B. Sarwer, PhD**
Associate Professor of Psychology in Psychiatry and Surgery
University of Pennsylvania School of Medicine
Director of Clinical Services
Center for Weight and Eating Disorders
Philadelphia, Pennsylvania

**Philip R. Schauer, MD**
Director, Advanced Laparoscopic and Bariatric Surgery
Cleveland Clinic
Professor of Surgery
Lerner College of Medicine
Cleveland, Ohio

**C. Daniel Smith, MD, FACS**
Professor and Chairman
Department of Surgery
Mayo Clinic and School of Medicine
Jacksonville, Florida

**CME SPONSOR**

**Robert J. Eckrich, MS, MT(ASCP)SBB**
Director, Education Programs
The Obesity Society
Silver Spring, Maryland

**Table 2**

**EMBRACE™ Scientific Agenda**

| Day 1 | |
|---|---|
| Who is the extremely obese person? | Patrick M. O'Neil, PhD |
| Medical and lifestyle management of the extremely obese patient | Robert F. Kushner, MD, MS |
| Psychosocial considerations in bariatric surgery: preoperative assessment and postoperative changes | David B. Sarwer, PhD |
| Surgical options for the extremely obese patient<br>• Gastric bypass & other malabsorptive surgeries<br>• Gastric banding surgery | <br>Philip R. Schauer, MD<br><br>Marc Bessler, MD, FACS |
| **Day 2** | |
| Bariatric surgery in adolescent patients | Thomas H. Inge, MD, PhD, FACS, FAAP |
| Setting realistic expectations: outcomes for bariatric surgery patients | Daniel B. Jones, MD, MS |
| Optimal bariatric care: pre- and postsurgery | Chris Nelson, MN, RN, FNP-C |
| Nutritional issues facing the bariatric surgery patient | Susan M. Cummings, MS, RD |
| Using a team approach to bariatric surgery (panel discussion) | Moderator:<br>C. Daniel Smith, MD, FACS |

*All presentations include Q&A discussions*

**References**

1. American Medical Association (AMA). State medical licensure requirements and statistics, 2007.
2. AMA Physician's Recognition Award and Credit System, Revised 2006.
3. AMA House of Delegates Policy #300.988.

# Multimedia in Surgical Education

Kevin McGovern

Since the days of the classical surgical theaters of the 19th century, surgical education has been based upon group learning. A senior surgeon or other health professional imparts his/her wisdom to one or more students; and eventually these students do the same with their students. Multimedia images have always played a strong role in supporting the transference of this knowledge. "Learning by seeing" remains at the forefront of surgical education.

One of the earliest surgical books was written by Serafeddin Sabuncuoglu in 1465. This book of pediatric surgery depicted existing concepts of that era, as well as new procedures developed by the author. So began the evolution of the visual image as an important tool in medical education. From DaVinci's early human dissections to the most well-known surgical atlases of the 20th Century by Netter, Zollinger, and others, visual images coupled with meaning, reflection, and understanding by the student have become an integral part of learning by seeing.

Surgical films debuted at the American College of Surgeons Clinical Congress in 1929. Collaboration with George Eastman led to an early recognition of quality in surgical filmmaking. Early films were often geared toward the general public, and shown around the world, to promote health and medical care. In 1950, the Ciné Clinic program was introduced, providing conference attendees the opportunity to see rare cases and new techniques with expert commentary by the surgeons. That program is still providing the same high-level quality of education for today's surgeons.

The introduction of television brought all the elements of motion pictures into the living rooms and work places of the modern world, and in the late 1970s, home video signaled the beginning of the modern communication age. Surgical teaching films viewed on a television, either by individuals or by groups, became a new standard for continuing education.

Today, the modern computer, and with it the World Wide Web, has once again changed the way people communicate and experience various media. Online reference Web sites, targeted, online, video-based education programs, and, indeed, e-mail communications have become the latest form of education and communication for the masses.

As media has evolved, the experience of surgical learning has evolved as well. While participation in surgery or caring for a patient can only be experienced through interaction with others, electronic communication, like the traditional book, allows students to study individually. Such individual learning, however, must be regulated to ensure that the educational content is valid and current.

### Surgical Education: See One, Do One, Teach One

The apprentice model of surgical education remains as strong as ever, with a vast array of distance-learning opportunities available to the contemporary surgical student. Surgical concepts, opinions, techniques, and data are so accessible, it is often difficult to assess their validity. Publishing multimedia, once the domain of specially trained technicians, is now used by much of the general public. Recorded video is particularly suited to laparoscopy, and in fact many operating rooms are equipped with state-of-the-art video production technology. Desktop publishing software makes it easy to create electronic slides, videos, Web sites, and printed publications. With the advent of the computer, Internet, and portable media players, a surgical student has instantaneous access to the precise information he/she is looking for at exactly the time it is needed.

Surgical associations such as the American College of Surgeons (ACS) and the Society of American Gastrointestinal Endoscopic Surgeons (SAGES) have begun to address the issue of validating surgical content through the development of distance-learning materials that are peer reviewed and approved by panels of expert surgeons.

### See One

The surgical atlas is a standard in surgical education. Within it, procedures are described, steps are explained and summarized, and detailed diagrams give visual examples of the written word. Adding a video to the techniques described makes the information come alive for the student. Take it one step further by adding a Web site that includes other viewpoints, commentary, activities, and perhaps a post-test, and the learning opportunities are limitless.

The ACS Video Library is a good example of how multimedia is used to enhance surgical education. Videos included in the library are part of a very unique collection of more than 1,000 titles organized by anatomy, procedure, and surgical technique. The strength of this library lies in the varied authorship of its content and the fact that each video is reviewed by the Committee on Video-Based Education under the guidance of the ACS Division of Education. The videos can be viewed on a variety of formats, including CD, DVD, streaming video, and podcast. Many surgical training programs are using the online version of the library for video lectures and are providing access to residents for independent study. The podcast version is distributed using a similar platform to iTunes. The videos are sorted by technique, e.g., *mobilizing the hepatic flexure* (the "song"), or by procedure, e.g., *right colectomy* (the "album").

**Do One**

While at this time there is no replacement for hands-on clinical experience, there are several skill-building simulators available that can enhance surgical skills and decision-making outside the operating room. Computer-based simulation is promising and, not surprisingly, most of these simulations have focused on minimally invasive procedures such as laparoscopy and interventional cardiology. Once the territory of science fiction, virtual reality (VR) came of age in the mid-1990s using what was then considered state-of-the-art computers. Today's VR systems often use off-the-shelf hardware and laptop computers. True-to-life computer graphics combined with tactile feedback from a human/computer interface has made VR a highly functional training tool. SimSuite® is one example of an immersive experience. Students are presented with a patient scenario and a functional mannequin patient within a catheterization laboratory configuration. Vital signs, ciné imaging, and catheter-based therapies all function in real-time. Immersion Medical produces a virtual laparoscopy simulator, a stand-alone system that provides procedure and skills training and records metrics for data analysis.

One interesting approach to surgical education that does not include computer-based simulation is the SAGES/ACS Fundamentals of Laparoscopic Surgery (FLS). This is a comprehensive curriculum that includes a multimedia-based education prestudy module, a hands-on, skills training component, and an assessment tool designed to teach the physiology, fundamental knowledge, and technical skills required in basic laparoscopic surgery.

The multimedia prestudy program covers didactics, interactive patient scenarios, and manual skills training. It is distributed as a CD-ROM or via a Web site, depending upon the learner's preference. It also includes printable text reviews and practice questions. The FLS Laparoscopic Trainer Box allows the user to practice technical skills and improve dexterity and psychomotor skills. Each skill used is directly transferable to laparoscopic skill and assessed for accuracy and timing.

The goal of FLS is to set the standard for laparoscopic surgery. Surgeons are required to continually document their competency in surgery. The FLS offers surgeons the appropriate tool to assess and document their own knowledge and skills in laparoscopy.

**Teach One**

The ultimate goal of surgical education is to impart sufficient knowledge and skills to surgeons so that they can provide safe and effective surgical care to their patients. Multimedia can have a profound impact on achieving this goal by embracing contemporary educational technologies and incorporating them appropriately into the curriculum of a surgical student in residency and beyond. The broad spectrum of teaching tools available today not only provides individuals with alternative methods of learning, it also expands the opportunities for what can be learned and from whom. There are pearls of wisdom to be gained from the great surgeons of the past and present and many have been captured through video imaging. The technology of today and tomorrow will not only preserve these pearls, but will allow future surgeons to continue learning from them for many years to come.

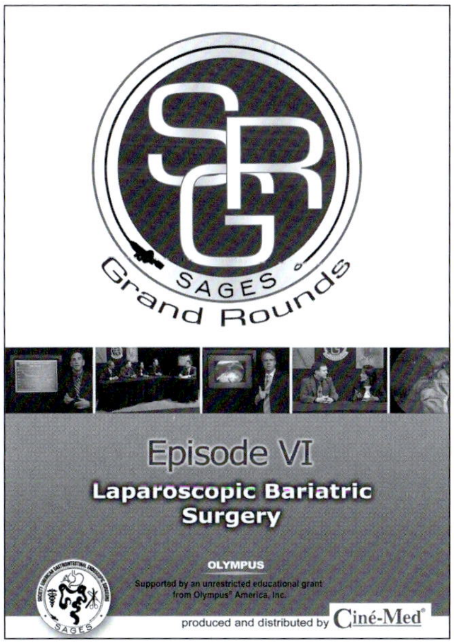
SRG
SAGES
Grand Rounds
Episode VI
Laparoscopic Bariatric Surgery
OLYMPUS
Supported by an unrestricted educational grant from Olympus® America, Inc.
produced and distributed by Ciné-Med®

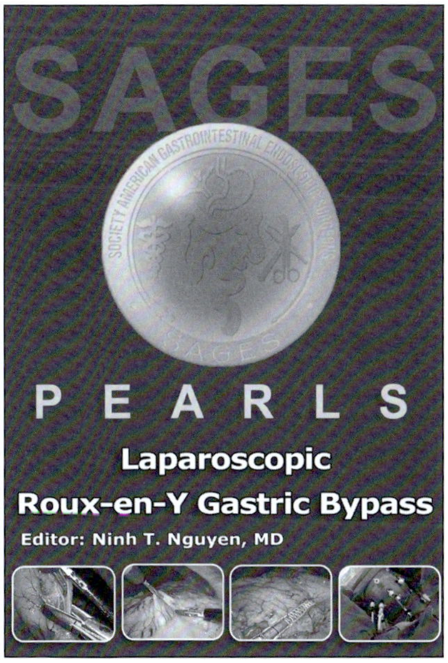
SAGES
PEARLS
Laparoscopic
Roux-en-Y Gastric Bypass
Editor: Ninh T. Nguyen, MD

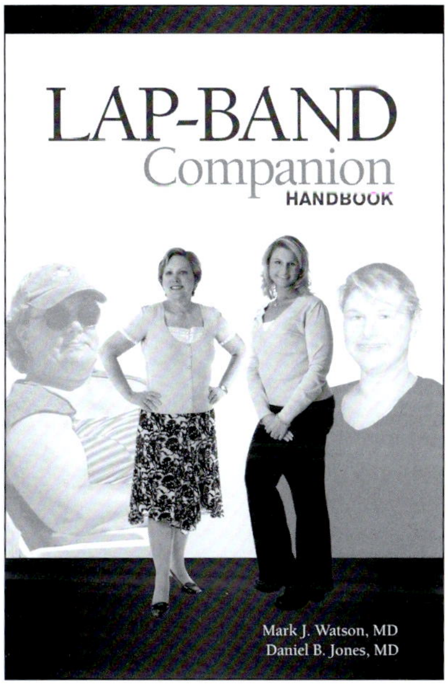
LAP-BAND
Companion
HANDBOOK
Mark J. Watson, MD
Daniel B. Jones, MD

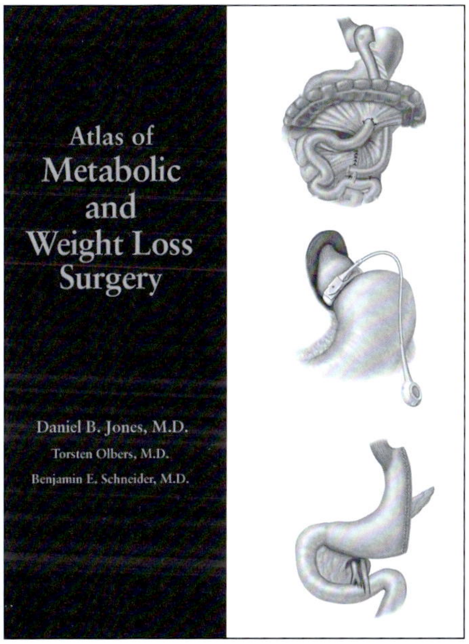
Atlas of
Metabolic
and
Weight Loss
Surgery
Daniel B. Jones, M.D.
Torsten Olbers, M.D.
Benjamin E. Schneider, M.D.

# Nurses: Creating a Professional Standard

Angi Walsh, RN, MA, CNOR

You've been reading about a number of obesity-related topics and are now wondering how I was selected to address the issue of bariatric education (for nurses) in this book. With more than 30 years experience as an operating room (OR) nurse, I have spent a lot of time in the role of preceptor, involved in a variety of specialty procedures and taking great pride in sharing acquired information with nursing colleagues. I spent 5 years teaching health education in high school, college, and community outreach programs, giving me credibility as an educator. Attaining a master's degree in education and critical and creative thinking earned me the ability to zero in on those specific aspects of the job that nurses do best and that add up to patient care.

Nursing has been in existence for many years and for most of that time was depicted as female-specific, with famous heroines such as Florence Nightingale and Clara Barton functioning without "formal education," but rather with on-the-job training.

The first formal training program for nurses was established in 1860, at the Florence Nightingale School in London. It took an additional 13 years for nurse training to come to the United States. In 1873, the first three nursing programs were introduced in the United States: at Bellevue Hospital in New York, New Haven Hospital in Connecticut, and Massachusetts General Hospital in Boston. Johns Hopkins Training School for Nurses became the first university program and opened in 1890.

**The Importance of Bariatric Training**

In order to identify why it's important to train nurses, we must first make a comparison between the didactic patterns that were present in nursing from the mid-19th through much of the 20th century, and the training available today. Early programs gave information to nurses based on previous practice. Now, in the 21st century, nurses are savvier; they want to know why something is important, where you obtain the evidence, what's in it for them, and how to apply the principles to their personal practice.

In preparation for this paper, I reviewed core curriculum requirements and outcome statements for 342 US nursing programs. The majority of programs did not include a course specifically addressing critical thinking skills and most programs no longer include a clinical rotation in the OR. Although both topics may be included as "electives" or built into a certain lesson plan, hands-on skills are an important component of any training program. Many adults have nontraditional learning styles — they want to learn new information by the most meaningful methods available.

There have been recommendations from different governing bodies for physicians who perform bariatric surgery. To quote a recommendation from the American College of Surgeons (ACS):

> "Bariatric surgery should be performed by a team of experienced surgeons, anesthesiologists, nurses, and nutritionists. Recovery room and nursing staff should be specifically trained in the management of the severely obese."

The key word listed in both sentences is "should," not "must." But working in a bariatric perioperative setting is the same as working in the setting of any other specialty, whether it is cardiology or ophthalmology. You don't put someone in a specialty and expect him or her to function at a proficient level. They could probably "wing it," but winging it doesn't produce safe patient outcomes. We have heard bariatric patients' horror stories of staff unaware of sensitivity issues or unable to provide basic care needs such as gowns that fit or furniture that can be used during their hospitalization. Thus, ensuring safe patient outcomes in bariatric surgery is an area that must be addressed during staff training.

**The Dedicated Bariatric Team**

While we do have a support team that begins the screening process for bariatric patients, during hospitalization the patients also have contact with the operating room and anesthesia personnel, nurses in the postanesthesia care unit (PACU), floor nurses, dieticians, and even housekeeping and x-ray transport services. All personnel must be educated on the safe care and handling of bariatric patients, as well as on the sensitivity issues that go along with such patients. Why is this important?

There are many health implications associated with obesity. Obesity does not occur just because an individual is lazy or overeats. It's a health issue that can arise out of heredity, medication use, lifestyle conditions, environment, and many other circumstances. Making negative comments about the obese is one of the few remaining socially acceptable activities based on bias. What then, does the medical staff that may have an obese person in its care need to know? Below is a checklist of subjects and actions with which bariatric care professionals should be familiar:

- Bariatric terminology
- Medical and surgical weight loss options for the bariatric patient
- Health implications of obesity
- Social and psychological impact of bariatric surgery
- Life changes brought on by bariatric surgery
- Dietary considerations for the bariatric patient
- Strategies for assessing the bariatric patient
- Bariatric patient management requirements
- Postoperative complications of bariatric surgery

Prior to giving my presentation at the conference on patient safety in obesity surgery at the Betsy Lehman Center in Boston (2005), I performed a MEDLINE and Cumulative Index to Nursing & Allied Health Literature (CINAHL) search for articles that specifically addressed training in this area for nurses. I found references that mentioned that it was important, but most of the literature only addressed what doctors do, how the surgery is done, and other technical issues. Few actually addressed nursing education. The Betsy Lehman Center for Patient Safety and Medical Error Reduction expert panel on perioperative nursing care of the weight loss surgery patient also found most evidence to be Category D (expert opinion).

**Competency-based Orientation and a Core Curriculum for Demonstration of Proficiency in Caring for Weight Loss Surgery Patients**

I would like to take this one step further and, as I am an "expert" on the types of nurse training that I do, recommend how a curriculum may be put together to train the staff with whom bariatric physicians work.

Recommendations exist from the bariatric community and other organizations sponsoring the surgeons with whom we work. At the time of my presentation, I had found that there were 1,435 bariatric surgeons who were active in the American Society for Metabolic and Bariatric Surgery (ASMBS) and about 395 nurses who worked with that group as well. At that time, about 140,000 bariatric procedures were being performed each year. We have had bariatric standards and recommendations from the Betsy Lehman report, the ACS, the ASMBS, the Association for Perioperative Registered Nurses (AORN) and the Massachusetts Nurses Association (MNA). At this writing, a certification exam is being developed by allied health members of the ASMBS. If each of those 1,435 doctors came in contact with one floor nurse and one recovery room nurse (not included here are any nurses, these doctors might have in their clinics), that's almost 3,000 nurses who would require training on the safe care and handling of bariatric patients. What I'm proposing is that we establish a partnership with physicians, setting standards for comprehensive training for bariatric nurses, and including a competency checklist to provide a way of validating the fact that the people we train are qualified for what they do.

**A Focus on Patient Education**

Our practice developed a brochure for our primary care physicians (PCPs) to show how our clinic operates using the multidisciplinary team (Figure 1). Using the nursing process, we illustrate how the whole team, starting with the PCP as a referral, focuses on the patient at the center, and the entire team contributes to the assessment and care of the patient.

**Figure 1**

Multidisciplinary Patient Education Model

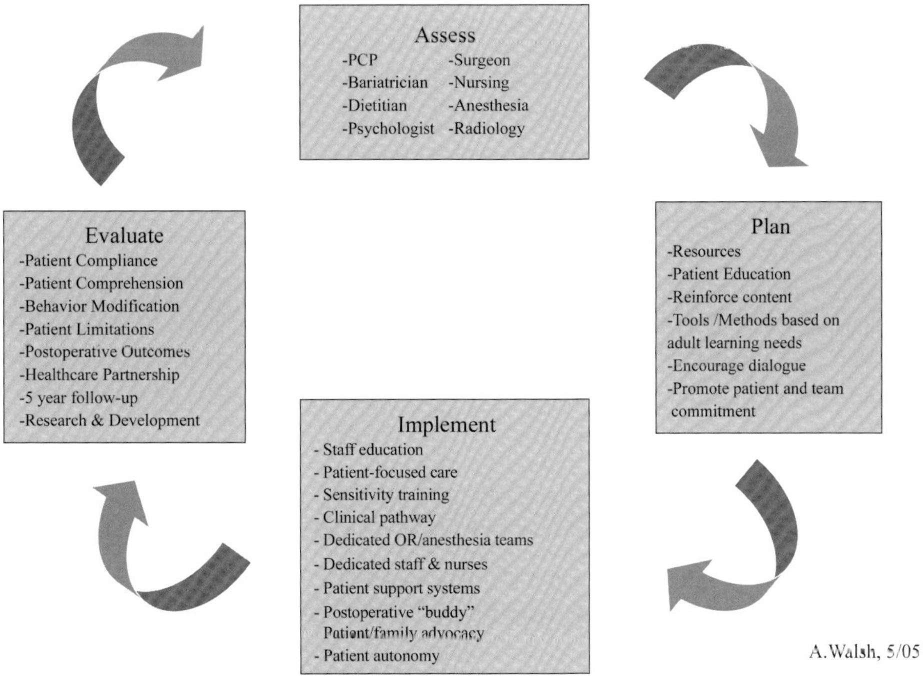


The patient comes into the program seeking a surgical alternative to his or her excessive weight and comorbid health issues. The patient is required to attend two surgery information seminars in order to be fully informed regarding the types of surgery available, possible outcomes, risks, benefits, as well as pre- and postoperative expectations, dietary considerations, and clinical follow-up. When the patient has completed the presurgical screening process and has decided on a procedure and surgeon, the team can create a plan of care using all available resources.

The patient education team is now in place. It is important to reinforce the content to the patient multiple times, because adults remember 80% of what they see, but only 35% of what they hear. That is, when patients come into a clinic and simply receive information, usually by the time they go back out to the front desk they've already forgotten how many appointments they have to make, who they're supposed to see next, and how soon they should come back. Thus, your information must be in a format carefully based on adult learning styles in order to reinforce all the information that you're giving. This requires both patient and team commitment.

In order to implement these standards in a given clinic or center, the entire staff must be educated not just the people in the clinic, but the nurses on the floors and in other disciplines. Sensitivity training is very important, as is ergonomic training. Injuries occur when patients are transported improperly, using the wrong type of equipment or supplies. OR staff is in serviced on proper use of bariatric equipment, beds, instruments, and supplies. To prevent injuries in the OR and in any dedicated bariatric unit, we use transfer devices.

Our clinic's staff acts as a resource to the OR and patient unit and our dietitians are liaisons to the hospital dietary department. I do rounds on the patients each day, setting up my patients with a post-op contact (a "bari-buddy"). We also try to offer everybody an e-mail address of certain patients who have volunteered their services. In order to conform to Health Insurance Portability and Accountability Act standards, bari-buddies are often people the patients have met at support groups, or a person who has had the same surgery or is in the same geographic location. They may call me or any of the doctors any time during the workday, but if they have questions on the weekends, nights or holidays, patients prefer not to have to bother us. They just want to know somebody can reassure them. Bari-buddies do not give medical advice, but they do supply needed support and they sign a confidentiality statement that is kept on file.

### Our Bariatric Center of Excellence

Our program has received Level 1a accreditation through the ACS as a bariatric Center of Excellence. We comply with National Institutes of Health (NIH) guidelines; do 5-year follow-ups on our patients; develop clinical pathways for consistency and planned outcomes; and do research and development through quality improvement activities and the National Surgical Quality Improvement Program (NSQIP) postoperative database.

### Special Considerations

All medical staff must be adequately prepared to take care of the morbidly obese population. They must be sensitive to the feelings of bariatric patients, be aware that there are HIPPA laws that must be followed, and include the patient and the family in all that they do in caring for the patient.

We have a "Persons of Size" committee at our hospital, which identified all the disciplines in the hospital and the adjustments that each had to make, as well as the training that we had to provide, in order to make sure that every department was capable of taking care of our patients. The task force also put together a policy for bariatric care standards, along with a summary of the kinds of equipment that would need to be available in the event a patient went to a floor other than one designated for surgery patients.

### Preoperative Assessment

Psychosocial, religious, and cultural sensitivity is very important because we serve an extremely diverse population and it cannot be assumed that all patients are going to have the same mental process as they approach this kind of surgery. The focus must always be on what the patient's individual needs are.

### Intraoperative Communication

Communication is always key. Nowadays, we use state-of-the-art endosuites, and voice-activated technology has taken away some of the things that the OR nurses used to do. However, it shouldn't take away the pattern of information exchange established by the team in the room. Each person must know what's happening as it's happening. No one can read anyone else's mind. As good as a team is, things do happen and they must be communicated so that all are on the same page. All staff must be expected to attend team training exercises for communication and patient safety.

### Postoperative Care

Clinical pathways are established so that you have a pattern in place as the patient comes through the system, the staff on the floor are clear as to which tests are to be done, and are familiar with the dietary advancement and discharge plan, etc. In order to maintain an open communication pattern, we must always make the needs of the patient clear to all departments.

### Discharge Planning

It is vital to make sure that patients have the equipment and supplies they will need at home. Is there an open wound that will require some kind of equipment or supplies? Many Medicare patients are required to have some kind of a prescription for their supplies. Is the patient routinely on antidepressants, oral agents (for diabetes, for example), or any other medications that will cause a problem if not resumed after surgery? Does the patient have the prescriptions, instructions, and basic information needed for a comfortable transition home?

### Training

Education reform in the last century was based on reassessing how people learn. John Dewey (1859-1952), a philosopher linked to a progressive education movement, believed that children learn in a certain way and often get bored if not kept stimulated. The teachers, he said, can't just take information, throw it out, and expect a child to sit there all day long, listening intently and absorbing the information. Both children and adults must have input into what they are learning. Two other individuals who have had impact in this regard are Malcolm Knowles (1913-1997) and Howard Gardner (born in 1943). Gardner identified multiple learning modes, noting that not everybody learns the same way. Some people are visual learners, some are auditory learners, and still others learn best by doing things hands-on. If you present things in a way that someone can relate to, they're going to learn better and retain that information. Knowles took this one step further when he said, "That's great, but adults learn differently than children." He created an adult learning theory that basically said that adults only learn what they think is important to them. Adults want to know

- Why they're using the information
- Why it's important
- How they will learn it
- How it should be applied

In 1984, in his book, *Andragogy in Action: Applying Modern Principles of Adult Learning*, Knowles said, "Adults are beginning to demand that their learning take place at a time, place, and pace that is convenient to them."

### Bariatric Team Partnership

We are very busy people. It is unrealistic to expect doctors to be everywhere and then also to be training all the staff, yet this is an important issue. I am very fortunate to work with physicians who have given me autonomy and the ability to develop a number of programs. In order for the system to work smoothly, a partnership with the team must be developed. Nurses will do more if they feel as though they're valued members of the team. They want to be able to apply their knowledge. When I was in the OR and I would scrub certain cases, nothing made me more frustrated than to be standing at the field ready to go, and having the surgeon say to me, "Just stand over there because I don't need you to do anything, just give me what I need." I would say, "But I can't anticipate your needs if I can't see what you're doing." The surgeon responded, "You don't need to."

This mentality has changed a lot as physicians have become more attuned to the fact that nurses want to be part of the team. They're excited about learning and are genuinely interested in seeing what the anatomy is and how procedures evolve. What's going to be the outcome, what's going to be the follow-up? There is more to this than just a patient coming in the door and having an operation, thanking the surgeon, going home and going on with his or her life.

### The Path to Nursing Education

There are three things that we need to consider. First, all nurses are adult learners. That's a given. Second, nurses vary in their professional experience. I'm not going to address a nurse who's been in practice for 30 years the same as I would a new graduate; they have different thoughts about their practice already. Third, as an instructor, I must know what the goals are of the people I am teaching. What benefits do they expect from learning from me? I'm not going to go into a room and start with a basic 101 course for somebody who has already been in practice for 20 or 30 years. They already know the basics; they just want to know the rest of the theory and to sharpen their hands-on skills.

In order to develop my curriculum, I must do a learner's needs assessment. The participants should identify why they're there, and what they want to get out of the program. I give a pretest to determine the basic knowledge of my students, followed by an icebreaker or other creative-thinking activity to stimulate group interaction. Activities are structured on a classroom format or as simulation labs, with perhaps some team training activities and a post-test to see how much knowledge was acquired during the session. I then perform an evaluation to find out how I can improve my programs.

**Figure 2**

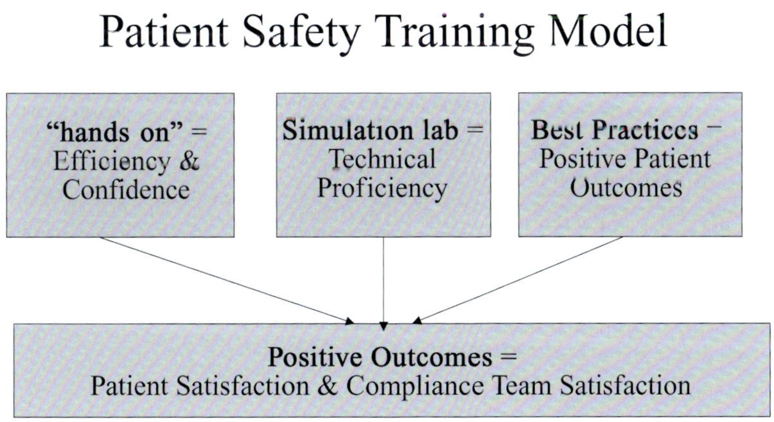


A patient safety training model I developed (Figure 2) shows the connection between what we know, what we learn, and how we can make improvements. As nurses, we require hands-on training, because this makes us more efficient and give us more confidence. In our skills and simulation center, I dedicate 2 days a week to working with the nursing staff in nursing and allied health education programs. I think it gives our nurses a greater appreciation for the fact that if you're scrubbed and you know what the instruments are and you know how to operate them, it makes for a more efficient and smooth case in all areas, because the doctors appreciate the team for providing safe patient care.

The simulation lab also provides technical proficiency. Nothing is more frustrating for a surgeon than to go into the OR and ask for a suture only to have you hand him the instrument and say, "I really don't know how to load this, I've never done it before." The surgeon then has to take time away from what he's doing, show you how to use it and hope that there's a small learning curve. If by the $10^{th}$ time a nurse has been in that same type of case, and still doesn't know how to do it, it's time to find another specialty.

**Best practices: a positive cycle**

Best practices give positive patient outcomes. Positive outcomes provide patients and their families with satisfaction and ensure increased compliance and better follow-up. Patients are going to come back to the clinic because they're excited to see you and to find out about the next step of their recovery. The whole team is going to be satisfied, because the doctors are going to go back to the OR where they will share the patient's experience with the team. "That patient we operated on 3 weeks ago came into clinic today. She or he has already lost 25 lbs and feels great!"

**Training methods**

Again, about 80% of people retain (i.e., learn) what they see. Thus, overhead or PowerPoint presentations and handouts are effective training tools. You can use video demonstrations and/or have activities that are instructor-led. Interaction is very good. Any type of learning through role-playing or interaction between people seems helpful in establishing a mental picture of what must be done in a given situation. Developing a Web-based, learning-specific program is also useful. For those who have difficulty with any of these methods, you can create a tool that can be used by students on their own.

Often I discuss with my groups whether they consider themselves "left- or right-brain" persons. I ask them to talk about their personal strengths or weaknesses. I'm very visual and very hands-on, so that's the way I teach, and I tend to assume that other people need that as well. But students may be more textbook-oriented and I must offer them references to use as well. The point is to give people a chance to acquire information in a variety of ways, to see which method works best for each student. What matters most is the end result: that we all have the same information when we finish.

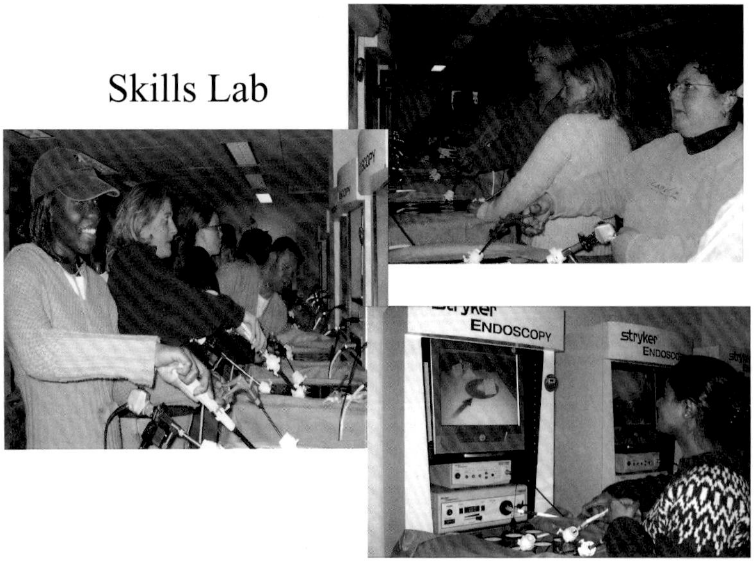


Pictured here are some of the nurses I've trained in our simulation lab. These students have a genuinely good time performing their skills and competing against each other. We also maintain a video library, established with the help of Ciné-Med, Inc., which provides in-depth information and demonstration of the bariatric program's processes and procedures. Our teleconference center allows us, at the push of a button, to tap into one of our ORs and have any number of medical professionals watch a hernia or a bariatric case—with the opportunity for the audience to interact with the OR staff without having to get up, get changed and go to the operating room.

I hold daylong workshops twice a year. I like to do a lot of different formats, because people who attend have different objectives. Breaking up the courses to provide small in-services for continuing education credits on a monthly or quarterly basis is also valuable, as more staff members are then able to take advantage of this training at a time when it's feasible for them to leave their units.

**More Teaching Techniques**

I frequently ask my learners to create a "manifesto," which is defined as thoughts or statements on a topic. For instance, below is a statement developed into a "manifesto."

> People are taught to live by the golden rule, *Do unto others*, when they are kids, but by the time they reach adulthood, it is long forgotten. As adults we have different standards that we have to live by. There are government standards, social standards, and guidelines that influence our daily lives. Our jobs have some standards that we have to live by because they have policies and procedures that have been established to make practice safe.

Another technique is the small group activity. I ask my students something like the following: "Reflect on essential components for nursing practice based on the things that you have learned in the workshop. Create a generic element for patient safety that could be applied to whichever unit you work in." This is followed by an open discussion, a flow-chart recording and a comparison of ideas.

**Recommendations**

I would make the following recommendations for ensuring optimum value to your students of this training:

1. Identify your target audience. There might be a group of learners from radiology, some floor nurses, and/or surgical techs. Try to put similar learning styles together because they're not going to have the same learning needs.
2. Be sure the material you are presenting can be applied to each particular practice. Often I'll invite patients who have had surgeries so that they can interact with the audience and pass on pieces of information that might be important to take back to the practice setting.
3. Utilize creative teaching methods. There is nothing more boring than to have someone stand at the front of the room, behind a podium, and just lecture without any interaction.
4. You have to be enthusiastic! I don't need to be a cheerleader, but I must at least embrace my specialty, so that people know I'm passionate about what I'm doing.

The fact is that nontraditional training methods provide a means for us to introduce information in a very relaxed atmosphere. We're using inanimate objects and simulators, virtual reality, and all kinds of new technology to help us prepare to be better at doing the work we do. Specialized education such as this brings us into a partnership with other disciplines. There are approximately 130 nursing specialty organizations at this time, of which only about 40 have formalized credentialing for those specialties. I am certified as a perioperative (OR) nurse and I'm hoping to be part of the first group of nurses to take the bariatric certification exam. Through our collective efforts to create patient safety standards and by obtaining certification for bariatric nursing, we can unite forces with our colleagues.

**Other Thoughts on Nurse Training for the Bariatric Arena**

- Bariatric training workshops should be standardized and presented in other facilities around the country.
- As a task force, we should maintain a book of standards to unify all bariatric practices.
- We must provide opportunities for nurses and allied health professionals to interact and improve their skills. We can assess our knowledge and competency because we'll have a formalized evaluation and checklist to reinforce our safety standards and best practices toward better patient outcomes.

**Suggested Reading**


1. Mulligan A, Young LS, Randall S, et al. Best practices for perioperative nursing care for weight loss surgery patients. *Obes Res*. 2005;13(2): 267-73.
2. Wittemore AD, Cella RJ, et al. Massachusetts Department of Public Health: Expert panel on bariatric surgery. Facility resources task group. 2004.
3. Lightizer B, et al. Persons of size task force final report. Beth Israel Deaconess Medical Center, Boston, MA. 2005.
4. AORN Bariatric Surgery Guideline. *AORN Journal*. 2004;79(5):1026-48.
5. Curley D. Patient safety considerations for bariatric programs. *Bariatrics Today*. 2005;2:22-3.
6. Knowles MS, et al. *Andragogy in Action: applying modern principles of adult education*. San Francisco, CA: Jossey Bass; 1984.
7. Knowles MS. *The Adult Learner*. Fifth ed. Woburn, MA: Butterworth-Heinemann; 1998.
8. Lillis K. A weighty problem: treating and transporting patients. *Healthcare Purchas News*. June 2002.
9. Batcheller J, et al. A practice model for patient safety: the value of the experienced registered nurse. *J Nurs Adm*. 2004;34:200-205.
10. Recommendations for facilities performing bariatric surgery. *Bull Am Coll Surg*. 2000; 85(9):20-3.
11. Nutting MA, Dock LL. *A History of Nursing*. Bristol, England: Thoemmes Press; 2000;v-xix.

# Preoperative Medical Evaluation

Edward A. Hatchigian, MD, MS

Weight loss surgery (WLS) has increased by significant number over the past 10 years. More and more obese individuals having tried numerous weight loss programs, products, medications (both prescription and/or over-the-counter), as well as popular diets and behavioral modalities, have been able to lose weight but unable to maintain. Therefore, they have reached the point that the surgical approach would be the most effective tool to achieve significant long-term results. To ensure patient safety and outcome of these individuals considering WLS, a comprehensive evaluation should be undertaken by a multidisciplinary screening approach. The first step in patient selection should be meeting the criteria of the body mass index (BMI) (Figure 1), which is calculated as weight in kilograms divided by height in meters squared, or estimated from pounds and inches using weight in pounds divided by height in inches squared and multiplied by 704.5.

**Figure 1**

| Body Mass Index | |
|---|---|
| <18.5 | Underweight |
| 18.5 - 24.9 | Normal Weight |
| 25.0 - 29.9 | Overweight |
| 30.0 - 34.9 | Class I Obesity |
| 35.0 - 39.9 | Class II Obesity (severe) |
| 40.0 & over | Class III Obesity (morbid) |

Those individuals with a BMI of 40 $kg/m^2$ and over have class III morbid obesity and would fulfill the criteria that has been established by the National Institutes of Health Evidence Report of 1998 (1) and used by third party payers for patient acceptance. Those individuals with BMI between 35 and 40 have class II severe obesity and should be considered for WLS if they have significant comorbid conditions that are associated with obesity such as diabetes, sleep apnea, reflux, hypertension, and osteoarthritis/DJD (Figure 2).

**Figure 2**

| Comorbid Conditions | |
|---|---|
| • Sleep apnea | • Coronary artery disease |
| • Asthma | • Cholelithiasis |
| • Dyslipidemia | • Venous ulcers/stasis |
| • Osteoarthritis/DJD | • Depression |
| • Hypothyroidism | • Hypertension |
| • Diabetes | • Polycystic ovary syndrome |

Once the candidate for WLS fulfils the criteria of the BMI, a thorough screening should be undertaken by a multidisciplinary team that includes medical, behavioral, and nutritional assessment. A multidisciplinary team for a WLS surgical program would include surgeons, internists/bariatric medical specialists, registered nurses, registered dietitians, psychiatrists/psychologists or social workers, and additional members such as exercise physiologists. The preoperative assessment should focus on those conditions that predispose patients to increased surgical risk such as age, (the older the individual the higher the risk), degree of obesity (the higher the BMI the greater the risk), and medical conditions such as cardiovascular factors (coronary artery disease, congestive heart failure, cardiomyopathy and arrhythmia, uncontrolled hypertension, and pulmonary hypertension); pulmonary factors (asthma/chronic obstructive pulmonary disease, obstructive sleep apnea, prior pulmonary embolus, and smoking); vascular factors (venous stasis, hypercoagulable states such as obesity, prior deep venous thromboses, family history of coagulopathy, and use of oral contraceptives); wound and nosocomial infections (BMI, central body fat distribution, and diabetes). Patients with unacceptable operative risk include those with unstable or severe coronary heart disease, severe pulmonary disease, and other conditions thought to seriously compromise anesthesia or wound healing (2). The goal of a comprehensive evaluation would be to minimize the operative risks. The major complications of WLS, especially the more aggressive "gold standard" Roux-en-Y gastric bypass procedure, include pulmonary embolism, respiratory failure, anastomotic leaks from the breakdown of suture or staple line, stomal obstruction, and bleeding(3). Some patients that present for WLS are often found to have undiagnosed conditions such as diabetes, hypothyroidism, hypertension, and sleep apnea. The preoperative assessment of the WLS patient (Figure 3) comprises a good history and physical exam.

**Figure 3**

## Preoperative Assessment

- History and physical exam
- ECG
- Laboratory tests
- Special laboratory tests
- Abdominal ultrasound r/o gallstones
- Pulmonary function tests
- Chest X-ray
- Echocardiogram
- Nuclear imaging study
- Sleep study
- Smoking cessation

The history should include not just past medical and surgical history, medications, allergies, social history such as tobacco, alcohol, caffeine, carbonated drinks, or recreational drug usage, family history, occupational history, but also a good summary of previous weight loss efforts by the patient such as commercial programs, weight loss products, diets (both commercial/individual), and medications for weight loss (both prescription and over-the-counter), as well as any form of physical activity and/or behavioral modification. Standard laboratory testing would include complete blood count (CBC)/differential, basic coagulation, electrolytes, chemistries, renal function, glucose, A1C, liver function tests (LFTs) including albumin and total protein, thyroid-stimulating hormone (TSH), iron profile, vitamin $B_{12}$, folic acid, vitamin D (25-hydroxy), lipid profile, and urinalysis. Special laboratory tests, for baseline purposes, may include: a *Helicobacter pylori* test, especially in patients with gastroesophageal reflux or history of peptic ulcer disease; C-reactive protein (CRP) for those with a strong family history of coronary artery disease and/or strong risk factors such as the metabolic syndrome; clotting factor studies for those who have history of/or strong risk of thromboembolic disease plus any patients that take medications requiring therapeutic levels of effectiveness such as digoxin, Dilantin, and Coumadin. Abdominal ultrasound is performed on all patients that have a gallbladder and often times gallstones are found and are removed during the Roux-en-Y gastric bypass procedure and recommended to be removed prior to having the adjustable lap band procedure. Pulmonary function test should be obtained for those with significant pulmonary issues such as asthma, dyspnea, and a strong smoking history. Echocardiograms are recommended for those who have heart murmurs, history of cardiomyopathy, and those who took the off-label prescription weight loss medication fenfluramine/phentermine (fen/phen) or Redux. It is strongly recommended that any patient with abnormal EKG, age over 60, and history of heart disease have a nuclear imaging study performed to evaluate cardiac risks/coronary artery disease. Patients who may at high risk for heart disease/myocardial infarction during noncardiac surgery should receive a beta blocker preoperatively to reduce the risk of perioperative event. Those individuals who state that they frequently snore, are fatigued during the day, and especially complain of waking up short of breath should be scheduled for a formal overnight polysomnography (sleep study). Those individuals who smoke are counseled to stop at least 6 to 8 weeks prior to surgery and to minimize weight gain often associated with smoking cessation—nicotine replacement patches and/or medications such as bupropion are recommended. All patients are encouraged to lose weight prior to surgery for two reasons, 1) to effectively change the consistency of the fatty liver to allow for manipulation of surgical instruments especially with the laparoscopic approach, and; 2) for psychological reasons to place the patient in the right frame of mind to facilitate the transition from pre- to postsurgery that for many can be an emotional roller-coaster ride.

All candidates for WLS are assessed preoperatively by a registered dietician. Their previous dietary habits are reviewed and they receive education and counseling for the new dietary requirements that they will have to adjust to postsurgically. They are also advised to take a daily multivitamin and other supplements that may be deemed necessary. All candidates are also evaluated for any behavioral and psychological issues, as there is a high incidence of depression, negative body image, eating disorders, and low quality of life in the severely obese individual that can be best evaluated by a multidisciplinary team that includes a licensed mental health provider (psychiatrist, psychologist, or social worker) who is experienced in the treatment of obese individuals(4).

In conclusion, WLS is currently the most effective treatment modality for managing severe obesity and its comorbid conditions. The best outcome for individuals going through WLS is through a dedicated multidisciplinary team that includes a spectrum of health-related disciplines that will provide a comprehensive medical screening and appropriate preoperative preparation, as well as perioperative and postoperative care. Collaboration from diverse disciplines such as anesthesiology, pulmonology, cardiology, and psychology are important in helping to integrate the multiple disciplines to achieve the successful outcome that is the goal of the team members.

**References**

1. National Institutes of Health. Clinical guidelines on the identification, evaluation and treatment of overweight and obesity in adults—the evidence report. *Obes Res*. 1998;6 (suppl 2):S51- S209 (Published correction appears in *Obes Res*. 1998;6:464.)
2. Saltzman E, Anderson W, Apovian CM, et al. Criteria for patient selection and multidisciplinary evaluation and treatment of the weight loss surgery patient. *Obes Res*. 2005; 13(2):234-43.
3. Steinbrook R. Surgery for severe obesity. *N Engl J Med*. 2004; 350(11):1075-9.
4. Greenberg I, Perna F, Kaplan M, Sullivan MA. Behavioral and psychological factors in the assessment and treatment of obesity surgery patients. *Obes Res*. 2005; 13(2):244-9.

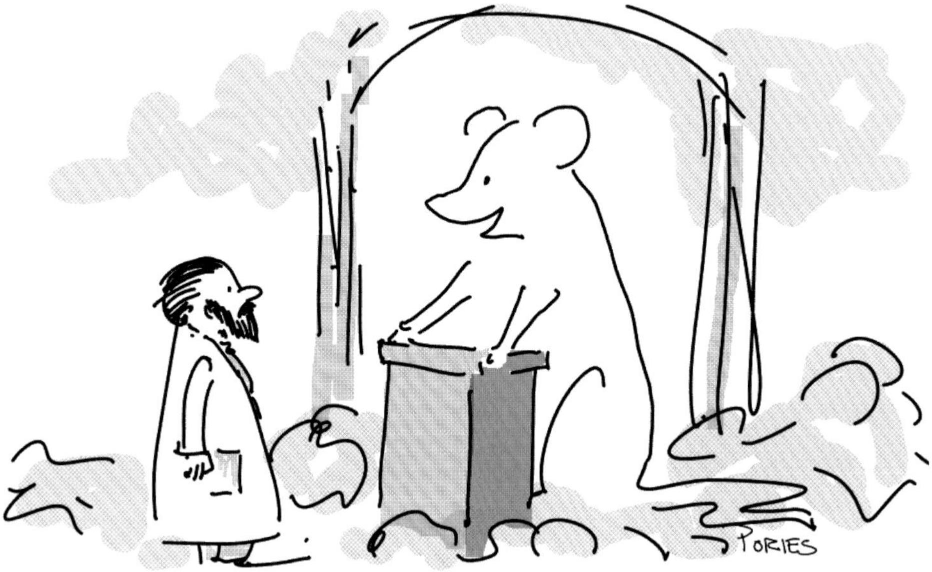


"Welcome. I'm Saint Peter and you must be Professor Franz, the famous experimental scientist...."

# Psychological Assessment

Isaac Greenberg, PhD
Ronna M. Casper, MEd, LCSW

Severe obesity is a serious chronic condition associated with a variety of life-threatening medical illnesses. It also has a major impact on mental health and quality of life (QOL). A higher-than-normal prevalence of psychopathology is seen in this population and there appears to be a direct relationship between body mass index (BMI) and the degree of psychosocial impairment. This impact on the overall QOL may have even more serious implications on public health than do the clear medical risks of obesity. Among the various psychological disorders seen in the obese, treatment-seeking population are a higher incidence of depression, anxiety, distorted body image, and eating disorders. This chapter reviews the complex psychological issues related to this procedure, offers recommendations regarding presurgical behavioral assessment, and reviews emerging data on the psychological impact of this important new treatment.

Severe obesity is a major health concern both in the United States and all over the world. Recent estimates suggest that up to 8% of total healthcare costs in Western countries are attributable to obesity. Furthermore, obesity is a health trend that is growing at an alarming rate.(1,2) The Third National Health and Nutrition Examination Survey (NHANES III) concluded that 32% of adults in the United States are overweight and 22.5 % are obese.(3) Numerous studies have demonstrated a direct relationship between increasing adiposity and mortality rates. Obese individuals are at increased risk for mortality and morbidity from cardiovascular disease, hypertension, type 2 diabetes, obstructive sleep apnea, lipid abnormalities, and stroke.(4,5) It now appears that cancer may be added to this list of the adverse health consequences of obesity.(6) In addition, obesity has numerous psychological effects that impact both QOL and, in some cases, the normal functioning of the affected individual.(7) Psychological and psychosocial consequences of obesity can impact medical issues, creating a vicious and deadly cycle.

Bariatric surgery is one treatment option increasingly being recommended for severely obese people who have had unsuccessful results with nonsurgical methods of weight reduction. In general, the BMI is used to define the degree of obesity and determine if the patient is an appropriate surgical candidate. Bariatric surgery includes procedures such as stomach stapling or banding and gastric bypass. This approach has emerged in recent years as the preferred treatment for severe obesity and has gained increased acceptance by the healthcare community and the public.(8) Mun et al(9) have recently published an excellent review of the surgical and medical options available to treat obesity.

While bariatric surgery is offering the hope of significant, sustainable weight loss to increasing numbers of patients with morbid obesity, the psychological ramifications of these procedures cannot be overstated. Patients who approach this treatment option carry the psychological consequences of years of obesity in complex interplay with factors such as social support systems, coping skills, psychiatric diagnoses, and more. Although these issues have not been well studied, there is an emerging body of research that can help clinicians plan treatment programs for these patients using comprehensive behavioral assessment as a cornerstone of treatment and provide needed psychological support both pre- and postoperatively to the patient and family.

## Public Perceptions and the Cycle of Failure

Virtually every patient who explores the option of bariatric surgery does so after undergoing countless failed attempts at sustained, significant weight loss. The data confirm that while patients may attain weight loss through nonsurgical methods, the maintenance of this loss is rarely achievable.(10) A recent 3-year study following weight changes in a community found that more than half the population in the study gained weight over the 3 years, while less than 5% actually lost any weight.(11) In small, well-controlled trials and in larger population studies, weight management seems to be resistant to change or control through behavioral, cognitive, nutritional, or "willpower" approaches.

There is an emerging understanding in health care that severe obesity is caused by a complex mixture of behavioral, genetic, and neurochemical factors.(12,13) Brownell(14) distinguishes between individual obesity and the environment that encourages it. Although treatments such as pharmacotherapy, behavior modification, and the use of support groups have produced increasingly better results, long-term success rates are still very discouraging.(11,15,16)

Certainly, the lack of sustained success at weight loss despite repeated efforts takes its psychological toll on patients. Add to this a public perception that directly blames individuals for their condition, and the results can be devastating. The notion that obesity is caused by poor willpower, a lack of effort, or a hidden agenda—while diminishing among those in health care—is still very much upheld in the popular press and among the public. This is in spite of all the data to the contrary, and even in spite of people's own personal failures to successfully maintain significant, meaningful weight loss.

Part of the reason for the persistence of this myth is that, at least in concept, the math seems simple: eat less food, burn more calories, and weight loss will be the reward. With so much medical and psychological gain waiting for the successful dieter, why wouldn't anyone succeed at this? This frame of references sets up a cycle of shame where society blames the obese for their affliction and in many, if not most cases, the obese blame themselves.

**Psychological Consequences of Obesity**

In what kind of environment does the obese person live? How is it different from the nonobese or normal-weight individual? How might this environment impact personality and psychological functioning?

Obese individuals are discriminated against(17) and this prejudice is seen even in the medical world.(18) Overweight females are also less likely to be married, have less education, and have lower household income then nonoverweight females.(19) Obese individuals have lower acceptance rates into prestigious colleges(20) and score significantly lower on QOL measures.(21) The literature on the psychosocial implications of obesity (especially in females) basically confirms what we generally suspect—that there is an enormous prejudice and discrimination built into most societies against the obese. This prejudice is immense, constant, and so pervasive as to be taken for granted. It is in this type of environment that obese children grow up and where obese adults must learn to function.

Many studies have attempted to measure the psychological status of obese individuals.(22,23) In one study(24), structured interviews were used to measure depression. The results showed that overweight and obese women (BMI >30 kg/m$^2$) were significantly more likely to have experienced major depression, suicidal ideation, and suicidal attempts in the recent past than nonobese women. Interestingly, this was not the case in men, where the opposite seemed to occur—i.e., obese men had a decreased risk of depression.

Overall, there appears to be a direct relationship between BMI and degree of QOL impairment. Severely obese people report significantly greater decrements in their QOL than persons with lower degrees of obesity. Clearly, the effect of obesity on public health goes far beyond the medical implications; there is also a significant decrease in functional status and well-being that may well eclipse the medical impact in the life of the obese individual.(25,26)

**Behavioral Assessment Prior to Bariatric Surgery**

Behavioral assessment prior to bariatric surgery and ongoing postoperative psychological care has quickly become the standard in the field. These procedures are designed to help ensure that patients choose a treatment approach that is likely to have the best results, measured not only by weight loss, but also by overall QOL.

**Rationale for Screening**

The complex psychological implications of severe obesity have already been noted. It has been estimated that up to 10% of patients who seek treatment are likely to have a clinically significant mood disorder that may require treatment before any weight loss program can be devised.(27) While one could well argue that an assessment of a patient's psychological makeup makes sense as part of the treatment of any serious, chronic health condition, there is a particularly strong case to be made for performing such an assessment prior to bariatric surgery.

For example, some evidence suggests that there may be unique psychological characteristics attached to obese people who seek treatment when compared with those who do not. In a study by Fitzgibbon et al(28), obese patients seeking treatment showed significantly higher pathology and distress scores than either nonobese or obese individuals who were not seeking treatment. This study supports what others have also suggested(29,30)—obese individuals seeking treatment may have more psychopathology than is seen in the general population.

Further, binge-eating disorder (described as the consumption of a large amount of food in a brief period of time, during which the individual experiences a perceived loss of control) is estimated to occur in approximately 15%(31) to 33%(32) of the obese population. This is much greater that what is seen in the general population and is correlated with a higher incidence of depression, lower self-esteem, symptoms of borderline personality disorder, and a higher incidence of all psychiatric disorders.(33)

It is important to note here that bariatric surgery is a life-altering procedure. It places significant demands on the coping skills of even the healthiest and most well-supported patients. The diet and lifestyle changes that the patient must adopt are profound and the patient's physical well-being, as well as long-term weight loss success, is dependent upon adherence to these changes. In addition, as major surgery, bariatric procedures are not without attendant, significant medical risks. For these reasons, most providers feel it is prudent to attempt to identify preoperatively those individuals with the highest psychiatric vulnerability.

While the research on the interplay between psychological factors and the eventual outcomes of bariatric surgery is in its infancy, there are indicative data that could help guide the preoperative assessment process. In a retrospective study, Delin et al(34) found several measures that they felt could predict better postoperative outcomes. Among these the most prominent was self-esteem, which related strongly to percent of excess weight lost. Delin et al concluded that those with low self-esteem could benefit from pre- and postoperative psychological intervention. There are numerous other studies referenced in this article that arrive at the same conclusion (e.g., 25,26). The weight of the data points to a mild effect of preoperative psychosocial status on post-op weight loss and psychological well-being.

The screening procedure, therefore, should be designed to assess each patient's strengths, as well as areas of vulnerability. In some cases, this screening may lead to exclusion from surgery due to the risk of both surgery and recurrent psychiatric complications. On the other hand, such careful screening may result in more prudent planning to support those at risk for recurrent psychiatric problems, so that they may receive the maximum benefits from bariatric surgery.

**Goals of the Behavioral Assessment**

A comprehensive behavior assessment constitutes the beginning of the treatment process for any obese patient. Wadden and Phelan(35) provide an excellent example of a behavioral assessment designed to help determine the best treatment option for a particular patient with obesity.

The goals of a comprehensive, presurgical assessment are somewhat different in that the treatment option has already been chosen. Through the assessment, we hope to identify those individuals who may require attention either before or after surgery to enhance their chances of success. Given the conflicting and short-term data available regarding psychological variables that may impact surgical outcome, the behavioral assessment should not be seen as an attempt to predict who will succeed and who will fail. Rather, it is done in an effort to enhance the postoperative success rate both in terms of total weight lost and optimal QOL indices.

An equally important goal of the preoperative psychological assessment is to gather information regarding the patient's understanding of obesity and its causes and to begin to dispel myths or misconceptions that may be present. Early in this process, we acknowledge that genetics and biology also play a role in the development of obesity. We explain that while the amount of weight lost, the ability to keep it off, and the willingness to take responsibility for making lifestyle changes all rest with the patient, it is the surgery that may set up the conditions for significant, lasting weight loss to occur. This is an entirely new possibility in the patient's life and it is this new promise and hope that we feel reinforces the preoperative changes that prepare the patient to benefit fully from the bariatric surgery.

We recommend that the behavior assessment be conducted by a trained mental health professional—a psychiatrist, psychologist, or social worker. The process may require 1 or 2 sessions to complete. Generally, the behavior assessment attempts to capture certain bits of information that will

- Give some insight into the psychological profile of the patient
- Have an impact on how we will design an optimal pre- and post-op support program
- Help the rest of the surgical team—nurses, physicians, surgeons—better understand the patient

Specifically, the goals of the intake evaluation are as follows:

1. Identify the relevant psychological, biological, genetic, and lifestyle factors that have contributed to the patient's history of obesity
2. Understand the patient's goals and expectations of the program
3. Define the core support systems that the patient relies on
4. Determine what coping strategies have been used by the patient when faced with adversity or challenges. Define strengths and weaknesses in the patient's ability to deal with the consequences of the surgery
5. Define an optimal program, either pre- or postoperative, that may support the patient in reaching identified goals
6. Encourage all patients to share fears and concerns about choosing this elective surgery; the reception they may receive when telling close family and friends that they are considering this; and the possible shame and humiliation they may feel in making this choice. Simply being an empathetic listener is an important part of the whole relationship between patient and interviewer(36)
7. Impart to the patient the highlights of the surgical program, program expectations and support systems available to program patients

**Components of the Screening Process**

An overview of the major components of the preoperative behavioral assessment is offered below. Examples of specific interview items appear in the Table. There are many ways to approach the intake process, and the operation continually evolves and changes as data accumulation and feedback impact the structure of the assessment.

**Lifestyle Issues**

The first part of the assessment is introductory in nature and is designed to obtain an understanding of each person's home environment. We like to get a general overview of the patient's present lifestyle. This includes marital and employment status, number of children, number and type of friends, family availability and support, and the degree of satisfaction with how life is going. We may learn more about which elements in the patient's life create satisfaction and contentment and which generate stress and upset. We try to find out how each person normally reacts to these issues—do they ever acknowledge the positive elements in their lives? How do they deal with the stressors?

All this should be undertaken in a friendly, nonthreatening context, which will allow us to gather insight into the patient's levels of stress, responsibility, stability, support systems, etc. Much of this information will influence decisions about the types of group participation we may require, whether family should be invited to meetings, and how best to communicate with the patient. Like everything else in this intake, the purpose is both to set the tone for a working relationship with the individual and to gather specific data that may help determine how the surgery might positively impact the person's life.

**Weight Loss and Weight History**

We also review the patient's weight and weight loss history. Most of this has been already reported on the intake forms we ask patients to fill out prior to the session or at home. We feel it is important to understand the patient's motives and goals in applying to a surgical program. We make several assumptions about most of our patients:

1. They've already tried many other weight loss programs and methods
2. They are within 10 to 15 pounds of their highest-ever weight
3. They've lost significant amounts of weight in the past and are very discouraged about nonsurgical weight loss programs

Since environment plays such a critical role in weight control, it is important to understand what kind of programs and behaviors have worked best with each person. While very few people successfully maintain a weight loss, the procedures that worked best (and worst) in the past may play an important role in future programs, including post-op maintenance strategies. It is, therefore, important to gather a detailed history of weight loss efforts and try to define what types of approaches and strategies produced the most successful outcomes, even if only for relatively brief intervals.

**Knowledge Base**

Obviously, before undertaking a major, potentially life-changing operation, the patient should know as much as possible about the surgery, its benefits and risks, as well as what our expectations are and the possible outcomes of the surgery. As part of the assessment, we talk with all patients about their goals and expectations, find out what they know about the surgery itself, and determine their sources of information. We invite all patients to attend an introductory group meeting where they can meet members of our staff and learn more about our surgical program. If possible, we encourage patients to attend such a meeting even before their first intake evaluation with us.

We suggest various books patients might want to look at, and recommend a wide variety of Web sites—including our own—ranging from government sites to chat rooms. The patient needs to fully understand not only the surgical issues, but also our support programs. If we are unsure about the level of the patient's commitment or knowledge base, we offer basic-skills groups to help sharpen behavioral, cognitive, and personal skills prior to the surgery and enhance the patient's chances for success postoperatively. These small, closed groups meet weekly for 8 weeks and focus on various specific issues such as stress management, behavior change, relapses, depression, eating in social situations, cognitive restructuring, and more.

**Psychological Assessment and Psychiatric Considerations**

This section of the interview deals with the psychological and psychosocial history of the patient. The surgery itself is a stressful episode. It also produces dramatic weight loss, which is very visible to others. Some patients (and much of the public) see the surgery as a sign of weakness because the patient could not accomplish the weight loss by so-called "willpower." Many patients are embarrassed that they must resort to surgery and tell very few others that they are undergoing weight reduction surgery. Friends and family will obviously be impacted by the dramatic weight loss. How well equipped is the patient to handle all this change? There are numerous underlying personality factors that may play a role, both in the short-term recovery from the surgery and in longer-term issues regarding sustaining the weight loss and deriving maximum benefits from it.

The assessment should also involve a comprehensive review of any major psychiatric disorders that may need to be treated before surgery is considered. The interviewer attempts to determine to what extent any significant psychiatric disorder or symptoms may interfere with the potential benefits of the surgery. What is the treatment history for this individual? What medications were used or are now being used? Are there compliance issues? Are there any ongoing or recurrent destructive behaviors we need to be aware of (a history of binge-eating, suicidal ideation or attempts, depression, bulimia, drug and alcohol use)? Does this person have a therapist? May we speak to the therapist? What kind of optimal support network can we design?

Since we are not conducting a formal clinical evaluation, determining whether the full, formal criteria of depression are met, as defined by the Diagnostic and Statistical Manual of Mental Disorders, 4th edition (DSM-IV)(37), is not our primary goal. Even the presence of any of the "Axis I" diseases may not necessarily rule out the surgical option, much depends on other factors such as support network, ability to follow instructions, social and lifestyle stability, etc. The results of the interview will, however, impact the course of treatment in terms of the recommendations made, the types of support groups in which the patient might need to participate, and the support mechanisms we might recommend, including an outside therapist.

Toward this end, part of the structured interview may include a test for depression, a test for anxiety, and general QOL questions. There are many depression tests to choose from, including the Beck Depression Inventory—II,(38) the Zung Depression Scale,(39) the Hamilton Depression Scale,(40) and others. Among anxiety scales there is a Zung version,(41) a Beck version,(42) and others. These should be filled out prior to the interview so that they may be discussed and reviewed during the initial meeting.

**Self-monitoring Logs**

As part of the behavioral assessment, we ask patients to start tracking their food intake. While they may have done this in the past, we need a more updated record to determine the types of food choices they make, the number of meals they eat, calorie intake, etc., so we may begin a behavior and nutrition intervention prior to the surgery. Patients are encouraged to keep these logs from the first visit right through to surgery. During any visit, professional staff members may review them with the patient.

There is ample evidence that calorie records generally reflect a significant under-reporting of intake.(43) The purpose of the self-monitoring logs is to simply get a rough snapshot of patterns regarding when patients eat, where, how often, what the hunger level is, and the pattern of exercise. From this information, new behavior patterns can be developed.

**Recommendations Following the Behavioral Assessment**

With the assessment data in hand, including scores on any depression and/or anxiety scales and input from any therapist the patient may be seeing, recommendations can be made to the treatment team. The recommendations for a particular person may include pre-op weight loss training, programs to sharpen skills that may be needed postoperatively, a strategy to increase knowledge about risks and benefits of surgery, or recommendations about helping the patient develop a more comprehensive support network. Frequent treatment team meetings are essential, as input from other members of the medical team may alter these observations.

**Psychological Changes Following Bariatric Surgery**

While there are as yet no definitive studies tracking psychological changes following bariatric surgery, there is a growing accumulation of data that suggest this type of surgery produces significant, positive psychosocial outcomes. These results seem to diminish a little over time; nevertheless, significant improvements are maintained compared with preoperative baseline measures or obese controls.

Since the weight loss is so rapid and spectacular in the first year or two following the surgery, many of the positive social changes and benefits of the weight loss may be reflecting these early and dramatic changes. After the first year or two, however, weight loss may stop and reverse to partial weight regain.(44) We may need to distinguish the early-onset, short-term changes in mental health from measures taken 2 or more years postoperatively.

Waters et al(45) followed 157 patients for up to 2 years to determine the effects of gastric bypass on various mental health indices. While there were significant improvements in scores for anxiety, depression, general health, positive well-being, self-control, and vitality after 6 and 12 months, it seems that after the postoperative euphoria and weight loss stabilized, so did measures of mental health, which returned to preoperative levels after the second year. They postulate that patients may come to depend on the medical and psychological supports from their clinic visits and that when the frequency of these visits decreases after the first 2 years, mental health improvement also reverses. In their follow-up of a larger sample of patients, they also found three suicides and two deaths due to alcohol abuse—a warning that this is a labile population that may require ongoing emotional support.

Since there appears to be a direct relationship between body weight and QOL(26,46), decreases in positive changes in mental health may simply reflect the stabilization, and even the weight regain, that is seen several years postoperatively.

The suggestion that the beneficial effects of bariatric surgery in terms of psychosocial functioning seem to decrease over time is intriguing. Is this a uniform finding or is there a differential outcome based on some pre-op/psychological profile? It suggests that further work needs to be done to determine if longer-term outcomes maintain their benefits. It also bolsters the case for research into the possible benefits of preoperative intervention.

Another behavior that seems to improve short term, and then fall back, is binge-eating. While there appears to be a decrease in binge-eating behavior in the short term following surgery(47), this change does not seem to hold when the measure is taken further out in time.(48) More long-term studies need to be done in this area since binge-eating seems to be associated with other psychopathologies.(33) A return to binge-eating behaviors post-op would not be a good prognosis for the maintenance of further positive changes.

Van Gemert(49) studied a group of 62 patients after bariatric surgery in which he measured this group's QOL vs QOL of 20 morbidly obese subjects who did not have the surgery. He, as have many other researchers, found that QOL measures such as mobility, energy, pain, and social isolation were all significantly below normal in the preoperative phase. In the first 2 years following surgery, the scores all approximated the normal values. Measures taken in this group more than 2 years post-op showed that QOL scores decreased somewhat over those taken sooner after surgery; however, these scores were still higher than scores in the control (nonsurgical) group. A prospective study by the same principle authors(49) confirmed these results, as have many other studies measuring QOL by various methods and through different surgical approaches.(50-53)

It is important to note that preliminary studies are suggesting that patients who undergo bariatric surgery may be at an increased risk for suicide. Suicide following gastric bypass occurs at 0.4% in the post-op population vs 0.03% to 0.01% in the general population.(54) Other causes of death in the post-op bariatric population include alcoholism and bulimia. These statistics are based on relatively small samples and need to be replicated in far larger studies. If replicated, however, the data suggest that a more comprehensive filtering procedure may be needed to identify those at risk.

## Conclusion

Given the extreme difficulties most severely obese patients have in losing weight and maintaining the loss using will-power and behavior modification (sometimes in combination with medications), surgical approaches to obesity seem to be very encouraging. Both from a medical perspective and a psychosocial analysis, the short- and long-term benefits of the surgery are significant. The effect of postsurgical weight loss on QOL is consistent and meaningful. Until other, less invasive approaches are developed to deal with the disease of severe obesity, a comprehensive approach, including bariatric surgery, may be the best hope of promoting significant enhancements in the QOL in this population.

**Table 1**
**Sample Interview Components for the Behavioral Assessment**

| Phase of interview | Sample components |
|---|---|
| **Introductory/lifestyle issues** | • Marital status, living condition<br>• Educational status<br>• Job status, work satisfaction<br>• Web of relationships |
| **Weight loss and weight history** | • How long have you struggled with obesity?<br>• What is the pattern of weight loss attempts?<br>• How much weight have you lost in the last 5 years?<br>• What is the most weight ever lost? How did you lose this weight? How long did you keep the weight off, this time or on other occasions?<br>• What do you consider your most successful method of weight loss thus far? Why do you think it was successful? |
| **Knowledge base regarding surgery** | • What have you read about this surgery? (Or: What do you know about this surgery?)<br>• Where do you get your information?<br>• What weight do you see yourself at 3 months after surgery? After 6 months? A year? After 2 years?<br>• How sure are you that this is the right approach for you?<br>• Why do you want to do this? What are the benefits for you?<br>• What do you see as the risks of this surgery for you?<br>• Who knows you are doing this? What reactions have you had from family and friends? |
| **Psychological history** | • Are you in therapy now? Have you been in the past?<br>• If you have a therapist, may we contact him/her?<br>• Do you take any psychotropic medicines or have you taken any in the past?<br>• Have you ever been hospitalized for a psychiatric problem?<br>• Have you ever thought about or attempted suicide?<br>• Do you have a history of bulimia? Binge-eating?<br>• Have you ever had a problem with depression or an anxiety disorder? Other psychiatric disorders?<br>• Do you use alcohol or illegal drugs? Have you used them in the past?<br>• Do you smoke? |

**References**


1. International Obesity Task Force. Managing the global epidemic of obesity: report of the WHO consultation on obesity. Geneva, Switzerland. World Health Organization; 1997.
2. Mokdad AH, Serdula MK, Dietz WH, et al. The spread of the obesity epidemic in the United States, 1991-1998. *JAMA*. 1999;282(16):1519-22.
3. Flegal KM, Caroll MD, Kuczmarski, RJ, et al. Overweight and obesity in the United States: prevalence and trends, 1960-1994. *Int J Obes Relat Metab Disord*. 1998;22(1):39-47.
4. Manson JE, Willett WC, Stampfer MJ, et al. Body weight and mortality among women. *N Engl J Med*. 1995;333(11):667-85.
5. Allison DB, Fontaine KR, Manson JE, Stevens J, Van Itallie TB. Annual death attributable to obesity in the United States. *JAMA*. 1999;282(16):1530-8.
6. Calle EE, Thun MJ, Petrelli JM, Rodriguez C, Heath CW Jr. Body-mass index and mortality in a prospective cohort of U.S. adults. *N Engl J Med*. 1999;341(15):1097-1105.
7. Fine JT, Colditz GA, Coakley EH, Mosley G, Manson JE, Willett WC, et al. A prospective study of weight change and health-related quality of life in women. *JAMA*. 1999;282(22): 2136-42.
8. National Heart, Lung, and Blood Institute (NHLBI). Clinical guidelines on the identification, evaluation and treatment of overweight and obesity in adults: the evidence report. *Obes Res*. 1998;6(suppl):51S-210S.
9. Mun EC, Blackburn GL, Matthews JB. Current status of medical and surgical therapy for obesity. *Gastroenterology*. 2001;120(3):669-81.
10. Perri MG, Corsica JA. Improving the maintenance of weight lost in behavioral treatment of obesity. In: *Handbook of Obesity Treatment*. Wadden TA, Stunkard AJ, eds. New York, NY: Guilford Press; 2002.
11. Crawford D, Jeffrey R, French S. Can anyone successfully control their weight? Findings of a three year community-based study of men and women. *Int J Obes Relat Metab Disord.*. 2000;24(9):1107-10.
12. Cardon LR, Carmelli D, Fabsitz RR, Reed T. Genetic and environmental correlations between obesity and body fat distribution in adult male twins. *Hum Biol*. 1994;66(3):465-79.
13. Popkin BM, Doak CM. The obesity epidemic is a worldwide phenomenon. *Nutr Rev*. 1998;56:106-14.
14. Horgen K, Brownell K. Confronting the toxic environment: environmental public health actions in a world crisis. In: *Handbook of Obesity Treatment*. Wadden TA, Stunkard AJ, eds. New York, NY: Guilford Press; 2002.
15. Perri MG. The maintenance of treatment effects in the long-term management of obesity. *Clin Psychol Science and Practice*. 1998;5:526-543.
16. Wilson,GT. Behavioral treatment of obesity: thirty years and counting. *Adv Behav Res Ther*. 1994;16:31-75.
17. Sobal J, Stunkard AJ. Socioeconomic status and obesity: a review of the literature. *Psychol Bull*. 1989;105(2):260-75.
18. Harris JE, Hamaday V, Mochan E. Osteopathic family physicians' attitudes, knowledge and self-reported practices regarding obesity. *J Am Osteopath Assoc*. 1999:99(7):353-65.
19. Gortmaker SL, Must A, Perrin JM, Sobol AM, Dietz WH. Social and economic consequences of overweight in adolescence and young adulthood. *N Engl J Med*. 1993;329(14):1008-12.
20. Pargaman D. The incidence of obesity among college students. *J Sch Health*. 1969; 39(9):621-7.

21. Sullivan M, Karlsson J, Sjöström L, et al. Swedish obese subjects (SOS). An intervention study of obesity: Baseline evaluation of health and psychosocial functioning in the first 1743 subjects examined. *Int J Obes Relat Metab Disord*. 1993;17(9):503-12.

22. Kral JG, Sjöström LV, Sullivan MB. Assessment of quality of life before and after surgery for severe obesity. *Am J Clin Nutr*. 1992;55(2 suppl):611S-614S.

23. Karlsson J, Sjöström L, Sullivan M. Swedish obese subjects (SOS). An intervention study of obesity: two-year follow-up of health-related quality of life (HQRL) and eating behavior after gastric surgery for severe obesity. *Int J Obes Relat Metab Disord*. 1998;22:113-126.

24. Carpenter KM, Hasin DS, Allison DB, et al. Relationships between obesity and DSM-IV major depressive disorder, suicide ideation, and suicide attempts: results from a general population study. *Am J Public Health*. 2000;90:251-257.

25. Glinski J, Wetzler S, Goodman E. The psychology of gastric bypass surgery. *Obes Surg*. 2001;11:581-588.

26. Wadden TA, Sarwer DB, Womble LG, et al. Psychosocial aspects of obesity and obesity surgery. *Surg Clin North Am*. 2001;81(5):1001-24.

27. Wadden TA, Anderson DA, Foster GD, Bennett A, Steinberg C, Sarwer DB. Obese women's perceptions of their physician's weight-management attitudes and practices. *Arch Fam Med*. 2000;9(9):854-60.

28. Fitzgibbon ML, Stolley MR, Kirschenbaum DS. Obese people who seek treatment have different characteristics then those who do not seek treatment. *Health Psychol*. 1993;12(5):342-5.

29. Friedman MA, Brownell KD. Psychological correlates of obesity: moving to the next research generation. *Psychol Bull*. 1995;117(1):3-20.

30. Fontaine KR, Bartlett SJ, Barofsky I. Health-related quality of life among obese persons seeking and not currently seeking treatment. *Int J Eat Disord*. 2000;27(1):101-5.

31. Stunkard AJ. Binge eating disorder and night eating syndrome. In: *Handbook of Obesity Treatment*. Wadden TA, Stunkard AJ, eds. New York, NY: Guilford Press; 2002:107-124.

32. Saunders R. Binge eating in gastric-bypass patients before surgery. *Obes Surg*. 1999;9(1):72-6.

33. Williamson DA, Martin CK. Binge eating disorder: a review of the literature after publication of DSM-IV. *Eat Weight Disord*. 1999;4(3):103-14.

34. Delin CR, Watts JM, Bassett DL. An exploration of the outcomes of gastric bypass surgery for morbid obesity: patient characteristics and indices of success. *Obes Surg*. 1995;5(2):159-70.

35. Wadden TA, Phelan S. Behavioral assessment of the obese patient. In: *Handbook of Obesity Treatment*. Wadden TA, Stunkard AJ, eds. New York, NY: Guilford Press; 2002:186-226.

36. Stunkard AJ. Talking with patients. In: *Obesity: Theory and Therapy*. Stunkard, AJ, Wadden, eds. New York, NY: Raven Press; 1993:355-363.

37. American Psychiatric Association. Diagnostic and Statistical Manual of Mental Disorders (DSM-IV), 4th ed. Washington, DC: American Psychiatric Association; 1994.

38. Beck AT, Steer RA, Brown GK. *Beck Depression Inventory II (BDI-II) Manual*. San Antonio. Harcourt Brace; 1996.

39. Zung WW, Richards CB, Short MJ. Self-rating depression scale in an outpatient clinic: further validation of the SDS. *Arch Gen Psychiatry*. 1965;13(6):508-515.

40. Hamilton M. A rating scale for depression. *J Neurol Neurosurg Psychiatry*. 1960;23:56-62.

41. Zung WW. A rating instrument for anxiety disorders. *Psychosomatics*. 1971;12(6):371-9.

42. Beck AT, Epstein N, Brown G, Steer RA. An inventory for measuring clinical anxiety: psychometric properties. *J Consult Clin Psychol.*1988;56(6):893-7.

43. Schoeller DA. Limitations in the assessment on dietary energy intake by self-report. *Metabolism.* 1995;44(2 suppl 2):18-22.

44. Powers PS, Rosemurgy A, Boyd F, Perez A. Outcome of gastric restriction procedures: weight, psychiatric diagnoses, and satisfaction. *Obes Surg.* 1997;7(6):471-7.

45. Waters GS, Pories WJ, Swanson MS, et al. Long-term studies of mental health after the Greenville gastric bypass operation for morbid obesity. *Am J Surg.* 1991;161(1):154-7.

46. Wadden TA, Stunkard AJ. Social and psychological consequences of obesity. *Ann Int Med.* 1985;103(6):1062-7.

47. Dymek MP, le Grange D, Neven K, Alverdy J. Quality of life and psychosocial adjustment in patients after Roux-en-Y gastric bypass: a brief report. *Obes Surg.* 2001;11(1):32-9.

48. Pekkarinen T, Koskela K, Huikuri K, et al. Long-term results of gastroplasty for morbid obesity: binge-eating as a predictor of poor outcome. *Obes Surg.* 1994;4(3):248-55.

49. Van Gemert WG, Adang EM, Greve JW, Soeters PB. Quality of life assessment of morbidly obese patients: effect of weight-reducing surgery. *Am J Clin Nutr.* 1998;67(2):197-201.

50. Danö P, Hahn-Pedersen J. Improvement of quality of life following jejunoileal bypass surgery for obesity. *Scand. J Gastroenterol.* 1977;12:769-74.

51. Hafner RJ, Watts JM, Rogers J. Quality of life after gastric bypass for morbid obesity. *Int J Obes.* 1991;15(8):555-60.

52. Choban PS, Onyejekwe J, Burge JC, et al. A health status assessment of the impact of weight loss following Roux-en-Y gastric bypass for clinically severe obesity. *J Am Coll Surg.* 1999;188(5):491-7.

53. Weiner R, Datz M, Wagner D, Bockhorn H. Quality-of-life outcome after laparoscopic adjustable gastric banding for morbid obesity. *Obes Surg.* 1999;9(6):539-45.

54. Hsu LK, Benotti P, Dwyer J, et al. Nonsurgical factors that influence the outcome of bariatric surgery: a review. *Psychosom Med.* 1998;60(3):338-346.

# Joslin Guidelines

Osama Hamdy, MD, PhD
Judy Giusti, MS, RD, LDN, CDE
Jo-Anne Rizzotto, MEd, RD, LDN, CDE

The new Joslin Diabetes Center nutrition guidelines are directed to overweight and obese people with type 2 diabetes, prediabetes (impaired glucose tolerance and impaired fasting glucose), or at risk for developing type 2 diabetes. In the United States, approximately 18 million people are currently diagnosed with diabetes and approximately 40 million are considered at risk for this chronic disease. About 40% of the nondiabetic U.S. population is still in the normal weight range (body mass index [BMI] 20-25 kg/m$^2$), while 60% are overweight, obese, or severely obese. In contrast, only 20% of diabetic patients are still in the normal weight range.

Thus, most diabetic patients are overweight, obese, or severely obese. The major clinical characteristics of this population are fasting and postprandial hyperglycemia, postprandial hypertriglyceridemia, insulin resistance, hyperinsulinemia, and low high-density lipoprotein (HDL). Meanwhile, their serum level of inflammatory cytokines like tumor necrosis factor-alpha (TNF-α), interleukin-6 (IL-6) and C-reactive protein (CRP) are increased. These proinflammatory cytokines predispose them to premature atherosclerosis and cardiovascular disease. However, diabetic patients continue to gain weight over time and have decreased energy expenditure. The United Kingdom Prospective Diabetes Study (UKPDS) also showed that weight gain in type 2 diabetics continues with most diabetes medications. If you add to these problems the increased serum level of low-density lipoprotein (LDL) and hypertension, you end up with a unique population at very high risk for coronary artery disease and stroke.

The current dietary guidelines recommend that 55% to 60% of daily caloric intake comes from carbohydrates. These recommendations date back to the late 1970s, when most clinicians agreed that the only way to reduce cardiovascular risk was to reduce dietary fat intake. At that time, carbohydrates were suggested as an alternative to reduced fat, while no strong evidence was available to suggest that this option carried less risk. Currently, nutritionists and diabetologists are still debating the value of such recommendations in the face of growing evidence that shows a strong link between weight gain, poor diabetes control, and increased carbohydrate intake.

One of the other major challenges for obesity management is physicians' inertia. Although most physicians agree that weight loss is fundamental in reducing cardiovascular complications in patients with type 2 diabetes, few are proactive in providing their patients with effective tools that may help them to lose weight. Although obese diabetic patients may not be able to achieve their ideal body weight even with significant effort, many can still lose 7% or more of their initial body weight if enrolled in a structured weight management program. Such modest weight loss improves insulin sensitivity and lipid abnormalities and may result in reduced risk for cardiovascular disease.

Dietary-intervention studies show that fad dietary programs can result in some weight loss that is not sustainable. More importantly, compliance to such diets decreases significantly over time. While weight loss is more significant at 6 months in patients who follow a strict, low-carbohydrate diet (<30 g/d), it is not better than reducing caloric intake by 500 kcal at 1 year of follow-up.

The Joslin Clinical Guidelines for Adults with Diabetes offers nutrition guidelines for overweight and obese adults with type 2 diabetes, prediabetes, and/or those at high risk for developing type 2 diabetes. As a weight management approach to assist healthcare providers in a clinical setting when counseling overweight or obese individuals, the guidelines recommend an individualized weight reduction plan, consisting of a relatively lower amount of carbohydrates and moderate in protein and fat with specific activity and behavior modification guidelines. These recommendations are quite different from the general dietary recommendations of the American Diabetes Association (ADA). The ADA guidelines have centered on hyperglycemia and cardiovascular risk factors such as hyperlipidemia and hypertension. The ADA recommends that individuals with prediabetes receive education to achieve weight loss of 5% to 10% of body weight and increase physical activity to 30 minutes a day, while stressing the importance of follow-up education to achieve success. The ADA guidelines also recommend a range of 45% to 65% of calories from carbohydrates and no more than 15% to 20% of calories from protein. The guidelines agree that the National Cholesterol Education Program (NCEP) recommendations for people with existing cardiovascular disease should apply to people with diabetes: 25% to 35% of calories should be from fat with <7% calories of saturated fat, 20% monounsaturated fat, and 10% polyunsaturated fat (and trans fat kept to a minimum).

As abdominal fat, and in particular visceral fat, is a major risk factor for type 2 diabetes, coronary artery disease, and hypertension, the Joslin guidelines target those people with

- BMI >25 kg/m$^2$
- Waist size of >40"/102 cm in men and >35"/88 cm in women with type 2 diabetes
- Prediabetes and at high risk for type 2 diabetes
- Metabolic syndrome
- First-degree relative with type 2 diabetes
- Confirmed diagnosis of insulin resistance

A BMI of >23 kg/m$^2$ and a waist size of >35"/90 cm in men and >31"/80 cm in women is used for the Asian population.

The goals of the Joslin guidelines are as follows:

- Improve metabolic control with weight loss and maintain achieved weight loss
- Prevent complications of diabetes by improving fasting and postprandial hyperglycemia
- Improve lipid profile and insulin sensitivity
- Improve body-fat distribution by reducing visceral fat
- Reduce cardiovascular risk by improving endothelial function and endothelial markers
- Reduce inflammatory cytokines and markers of inflammation and increased coagulation
- Improve blood pressure to decrease the risk of cardiovascular and renal complications
- Enhance thermogenesis and maintain lean body mass
- Provide a balanced meal plan to include carbohydrate, protein, and fat
- Improve overall health through physical activity
- Prevent and treat the chronic complications of diabetes

**Weight Loss**

The Joslin guidelines are based on the premise that successful weight loss can be achieved by a modest lowering of total caloric intake and percentage of caloric intake from carbohydrates, while changing the type of carbohydrate one eats, in addition to modestly raising protein, eating heart-healthy fats, increasing fiber intake, and increasing regular physical activity. It has been demonstrated that relatively higher protein diets can increase satiety, improve insulin sensitivity, reduce fasting insulin levels, and improve blood glucose control with an energy-restricted meal plan (500 kcal/d).

A modest weight loss of 5% to 10% of body weight is encouraged. This is supported by previous research in the Diabetes Prevention Program (DPP) that demonstrated that lifestyle changes with a 7% weight loss delayed the development of type 2 diabetes in high-risk individuals by 58%, over an average duration of 3 years, as compared with the placebo group. The Joslin nutrition guidelines recommend that individuals eat 250 to 500 fewer calories a day, through an individualized and structured meal plan. Total calories should not be less than 1,000 to 1,200 for women and 1,200 to 1,600 for men.

Meal replacements (MRs) in the form of shakes, bars, or ready-to-mix powders can be incorporated into a weight loss meal plan, and can be helpful for some individuals to initiate weight loss. Meal replacements are a successful adjunct therapy for weight loss and may be a convenient way for obese individuals to adhere to an energy-restricted meal plan. The guidelines emphasize making lifestyle changes and setting short-term and long-term goals that are realistic and achievable.

### Macronutrients

#### Carbohydrates

In the past, recommendations for carbohydrate intake were higher due to the concern about too much fat being linked to cardiovascular disease (CVD). In the early 70s, there was great concern about the link between eating fat and CVD. As a result, the message was to cut down on fat and replace it with carbohydrates. Research identified later that it is the saturated fat and trans fat that contributes to CVD and not all other types of fat. While Americans are eating less fat than they did years ago, carbohydrate consumption has increased tremendously over the last few decades and Americans continue to get heavier as a result. Short-term data have demonstrated that successful weight loss can occur with a relatively lower-carbohydrate, higher-protein, and higher-fat approach.

The Joslin guidelines carbohydrate recommendations are based on reducing overall daily carbohydrate intake to about 40% of total calories. Total carbohydrate intake should not be less than 130 g/d, based on the recommendations of the National Academy of Sciences Food and Nutrition Board, because the brain and central nervous system use glucose as their primary energy source. The guidelines recommend that when planning meals for weight loss, the glycemic index (GI) and glycemic load (GL) should be taken into consideration. The GI and the GL of foods look at individual foods, how quickly the body absorbs them, how much carbohydrate a serving contains, and the impact on blood glucose. The GI/GL concept is an important factor that patients should apply in their daily selection of carbohydrates. Foods with a low GI or a low GL are less likely to cause a sharp rise in blood glucose after eating.

While the concept of GI and GL is still controversial, the Joslin guidelines recommend individuals choose foods with a lower GI. Examples of favorable carbohydrates are: unprocessed whole grain starches, cereals containing oats and barley, legumes, fruits and vegetables. The ADA, in its analysis of randomized controlled trials of the effects of GI on overall blood glucose control, has suggested that the GI may be of additional benefit rather than considering total carbohydrate alone. Further investigation is warranted regarding the GL and mixed meals on blood glucose control.

#### Fiber

Evidence from both epidemiological and short-term experimental studies suggest that fiber plays a role in weight loss and can assist with insulin resistance and cholesterol lowering. It was observed in a large prospective cohort study that women who consumed more whole grains consistently had a 49% lower risk of major weight gain compared with women who ate less whole grains. Joslin's guidelines encourage eating 20 to 35 g of fiber per day and up to 50 g of fiber per day if tolerated. Fiber is found in whole grain foods, fruits and vegetables, and legumes. The benefits of adding fiber to a healthy meal plan are many. In addition to keeping your digestive tract running smoothly, it helps you feel full, it improves glycemic control, and decreases hyperinsulinemia. In a recent study, fiber intake was determined from dietary records for 2,532 men and 3,429 women. In those with the highest total dietary fiber intake there was a lower risk of: overweight, elevated waist-to-hip ratio, high blood pressure, and high cholesterol. Research findings suggested that 25 g of total dietary fiber per day is the minimum intake required to achieve a significant protective effect against cardiovascular disease; however, total dietary fiber intakes of 30 to 35 g per day will provide an even greater protective effect. Another study also demonstrated that higher levels (50 g/day) of fiber can lower plasma lipid concentrations in patients with type 2 diabetes. Fiber supplements (e.g., psyllium, B-glucan) may be needed to reach higher intakes, although natural sources of fiber like fruits and vegetables are usually preferable.

#### Protein

The Joslin guidelines recommend 20% to 30% of daily calories should come from protein. This is a range of protein based on calorie consumption. Someone who is eating a higher amount of calories would be in the 20% range, while someone eating fewer calories would be in the 30% range. For instance, a meal plan of 1,200 calories would provide 81 g of protein or 30% of calories, while a meal plan of 1,800 calories would provide 120 g of protein or 20%. The amount of protein is based on an individual's total daily calories and proportional to carbohydrate and fat calculations (see Table 1). These recommendations are for people with normal kidney function. Those people with microalbuminuria or impaired renal function should not follow the higher protein recommendation.

Adequate protein combined with resistance exercise helps to maintain lean body mass during weight loss. Clinical trials have shown that increasing protein from 15% to 30% of calories enhances weight loss. In addition, insulin sensitivity is increased, with greater reduction of A1C. Systolic and diastolic blood pressure and LDL cholesterol decrease significantly. One study demonstrated that an increased protein intake in persons with type 2 diabetes resulted in a 40% decrease in the mean 24-hour glucose response.

Another study found a 5.7% reduction in LDL cholesterol in subjects following a high protein (HP), energy-restricted diet of 28% protein, 42% carbohydrate, and 28% fat (8% saturated fatty acids, 12% monounsaturated fatty acids, 5% polyunsaturated fatty acids.) This was compared with a group following a low protein (LP), energy-restricted diet of 16% protein, 55% carbohydrate, and 26% fat (8% saturated fatty acids, 11% monounsaturated fatty acids, 5% polyunsaturated fatty acids). The LP diet resulted in only a 2.7% reduction in LDL cholesterol. Lean sources of protein are encouraged. These include fish, turkey, chicken, low-fat dairy, and vegetarian proteins such as tofu, beans, and peas. Foods high in saturated fat, including beef, pork, lamb, and high-fat dairy products (e.g., whole milk, yogurt), should be consumed only in small amounts.

**Fat**

The Joslin guidelines for fat recommend 30% to 35 % of total caloric intake. Saturated fat should be limited to <10% of total caloric intake, or <7% in individuals with LDL cholesterol >100 mg/dL. Polyunsaturated fat should comprise up to 10% of total calories, and monounsaturated fat up to 15% to 20% of total calories. Joslin emphasizes increasing Omega 3 fats and a high intake of monounsaturated and polyunsaturated fat. Sources of omega-3 fats include fatty types of fish such as salmon, mackerel, lake trout, herring, and sardines, as well as walnuts, flaxseed, and soy. Foods high in monounsaturated fat include olive oil, canola oil, peanut oil, avocados and nuts. Foods high in trans fats (e.g., fast foods, commercially baked goods, some margarines) should be avoided.

**Physical Activity**

The Joslin guidelines recommend that physical activity should be an integral part of a weight loss program. Research has shown that increasing physical activity can improve blood glucose, help prevent coronary artery disease and CVD. Specifically, the guidelines agree with the 2005 Dietary Guidelines for Americans—60 to 90 minutes of activity most days of the week. Recommended activities include: walking, biking, swimming, or dancing, with a minimum of 150 to 175 minutes of moderate physical activity a week. Physical activity should include not only cardiovascular activities and stretching for flexibility, but also resistance activities to maintain or increase lean body mass. Physical activity is an important part of any weight loss program, and is essential in maintaining weight loss.

**Implementation of Joslin Guidelines**

Successful implementation of the Joslin guidelines has been shown in the Joslin Clinic Why WAIT? (Weight Achievement and Intensive Treatment) program. A 12-week, multidisciplinary, weight reduction, and intensified diabetes management program geared for clinical practice, the program is staffed by a physician, nurse practitioner, dietitian, exercise physiologist, and behavioral psychologist.

**Results**

Over a 15-month period, 5 groups of patients were enrolled in the Why WAIT? program—a total of 62 participants (22 men, 40 women) with an average age of 56.1±1.4 years (mean±SE), average diabetes duration of 7.2±0.8 years, and average BMI of 37.8±0.64 kg/m$^2$. Patients with renal impairment or severe microalbuminuria and patients unable to exercise were excluded. The program included: a once-weekly didactic session; a change of diabetes medications to enhance weight reduction; modest caloric reduction of 500 kcal/d; and, modified dietary intervention using regular food and meal replacement containing about 40% carbohydrates, 20% to 30% protein, and 30% to 35% fat. It also included a graded and balanced exercise intervention that gradually increased from 20 to 30 minutes per day, 3 to 4 times per week, up to 45 to 60 minutes per day, 6 times per week. The behavioral modification included a once-a-week group discussion coached by a psychologist. Following the initial 12 weeks, participants were offered a monthly support session aimed at maintaining the achieved weight loss. After the initial 12 weeks, participants lost an average of 23.5±1.2 lbs or 9.8±0.4% ($P$<.001) of their initial body weight and 18.0±2.1% ($P$<.001) of their initial body fat. Waist circumference decreased by 3.5+0.34 inches ($P$<.001), and A1c dropped from 7.3±0.16% to 6.4±0.11% ($P$<.001). Total cholesterol decreased by 12.2±12.9% ($P$<.001), triglyceride by 10.9±7.8% ($P$=.01), and LDL by 11.5±3.1% ($P$<.001). C-reactive protein decreased significantly from 6.0±0.85 to 4.2±0.65 mg/L ($P$=.002) and was found to correlate with percentage weight reduction and fat loss ($P$<0.05). Those who completed 1 year follow-up were able to maintain the achieved weight loss and the metabolic improvements. We conclude that application of this weight management program in routine diabetes practice is a valid option. Long-term benefits were maintained for 1 year. This model can be disseminated for application in routine diabetes practice.

**Table 1**

**Suggested Macronutrient Distribution According to Joslin Clinical Guideline**

| Calorie Level | Carbohydrate | | Protein | | Fat | |
|---|---|---|---|---|---|---|
| | Grams | % | Grams | % | Grams | % |
| 1,000 | 130 | 52 | 60 | 24 | 27 | 24 |
| 1,200 | 130 | 43 | 81 | 27 | 40 | 30 |
| 1,500 | 150 | 40 | 113 | 30 | 50 | 30 |
| 1,800 | 180 | 40 | 120 | 27 | 68 | 33 |
| 2,000 | 200 | 40 | 130 | 26 | 75 | 34 |



**Suggested Readings**

1. National Institute of Diabetes and Digestive and Kidney Diseases. National Diabetes Statistics fact sheet: general information and national estimates on diabetes in the United States, 2005. Bethesda, MD: US Department of Health and Human Services, National Institute of Health, 2005. Accessed February 27, 2006.
2. Joslin Diabetes Center & Joslin Clinic: Clinical Nutrition Guideline for Overweight and Obese Adults with Type 2 Diabetes, Pre-diabetes or at High Risk for Developing Type 2 Diabetes. Available at: http://www.joslin.org/managing_your_diabetes_joslin_clinical_guidelines.asp. Accessed August 21, 2007.
3. US Department of Health and Human Services and the Department of Agriculture: 2005 Dietary Guidelines for Americans. 6th ed. January 12, 2005. Accessed April 22, 2006.
4. Sheard N, Clark N, Nathaniel G, Brand-Miller J C, et al. Dietary Carbohydrate (Amount and Type) in the Prevention and Management of Diabetes: A statement by the American Diabetes Association. *Diabetes Care*. 2004;27(9):2266-2271.
5. American Diabetes Association (ADA). Standards of medical care in diabetes—2006 (position statement). *Diabetes Care*. 2006; 29(suppl. 1)S4-S42.
6. Johnston CS, Tjonn SL, Swan PD. High-protein, low-fat diets are effective for weight loss and favorably alter biomarkers in healthy adults. *J Nutr*. 2004;134(3):586-91.
7. Diabetes Prevention Program Research Group (DPP). Reduction in the incidence of type 2 diabetes with lifestyle intervention with Metformin. *N Engl J Med*. 2002;346(6):393-403.
8. Yip I, Go VL, DeShields S, Saltsman P, et.al. Liquid meal replacements and glycemic control in obese type 2 diabetes patients. *Obes Res*. 2001;9(suppl 4):341S-347S.
9. McAuley KA, Hopkins CM, Smith KJ, et al. Comparison of high-fat and high-protein diets with a high-carbohydrate diet in insulin-resistant obese women. *Diabetologia*. 2005;48(1):8-16.

10. Institute of Medicine of the National Academies. Dietary Reference Intakes for Energy, Carbohydrate, Fiber, Fat, Fatty Acids, Cholesterol, Protein, and Amino Acids (Macronutrients). Washington, DC: National Academy Press; 2002.

11. Ludwig DS. Dietary glycemic index and obesity. *J Nutr*. 2000;130(2S Suppl):280S–283S.

12. American Diabetes Association (ADA). Dietary carbohydrate (amount and type) in the prevention and management of diabetes (ADA Statement). *Diabetes Care*. 2004;27(9): 2266-71.*

13. Liu S, Willett WC, Manson JE, Hu FB, Rosner B, Colditz G, Relation between changes in intakes of dietary fiber and grain products and changes in weight and development of obesity among middle-aged women. *Am J Clin Nutr*. 2003;78(5): 920-7.

14. Lairon D, Arnault N, Bertrais S, et al. Dietary fiber intake and risk factors for cardiovascular disease in French adults. *Am J Clin Nutr*. 2005;82(6):1185-94.

15. Chandalia M, Abihimanyu G, Lutjohann D, et al. Beneficial effects of high dietary fiber intake in patients with type 2 diabetes mellitus. *N Engl J Med*. 2000;342(19):1392-8.

16. Gannon MC, Nuttall FQ, Saeed A, et al. An increase in dietary protein improves the blood glucose response in persons with type 2 diabetes. *Am J Clin Nutr*. 2003;78(4):734-41.

17. Parker B, Noakes M, Luscombe N, et al. Effect of a high-protein, high-monounsaturated fat weight loss diet on glycemic control and lipid levels in type 2 diabetes. *Diabetes Care*. 2002; 25(3):425-30.

18. Klein, S, Sheard NF, Pi-Sunyer X, et al. Weight management through lifestyle modification for the prevention and management of type 2 diabetes: rationale and strategies: a statement of the American Diabetes Association, the North American Association for the Study of Obesity, and the American Society for Clinical Nutrition. *Diabetes Care*. 2004;27(8):2067-73.

19. Wing RR, Phelan S. Long-term weight loss maintenance. *Am J Clin Nutr*. 2005;82(1 suppl):222S-225S.

20. Hamdy O, Carver C, Grant G, et al. Weight achievement and intensive treatment (Why WAIT?): an innovative, multidisciplinary clinical-practice program for weight control in obese diabetic patients. [Abstract taken from ADA 66th Annual Meeting, June 2006].

21. Clinical Nutrition Guideline Appendix A: Suggested Macronutrient Distribution According to Clinical Guideline. Available at: http://www.joslin.org/759_joslin_clinical_guidelines.asp. Accessed March 31, 2006.

*This paper discusses the glycemic index (GI) and glycemic load (GL). It evaluated current research and the use of the GI and GL on glucose control and insulin production.

# Nutrition Assessment

Susan Cummings, MS, RD

Medical nutrition therapy (MNT) is the nutritional treatment necessary to manage or treat a condition, illness, or injury. It incorporates a thorough nutrition assessment, an individualized care plan designed for each patient followed by the provision of diet counseling to implement the care plan, and monitoring and adjustments of the care plan and nutrition therapy as needed. This chapter will focus on the nutritional assessment for patients considering bariatric surgery.

A thorough nutritional assessment: 1) identifies nutritional risks and complications, 2) provides baseline data with which to measure treatment outcomes, and 3) guides treatment recommendations. Expert opinion suggests that registered dietitians (RDs) are best qualified to provide nutritional care, including preoperative assessment and postoperative education, counseling, and follow-up.(1) Although there are no data that provide information regarding behavioral and/or lifestyle contraindications for weight loss surgery (WLS), the decision to recommend this surgery requires assessing the risk-benefit ratio. A thorough nutrition evaluation takes into consideration medical and psychological factors and identifies nutritional risks and complications, including micronutrient deficiencies and nutrition-related comorbidities that have a significant relationship to food choices and food-related behaviors, such as metabolic syndrome, diabetes, and hyperlipidemia. A patient's lifestyle, work hours, meal structure, sleep pattern, access to healthy foods, psychosocial status, support systems, motivation, and readiness are all considered in the nutrition assessment.

**Presurgery Nutrition Assessment—Anthropometrics**

Clinically useful measures of body weight are those that are highly correlated with risks of physical health and are noninvasive, easy to use and inexpensive, as well as reliable and capable methods for reflecting short- and long-term changes in body fat.(2) The standard measurement for weight status is body mass index (BMI), estimated by weight (kg) divided by height ($m^2$). The BMI chart is available on the following page. Office scales should be able to weigh patients who are greater than 350 lbs and be calibrated on a regular basis. The designated professional(s) doing the anthropometric measurements should be trained to use techniques that have been standardized and should be nonjudgmental and sensitive to the patient's privacy. Emotional attachments to weight should be taken into consideration. Ideally, the scale is kept in a private location.

It is advisable to determine a specific protocol for all anthropometric measurements, i.e., when measuring weight, a protocol should ensure clinical consistency such as street clothes with or without shoes. Weights should be recorded to the nearest 0.1 kg.

Height should be measured every 5 years and, as with weight, techniques for measuring height should be standardized. The patient should be instructed to stand with heels together, weight evenly distributed on both feet, and head positioned with the line of vision horizontal to the floor. The patient should be instructed to remove hair ornaments. Lower the headboard (if using a stadiometer) or bar (if using a balance scale) to the most superior point on the head, exerting pressure to compress the hair When using a bar attached to a scale, the bar should be straight and perpendicular to the floor. Record the height measurement to the nearest 0.1 cm.

**BMI Chart (lbs)**

| BMI | 23 | 24 | 25 | 26 | 27 | 28 | 29 | 30 | 31 | 32 | 33 | 34 | 35 |
|---|---|---|---|---|---|---|---|---|---|---|---|---|---|
| Height (inches) | Body Weight (pounds) | | | | | | | | | | | | |
| 58" (4′10") | 110 | 115 | 119 | 124 | 129 | 134 | 138 | 143 | 148 | 153 | 158 | 162 | 167 |
| 60" (5′) | 118 | 123 | 128 | 133 | 138 | 143 | 148 | 153 | 158 | 163 | 168 | 174 | 179 |
| 62" (5′2") | 126 | 131 | 136 | 142 | 147 | 153 | 158 | 164 | 169 | 175 | 180 | 186 | 191 |
| 64" (5′4") | 134 | 140 | 145 | 151 | 157 | 163 | 169 | 174 | 180 | 186 | 192 | 197 | 204 |
| 66" (5′6") | 142 | 148 | 155 | 161 | 167 | 173 | 179 | 186 | 192 | 198 | 204 | 210 | 216 |
| 68" (5′8") | 151 | 158 | 164 | 171 | 177 | 184 | 190 | 197 | 203 | 210 | 216 | 223 | 230 |
| 70" (5′10") | 132 | 167 | 174 | 181 | 188 | 195 | 202 | 209 | 216 | 222 | 229 | 236 | 243 |
| 72" (6′) | 169 | 177 | 184 | 191 | 199 | 206 | 213 | 221 | 228 | 235 | 242 | 250 | 258 |
| 74" (6′2") | 179 | 186 | 194 | 202 | 210 | 218 | 225 | 233 | 241 | 249 | 256 | 264 | 272 |
| 76" (6′4") | 189 | 197 | 205 | 213 | 221 | 230 | 238 | 246 | 254 | 263 | 271 | 279 | 287 |

### Criteria for Surgery

The National Institutes of Health (NIH) Consensus Development Conference on Gastrointestinal Surgery for Severe Obesity patient-selection criteria for bariatric surgery includes a BMI $\geq$40 kg/m$^2$, or BMI $\geq$35 in the presence of significant comorbidities.(3) In addition, the recommendation is for patients to be well-informed and motivated and that previous nonsurgical approaches to long-term weight loss have failed. Recently, the Centers for Medicare & Medicaid Services (CMS) determined that the evidence is adequate to conclude that open and laparoscopic Roux-en-Y gastric bypass (RYGB), laparoscopic adjustable gastric banding (LAGB), and open and laparoscopic biliopancreatic diversion with duodenal switch (BPD/DS) are reasonable and necessary for Medicare beneficiaries who have a BMI $\geq$35, have at least one comorbidity related to obesity, and have been previously unsuccessful with medical treatment for obesity. Therefore, a patient's weight and dieting history must be part of the presurgical nutrition assessment and can be obtained through a questionnaire given to the patient prior to the nutrition visit (Table 1). The dietitian and other healthcare professionals can then review the information for accuracy during the interview.

### Weight History

Although there are data to suggest genetics have an influence on biological determinants of obesity (such as resting energy expenditure, diet-induced thermogenesis, and metabolic responses to overeating), there are no accurate ways to measure an individual's genetic predisposition to obesity. There are variables, however, that may suggest a patient's predisposition to obesity based on genetic influences. These variables include age of onset of obesity and family weight history. It is important to note, however, that since obesity is a polygenetic disorder, individuals have varying degrees of genetic influences.

### Age of Onset of Obesity

Childhood or adolescent onset may be indicative of a strong genetic predisposition to obesity. Fat-cell proliferation in childhood and/or adolescence may lead to hyperplastic obesity (increase in fat cell numbers) versus hypertrophic obesity (increase in fat-cell size without excessive numbers). Patients with hypertrophic obesity have a reasonable prognosis for reaching average weight or normal BMI after weight loss efforts because hypertrophy is reversible.(4) However, hyperplastic obesity does not seem to be reversible.(5) Individuals with severe, hyperplastic obesity are likely to have 2 to 3 times the normal number of fat cells and a fat mass that is increased by the same proportion.(6) These may be the patients who do not reach a normal BMI after WLS. This is important information to share with patients, as patient expectations are often unrealistic or unsubstantiated. Many patients believe that they will lose 100% of their excess body weight. Fourteen years of data on patients undergoing RYGB show mean weight losses of 65% of excess body weight, with a regain of about 10% to 15% in the first 2 to 5 years.(7) Currently, there are no data to predict which patient characteristics are predictive of weight loss postsurgery. Family weight history, particularly immediate family (parents and siblings), may give additional information on genetic and/or environmental influences. Data from adoption studies suggest that genetic factors may account for an estimated 40% to 70% of the variance in body weight.(8)

**Dieting history**

Previous dieting attempts can be categorized as: commercial diet programs, with or without meal replacements; medically supervised diet programs, including prescribed weight loss medications; previous nutritional programs with an RD; and self-directed diets, including over-the-counter weight loss aids and/or nutritional supplements. Patients should be asked for the dates (or at what age) they participated in these programs; how many times they participated in the program (re-enrollments); how much weight was lost and how much regained; and how long they were able to maintain the weight loss. Since failure of previous nonsurgical weight loss programs is required by insurance carriers, this information should be well documented and included in the letter of medical necessity sent to the patient's insurance provider. Some insurance providers require a recent, 3-to-6-month, medically supervised weight loss program and in such cases, a physician or dietician can partner to provide a program through individual visits. Alternatively, based on the number of patients seeking help with weight loss, it may be more resource-efficient to design ongoing nutrition groups led by a an RD. The physician or dietician should provide documentation of patient participation and the patients' weights at each visit.

Additional probing questions about dieting history that may help to identify postoperative challenges include:

- What made maintenance difficult? What were the triggers to weight regain after dieting attempts?
- Has the patient been or is the patient on medications that increase hunger and/or cravings (specifically weight-promoting psychopharmacological medications)?
- Can any weight-promoting medications be changed to less weight-promoting medications?
- Has the patient been on weight loss medications that did or did not work?
- What are the learned and cognitive influences guiding eating behaviors?
- Were there emotional triggers to weight regain? Did the patient start to binge-eat? Is there a history of binge-eating? Does the patient meet the criteria for binge-eating disorder (BED)?

**Assessing for eating disorders**

Established eating behavior assessment tools include the Dutch Eating Behavior Questionnaire;(9) the Three-Factor Eating Questionnaire;(10) the Binge-Eating Survey;(11) and the Questionnaire on Eating and Weight Patterns (QEWP-R).(12) These questionnaires can be easily administered. Binge-eating disorder can also be assessed through a patient interview.

Binge-eating disorder is characterized by recurrent episodes of binge-eating associated with subjective and behavioral indicators of impaired control over, and significant distress about, the binge-eating without the presence of inappropriate compensatory behaviors, inducing purging, fasting, or compulsive exercising. A binge comprises at least two elements: one subjective (a sense of loss of control) and the other objective (the actual amount of food consumed).(13) There is uncertainty of what the amount of food eaten should be in order for an event to be considered a binge; however, it is described as an amount that is definitely larger than most people would eat.

Screening questions (13) for BED would include:

- Are there times when you cannot stop eating?
- Are you eating unusually large amounts of food in a short time period?
- Do you ever feel extremely guilty or depressed afterward?
- Do you feel more determined to diet afterward?

The belief that dieting is a risk factor for BED appears to be incorrect and has been rejected by the National Task Force on the Prevention and Treatment of Obesity, which has concluded that empirical studies do not support the belief that dieting induces binge-eating in adults with obesity who seek weight reduction.(14,15)

Night-eating syndrome (NES) was first noted in 1955 and is described as a stress-related eating, sleeping, and mood disorder associated with disordered neuroendocrine function.(16) It follows a characteristic circadian pattern and is characterized by morning anorexia and evening hyperphagia and insomnia, often with depression. Night-eating syndrome is uncommon in the general population and although present in nonobese persons, is more common in persons with obesity. Prevalence of NES increases with increasing weight and the syndrome appears to be a unique combination of eating, sleeping, and mood disorders. It differs from BED in that there is far greater frequency of nighttime awakenings and less food is ingested at these times. Information about the prognosis and treatment of NES is limited and more research on the syndrome is warranted.

**Determining the Patient's Current Eating Patterns**

An assessment of eating patterns will help identify problematic eating behaviors that may lead to overeating, under-eating, and/or poor food choices triggered by a chaotic, stressful life style or patient's inability to plan and prepare healthy meals and/or snacks. Presurgery guidance in structuring meals and snacks, making time for procuring healthy foods, practicing mindful eating, and paying attention to hunger and satiety are useful strategies when preparing for WLS.

Questions to ask regarding meal and snacking patterns include:

- Does the patient skip meals? Is the patient a "chronic snacker/picker?"
- When and what time of day are most calories consumed? During meals? When snacking? When drinking beverages? During the day or evening?
- How much control does the patient have over his/her food choices?
- Who shops and prepares the food?
- How many meals a week/month are eaten out?
- What types of restaurants does the patient frequent?
- Does the patient consume large amounts of high-calorie beverages?

**Assessing the Patient's Energy Expenditure**

Total energy expenditure (TEE) is estimated using predictive equations for resting metabolic rate and adding an activity factor. The Mifflin-St Jeor equation using actual weight may be the most accurate for estimating resting metabolic rate (RMR) for overweight and obese individuals. The equation was tested only on Caucasian subjects and, thus, may not be accurate for other groups. Research on predictive equations separating obese from nonobese subjects is limited.(17) The Mifflin-St Jeor equation for energy assessment, or basal metabolic rate (BMR), is as follows:

Male: $BMR = 10 \times weight + 6.25 \times height - 5 \times age + 5$

Female: $BMR = 10 \times weight + 6.25 \times height - 5 \times age - 161$

Once the BMR is calculated, an activity factor is assigned based on the patient's reported activity. Total energy expenditure is estimated by multiplying the BMR by the physical activity level (PAL). These levels were developed based on doubly labeled water (DLW) studies (18) and are as follows:

- Sedentary 1.2 (chair-bound or bed-bound)
- Lightly active 1.4-1.5 (sedentary job, little or no strenuous leisure activity)
- Moderately active 1.5 (moderate exercise/sports 3-5 days a week)
- Extremely active 1.6 (hard exercise/sports 6-7 days a week)
- Extra active 1.9 (very hard exercise/sports and physical job)

**Caloric and Nutritional Intake**

Patients can be asked to keep a food diary for 1 day or to recall what they have eaten in the past 24 hours. The dietician will review this recall with them and probe to ensure that all foods, beverages, and portions are recorded. In addition, it is essential to obtain the following information from the patient:

- How do meals vary day to day or on weekends?
- What food allergies or intolerances does the patient have?
- In terms of alcohol consumption, what does the patient drink, how often, and how many drinks, on average, each time?

- Does the patient use dietary and/or herbal supplements and if so, what type and dose?
- Does the patient use meal replacements such as protein shakes, bars, or frozen meals?

An RD can estimate caloric intake and percent of calories from carbohydrate, protein, and fat and then assess the nutritional adequacy of the diet. Patients tend to underestimate portions and total caloric intake (19); therefore, there may be discrepancies between the intake reported and estimated calorie needs. In this case, it is useful to ask additional probing questions such as: Do you pick while cooking? Do you eat off of your children's plates? What size glass or paper cups do you tend to drink from? If I looked in your refrigerator and freezer, what would I see? If I looked in your food cabinets, what foods would I see? Are there snacks available at work and do you tend to eat them? Additional probing questions may be to ask about added fats, added sugar, and hidden calories.

Early, post-WLS patients will be challenged to make the time to eat in a slow, mindful manner, to procure nutrient-dense foods and appropriate, noncarbonated, noncaloric clear liquids, and to take vitamin and mineral supplements. Therefore, eliciting information about the patient's ability to procure healthy foods and supplements and who does the grocery shopping and meal preparation is important. If the patient is not the shopper or preparer, than educating the appropriate individual and making sure that the patient will have access to the appropriate foods, fluids, and supplements is essential. Presurgical nutrition education for all patients and their families will help prepare patients for the early postoperative challenges and long-term nutritional needs following WLS.

**Nutritional Status: Presurgery Laboratory Workup**

Nutritional screening labs, prebariatric surgery, should include: $B_{12}$, folate, iron studies, including hemoglobin/hematocrit, total iron-binding capacity (TIBC) and ferritin, parathyroid hormone, 25-hydroxy vitamin D, serum calcium, folic acid, thiamin ($B_1$), and vitamin K. Obtaining baseline micronutrient status and repleting those that are deficient is essential prior to WLS. Additional presurgical nutritional labs include fasting blood glucose, A1C, and lipid profile. Successful patient outcomes include resolved and/or significant improvement in comorbidities such as diabetes and hyperlipidemia.

Patients undergoing WLS are at risk for deficiencies in iron, $B_{12}$, and vitamin D, and impaired calcium absorption and should be informed that a lifetime of postsurgical nutritional supplementation is essential(20,21,22,23,24) (See Table 2). Patients, especially postmenopausal women, should be advised to get a baseline bone density test presurgery and every 2 years thereafter.

**Physical Activity**

An individual's activity and the effect of that activity on TEE can vary daily. In order to calculate TEE, an assumption must be made about PALs. Nonexercise activity thermogenesis (NEAT) is the cumulative energy expended during all activities of daily living (ADL), excluding formal, purposeful exercise programs, RMR, and diet-induced thermogenesis.(25) It is highly variable among individuals and there is evidence suggesting that it is critical in determining a person's susceptibility to body-fat deposition, and thus, is a major factor in human obesity. A variety of factors influence nonexercise activity, including occupation, environment, education, genetics, age, gender, and body composition, but little is known about the magnitude of effect.(26) Assessing a patient's nonexercise activity is part of a total obesity assessment. Providing or encouraging patients to purchase activity pedometers to assess daily activity is useful. Questionnaires regarding hours of day spent in sedentary activity (sleeping, sitting, watching television, at the computer, etc.) are also useful in assessing ADL.

An assessment of physical activity may identify those patients who may benefit from a presurgical physical therapy referral. To reduce the risk of deep vein thrombosis (DVT), patients are encouraged to be mobile immediately after surgery. Patients should be aware of the risks of developing blood clots by sitting or reclining for long hours without movement after surgery. Assisting the sedentary patient in setting activity goals in preparation for postsurgical mobility may help to reduce these risks.

### Motivation

Patients vary in their commitment and the extent to which they are ready to tolerate the discomfort associated with change. They also vary in the key features of the weight problem that concerns them. Some may be motivated by health, others by appearance. Some hope to solve life problems, which may need to be identified and dealt with prior to any weight loss attempts. Many patients want to lose weight; however, we cannot assume that all patients are equally ready to make significant and sustained alterations in their behavior. Identifying and helping individuals to clarify what their motivation is and what commitments they are willing to make is a very important component of the comprehensive evaluation.

### Assessing Readiness

The stages-of-change model identifies a sequence of stages.(27) It is useful to identify what stage of change the patient is in for each new behavior. If an individual hasn't even thought about increasing physical activity (precontemplation stage), he/she is not likely to take a successful action step without first moving toward contemplation and identifying his/her intrinsic motivation to make the change and then preparing to actually make a sustainable change. The following is a list of the stages of change and suggestions that response providers can make at each stage:

- Precontemplation

  Patient is not currently considering change

  *Personalize risk*
- Contemplation

  Patient is thinking about it

  *Help to problem solve*
- Preparation

  Some experience with change: patient is trying to change; getting ready

  *Give direction and support*
- Action

  Practicing new behavior regularly for 3 to 6 months

  *Reinforce healthy behaviors*
- Maintenance

  Patient shows continued commitment to sustaining new behavior

  *Provide relapse strategies*

### Assessing Barriers to Treatment

What role does the patient's weight play? For some individuals, weight may be perceived as a protection. There may be fears associated with losing the weight, i.e., that becoming thinner will make the person more vulnerable. Assessment of a patient's belief that he/she will be able to make the required nutritional changes after WLS is an important component of a thorough presurgical assessment. Patients should be asked questions like, "How confident are you in your ability to make the necessary nutritional changes after the surgery?" Answers may help identify issues that can be worked through prior to surgery and can illuminate need for additional presurgical preparation and nutritional education.

Support systems for patients after WLS are key. Patients should be able to identify who in their life will provide support and be available to assist them as needed. If a patient lacks support and is unable to care for him-/herself—especially if he/she should develop complications—arrangement for postsurgical rehabilitation is indicated.

### The Dietitian's Role in the Evaluation and Assessment Phase

Dietitians are uniquely trained to assess and monitor the physiological changes that occur in a patient's nutritional status and to educate, guide, and support patients in the challenges of behavioral change. A pre- and postsurgical medical team consisting of a physician, RD, mental health provider, and physical therapist or exercise physiologist can provide the preoperative assessments, identify risks and benefits, and increase patient safety by using this evaluation to prepare patients for WLS and postsurgical challenges.

**References**


1. Saltzman E, Anderson W, Apovian CM, Boulton H, Chamberlain A, Cullum-Dugan D, Cummings S, et al. Criteria for patient selection and multidisciplinary evaluation and treatment of the weight loss surgery patient. *Obes Res*. 2005;13(2):234-43.
2. Cummings S, Parham ES, Strain GW. Position of the American Dietetic Association: weight management. *J Am Diet Assoc*. 2002;102(8):1145-55.
3. NIH Conference. Gastrointestinal surgery for severe obesity: Consensus Development Conference Panel. *Ann Intern Med*. 1991;115(12):956-61.
4. Krotkiewski M, Sjöström L, Björntorp P, Carlgren G, Garellick G, Smith U. Adipose tissue cellularity in relation to prognosis for weight reduction. *Int J Obes*. 1977;1(4):395-416.
5. Naslun I, Hallgren P, Sjöström L. Fat cell weight and number before and after gastric surgery for morbid obesity in women. *Int J Obes*. 1988;12(3):191-7.
6. Wadden TA, Strunkard AJ, eds. *Handbook of Obesity Treatment*; Guilford Press, 2003.
7. Pories WJ, Swanson MS, MacDonald KG, et al. Who would have thought it? An operation proves to be the most effective therapy for adult-onset diabetes mellitus. *Ann Surg*. 1995;222(3):339-50; discussion 350-2.
8. Stunkard AJ, Harris JR, Pedersen NL, McClearn GE. The body-mass index of twins who have been reared apart. *N Engl J Med*. 1990;322(21):1483-7.
9. van Strien T, Frijters JER, Bergers GPA, Defares PB. The Dutch Eating Behavior Questionnaire (DEBQ) for assessment of restrained, emotional and external eating behavior. *Int J Eat Dis*. 1986;5(2):295-315.
10. Stunkard AJ, Messick S. The three-factor eating questionnaire to measure dietary restraint, disinhibition and hunger. *J Psychosom Res*. 1985;29(1):71-83.
11. Gormally J, Black S, Daston S, Rardin D. The assessment of binge eating severity among obese persons. *Addict Behav*. 1982;7(1):47-55.
12. Yanovski SZ. Binge eating disorder: current knowledge and future directions. *Obes Res*. 1993;1(4):306-24.
13. Wilfley DE, Wilson GT, Agras WS. The clinical significance of binge eating disorder. *Int J Eat Disord*. 2003;34(suppl):S96-S106.
14. National Task Force on the Prevention and Treatment of Obesity, National Institutes of Health. Dieting and the development of eating disorders in overweight and obese adults. *Arch Intern Med*. 2000;160(17):2581-9.
15. Stunkard AJ, Allison KC. Binge eating disorder: disorder or marker? *Int J Eat Disord*. 2003;34(suppl):S107-S16.
16. Stunkard AJ, Allison KC. Two forms of disordered eating in obesity: binge eating and night eating. *Int J Obes Relat Metab Disord*. 2003;27(1):1-12.
17. Mifflin MD, St Jeor ST, Hill LA, Scott BJ, Daugherty SA, Koh YO. A new predictive equation for resting energy expenditure in healthy individuals. *Am J Clin Nutr*. 1990;51(2):241-7.
18. Scrimshaw NS, Waterlow JC, Schürch B, eds. Proceedings of an International Dietary Energy Consultative Group workshop held in London, England, October 31 to November 4, 1994.
19. Braam LA, Ocké MC, Bueno-de-Mesquita HB, Seidell JC. Determinants of obesity-related underreporting of energy intake. *Am J Epidemiol*. 1998;147(11):1081-6.
20. Halverson JD. Micronutrient deficiencies after gastric bypass for morbid obesity. *Am Surg*. 1986;52(11):594-8.

21. Avinoah E, Ovnat A, Charuzi I. Nutritional status seven years after Roux-en-Y gastric bypass surgery. *Surgery*. 1992;111(2):137-42.

22. Brolin RE, Gorman RC, Milgrim LM, Kenler HA. Multivitamin prophylaxis in prevention of post-gastric bypass vitamin and mineral deficiencies. *Int J Obes*. 1991;15(10):661-7.

23. Brolin RE, Gorman JH, Gorman RC, et al. Prophylactic iron supplementation after Roux-en-Y gastric bypass: a prospective, double-blind, randomized study. *Arch Surg*. 1998;133(7):740-4.

24. Brolin RE, Gorman JH, Gorman RC, et al. Are vitamin $B_{12}$ and folate deficiency clinically important after Roux-en-Y gastric bypass? *J Gastrointest Surg*. 1998;2(5):436-442.

25. Kotz CM, Levine JA. Role of non-exercise activity thermogenesis (NEAT) in obesity. *Minn Med*. 2005;88(9):54-7.

26. Levine JA. Non-exercise activity thermogenesis (NEAT): environment and biology. *Am J Physiol Endocrinol Metab*. 2004;286(5):E675-85.

27. Prochaska, JO, DiClemente CC. Transtheoretical therapy toward a more integrative model of change. *Psychotherapy: Theory, Research and Practice*. 1982;19(3):276-88.

Table 1

# NUTRITION ASSESSMENT PREBARIATRIC SURGERY

**Patient Name:** ______________________________ **Patient hospital number:** ____________

**Age:** ______________ **Birth date:** ______________ **Date of evaluation:** ____________

**Obesity co-morbidities**

- ☐ Type 1 or type 2 diabetes
- ☐ Hypertension
- ☐ Asthma/SOB
- ☐ Cancer
- ☐ Anorexia or bulimia
- ☐ Binge or emotional eating
- ☐ Cardiovascular disease
- ☐ Liver/Renal disease
- ☐ GERD
- ☐ Sleep apnea
- ☐ Depression
- ☐ Chronic back pain
- ☐ Arthritis
- ☐ Edema
- ☐ Hyperlipidemia
- ☐ Metabolic syndrome
- ☐ Gallbladder disease
- ☐ Other:

---

**Significant family medical history:**

---

**Psychosocial history:**
Employment:
Medical insurance:
Lives with:
Married/divorced/single
Children and ages:

---

*Primary care physician*
**Phone:**
**Fax:**
**E-mail:**

*Address*

---

**Height:** __________(inches) (cm)
**Weight:**__________(lbs.) (kg)
**Estimated energy expenditure:**
**Mifflin-St Jeor**
**Men RMR:** ____________________
**(9.99 x wt (kg) + (6.25 X ht(cm) – (4.02 X age) + 5**
**Women RMR:** ____________________
**(9.99 X wt kg) + (6.25 x ht cm) – (4.92 x age) – 161**

**Body mass index (BMI)**
**Obesity classification: I II III**

---

**Weight history:**
Lowest adult weight? _____ age:______
Highest adult weight? _____ age: ______
Usual adult weight? (w/o dieting/5 y or more?)

***Lowest***
How achieved? ________________
How long at lowest weight? ______
**Highest**
Triggers/known causes? ________________
How long at highest weight? ______

---

**Family weight history:**

**Mother:**
- ☐ weight normal
- ☐ overweight
- ☐ obesity

**Father:**
- ☐ weight normal
- ☐ overweight
- ☐ obesity

**Sibling 1: male or female?**
- ☐ weight normal
- ☐ overweight
- ☐ obesity

**Sibling: 2: male or female?**
- ☐ weight normal
- ☐ overweight
- ☐ obesity

**Sibling 3. male or female?**
- ☐ weight normal
- ☐ overweight
- ☐ obesity

**Sibling 4: male or female?**
- ☐ weight normal
- ☐ overweight
- ☐ obesity

| **Previous weight loss medications:** | **Medication** | **Medication** |
|---|---|---|
| Who prescribed? | | |
| What dose? | | |
| How long on medication? | | |
| Weight loss on medication? | | |
| How long maintained weight loss? | | |

**Meal replacements / liquid diets**
Type?
When?
How much lost?
How long maintained?

**Weight loss programs?**
- ☐ Weight Watchers
- ☐ Jenny Craig
- ☐ LA Weight Loss
- ☐ TOPS
- ☐ Overeaters Anonymous
- ☐ Nutri Systems
- ☐ Other:

Year
Weight lost/regained?

**Previous dietitian counseling?**
Where:
Weight lost?
How long maintained?

**Hospital-based nutrition, behavior modification program**

Name: ______________________ Year: ______________

Name: ______________________ Year: ______________

**24-hour recall/ frequency**
Start with time patient wakes, first beverage or food and go through day asking for usual and typical variations. Include how weekends may vary.

☐ **Lactose intolerant?**

| TIME | FOOD/BEV | AMOUNT |
|---|---|---|
| | | |

**Religious / cultural food:** **Describe:**

**Food allergies?**______________ **Describe:**

**Alcohol intake?**______________
**What type?**

**How often?**
**How many alcoholic drinks?**
**Per day?**
**Per week?**
**Per month?**

**Dining out:**

| | | | |
|---|---|---|---|
| Sit-down restaurants? | How often | ___ per week | ___ per month |
| Fast-food restaurants? | How often | ___ per week | ___ per month |
| Order out / take home foods | How often | ___ per week | ___ per month |

**Meets criteria for binge-eating disorder?** ☐ **Yes** ☐ **No**
**Describe:**

Grazing/night eating? ☐ Yes ☐ No
Describe:

---

Do you feel you have strong, frequent feelings of hunger relative to others? ☐ Yes ☐ No

Do you feel it takes an unusually large amount of food for you to feel comfortably full? ☐ Yes ☐ No

**Most days do you eat until:** You are comfortable? ☐ Yes ☐ No
Very full? ☐ Yes ☐ No
Stuffed? ☐ Yes ☐ No

**Activities of daily living**
☐ Sedentary
☐ Moderately active
☐ Very active
Describe:

**What is your motivation for weight loss surgery?**
Describe:

| Laboratory data: ☐Per patient ☐Per report | Date: | Glucose | Vit D | PTH | B12 | Iron | Ferritin | TIBC | Ca | Hb/Hct |
|---|---|---|---|---|---|---|---|---|---|---|
| | TG | | | | | | | | | |
| | LDL: | HbA1C | | | | | | | | |
| | HDL: | | | | | | | | | |
| Medications: | Type | Dose | Prescribed by | How long? | Vitamins / supplements: list | | | | | |

Patient's **response to:**

**Patient's expectations of postsurgical eating habits:**

**Are you confident in your ability to make these changes?**
☐ Realistic
☐ Does not seem to envision changes in diet / behavior

**How do you think you will deal with your dietary restrictions?**
☐ Realistic
☐ Does not seem to envision changes in diet / behavior

**If you have a history of emotional eating or eating out of boredom, how will you handle these after surgery?**
☐ Realistic
☐ Does not seem to envision changes in diet / behavior

**List behaviors or food changes that patient thinks will be a challenge to manage after surgery:**

**Patient identified the following person(s) who will be his/her support after weight loss surgery:**

**Patient has attended surgical orientation**
Yes or No
**If no, patient will attend orientation:**
Date: ______________________

---

**DIETITIAN'S ASSESSMENT:**

**Patient deemed nutritionally appropriate to proceed:**
☐ **Yes**
☐ **Contingencies**
☐ **No**

**Contingencies (if any):**

☐ **Referral to appropriate discipline and re-evaluate at a later date as indicated**

**Date:**
**RD (print name:)** ______________________
**RD: contact information:** **office phone:** ______________________
**fax:** ______________________
**e-mail:** ______________________
**RD mailing address:** ______________________
**RD signature:** ______________________

**Table 2**
**Micronutrient Deficiencies Table**

| Nutrient | Normal | Notes | Supplement Daily |
|---|---|---|---|
| **Vitamin D**<br>Vit D 25-OH | 20-46.7 mg/dL<br><br>**RDI's:**<br>Ages 19-50:<br>200 IU/day<br>Ages 51-69:<br>400 IU /day<br>Ages 70+:<br>600 IU/day | **Normal anatomy:**<br>• Vitamin D is absorbed primarily in the proximal part of the small bowel<br>• Vitamin D is needed to maintain normal blood levels of calcium and phosphorous; it aids in absorption of calcium, promotes bone mineralization and prevents rickets in children and osteomalacia in adults<br>• Activity is primarily in intestines, kidney, and bone<br>• Vitamin D deficiency is an epidemic in United States; test pre-gbp surgery and replete as needed.<br>**(>30 is optimal for bone health)**<br>**Markers for vitamin D deficiencies:**<br>• 25-hydroxy vitamin D: most accurate measure of vitamin D stores<br>• PTH: increased in D deficiency<br>• AlkPhos increased in vitamin D deficiency<br>• Serum phosphorous low in vitamin D deficiency | 400-600 IU/day; (calcium supplement with vitamin D)<br><br>**Food sources:**<br>• Cod liver oil, 1 tbs: 1,360 IU<br>• Salmon, cooked, 3 1/2 oz: 360 IU<br>• Milk, nonfat, reduced fat, and whole, vitamin D fortified, 1 c: 98 IU<br>• Margarine, fortified, 1 tbs: 60 IU<br>• Dry cereal, vitamin D fortified w/10% of the recommended daily value, 3/4 c: 40-50 IU (other cereals may be fortified with more or less vitamin D)<br>• Egg, 1 whole (vitamin D is present in the yolk): 25 IU |

| Nutrient | Normal | Notes | Supplement Daily |
|---|---|---|---|
| **Calcium** | **Serum calcium:** 9-10.5 mg/dL<br><br>**Ionized calcium:** 4.5-5.6 mg/dL<br><br>**RDA:** 1200 mg/d | **Normal anatomy**: absorbed in duodenum, proximal gut<br>**GBP**: most of absorption area bypassed<br>**Low serum calcium**<br>• May be low due to poor absorption and/or malnutrition<br>• Half of calcium in the blood is bound to albumin. The other half is free floating "ionized" calcium<br>**Marker**:<br>Bone density studies should be recommended at baseline and every 2 years post-gbp, especially in postmenopausal women and high-risk patients. | 1000 – 1500 mg/day, divided doses<br><br>**Chewable or liquid** calcium in the first month; may switch to pill thereafter<br><br>Calcium citrate is the preferable source of supplemental calcium after gbp (*always take in divided doses*) |
| **Vitamin $B_{12}$**<br>cobalamin | 160-950 pg/mL<br><br>RDA: 2.5 ug/d | **Normal anatomy**:<br>• $B_{12}$ is used to convert inactive folate to active folate<br>• Intrinsic factor (IF), which is secreted by the stomach, is necessary for absorption<br>• Gastric acid also assists in $B_{12}$ absorption by detaching $B_{12}$ from its binding protein<br>**Gastric bypass**:<br>• The major part of the stomach (gastric remnant) is bypassed<br>• Insufficient secretion of IF and decreased $B_{12}$–IF complex formation is due to poor mixing beyond the jejunojejunal junction<br>• Proteolytic destruction of intrinsic factor has been cited as cause of altered absorption of $B_{12}$ after gbp surgery. (Behrns et al) | 350 mcg/day<br>May take sublingually |

| Nutrient | Normal | Notes | Supplement Daily |
|---|---|---|---|
| **Folic Acid** | 3.1 – 17.4 ng/mL<br>or<br>11-57 mmol/L<br><br>RDA: 400 mcg/d | **Normal anatomy:**<br>• Absorbed in duodenum and most efficiently in the jejunum<br>• A coenzyme involved in transferring carbons within cells and in amino acid metabolism<br>**Gastric bypass:**<br>• Folic acid deficiency post-gbp is not prevalent<br>• Deficiency can cause megaloblastic anemia. Signs/symptoms include red tongue, anemia, GI disturbances, and diarrhea | • 400 mcg/day; daily multivitamin or prenatal multivitamin usually adequate<br><br>• Supplementation of folic acid should always include $B_{12}$; folic acid can mask $B_{12}$ deficiency<br><br>• Upper limit for supplementation is 1000 mcg/day male and female |
| **Thiamin $B_1$** | **Female:**<br>30 – 160 mcg/dL<br>**Male:**<br>30 – 300 mcg/dL<br><br>**RDA:**<br>adults 1.2 mg | **Normal anatomy:**<br>• Absorbed primarily in proximal gut<br>• Acts as a coenzyme in reactions that remove $CO_2$<br><br>**Gastric bypass**<br>• Prime absorptive area bypassed<br>• Scattered reports of beriberi after gbp<br>• Patients frequently have vomiting<br>• Thiamine deficiency has been described after vbg<br>Acute Post-Gastric Reduction Surgery (APGARS) neuropathy (approx 40% thought to be due to thiamine deficiency) | Multivitamin with 100% RDA for thiamine |

| Nutrient | Normal | Notes | Supplement Daily |
|---|---|---|---|
| **Vitamin K** | **DRI:**<br>Females: 120 mcg/d<br><br>Males: 90 mcg/day | **Normal anatomy:**<br>• Vitamin K is found in a number of foods, however, the **chief source of vitamin K** is **synthesis by bacteria in the large intestine** and, in most cases, absence of dietary vitamin K is not at all deleterious. **Vitamin K is a fat-soluble vitamin** and both dietary and microbial vitamin K are absorbed into intestinal lymph along with other lipids<br>• Vitamin K is involved in making proteins that are involved in blood clotting and coagulation<br>**Gastric bypass**:<br>Bypassing the duodenum may result in lipid malabsorption in the small intestine and lead to defects in absorption of vitamin K.<br>**Markers:**<br>**Prothrombin time** (PT): 11.3-13.3 s<br>**PTT**: 22-35 s | • Multivitamin with vitamin K or calcium supplement with vitamin K<br><br>• Food sources: green vegetables (collards, spinach, salad greens, broccoli), brussels sprouts, cabbage, plant oils, and margarine |

| Nutrient | Normal | Notes | Supplement Daily |
|---|---|---|---|
| **Iron** | Female:<br>30-160 mg/dl<br><br>Male:<br>30-300 mg/dl<br><br>RDA: 18 mg/d | **Normal anatomy**:<br>• Iron absorption occurs predominantly in the duodenum and upper jejunum<br>• Despite the fact that iron is the second most abundant metal in the earth's crust, iron deficiency is the world's most common cause of anemia.<br>• The physical state of iron entering the duodenum greatly influences its absorption. At physiological pH, ferrous iron ($Fe^{2+}$) is rapidly oxidized to the insoluble ferric ($Fe^{3+}$) form. Gastric acid lowers the pH in the proximal duodenum, enhancing the solubility and uptake of ferric iron.<br>**Gastric bypass**: The gastric remnant is bypassed and gastric-acid production needed in iron absorption is reduced substantially.<br>**Markers:**<br>**TIBC:** (measures all protein available to bind mobile iron), number of cells not bound with iron 228-428 mcg/dl<br>**Ferritin**: measure of stored iron<br>Female: 12-300 ng/ml<br>Male: 30-300ng/ml<br>Increased levels of ferritin can be a sign of iron | Multivitamin with iron<br>**Inhibitors** of iron absorption: phytates, tannins and antacids<br>**Facilitators** of iron absorption: ascorbic acid (vitamin C) and amino acids<br><br>**Pregnancy**<br>**Non-RYGP**<br>30 mg/d<br>60 mg/d if low entering preg.<br>**Post-RYGB**<br>• Prenatal vitamin (30 mg/d) plus supplement up to 100 mg/total/day) |

**References:**


1. Marcason W. What are the dietary guidelines following bariatric surgery? *J Am Diet Assoc*. 2004;104(3):487-8.
2. Halverson JD. Micronutrient deficiencies after gastric bypass for morbid obesity. *Am Surg*. 1986;52(11):594-8.
3. Avinoah E, Ovnat A, Charuzi I. Nutritional status seven years after Roux-en-Y gastric bypass surgery. *Surgery*. 1992;111(2):137-42.
4. Brolin RE, Gorman RC, Milgrim LM, Kenler HA. Multivitamin prophylaxis in prevention of post-gastric bypass vitamin and mineral deficiencies. *Int J Obes Relat Metab Disord*. 1991;15(10):661-7.
5. Brolin RE, Gorman JH, Gorman RC, et al. Prophylactic iron supplementation after Roux-en-Y gastric bypass: a prospective, double-blind, randomized study. *Arch Surg*. 1998;133(7):840-4.
6. Rhode BM, Shustik C, Christou NV, MacLean LD. Iron absorption and therapy after gastric bypass. *Obes Surg*, 1999;9(1):17-21.
7. Rhode BM, Arseneau P, Cooper BA, Katz M, Gilfix BM, MacLean LD. Vitamin $B\text{-}_{12}$ deficiency after gastric surgery for obesity. *Am J Clin Nutr*. 1996;63(1):103-9.
8. Schilling RF, Gohdes PN, Hardie GH. Vitamin $B_{12}$ deficiency after gastric bypass surgery for obesity. *Ann Intern Med*. 1984;101(4):501-2.
9. Brolin RE, Gorman JH, Gorman RC, et al. Are vitamin $B_{12}$ and folate deficiency clinically important after Roux-en-Y gastric bypass? *J Gastrointest Surg*. 1998;2(5):436-42.
10. Goode LR, Brolin RE, Chowdhury HA, Shapses SA. Bone and gastric bypass surgery: effects of dietary calcium and vitamin D. *Obes Res*. 2004;12(1):40-7.
11. Shaker JL, Norton AJ, Woods MF, Fallon MD, Findling JW. Secondary hyperparathyroidism and osteopenia in women following gastric exclusion surgery for obesity. *Osteoporos Int*. 1991;1(3):177-81.

# Anesthetic Considerations

Stephanie B. Jones, MD

This chapter addresses the perioperative implications of anesthesia and bariatric surgery. Why is this important? There is a frightening increase in obesity across the country. From 1991 to 2001, the prevalence of obesity in Massachusetts, a relatively "thin" state by US standards, increased from the 10% to 14% range, to 15% to 19%. Consequently, anesthesiologists must care for "patients of size" on a frequent basis, not only during bariatric surgery. The obese patient may develop cholelithiasis, require joint replacement for weight-related degenerative joint disease, or simply need a basic procedure such as a breast biopsy or knee arthroscopy. Although some of the issues addressed are specific to weight loss surgery (WLS), most are applicable to any obese patient entering the operating room.

The anesthesia task force of the Massachusetts Expert Panel on Weight Loss Surgery, sponsored by the Betsy Lehman Center for Patient Safety, is composed of 8 anesthesiologists who regularly care for bariatric patients. We were chartered with evaluating the available literature in order to create guidelines for anesthetic care of the bariatric patient. The quantity and quality of literature specifically addressing obesity and anesthesia is limited, thus the recommendations were predominantly consensus-based. Happily, agreement was fairly easily reached, not always the case amongst a group of physicians—even those accustomed to caring for a particular patient population.

The number of bariatric procedures performed per year is increasing at an exponential rate. This is because WLS is clearly a beneficial procedure. Flum et al calculated a 30-day mortality after bariatric surgery of about 2%, but the adjusted hazard for death was 33% lower 1 year after surgery. Christou et al showed an 89% decreased relative mortality risk at 5 years, comparing operated with nonoperated patients. The study has some limitations, but it does give the sense that there is good reason to accept the perioperative risks inherent to WLS.

The long-term decrease in mortality following WLS is presumably due to resolution of obesity-related diseases. The majority of patients will experience improvement in conditions such as gastroesophageal reflux disease (GERD), type 2 diabetes, obstructive sleep apnea (OSA), and hypertension. With weight loss and fewer comorbid conditions, anesthetic risk during future procedures may be reduced as well.

Most bariatric patients have extensive preoperative assessments prior to presenting for surgery. Issues of specific concern to the anesthesiologist, such as the airway exam and potential for difficult intravenous access, are added to the existing database during the preanesthetic visit. Obese patients may, of course, present for other surgical procedures, in which case more data gathering may be necessary. It can be difficult in the obese population to use some of the traditional markers for cardiac disease. Exercise tolerance may be an unreliable predictor if weight impairs mobility. A sedentary lifestyle may not induce angina, nor can exertional shortness of breath be assessed. Patients may sleep semi-recumbent due to restrictive pulmonary physiology or GERD, masking signs of heart failure such as orthopnea or paroxysmal nocturnal dyspnea. Lower extremity edema may be obscured by venous stasis. As a result, the threshold to refer for cardiac testing is often lower.

The principle of current anesthesia preoperative assessment is selective testing. Most bariatric patients will have an electrocardiogram (EKG) because of the difficulty in assessment of cardiac disease, as noted above. Chest x-rays are typically low yield unless indicated by a finding on history or physical examination, such as signs of heart failure. Is a polysomnography study to test for OSA needed for all WLS patients? As many as 90% of WLS patients may have sleep apnea, the majority undiagnosed. At a minimum, patients should be screened for OSA using clinical criteria during the preanesthetic evaluation, so that appropriate precautions may be taken during intraoperative and postoperative care. Formal testing of those deemed to be high risk allows initiation of continuous positive airway pressure (CPAP) or other therapy, if indicated. No studies currently demonstrate a positive effect of preoperative CPAP on perioperative morbidity, but it intuitively makes sense. A diagnosis of severe OSA might warrant checking a baseline arterial blood gas (ABG), looking for hypoxic hypoventilation (Pickwickian) syndrome. This data may also be useful if difficulty weaning from the ventilator is anticipated due to extreme body mass index

(BMI) or underlying respiratory disease. Further tests are selected based upon surgical complexity, history, and physical exam. For example, a hemoglobin level should be obtained if anemia is suspected or significant blood loss is anticipated; glucose for diabetic patients; blood urea nitrogen (BUN), creatinine, and potassium for patients with known or suspected renal disease. The majority of WLS patients will have full laboratory testing during their presurgical evaluation, and results obtained within 6 months of surgery should be acceptable barring significant interval changes in medical condition.

In the immediate preoperative period, attention must be paid to several issues. Sedatives such as midazolam should be administered cautiously in patients with OSA, as increased sensitivity to these agents may precipitate airway obstruction. Conflicting data exist on aspiration risk in the obese. The prevailing dogma has been that obesity increases the incidence of aspiration. More recent data suggest that this may not be the case, but that difficulty with airway management leads to gastric distention and subsequent regurgitation. Many patients who present for surgery already take a proton pump inhibitor or $H_2$-receptor blocker for symptomatic GERD. Untreated patients with symptomatic reflux may benefit from an intravenous $H_2$ blocker or oral sodium bicitrate, a nonparticulate antacid.

Weight loss surgery patients are at significant risk for perioperative deep venous thrombosis (DVT) and pulmonary embolism (PE). DVT prophylaxis may include subcutaneous unfractionated or low molecular-weight heparin, sequential compression boots, or a combination of these. Postoperative wound infection is another relatively common occurrence due to poor oxygenation of fatty tissue. Prophylactic antibiotics should be administered prior to and within 30 minutes of incision.

Intraoperatively, the American Society of Anesthesiologists (ASA) standard monitors should be used for all patients undergoing WLS. Invasive arterial blood pressure measurement is occasionally cited as necessary when a noninvasive cuff cannot fit a conically shaped upper arm. For most patients, noninvasive monitoring at an alternative site, such as the forearm, is an adequate solution. Newer devices that noninvasively monitor radial-artery blood pressure are another, albeit more expensive, option. An arterial catheter may be indicated for other reasons, such as monitoring ABG data. Central venous access is sometimes needed for a patient with insufficient peripheral venous access. Monitoring of central venous pressures is not of particular utility, especially during laparoscopic procedures. Abdominal insufflation pressure is transmitted to the thorax, artifactually increasing the measured venous pressure. Frequent position changes during these procedures will further alter measured pressure.

Insufflation pressure and position changes will also affect pulmonary artery pressures measured via a pulmonary artery (PA) catheter, but cardiac output data can still be obtained. Fortunately, WLS patients are rarely sick enough to justify PA catheter monitoring, but there are certainly cases where WLS is planned as a last ditch effort for someone with severe cardiac dysfunction. The possible benefit of a PA catheter must be weighed against the risks, including difficulty with insertion or risk of PA rupture if the patient has developed pulmonary hypertension from severe OSA. As the use of transesophageal echocardiography (TEE) becomes more prevalent during noncardiac surgery, patients such as these may benefit. With TEE, the patient's cardiac response to abdominal insufflation and position changes can be observed and postoperative care and monitoring planned utilizing this information.

Anesthesiologists realize that a morbidly obese patient can potentially present a difficult airway. However, weight or BMI alone is not predictive of difficult intubation. Positive predictors include a large neck, measured by circumference or ultrasound depth of pretracheal tissue, and a Mallampati classification of 3 or 4. The Mallampati classification has relatively poor sensitivity and specificity, but if the view of the soft palate is limited (class 3) or nonexistent (class 4), extra care should certainly be taken to ensure safe airway management. Mask ventilation may also be problematic, especially if the patient has OSA, due to collapse of excess oropharyngeal soft tissue following induction of anesthesia.

Difficult intubation and difficult mask ventilation in a morbidly obese patient can lead to catastrophe, as the oxygen saturation will decrease more rapidly than in an otherwise healthy individual with a lower BMI. This leaves less time to secure the airway. Two factors contribute to rapid desaturation: decreased oxygen supply and increased oxygen demand. Decreased supply is primarily related to a decreased functional residual capacity (FRC) in the lungs. Oxygen in the FRC is available to the patient during the apneic period. The purpose of preoxygenating prior to induction is to maximize this reserve. The time available before desaturation can be increased by preoxygenating and inducing the patient in a 25- to 30-degree head-up position. Another study lengthened this "safe apnea period" by using CPAP during induction. Both these maneuvers presumably increase the FRC and consequently the amount of lung volume available to preoxygenate. Increased demand results simply from the larger mass of tissue requiring oxygenation. Cardiac output is elevated and the already decreased supply of oxygen is used up more quickly.

The most conservative approach to securing the airway is via awake fiber-optic intubation. Excellent topical anesthesia and patient education are the keys to ensuring patient cooperation with this technique, particularly given that OSA may make the use of intravenous sedation risky. The same excessive soft tissue that creates difficulty with direct laryngoscopy and mask ventilation may obscure the view through the bronchoscope—this is not a case for the occasional fiber-optic scope user. For the majority of WLS patients, assuming an otherwise reasonable airway exam, I typically use a rapid-sequence induction with propofol or etomidate and succinylcholine. The patient should be ramped up somewhat on blankets to optimize the "sniffing position," with the chin above the level of the chest (Figure 1). This may help facilitate insertion of the laryngoscope blade into the mouth and, at least in theory, better align the view between the oropharynx and larynx. We have a dedicated difficult-airway cart present in our bariatric operating rooms and I always have an extra pair of hands in the operating room should immediate assistance become necessary.

**Figure 1a**

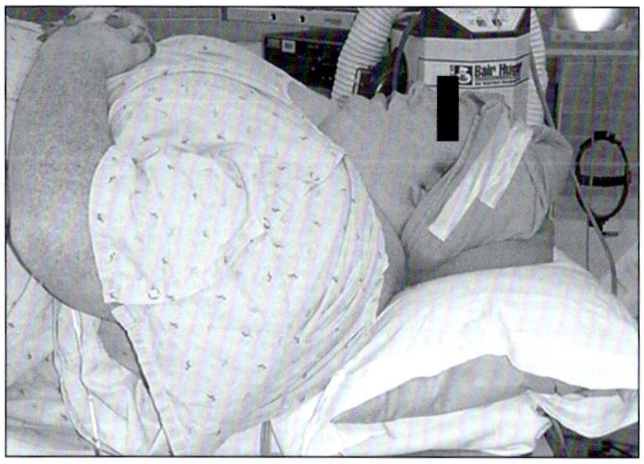

**Figure 1b**

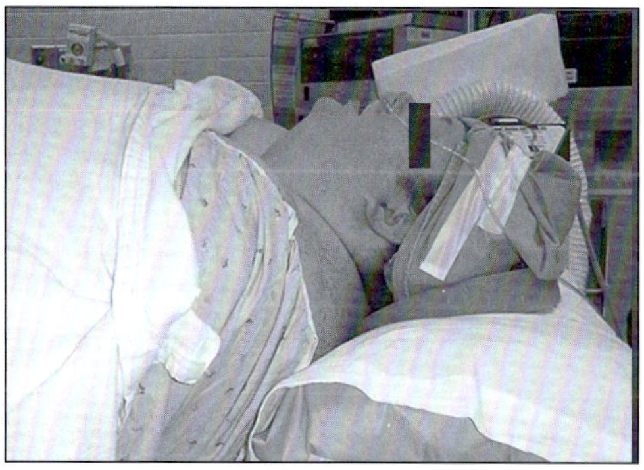

Figure 1a and 1b: patient with BMI of 54, in fully supine (a) and "ramped" (b) position for intubation. Note chin positioned above chest and head in "sniff" position.

A variety of airway tools are available to help secure a difficult airway. Examples range from the intubating bougie or Eschmann stylet (Figure 2), to intubating laryngeal mask airways (LMA) (Figure 3), to fiber-optic bronchoscopes. Relatively simple devices often work well in the obese patient, as there is usually not an anatomic abnormality, per se, but rather soft tissue obscuring visualization. A quick attempt to locate the trachea with an Eschmann stylet will frequently be successful in practiced hands and takes very little time. The intubating LMA (Fastrach™) is another fairly low-tech choice that requires some practice, but is easy to learn and use. It is a specially designed LMA that facilitates either blind or fiber-optic intubation. It offers the additional benefit of ventilation through the LMA prior to passage of the endotracheal tube, if necessitated by falling saturation levels. Regardless of the devices selected, the key is to have them readily accessible in the operating room and to be comfortable with their use.

**Figure 2**

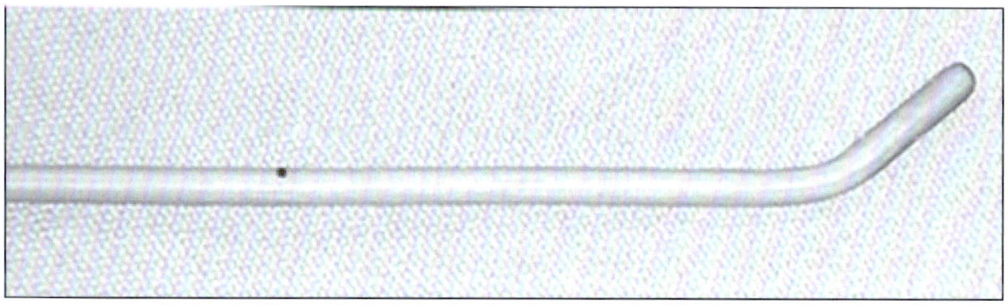

**Figure 3**

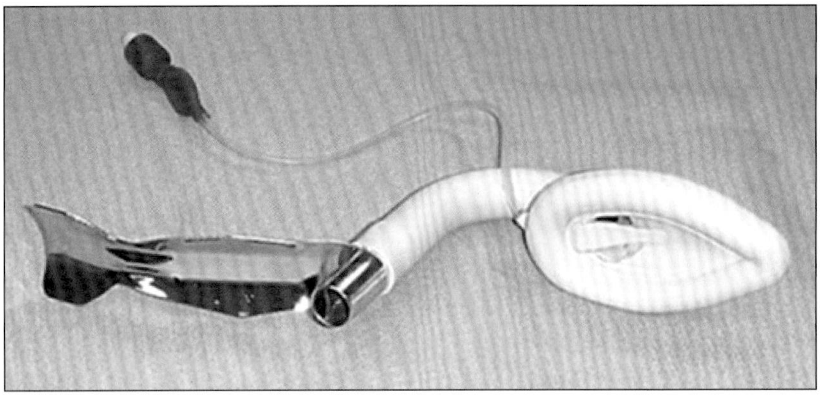

**Figure 4. Intubating (Fastrach™) LMA**

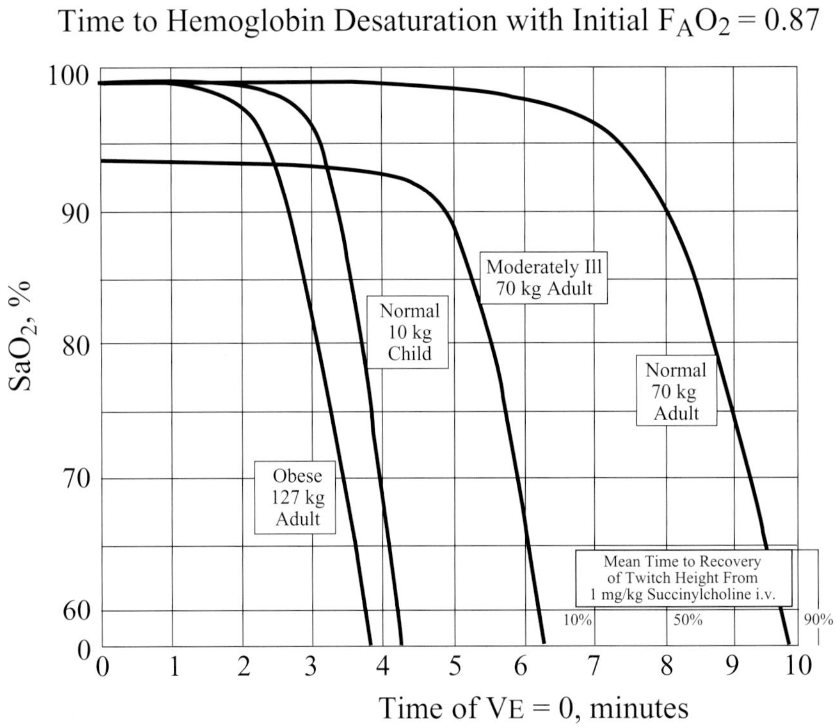


From Benumof JL, et al. *Anesthesiology* 1997;87:979-82

Once endotracheal intubation is achieved, the next potential problem involves mechanical ventilation of a patient with restrictive respiratory mechanics. Ventilation-perfusion mismatch is exacerbated by supine or Trendelenburg (head down) positioning, as well as by mechanical pressure from the pneumoperitoneum. Peak inspiratory pressures are typically elevated, but may be improved with the use of pressure-control ventilator settings instead of the more typical volume control. If oxygenation is suboptimal, positive end expiratory pressure (PEEP) may improve alveolar exchange. However, if the addition of PEEP decreases venous return and cardiac output, there may be no net-positive effect on oxygen levels.

Obese patients need to be well secured to the operating table to avoid shifting with table position changes. This can be accomplished with the use of a beanbag, footboard, belts, or some combination of these. The risk of postoperative neuropathy is increased, particularly ulnar neuropathy in men due to pressure at the ulnar groove. Care should be taken to pad pressure points, although it is unclear how much this reduces the overall incidence. Another possible pressure neuropathy is at the lateral femoral cutaneous nerve, following prolonged side tilt against a tightened belt. A second injury source, aside from pressure, is stretch. The brachial plexus is vulnerable when the patient is ramped up on blankets for intubation, leaving the arms hanging without support. The arm boards should have blankets or other padding added to eliminate the height difference. The brachial plexus may be stretched backwards if the arm slips off the arm board; the sciatic nerve, if a leg slips sideways off the table. The peroneal nerve may be stretched during prolonged dorsiflexion against a footboard. Thankfully, most perioperative neuropathies are self-limiting and will resolve within weeks or months.

There are limited data available specifically concerning pharmacokinetics and pharmacodynamics of anesthetic drugs in the morbidly obese. Approximately 20% to 30% of bariatric patients will have elevated liver function test values, although this seems to have little effect on anesthetic drug metabolism. Renal metabolism of drugs tends to be more rapid due to increased renal blood flow and glomerular filtration rate. Highly lipophilic drugs such as sodium pentathol and benzodiazepines have an increased volume of distribution. Thus, a higher dose calculated using actual body weight will be needed and the effects will last longer. Less lipophilic medications, such as nondepolarizing muscle relaxants, should be dose-based according to lean body mass (LBM), which equals ideal body weight, plus approximately 20% to 40%, the extra percentage accounting for the lean weight portion of total weight gain. The newer, less-soluble inhalational agents, sevoflurane and desflurane, are typically selected to speed emergence time. Studies tend to favor desflurance slightly with respect to various measures of emergence, although other studies have shown no significant difference between the two. I believe it primarily comes down to the personal preference of the anesthesiologist, particularly if total anesthetic time is under 2 hours. Isoflurane and other older agents are more lipid soluble and will continue to leach from fat stores after emergence; isoflurane has been shown to delay emergence and postanesthesia care unit (PACU) discharge compared with the shorter-acting agents.

Pulmonary function will decrease postoperatively. Open procedures will cause a greater decrease in forced vital capacity (FVC) and forced expiratory volume in 1 second (FEV1) when compared with laparoscopy, but postlaparoscopic measurements will still be below baseline. Patients that use CPAP at home for OSA should bring their equipment and have it available in the PACU. Patients who are naïve to CPAP may not tolerate it well, but it should certainly be considered for those with clinical signs of OSA in the perioperative period. There were anecdotal reports several years ago attibuting anastamotic leak to entrainment of air into the stomach during CPAP therapy, but subsequent studies have refuted this. Postoperative incentive spirometry has not specifically been shown to decrease postoperative pulmonary morbidity in bariatric patients, but it certainly can't hurt.

Consideration should be given to epidural analgesia for open procedures. Placement can be technically difficult in larger patients. There is a higher failure rate after successful placement, as the increased distance between the epidural space and skin can lead to dislodgment of the catheter with soft tissue shearing during patient transfer or other movement. A few centers that predominantly perform open procedures have the catheter placed under fluoroscopic guidance by the pain service, and then tunneled under the skin for extra security. Epidural analgesia might potentially delay ambulation, depending upon the medications administered, and early ambulation is an important tool for preventing DVT and PE and reducing pulmonary morbidity.

Nonopioid adjuncts should be used for pain management whenever practical, in order to reduce the amount of narcotics required and their accompanying side effects. Options include local anesthetic wound infiltration, intravenous ketorolac or COX-2 inhibitors, or newer agents such as dexmedetomidine. Some surgeons are uncomfortable with ketorolac due to potential platelet inhibitory effects, and I tend to limit its use to gastric banding rather than bypass procedures. Introduction of parenteral COX-2 inhibitors, with a better platelet profile, appears to have been delayed by reports of significant cardiac side effects with long-term use of certain oral formulations. It is unclear when or whether this class of drugs will be available for use in the operating room. Dexmedetomidine acts at the alpha-2 receptor and while mildly sedating, maintains respiratory rate. It has been used more often in patients undergoing open procedures as a continuous infusion intra- and postoperatively, and has been shown to reduce narcotic requirements.

It is important to treat postoperative nausea and vomiting (PONV) aggressively. Laparoscopic procedures place the patient at increased risk of PONV, so antiemetic prophylaxis should be routinely administered. Active retching may disrupt fresh anastomoses after a gastric bypass or herniate the stomach through a gastric band and must be treated promptly.

Finally, the entire perioperative team must recognize that these are technically demanding procedures performed on a population with significant risk of perioperative morbidity. Continuous communication amongst all personnel pre-, intra- and postoperatively is essential to the safe care of the bariatric patient.

**Suggested Reading**

1. Arain SR, Ruehlow RM, Uhrich TD, Ebert TJ. The efficacy of dexmedetomidine versus morphine for postoperative analgesia after major inpatient surgery. *Anesth Analg*. 2004;98(1):153-8.
2. Gross JB, Bachenberg KL, Benumof JL, et al. Practice guidelines for the perioperative management of patients with obstructive sleep apnea: a report by the American Society of Anesthesiologists Task Force on Perioperative Management of patients with obstructive sleep apnea. *Anesthesiology*. 2006;104(5):1081-93.
3. Benumof JL. Obstructive sleep apnea in the adult obese patient: implications for airway management. *Anesthesiol Clin North America*. 2002;20(4):789-811.
4. Brodsky JB, Lemmens HJ, Brock-Utne JG, Vierra M, Saidman LJ. Morbid obesity and tracheal intubation. *Anesth Analg*. 2002;94(3):732-6.
5. Cheymol G. Effects of obesity on pharmacokinetics: implications for drug therapy. *Clin Pharmacokinet*. 2000;39(3):215-31.
6. Christou NV, Sampalis JS, Liberman M, et al. Surgery decreases long-term mortality, morbidity, and healthcare use in morbidly obese patients. *Anal Surg*. 2004;240(3):416-23.
7. El-Dawlatly AA, Al-Dohayan A, Abdel-Meguid ME, El-Bakry A, Manaa EM. The effects of pneumoperitoneum on respiratory mechanics during general anesthesia for bariatric surgery. *Obes Surg*. 2004;14(2):212–5.
8. Flum DR, Dellinger EP. Impact of gastric bypass operation on survival: a population-based analysis. *J Am Coll Surg*. 2004;199(4):543-51.
9. Gander S, Frascarolo P, Suter M, Spahn DR, Magnusson L. Positive end-expiratory pressure during induction of general anesthesia increases duration of nonhypoxic apnea in morbidly obese patients. *Anesth Analg*. 2005;100(2):580-4.
10. Hallowell PT, Stellato TA, Schuster M, et al. Potentially life-threatening sleep apnea is unrecognized without aggressive evaluation. *Am J Surg*. 2007;193(3):364-7.
11. Huerta S, DeShields S, Shpiner R, et al. Safety and efficacy of postoperative continuous positive airway pressure to prevent pulmonary complications after Roux-en-Y gastric bypass. *J Gastrointest Surg*. 2002;6(3):354-8.
12. Lattimore JD, Celermajer DS, Wilcox I. Obstructive sleep apnea and cardiovascular disease. *J Am Coll Cardiol*. 2003;41(9):1429-37.
13. Mokdad AH, Ford ES, Bowman BA, et al. Prevalence of obesity, diabetes, and obesity-related health risk factors, 2001. *JAMA*. 2003;289(1):76-9.
14. O'Keeffe T, Patterson EJ. Evidence supporting routine polysomnography before bariatric surgery. *Obes Surg*. 2004;14(1):23–6.
15. Ogunnaike BO, Jones SB, Jones DB, Provost D, Whitten CW. Anesthetic considerations for bariatric surgery. *Anesth Analg*. 2002; 95(6):1793-805.
16. Pelosi P, Ravagnan I, Giurati G, et al. Positive end-expiratory pressure improves respiratory function in obese but not in normal subjects during anesthesia and paralysis. *Anesthesiology*. 1999;91(5):1221-31.
17. Ramaswamy A, Gonzalez R, Smith CD. Extensive preoperative testing is not necessary in morbidly obese patients undergoing gastric bypass. *J Gastrointest Surg*. 2004;8(2):159-64.

18. Sawyer RJ, Richmond MN, Hickey JD, Jarratt JA. Peripheral nerve injuries associated with anaesthesia. *Anaesthesia*. 2000;55(10):980–91.

19. Schumann R, Jones SB, Ortiz VE, et al. Best practice recommendations for anesthetic perioperative care and pain management in weight loss surgery. *Obes Res*. 2005;13(2):254-66.

20. Schumann R, Shikora S, Weiss JM, Wurm H, Strassels S, Carr DB. A comparison of multimodal perioperative analgesia to epidural pain management after gastric bypass surgery. *Anesth Analg*. 2003;96(2):469–74.

21. Siyam MA, Benhamou D. Difficult endotracheal intubation in patients with sleep apnea syndrome. *Anesth Analg*. 2002;95(4):1098-102.

22. Sprung J, Whalley D, Falcone T. The effects of tidal volume and respiratory rate on oxygenation and respiratory mechanics during laparoscopy in morbidly obese patients. *Anesth Analg*. 2003:97(1):268–74.

23. Strum EM, Szenohradszki J, Kaufman WA, et al. Emergence and recovery characteristics of desflurane versus sevoflurane in morbidly obese adult surgical patients: a prospective, randomized study. *Anesth Analg*. 2004; 99(6):1848-53.

24. Whalen FX, Gajic O, Thompson GB, et al. The effects of the alveolar recruitment maneuver and positive end-expiratory pressure on arterial oxygenation during laparoscopic bariatric surgery. *Anesth Analg*. 2006;102(1):298-305.

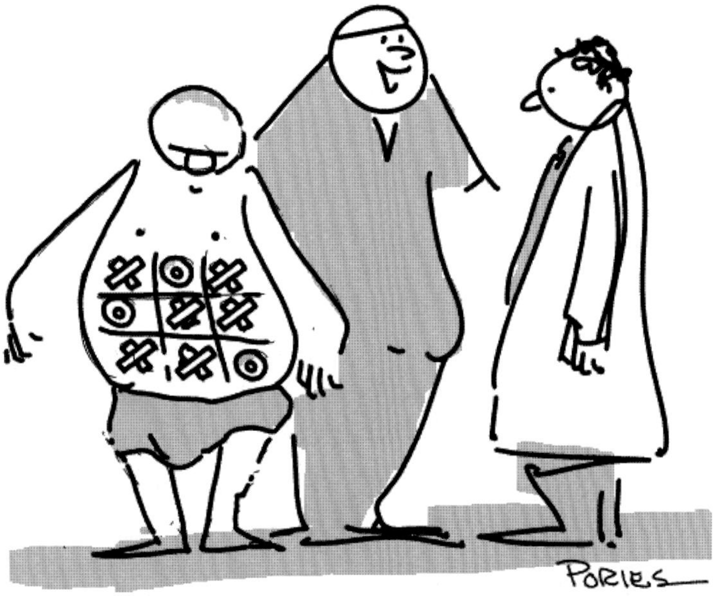


"We use nine ports."

# Laparoscopic Gastric Bypass

Tracy Pitt, DO
Stacy Brethauer, MD
Philip Schauer, MD

In 1967, Mason and Ito were the first to report gastric bypass (partial gastrectomy with loop gastrojejunostomy (GJ)) as a means of weight reduction.(1) This concept developed subsequent to the observation that patients undergoing partial gastrectomy secondary to peptic ulcer disease, for example, had poor weight gain. This procedure then fell out of favor because of resulting severe bile reflux. Gastric bypass was further modified in 1977 by Alden to include a transverse gastric staple line, without resection of the gastric remnant, and a loop gastrojejunostomy (GJ).(2) This was again associated with complications that led to other innovations. The gastric bypass was modified by Griffin et al in 1977(3) to include a Roux limb anastomosis, followed by several innovations, including the long Roux-limb bypass (RYGB) for super-obese patients introduced by Brolin et al in 1992.(4)

In 1994, Wittgrove, Clark, and Tremblay were the first to report that laparoscopic Roux-en-Y gastric bypass (LRYGB) was feasible.(5) These investigators utilized an EEA stapler with transoral anvil placement to create the GJ. Other authors have subsequently described techniques for transgastric anvil placement.(6) In 2000, Higa and Boone described the first laparoscopic hand-sewn GJ.(7) From 1999 to 2000, several authors, including Wittgrove, Nguyen, DeMaria, and Schauer, presented large case series that demonstrated laparoscopic gastric bypass to be both feasible and safe.(8-12) [Figures 1 a-d]

**Figure 1a. Creation of the 15- to 30-cc gastric pouch using a laparoscopic linear stapler**

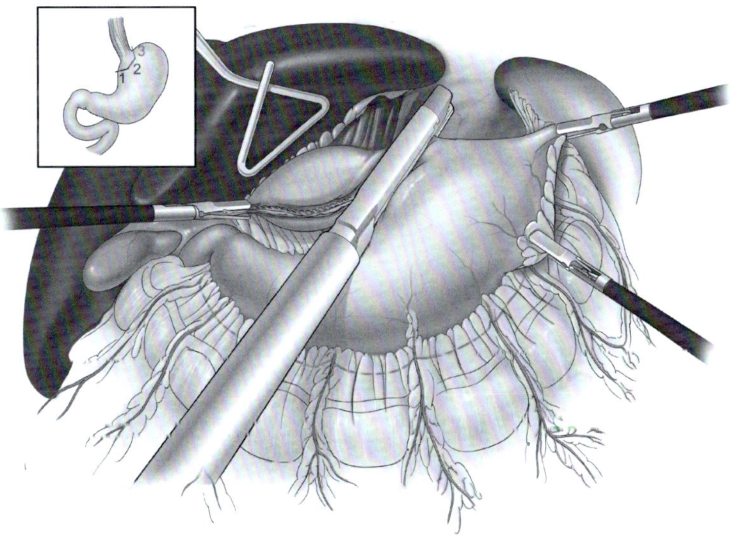

Figure 1b. Creation of the gastrojejunostomy using a linear stapler

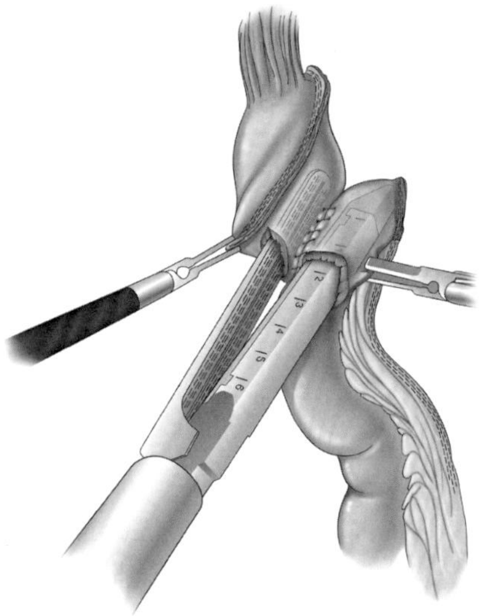

Figure 1c. Creation of the jejunojejunostomy using a laparoscopic linear stapler

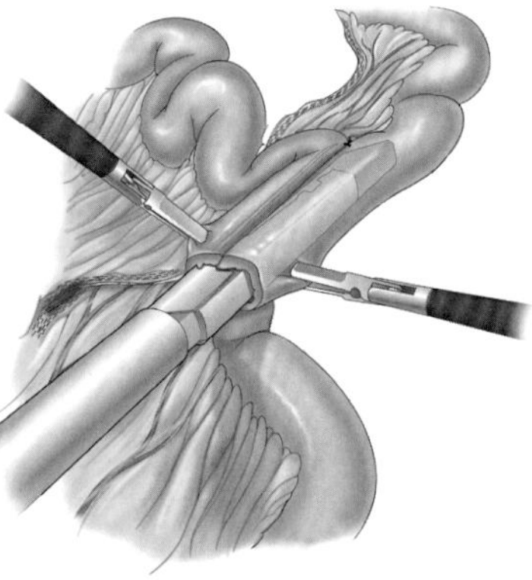

Figure 1d. Final anatomical arrangement of a completed laparoscopic Roux-en-Y gastric bypass

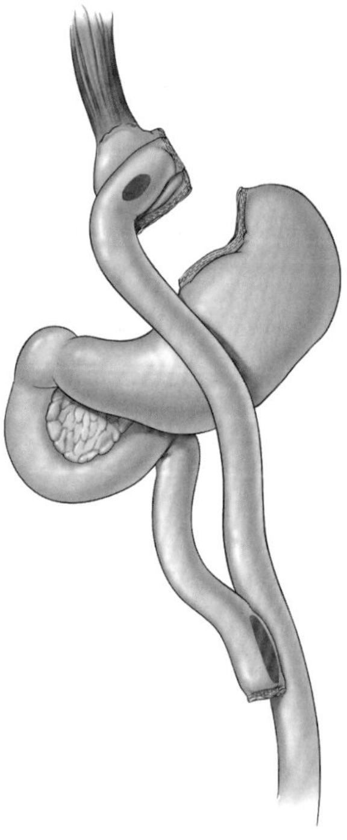

### Open vs. Laparoscopic Gastric Bypass Surgery

Pories et al showed early on that open gastric bypass could be performed safely with a mortality of 1.2% and sustained weight loss up to 10 years, and offered improvement or resolution of type 2 diabetes in 95% of patients.(13) During the 1980s and 1990s, open gastric bypass surgery emerged as the benchmark against which the laparoscopic approach was to be compared.

Since Wittgrove's first description of LRYGB, it has become the most commonly performed weight loss procedure in the United States (80% to 90% of all weight loss surgeries).(14) Subsequently, there have been several large series of laparoscopic RYGB,(8,9,12,15-17) and three randomized controlled trials(18-20) comparing LRYGB with open RYGB. Lujan et al showed that the laparoscopic approach to gastric bypass was associated with a shorter operating time, fewer complications, and a shorter hospital stay.(18) Westling et al found that patients in the laparoscopic group required less pain medication, had a shorter hospitalization, and required fewer sick days; however, their operating time was significantly longer than in the open group.(20) Nguyen et al found that patients in the laparoscopic group had significantly longer operating time but operative blood loss, hospital stay, and return to normal activities were significantly improved.(19) Furthermore, the laparoscopic group showed no difference in the rate of complications compared with the open group, while its quality-of-life scores were better than those of the open group.(19) Taken together, these results show that the laparoscopic approach can be performed safely and is associated with less pain, shorter hospital stay, decreased wound complications, and fewer incisional hernias than open RYGB. The benefits of laparoscopy in general have been conclusively demonstrated and appear to apply in the arena of bariatric surgery as well.

### Complications

There is no doubt that bariatric surgery is associated with complications and one must ensure that patients and family are well informed regarding those risks. The risks and benefits of laparoscopic RYGB must be evaluated for each person considering surgery. This discussion should not only consider the short-term risks of the surgery, but also the long-term risks of continued obesity and obesity-related illness that can decrease life expectancy.(21)

The most common complications associated with laparoscopic RYGB include: gastrointestinal bleeding (0.8-4.4%), anastomotic leak (0.7-5.1%), wound infection (0.1-5%), thromboembolism (0.4-1.1%), stomal stenosis/stricture (1.6-14.4%), gastrogastric fistula/marginal ulcer (0.4-5.1%), intestinal obstruction (0.2-4.5%), cholelithiasis requiring removal of the gallbladder (1.4-2.1%), and nutritional deficiencies (23.8% in one study including iron deficiency, anemia, hypokalemia, hypomagnesemia, and protein-calorie malnutrition).(8,9,12,16,22-25) Most of the complications discussed in the referenced articles include both major and minor complications that do not require surgery and have no long-term effects.

Anastomotic leak is a dreaded complication after RYGB and carries a mortality rate of up to 30% when it occurs. Leakage from the gastrojejunal (GJ) anastomosis can be contained or can result in diffuse peritonitis. A technical failure at the anastomosis will present in the early postoperative period with rapid clinical deterioration, but most leaks occur around postoperative day 5 and result from perforation of an ischemic area at the anastomosis. In a retrospective review by Sugerman et al, 5.3% of patients were identified to have a leak—77% were identified within 1 week, all leaks were identified within 28 days; and upper gastrointestinal (UGI) series was diagnostic in all patients after >1 contrast studies.(26) Major complications often present with subtle findings in these patients and confirmatory physical exam findings (peritoneal irritation) are the exception rather than the rule when an abdominal catastrophe is developing. Often, one of the first signs that leak has occurred is sustained tachycardia (heart rate >120 beats/min).(27) Other signs include tachypnea, increasing pain, decreased urine output, hypotension, and/or increasing drain output. When this entity is suspected, a water-soluble contrast study is the first diagnostic test utilized. Computed tomography can also be helpful for the identification of free fluid or abscesses. Depending on the imaging characteristics and the patient's clinical condition, operative intervention vs. conservative therapy is implemented. At the other extreme of the spectrum, some leaks are subclinical and require no operative intervention. These are identified to be contained leaks with no clinical signs of patient distress. However, it cannot be understated that a high index of suspicion and diligent patient evaluation are necessary for the identification of a gastrointestinal (GI) leak.

Gastrointestinal bleeding, either intraluminal or intraperitoneal, most often occurs at the staple line, a trocar site, or from omental vessels. Bleeding may be classified as early (<48h) or late (>48h). Staple-line bleeding can occur at the GJ, the jejunojejunostomy, or the gastric staple line (pouch or bypassed portion). Intraperitoneal bleeding is suggested by systemic signs of hemorrhage, no intraluminal signs of bleeding, or bloody drain output. In one retrospective review, 85% of patients with GI hemorrhage after laparoscopic RYGB were managed conservatively (fluids, blood products as needed, discontinuation of heparin) while only 15% required operative exploration.(25) Reoperative intervention is warranted in patients who are actively bleeding (<6h postoperatively with rapidly falling hematocrit despite resuscitation) and includes endoscopic (for pouch or anastomotic bleeding) or surgical techniques (excluded stomach, intraperitoneal), depending upon the presumed source of the bleeding.(28)

Prevention of intraoperative bleeding may be accomplished by using smaller staple heights (3.5 mm blue load for the GJ and 2.5 mm white load for jejunojejunostomy), over-sewing of the staple line, and/or the use of staple line reinforcement.(28) Angrisani et al showed that fewer hemostatic clips were needed and no postoperative transfusions were required in a cohort in which bovine pericardial buttressed staple lines were created.(29)

Wound infections at the port sites are most often mild and easily treated with antibiotics or local wound drainage. In one study of 275 patients, the authors noted a 22% wound infection rate during the first 50 procedures. These occurred at the left upper quadrant (LUQ) trocar site where the end-to-end anastomosis (EEA) stapler handle was placed into the abdomen. The infection rate decreased to 10% when routine bowel preps were started, then decreased to 1.5% with use of the gastrointestinal anastomosis (GIA) stapler for linear anastomosis.(8) These complications have not been reported to contribute to mortality and contribute little to the patient's postoperative morbidity. There is ample evidence to support the use of prophylactic antibiotics perioperatively for laparoscopic RYGB.(30)

Venous thromboembolism (VTE) is second only to leaks as a cause of mortality in the postoperative patient. The incidence is <1% in recent publications, however, the mortality for patients with pulmonary embolism (PE) ranges from 27% to 66%.(31-34) Since obesity is considered a risk factor for pulmonary embolism in all surgical disciplines, preventing this complication is an important part of the bariatric surgeon's perioperative care. One study has identified body mass index (BMI) >50 kg/m$^2$, obesity hypoventilation syndrome, and chronic venous insufficiency as risk factors for PE.(32) In bariatric patients who develop PE, one third will experience this after hospital discharge.(32) Therefore, extended prophylaxis for VTE may be warranted in very high-risk patients. Any patient who develops hypoxia, tachypnea, dyspnea, chest pain, or new arrhythmia postoperatively must be evaluated for deep vein thrombosis and/or pulmonary embolism (DVT/PE). Currently, the American College of Chest Physicians (ACCP) provides no specific recommendations for thromboprophylaxis in bariatric surgery patients and, while VTE prophylaxis is universally recommended, there is no consensus among bariatric surgeons regarding an optimal regimen or duration of prophylaxis.(35) In general, these patients should receive thromboprophylaxis according to the ACCP guidelines with low-dose unfractionated heparin or low molecular weight heparin (LMWH) (grade 1A evidence), with the addition of leg compression devices if multiple risk factors are present (grade 1C). There are several studies demonstrating the effectiveness of adjusted-dose unfractionated heparin and LMWH in bariatric surgery patients.

Anastomotic stricture at the GJ occurs in up to 15% of patient after laparoscopic RYGB. Most strictures either result from ischemia at the anastomosis (tension on the Roux limb) or are associated with a marginal ulcer. This complication has been reported with all techniques for creation of the GJ (linear staple, circular staple, hand-sewn), but it is more common with the circular-stapled anastamosis.(8,9,16) Patients typically present within 3 months of surgery with nausea, emesis, pain/discomfort, regurgitation of saliva, and dysphagia. This complication can lead to multiple hospital admissions, dehydration, and nutritional deficiencies and may even require revisional bariatric surgery, thereby resulting in increased costs, increased morbidity, and the potential mortality associated with revisional surgery. Most often, strictures can be successfully treated with endoscopic balloon dilation. Ngyuen et al retrospectively evaluated 185 patients, 15.7% of whom developed strictures at the GJ. The median time to symptoms was 46 days and all patients responded favorably to balloon dilation, although 17% required >1 dilation. There were no surgical revisions necessary.(36) In a large retrospective review by Carrodeguas et al, 94 of 1,291 patients developed a stricture following laparoscopic RYGB. All patients were successfully dilated endoscopically to 10 to 16.5 mm in ≤4 sessions, with two perforations, one requiring operative revision.(37) Finally, Barba et al showed endoscopic balloon dilation of anastamotic strictures to be safe and effective.(38)

Marginal ulcers at the GJ may be related to tension or ischemia on the anastomosis, and have also been associated with the presence of foreign material (staples or nonabsorbable suture), nonsteroidal use, excessive acid exposure in the gastric pouch (gastrogastric fistula), and smoking. Marginal ulcers often present with chronic pain, nausea, bleeding, and, rarely, perforation. When suspected, these pathologies are identified through endoscopy. Most often, they respond to proton pump inhibitor therapy without adverse consequences. Dallal et al found that of 201 gastric bypass patients, 3.5% had developed ulcer disease. One of 7 (14%) required reoperation; however, the remaining patients' symptoms and ulcer disease resolved with medical therapy. There was no postoperative mortality or long-term morbidity associated with this problem.(39)

Gastrogastric fistula was found in 1% of all LRYGB patients and in 19% of patients with marginal ulcer, indicating that a gastrogastric fistula can complicate or contribute to a marginal ulcer.(40) Gastrogastric fistulas form secondary to dehiscence of a staple line or after a leak from the GJ or pouch. When gastrogastric fistulas and refractory ulcers coexist, there is a greater likelihood that surgical correction will be needed.(40)

Intestinal obstruction after LRYGB is most often due to an internal hernia, but obstruction can also be related to adhesion after laparoscopy. The most common presenting symptom in these patients is nausea, emesis, and/or abdominal pain.(41) Some patients may present with chronic abdominal pain as a symptom of obstruction.(42) Thus, diligence and persistence are important when evaluating intermittent abdominal pain, as this may represent intermittent obstruction of an internal hernia through a mesenteric defect. Often, diagnostic laparoscopy for chronic abdominal pain with no clear etiology will reveal an internal hernia that potentially obstructs intermittently, causing the patients chronic symptoms. Higa et al evaluated 1,040 patients and identified an obstruction rate of 2.5% due to internal hernia. They noted, however, that this rate decreased with routine closure of the mesenteric defects using nonabsorbable suture material.(23) Blachar et al found that 4.5% of patients presented with intestinal obstruction. Approximately 60% were due to internal hernia and were diagnosed an average of 235 days postoperatively while 40% were due to adhesions diagnosed an average of 90 days postoperatively.(22) Interestingly, bowel obstructions that occur early (<1 month) are more likely to require surgical intervention and resection, whereas those occurring late (>1 month) are more likely to respond to conservative measures.(41) Radiographic studies were used by Hwang et al to evaluate intestinal obstruction in 64% of suspected small bowel obstruction cases, with a positive finding in 86% of patients. Of patients with suspected obstruction, 36% were diagnosed intraoperatively during exploratory surgery for acute pain.(41) Intestinal obstruction can be diagnosed using upper gastrointestinal (UGI) series or computed tomography with accuracy.(22)

Weight loss following gastric bypass is accompanied by a rise in the incidence of gallstones, with 38% to 52% of patients developing stones within 1 year of surgery. One study found that 1.4% of patients required surgery after gastric bypass for symptomatic cholelithiasis, and Higa et al noted a 2.1% incidence of laparoscopic cholecystectomy in their series.(8,16) Currently, there is no consensus regarding prophylactic cholecystectomy and this decision is at the discretion of the operating surgeon.(43) Some authors propose performance of laparoscopic cholecystectomy for the presence of stones identified preoperatively and others recommend resection postoperatively for symptomatic cholelithiasis. Others have advocated that routine prophylactic cholecystectomy be performed. Fobi et al retrospectively found an incidence of gallbladder pathology in 86% of patients undergoing weight reduction surgery and prophylactic cholecystectomy.(44) The prophylactic use of oral ursodiol at 600 mg daily for the first 6 months after LRYGB significantly reduces incidence of gallstone formation after gastric bypass (2% vs 32% in placebo, $P<.01$).(45)

Severe nutritional deficiencies are relatively uncommon after proximal gastric bypass, but are more commonly associated with distal gastric bypass or biliopancreatic diversion. In one study, iron deficiency was noted in 9.8% of patients and anemia in 8%, while hypokalemia, hypomagnesemia, and protein-calorie malnutrition were found in 5%, 0.7%, and 0.3%, respectively.(8) Iron deficiency occurs in 6% to 50% of patients following gastric bypass, owing to the bypass of the primary site of absorption (duodenum and jejunum).(46,47) Protein malnutrition occurs infrequently with proximal gastric bypass.(4,48-50) Vitamin $B_{12}$ and folate are also found to be deficient in 36% of these patients, potentially due to the lack of sufficient intrinsic-factor secretion from the bypassed gastric parietal cells.(51) Halverson identified a 67% vitamin $B_{12}$ deficiency and 38% folate deficiency after gastric bypass.(47) Bone turnover and bone demineralization are higher in bypass patients compared with patients using standard obese controls.(52) Therefore, calcium and vitamin D supplementation is protective against bone demineralization and osteopenia. The recommended prophylaxis in gastric bypass patients includes one multivitamin daily, iron 320 mg twice daily, oral $B_{12}$ 500 mcg/day, folate 400-1000 mcg/day, and calcium 1200 mg to 1500 mg/day with vitamin D 400 IU/day.(53)

### Mortality

The mortality associated with gastric bypass ranges from 0% to 1.4% in most studies.(8,9,12,17,23,24,33,54,55) In one large retrospective review of 1,067 patients by Livingston et al, there were 14 deaths (1.3%). The causes of mortality included 6 pulmonary emboli, 3 due to sepsis of unknown origin, 1 leak, 2 organ system failures, and 2 due to UGI hemorrhage.(33) Variables that have been shown to be related to increased mortality include male gender, advanced age, need for reoperation, surgeon inexperience, and Medicaid insured (versus privately insured).(21,54,56)

### Life Expectancy

In Christou's observational cohort study, 5-year mortality in the bariatric surgical group was 0.68% compared with 16.2% in the medically managed obese patients (89% relative risk reduction).(57) Flum et al evaluated survival after gastric bypass in a retrospective cohort study and found a 27% reduction in 15-year mortality in morbidly obese patients who underwent gastric bypass versus those who did not. After the surgical patients reached the first postoperative year, the long-term survival advantage increased to 33%.(21) The Swedish obese subjects intervention trial has recently presented survival results with a 5-year to 18-year follow-up.(58) The researchers reported an adjusted risk reduction of 31.6% in the surgery group, which was statistically significant ($P$=.008).(58) Another group recently presented its data for 8,172 gastric bypass patients and identified an all-cause total mortality reduction of 40% ($P$<.0001) and a 53% reduction when external deaths were excluded ($P$<.0001). These studies show that the mortality rate associated with bariatric surgery is low and, in fact, is significantly lower than the rate in medically treated cohorts who do not receive surgery.

### Weight Loss

When considering outcomes for bariatric surgical procedures, the percent excess weight loss (%EWL) is most often used to rate the success of a procedure. For restrictive procedures such as the LAP-BAND, %EWL is generally quoted to be 40 to 60.(59,60) Results from studies evaluating the malabsorptive procedures indicate that %EWL is approximately 70 to 80.(61,62) Malabsorptive procedures carry a higher rate of perioperative and long-term complications. The %EWL most often cited for LRYGB ranges from 70 to 80.(7-9,12,24) laparoscopic RYGB has consistently shown effective weight loss with long-term durability. (Table 1)

### Comorbidity Resolution

Comorbidities associated with obesity are many and result in poor long-term outcomes and decreased life expectancy compared with normal weight patients. Furthermore, the effects of obesity on quality of life, medical costs, and survival cannot be underestimated.(63)

The effects of weight loss surgery on the associated comorbidities has been extensively studied and documented in the literature. Type 2 diabetes and hypertension (HTN) are the most common and most studied comorbidities. In a retrospective review of 500 LRYGB patients, Wittgrove et al identified an overall decrease in comorbidities of 96%.(9) Type 2 diabetes resolved in 98%, hypertension in 92%, gastroesophageal reflux disease (GERD) in 98%, and obstructive sleep apnea (OSA) in 92%. In a prospective review of 275 patients, the effects of laparoscopic RYGB on comorbidities were reported to be resolved or improved in 100% of type 2 diabetes, 88% of HTN, 96% of dyslipidemia, 96% of GERD, 88% of osteoarthritis, and 93% of OSA patients.(8) DeMaria et al prospectively followed 281 patients and identified resolution of type 2 diabetes in 93%, HTN in 52%, GERD in 95%, incontinence in 88%, and orthopedic problems in 76%. Similarly, Sugerman et al found an improvement or resolution of diabetes in 83% and HTN in 69%, with an associated greater %EWL in the patients with comorbidity resolution.(55) Dyslipidemia was also improved across the board, affecting 70% of patients. Total cholesterol, triglycerides, and low-density lipoprotein (LDL) levels were all decreased while high-density lipoprotein (HDL) levels improved. Hypertension improved in 61.7% and OSA in 85.7% of patients. The Swedish Obese Subjects (SOS) study showed that resolution in comorbidities including diabetes, dyslipidemia, HTN, and hyperuricemia was durable out to 10 years for gastric bypass.(64)

Another comorbidity resulting from obesity is nonalcoholic fatty liver disease (NAFLD), which can range in severity from steatosis to hepatitis to cirrhosis. In a population-based cohort study, NAFLD was associated with an increased risk of mortality versus population controls,(65) and it has been shown that gastric bypass surgery can improve the early changes associated with NAFLD.(66) A prospective study evaluated the degree of steatosis using intraoperative and postoperative liver biopsy. As a result of the investigation, the researchers found that the degree of steatosis and inflammation decreased by 30% in patients after LRYGB.(67)

The concept of "the metabolic syndrome" is an area of great interest and investigation. Metabolic syndrome has been defined by several organizations and includes type 2 diabetes or insulin resistance, central obesity, dyslipidemia, and HTN.(68-70) The significance of this syndrome is its relationship with increased cardiovascular mortality. Again, the beneficial effects of gastric bypass surgery with regard to improvement or resolution of the metabolic syndrome have been shown.(67,71,72)

Much of the comorbidity resolution is directly related to the weight loss achieved from the surgery, however weight loss does not account for all of the benefits. There are numerous neurohumoral pathways that are involved and not yet understood. The effects of LRYGB on gut hormones, glucose metabolism, and appetite is an area of active research. To date, however, the overwhelming benefit of weight loss surgery with respect to comorbidity resolution has been conclusively demonstrated and the significance is obvious.

**Quality of Life**

Obesity has multiple adverse effects on a patient's sense of well-being, physical functioning, and overall quality of life (QOL). Many tasks, such as riding in a car, flying in a plane, going to the mall, or even tying one's shoe laces may be nearly impossible for patients with severe obesity. Several studies have addressed the effect of bariatric surgery on patients' QOL.(73-77) In a cross-sectional cohort study with a follow-up period of 13 years, there were significant improvements in QOL scores (SF-36) in postsurgical patients.(74) The SF-36 form scores several aspects of life, including physical functioning, physical role, bodily pain, general health, vitality, social functioning, emotional role, and mental health. Boan et al evaluated binge-eating disorder in postbariatric surgery patients, comparing their results with normal population controls and found significantly improved binge-eating scores, as well as a decrease in the patients' sense of hunger and improvements in their QOL.(73) Another interesting study showed that the rate of gainful employment at 5-years postsurgery was 16%.(77) Overall, weight loss surgery had a huge impact on a patient's QOL and sense of well-being.

**Cost**

The direct and indirect costs of morbid obesity are high. Most costs are related to the chronic comorbidities of diabetes, HTN, and cardiovascular disease, and in 2000, the Centers for Disease Control (CDC) estimated the total cost of obesity at $117 billion per year.

Several studies have evaluated the cost-effectiveness of bariatric surgery. Sampalis et al compared long-term healthcare costs related to 1,035 patients who underwent bariatric surgery with those related to 5,746 age- and gender-matched obese individuals as controls.(78) The majority of surgery performed was open RYGB (79%), and the group that received surgery had lost 67% of their excess body weight at 5-year follow-up. At 3.5 years, the cost of their RYGB surgery was compensated for by a reduction in their total healthcare costs. At 5 years, there was a 29% reduction in combined healthcare costs for the surgical group.

Medication cost, specifically for hypertension and diabetes medications, are reduced by as much as 77% after bariatric surgery.(79) Snow et al(80) found that, after LRYGB the savings in drug costs at 32 months postsurgery was equal to the cost of the surgery. The SOS trial compared the use of pharmaceuticals by 510 surgically treated patients and 455 medically treated patients with pharmaceutical use by 958 normal weight reference individuals. At 6 years, surgical patients had a significant reduction in costs for diabetes and cardiovascular medications, but this was offset by increased use of gastrointestinal medication and nutritional supplements.(81) Overall, it appears that the initial cost of surgical intervention is at least balanced, if not reduced, by the cost of long-term medical care.

## Conclusion

Based on the evidence, one can draw the following conclusions:

- The operative mortality rate (0.03% to 1.0%) for gastric bypass appears to be quite understandable, considering the high-risk nature of these patients
- Complication rates after LRYGB (3% to 10% perioperatively and 5% to 15% long-term) are also understandable, considering the poor long term outcome associated with obesity.
- The %EWL (at 65 to 80) is substantial after LRYGB.
- Comorbidity resolution and QOL are significantly improved after LRYGB and these effects appear to be durable.

In summary, LRYGB is a safe, effective, long-term treatment option for morbid obesity and obesity-related diseases.

**Table 1**

**Laparoscopic Roux-en-Y gastric bypass: outcomes**

| **Study demographics** | | | **Complications** | | | | |
|---|---|---|---|---|---|---|---|
| **Author** | N | Year | Major (%) | Minor (%) | Total (%) | %EWL | Mortality (%) |
| **Christou**[57] | 1,035 | 2004 | — | — | — | 67.1 | 0.7 |
| **Flum**[21] | 3,328 | 2004 | — | — | — | — | 1.9 |
| **Perugini**[24] | 188 | 2003 | — | — | 25.5 | 61 | 1.1 |
| **Papasavas**[17] | 116 | 2002 | — | — | 23.3 | 77 | 0.9 |
| **DeMaria**[12] | 281 | 2002 | — | — | — | 70 | 0 |
| **Blachar**[22] | 463 | 2002 | 9.5 | 6.7 | 16.2 | — | 0.4 |
| **Higa**[16] | 1,500 | 2001 | — | — | 14.8 | 69 | 0.2 |
| **Higa**[23] | 1,040 | 2000 | — | — | 14.7 | 70 | 0.5 |
| **Schauer**[8] | 275 | 2000 | 3.3 | 27 | 30.3 | 77 | 0.4 |
| **Wittgrove and Clark**[9] | 500 | 2000 | — | — | — | 70 | 0 |

## References


1. Mason EE, Ito C. Gastric bypass in obesity. *Surg Clin North Am*. 1967;47(6):1345-51.
2. Alden JF. Gastric and jejunoileal bypass: a comparison in the treatment of morbid obesity. *Arch Surg*. 1977;112(7):799-806.
3. Griffen WO Jr, Young VL, Stevenson CC. A prospective comparison of gastric and jejunoileal bypass procedures for morbid obesity. *Ann Surg*. 1977;186(4):500-9.
4. Brolin RE, Kenler HA, Gorman JH, Cody RP. Long-limb gastric bypass in the super-obese: a prospective randomized study. *Ann Surg*. 1992;215(4):387-95.
5. Wittgrove AC, Clark GW, Tremblay LJ. Laparoscopic gastric bypass, Roux-en-Y: preliminary report of five cases. *Obes Surg*. 1994;4(4):353-57.
6. de la Torre RA, Scott JS. Laparoscopic Roux-en-Y gastric bypass: a totally intra-abdominal approach—technique and preliminary report. *Obes Surg*. 1999;9(5):492-8.
7. Higa KD, Boone KB, Ho T, Davies OG. Laparoscopic Roux-en-Y gastric bypass for morbid obesity: technique and preliminary results of our first 400 patients. *Arch Surg*. 2000;135(9):1029-33; discussion 1033-4.

8. Schauer PR, Ikramuddin S, Gourash W, Ramanathan R, Luketich J. Outcomes after laparoscopic Roux-en-Y gastric bypass for morbid obesity. *Ann Surg*. 2000;232(4):515-29.

9. Wittgrove AC, Clark GW. Laparoscopic gastric bypass: Roux-en-Y, 500 patients: technique and results, with 3-60 month follow-up. *Obes Surg*. 2000;10(3):233-9.

10. Nguyen NT, Ho HS, Mayer KL, Palmer L, Wolfe BM. Laparoscopic Roux-en-Y gastric bypass for morbid obesity. *JSLS*. 1999;3(3):193-6.

11. Nguyen NT, Ho HS, Palmer LS, Wolfe BM. Laparoscopic Roux-en-Y gastric bypass for super/super obesity. *Obes Surg*. 1999;9(4):403-6.

12. DeMaria EJ, Sugerman HJ, Kellum JM, Meador JG, Wolfe LG. Results of 281 consecutive total laparoscopic Roux-en-Y gastric bypasses to treat morbid obesity. *Ann Surg*. 2002;235(5):640-5; discussion 645-7.

13. Pories WJ, MacDonald KG Jr, Morgan EJ, et al. Surgical treatment of obesity and its effect on diabetes: 10-y follow-up. *Am J Clin Nutr*. 1992;55(2 Suppl):582S-585S.

14. Samuel I, Mason EE, Renquist KE, Huang YH, Zimmerman MB, Jamal M. Bariatric surgery trends: an 18-year report from the International Bariatric Surgery Registry. *Am J Surg*. 2006;192(5):657-62.

15. Abdel-Galil E, Sabry AA. Laparoscopic Roux-en-Y gastric bypass—evaluation of three different techniques. *Obes Surg*. 2002;12(5):639-42.

16. Higa KD, Ho T, Boone KB. Laparoscopic Roux-en-Y gastric bypass: technique and 3-year follow-up. *J Laparoendosc Adv Surg Tech A*. 2001;11(6):377-82.

17. Papasavas PK, Hayetian FD, Caushaj PF, et al. Outcome analysis of laparoscopic Roux-en-Y gastric bypass for morbid obesity. The first 116 cases. *Surg Endosc*. 2002;16(12):1653-7.

18. Lujan JA, Frutos MD, Hernandez Q, et al. Laparoscopic versus open gastric bypass in the treatment of morbid obesity: a randomized prospective study. *Ann Surg*. 2004;239(4):433-7.

19. Nguyen NT, Goldman C, Rosenquist CJ, et al. Laparoscopic versus open gastric bypass: a randomized study of outcomes, quality of life, and costs. *Ann Surg*. 2001;234(3):279-89; discussion 289-91.

20. Westling A, Gustavsson S. Laparoscopic vs open Roux-en-Y gastric bypass: a prospective, randomized trial. *Obes Surg*. 2001;11(3):284-92.

21. Flum DR, Dellinger EP. Impact of gastric bypass operation on survival: a population-based analysis. *J Am Coll Surg*. 2004;199(4):543-51.

22. Blachar A, Federle MP, Pealer KM, Ikramuddin S, Schauer PR. Gastrointestinal complications of laparoscopic Roux-en-Y gastric bypass surgery: clinical and imaging findings. *Radiology*. 2002;223(3):625-32.

23. Higa KD, Boone KB, Ho T. Complications of the laparoscopic Roux-en-Y gastric bypass: 1,040 patients—what have we learned? *Obes Surg*. 2000;10(6):509-13.

24. Perugini RA, Mason R, Czerniach DR, et al. Predictors of complication and suboptimal weight loss after laparoscopic Roux-en-Y gastric bypass: a series of 188 patients. *Arch Surg*. 2003;138(5):541-5; discussion 545-6.

25. Mehran A, Szomstein S, Zundel N, Rosenthal R. Management of acute bleeding after laparoscopic Roux-en-Y gastric bypass. *Obes Surg*. 2003;13(6):842-7.

26. Carucci LR, Turner MA, Conklin RC, DeMaria EJ, Kellum JM, Sugerman HJ. Roux-en-Y gastric bypass surgery for morbid obesity: evaluation of postoperative extraluminal leaks with upper gastrointestinal series. *Radiology*. 2006;238(1):119-27.

27. Hamilton EC, Sims TL, Hamilton TT, Mullican MA, Jones DB, Provost DA. Clinical predictors of leak after laparoscopic Roux-en-Y gastric bypass for morbid obesity. *Surg Endosc*. 2003;17(5):679-84.

28. Nguyen NT, Longoria M, Chalifoux S, Wilson SE. Gastrointestinal hemorrhage after laparoscopic gastric bypass. *Obes Surg*. 2004;14(10):1308-12.

29. Angrisani L, Lorenzo M, Borrelli V, Ciannella M, Bassi UA, Scarano P. The use of bovine pericardial strips on linear stapler to reduce extraluminal bleeding during laparoscopic gastric bypass: prospective randomized clinical trial. *Obes Surg*. 2004;14(9):1198-202.

30. Forse RA, Karam B, MacLean LD, Christou NV. Antibiotic prophylaxis for surgery in morbidly obese patients. *Surgery.* 1989;106(4):750-6; discussion 756-7.

31. Brolin RE. Update: NIH consensus conference. Gastrointestinal surgery for severe obesity. *Nutrition*. 1996;12(6):403-4.

32. Carmody BJ, Sugerman HJ, Kellum JM, et al. Pulmonary embolism complicating bariatric surgery: detailed analysis of a single institution's 24-year experience. *J Am Coll Surg*. 2006;203(6):831-7.

33. Livingston EH, Arterburn D, Schifftner TL, Henderson WG, DePalma RG. National Surgical Quality Improvement Program analysis of bariatric operations: modifiable risk factors contribute to bariatric surgical adverse outcomes. *J Am Coll Surg*. 2006;203(5):625-33.

34. Sapala JA, Wood MH, Schuhknecht MP, Sapala MA. Fatal pulmonary embolism after bariatric operations for morbid obesity: a 24-year retrospective analysis. *Obes Surg*. 2003;13(6):819-25.

35. Sauerland S, Angrisani L, Belachew M, et al. Obesity surgery: evidence-based guidelines of the European Association for Endoscopic Surgery (EAES). *Surg Endosc*. 2005;19(2):200-21.

36. Nguyen NT, Stevens CM, Wolfe BM. Incidence and outcome of anastomotic stricture after laparoscopic gastric bypass. *J Gastrointest Surg*. 2003;7(8):997-1003; discussion 1003.

37. Carrodeguas L, Szomstein S, Zundel N, Lo Menzo E, Rosenthal R. Gastrojejunal anastomotic strictures following laparoscopic Roux-en-Y gastric bypass surgery: analysis of 1291 patients. *Surg Obes Relat Dis*. 2006;2(2):92-7.

38. Barba CA, Butensky MS, Lorenzo M, Newman R. Endoscopic dilation of gastroesophageal anastomosis stricture after gastric bypass. *Surg Endosc*. 2003;17(3):416-20.

39. Dallal RM, Bailey LA. Ulcer disease after gastric bypass surgery. *Surg Obes Relat Dis*. 2006;2(4):455-9.

40. Gumbs AA, Duffy AJ, Bell RL. Incidence and management of marginal ulceration after laparoscopic Roux-Y gastric bypass. *Surg Obes Relat Dis*. 2006;2(4):460-3.

41. Hwang RF, Swartz DE, Felix EL. Causes of small bowel obstruction after laparoscopic gastric bypass. *Surg Endosc*. 2004;18(11):1631-5.

42. Lauter DM. Treatment of nonadhesive bowel obstruction following gastric bypass. *Am J Surg*. 2005;189(5):532-5; discussion 535.

43. Mason EE, Renquist KE. Gallbladder management in obesity surgery. *Obes Surg*. 2002;12(2):222-9.

44. Fobi M, Lee H, Igwe D, et al. Prophylactic cholecystectomy with gastric bypass operation: incidence of gallbladder disease. *Obes Surg*. 2002;12(3):350-3.

45. Sugerman HJ, Brewer WH, Shiffman ML, et al. A multicenter, placebo-controlled, randomized, double-blind, prospective trial of prophylactic ursodiol for the prevention of gallstone formation following gastric-bypass-induced rapid weight loss. *Am J Surg*. 1995;169(1):91-6; discussion 96-7.

46. Brolin RE, Gorman RC, Milgrim LM, Kenler HA. Multivitamin prophylaxis in prevention of post-gastric bypass vitamin and mineral deficiencies. *Int J Obes*. 1991;15(10):661-7.

47. Halverson JD. Micronutrient deficiencies after gastric bypass for morbid obesity. *Am Surg*. 1986;52(11):594-8.

48. Brolin RE, LaMarca LB, Kenler HA, Cody RP. Malabsorptive gastric bypass in patients with superobesity. *J Gastrointest Surg*. 2002;6(2):195-203; discussion 204-5.

49. Kalfarentzos F, Dimakopoulos A, Kehagias I, Loukidi A, Mead N. Vertical banded gastroplasty versus standard or distal Roux-en-Y gastric bypass based on specific selection criteria in the morbidly obese: preliminary results. *Obes Surg*. 1999;9(5):433-42.

50. Skroubis G, Sakellaropoulos G, Pouggouras K, Mead N, Nikiforidis G, Kalfarentzos F. Comparison of nutritional deficiencies after Roux-en-Y gastric bypass and after biliopancreatic diversion with Roux-en-Y gastric bypass. *Obes Surg*. 2002;12(4):551-8.

51. Marcuard SP, Sinar DR, Swanson MS, Silverman JF, Levine JS. Absence of luminal intrinsic factor after gastric bypass surgery for morbid obesity. *Dig Dis Sci*. 1989;34(8):1238-42.

52. Coates PS, Fernstrom JD, Fernstrom MH, Schauer PR, Greenspan SL. Gastric bypass surgery for morbid obesity leads to an increase in bone turnover and a decrease in bone mass. *J Clin Endocrinol Metab*. 2004;89(3):1061-5.

53. Shah M, Simha V, Garg A. Review: long-term impact of bariatric surgery on body weight, comorbidities, and nutritional status. *J Clin Endocrinol Metab*. 2006;91(11):4223-31.

54. Livingston EH, Huerta S, Arthur D, Lee S, De Shields S, Heber D. Male gender is a predictor of morbidity and age a predictor of mortality for patients undergoing gastric bypass surgery. *Ann Surg*. 2002;236(5):576-82.

55. Sugerman HJ, Wolfe LG, Sica DA, Clore JN. Diabetes and hypertension in severe obesity and effects of gastric bypass-induced weight loss. *Ann Surg*. 2003;237(6):751-6; discussion 757-8.

56. Poulose BK, Griffin MR, Moore DE, et al. Risk factors for post-operative mortality in bariatric surgery. *J Surg Res*. 2005;127(1):1-7.

57. Christou NV, Sampalis JS, Liberman M, et al. Surgery decreases long-term mortality, morbidity, and health care use in morbidly obese patients. *Ann Surg*. 2004;240(3):416-23; discussion 423-4.

58. Sjöström L. Soft and hard endpoints over 5 to 18 years in the intervention trial Swedish Obese Subjects (Abstract). *Obes Rev*. 2006;7(suppl. 2):27.

59. Parikh MS, Shen R, Weiner M, Siegel N, Ren CJ. Laparoscopic bariatric surgery in super-obese patients (BMI>50) is safe and effective: a review of 332 patients. *Obes Surg*. 2005;15(6):858-63.

60. Ponce J, Paynter S, Fromm R. Laparoscopic adjustable gastric banding: 1,014 consecutive cases. *J Am Coll Surg*. 2005;201(4):529-35.

61. Hess DS, Hess DW. Biliopancreatic diversion with a duodenal switch. *Obes Surg*. 1998;8(3):267-82.

62. Rabkin RA, Rabkin JM, Metcalf B, Lazo M, Rossi M, Lehmanbecker LB. Laparoscopic technique for performing duodenal switch with gastric reduction. *Obes Surg*. 2003;13(2):263-8.

63. Mensah GA, Mokdad AH, Ford E, et al. Obesity, metabolic syndrome, and type 2 diabetes: emerging epidemics and their cardiovascular implications. *Cardiol Clin*. 2004;22(4):485-504.

64. Sjöström L, Lindroos AK, Peltonen M, et al. Lifestyle, diabetes, and cardiovascular risk factors 10 years after bariatric surgery. *N Engl J Med*. 2004;351(26):2683-93.

65. Adams LA, Lymp JF, St Sauver J, et al. The natural history of nonalcoholic fatty liver disease: a population-based cohort study. *Gastroenterology*. 2005;129(1):113-21.

66. Silverman EM, Sapala JA, Appelman HD. Regression of hepatic steatosis in morbidly obese persons after gastric bypass. *Am J Clin Pathol*. 1995;104(1):23-31.

67. Mattar SG, Velcu LM, Rabinovitz M, et al. Surgically-induced weight loss significantly improves nonalcoholic fatty liver disease and the metabolic syndrome. *Ann Surg*. 2005;242(4):610-7; discussion 618-20.

68. Executive Summary of The Third Report of The National Cholesterol Education Program (NCEP) Expert Panel on Detection, Evaluation, and Treatment of High Blood Cholesterol in Adults (Adult Treatment Panel III). *JAMA*. 2001;285(19):2486-97.

69. Alberti KG, Zimmet PZ. Definition, diagnosis and classification of diabetes mellitus and its complications. Part 1: diagnosis and classification of diabetes mellitus provisional report of a WHO consultation. *Diabet Med*. 1998;15(7):539-53.

70. Balkau B, Charles MA. Comment on the provisional report from the WHO consultation. European Group for the Study of Insulin Resistance (EGIR). *Diabet Med*. 1999;16(5):442-3.

71. Lee WJ, Huang MT, Wang W, Lin CM, Chen TC, Lai IR. Effects of obesity surgery on the metabolic syndrome. *Arch Surg*. 2004;139(10):1088-92.

72. Madan AK, Orth W, Ternovits CA, Tichansky DS. Metabolic syndrome: yet another co-morbidity gastric bypass helps cure. *Surg Obes Relat Dis*. 2006;2(1):48-51; discussion 51.

73. Boan J, Kolotkin RL, Westman EC, McMahon RL, Grant JP. Binge eating, quality of life and physical activity improve after Roux-en-Y gastric bypass for morbid obesity. *Obes Surg*. 2004;14(3):341-8.

74. de Zwaan M, Lancaster KL, Mitchell JE, et al. Health-related quality of life in morbidly obese patients: effect of gastric bypass surgery. *Obes Surg*. 2002;12(6):773-80.

75. Dymek MP, Le Grange D, Neven K, Alverdy J. Quality of life after gastric bypass surgery: a cross-sectional study. *Obes Res*. 2002;10(11):1135-42.

76. Kolotkin RL, Crosby RD, Pendleton R, Strong M, Gress RE, Adams T. Health-related quality of life in patients seeking gastric bypass surgery vs non-treatment-seeking controls. *Obes Surg*. 2003;13(3):371-7.

77. Velcu LM, Adolphine R, Mourelo R, Cottam DR, Angus LD. Weight loss, quality of life and employment status after Roux-en-Y gastric bypass: 5-year analysis. *Surg Obes Relat Dis*. 2005;1(4):413-6; discussion 417.

78. Sampalis JS, Liberman M, Auger S, Christou NV. The impact of weight reduction surgery on health-care costs in morbidly obese patients. *Obes Surg*. 2004;14(7):939-47.

79. Craig BM, Tseng DS. Cost-effectiveness of gastric bypass for severe obesity. *Am J Med*. 2002;113(6):491-8.

80. Snow LL, Weinstein LS, Hannon JK, et al. The effect of Roux-en-Y gastric bypass on prescription drug costs. *Obes Surg*. 2004;14(8):1031-5.

81. Narbro K, Agren G, Jonsson E, Naslund I, Sjostrom L, Peltonen M. Pharmaceutical costs in obese individuals: comparison with a randomly selected population sample and long-term changes after conventional and surgical treatment: the SOS intervention study. *Arch Intern Med*. 2002;162(18):2061-9.

# Laparoscopic Adjustable Band

Christine Ren, MD

The adjustable gastric band is an implantable device that is placed around the stomach circumferentially just below the gastroesophageal (GE) junction.

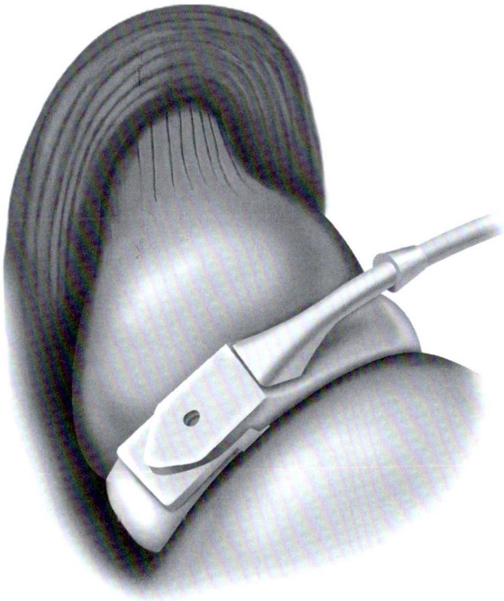

This is a schematic of where the band actually lies, and the 2 portions of the band that are incorporated within this system. There is a ring-like portion of the band that has an inflatable balloon internally, connected to hollow tubing that goes into a standard Mediport® implanted in the abdomen, underneath the skin. The reason only this product line is being shown is because it is presently the only lap-band product available in the United States that has been approved by the US Food and Drug Administration (FDA). There are several other bands that are available internationally and one that will be available on the market here in the United States within several years.

This device works to help weight loss by doing several things. Primarily, it creates a gastric pouch very high up, just below the GE junction, by constricting the stomach and creating a 12-mm stoma which is later adjusted and made smaller. After surgery, patients experience early satiety. They have a decreased appetite and must undergo behavior modification, learning to eat slower and to take the time to make healthy food choices. This results in patients making a dietary modification. As with any other operation, including gastric bypass, the success of gastric banding depends as much on the patient as it does on the operation. Healthy food choices and exercise continue to play a role in optimal outcome.

This operation is the most common bariatric operation performed in the world and certainly outside the United States. In the past 13 years, more than 180,000 bands have been placed. In the United States, we're getting more and more experienced at performing the procedure and will be looking forward to seeing other new devices that will help improve it.

During the procedure, the stomach is retracted caudad, and the angle of His is then mobilized. We then go to the lesser curvature of the stomach where the pars flaccida is divided, the right crus is identified as a landmark, and where the peritoneum is then opened up. This is a point of entry where our instrument will then be placed behind the stomach, passed behind posteriorly so that it comes out at the angle of His.

The band tubing is then grasped and literally wrapped around the upper portion of the stomach. There is a locking mechanism in this band, which is quite easy to maneuver.

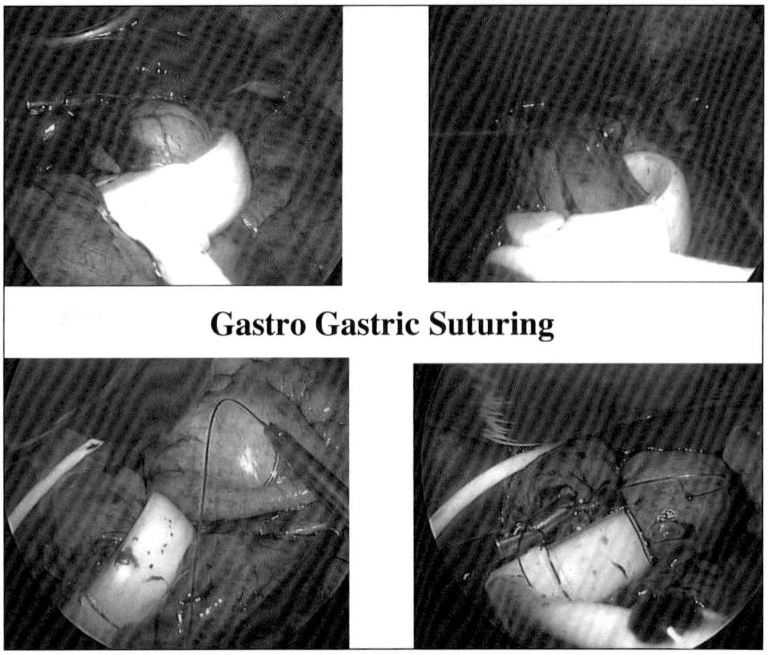

Gastro Gastric Suturing

Once the band is wrapped circumferentially around the stomach, it is kept in place by suturing the stomach to itself, over the band, with a permanent suture. The tubing is connected to a port that is secured to the rectus fascia underneath the skin and subcutaneous fat.

The operation takes about an hour to perform. It's usually an overnight stay; however, many surgeons are doing this quite safely as an outpatient operation. Most patients go back to work in about 3 days and the follow-up is much more intensive, particularly in our program at New York University (NYU). We like to see our patients every month for the first year (but many surgeons see them every 2 months for the first year), every 3 months for the second and third year, and then once or twice a year for life. The most important reason for seeing these patients afterward is not only to help them through the postoperative process of how to live with the band, how to eat with it, and how to use it as a tool, but more importantly so that the band may be tightened. This tightening is done as a 5-minute office procedure or in the radiology suite where the reservoir port is accessed with a nonspring needle (a Huber needle) and saline is injected into the port in order to tighten the band. About 5 "tightenings" (also known as adjustments) per year are required. This can go on for about 2 or 3 years in order to tailor the band tightness to each person.

We are looking for a gradual weight loss. There is no plummeting of weight after this operation; it is more of a slow weight loss of about 1 to 2 lbs a week, which continues for 2 to 3 years. By 2 years, most patients lose on average 50% to 65% of excess weight. However, there are 3 vital components of success for this operation. The technique is about 30% of the success, but the follow-up and adjustments must also be on target. Without all three, the gastric band is ineffective. I must stress this as the most important point, because I think that too often, many programs are missing one of these components. And if you miss one, your operation has only two thirds of a chance for ultimately being a success.

All of the long-term studies that we have came out of Europe and Australia, primarily because the band has been used in those areas for a much longer period of time. What we see in the papers that have very large numbers (in the hundreds) is a gradual excess weight loss of about 40% to 45% in the first year. Then, there is gradually more, up to the point where by 7 or 8 years weight loss is in the 55% to 60% range. Therefore, it is a durable operation. In the United States, we have had several papers come out with up to 3-year follow-up, and the weight loss is similar. In the first year, there is anywhere between 38% and 50% excess weight loss, and by 3 years, the excess weight loss is anywhere up to 60%.

In the mid-1990s, the FDA trial was a study of 300 patients using an older technique. The results, although very good compared with medical weight loss, were actually much less than what it is typical now. I think this shows that this operation is susceptible to a learning curve just like gastric bypass and all of the other operations that we speak about today.

Along with the weight loss after gastric banding, one sees the benefits of reduction of comorbidities. The overall resolution in improvement of comorbidities is seen in all medical areas, including hypertension, hyperlipidemia, diabetes, asthma, reflux and sleep apnea.

## Weight Loss and Diabetes After Laparoscopic Adjustable Gastric Band

- 1 year post-op: 44.3% EWL (BMI= 36.4)
- 30% improvement in insulin sensitivity
- 20%-30% improvement in beta-cell function

Dixon showed that at 1 year, with 44% excess weight loss from gastric banding, there is a 30% improvement in insulin sensitivity and a 20% to 30% improvement in beta-cell function, particularly in patients who have had diabetes for less than 7 years in duration.

In addition, 2 years after surgery with the 51% excess weight loss, we find that 65% of patients are cured of diabetes, meaning all insulin or oral medications are discontinued. This is independent of the patients who have an improvement of their diabetes.

There are complications involved with this operation, although very large series that we have in the literature show the mortality rate as extremely low. Most studies have zero mortality. There are several papers that have occasional mortality, up to 1.2%, depending on the number of patients in the study. The complication rates vary anywhere between 1% and 8%. We do have an incidence of band slippage, where the stomach herniates up through the band, the band slides down further onto the stomach, and pouch dilatation occurs, causing excessive heartburn, reflux, and weight regain. This happens in 2% to 14% of patients. The 14% end of the range is much more prevalent when the older technique (perigastric) is used for this operation. As the techniques have been modified, the slip rate has come down to about 3% to 5%.

Occasionally, the band does erode into the stomach, which then requires that the band be removed. This occurs in 0% to 3% of instances. Since the band is a device, you can have device failures such as a break or leak in the tubing, or the port may flip up to 10% of the time. Band removal occurs in patients who cannot tolerate restriction, or where the band is not providing appropriate weight loss. Up to 5% of bands will require removal.

In our early experience right after the FDA approved the LAP-BAND, there were four centers in the United States that actually collated their data together. After 1 year, 115 patients were evaluated and found to have a total complication rate (both early and late) of 20%. Specifically, early complications included 5 wound infections, 2 stomal obstructions, and less than 1% bleeding. There was less than 1% gastric pouch dilatation and a 2% slip rate. Out of the 115 patients, only 1 had erosion and 7% had tube disconnection. Two of these bands had to be removed. There was a 13% reoperation rate, the majority being performed laparoscopically, on an outpatient or overnight-stay basis.

There is a concern about esophageal dilatation with this operation. Dr. Horgan at the University of Illinois looked at 200 of his patients, performing manometry and fluoroscopy on all of them, and found that no patients had any esophageal dysmotility or aperistalsis 1 year after surgery.

Is this operation applicable to the masses, to all the community surgeons, and to all academic centers? In Italy, there is a national registry of surgeons who perform gastric banding at a total of 27 centers. These surgeons collected almost 2,000 patients and found that they typically started with a body mass index (BMI) of 43.7 kg/m$^2$ and went down to a BMI of 32 at 6 years. They found that there was a 0.5% mortality, most commonly from cardiac complications or pulmonary emboli, and that there was about a 10% short- and long-term complication rate mostly due to tubing and/or port malfunctioning that required replacement, or that there was a gastric pouch dilation with gastric prolapse, which had a 5% incidence. There was a band erosion rate of 1%; however, in view of almost 2,000 patients, we can see that this is a safe and effective operation on a broad scale.

In our own practice at NYU, we perform all three operations laparoscopically: gastric banding, gastric bypass, and biliopancreatic diversion with duodenal switch (BPD/DS). We compared 697 total operations, breaking them down and looking at their complication rates. We found that when we looked at both early and late complications, the gastric band does continue to have a lower complication rate compared with the other bypass operations. However, when you look at the severity of complications, we find that all operations really have a very low severe-complication rate, specifically Grade 3 and Grade 4, which represent organ resection or irreversible disability or death. The gastric banding has a 0.23% severe-complication rate, significantly lower than the gastric bypass and BPD/DS.

So what we've found is that gastric banding does carry a risk of complications, but they're usually of a low grade of severity and are rarely fatal. These complications are easily treated, and we usually can revise the band or simply take it out. There is no permanent alteration of the patient's anatomy. If there is poor weight loss, then the band is a revisable situation.

Long term, what not many people talk about is the nutritional implications of our bariatric operations. We see that the LAP-BAND really carries no nutritional sequelae because there is no malabsorption or malnutrition. That's an advantage.

An interesting study was presented in April 2005 at the Society for American Gastrointestinal and Endoscopic Surgery (SAGES) meeting. It was a prospective, nonrandomized study by Beslar et al that looked at more than 200 laparoscopic gastric bypasses and 160 gastric bandings. What they found was that although the groups were very comparable as far as gender, BMI, age, and preoperative comorbidity were concerned, there was a difference in early complications. The LAP-BAND had a 0.6% complication rate in the first 30 days, and the gastric bypass had a 5.2% complication rate. However, when the late complications were looked at, there was a higher complication rate after gastric banding than after gastric bypass. Therefore, the complication rates overall were comparable.

When they recorded the percent excess weight loss from 3 to 24 months, the researchers found that at 2 years, the weight loss with gastric banding was 48%, which was lower than with gastric bypass. However, interestingly, the resolution of comorbidities, including hypertension, diabetes, urinary stress incontinence, asthma, gastroesophageal reflux, and chronic low back pain, was exactly the same with both operations, regardless of the fact that the weight loss was lower with the gastric banding.

So why do patients have bariatric surgery? Well, a study out of Australia shows that most people have surgery because they have ill health or they have fear of deteriorating future health. What we at NYU looked at was, "What does the patient think? What are his or her concerns over surgery?" Not surprisingly, after surveying 470 consecutive patients prior to surgery and asking them which operation they chose, 81% of our patients chose gastric banding. Of course, that's extremely biased, because our program is known for excelling in LAP-BANDS, so it was not a surprise. But when asked why they chose gastric banding, patients, by a 43% margin, said safety was their leading concern.

In conclusion, the LAP-BAND is a safe operation because there is no bowel anastomosis, no bowel surgery, and no malabsorption. The short- and long-term complications are low with this operation. The band is adjustable and can be tightened or loosened according to the clinical status of the patient. It is reversible if it does not work, or if it is not tolerated by the patient, and it is revisable. If there are any complications, they are fixable. And, if the weight loss is inadequate, the band can be revised to a different operation. No bridges are burned. But what we also know is that the complications are qualitatively less severe and less costly than the other surgical procedures, and can be fixed with a minimum morbidity. Gastric banding is a safe surgical option, and the long-term weight loss of 55% excess weight does result in improvement of comorbidities. There are no nutritional risks involved. This is an operation that may be applicable to the masses—to the public healthcare crisis that we have. Finally, the midterm results here in the United States are comparable to the ones seen over a longer period of time internationally.

### Suggested Reading


1. Chapman AE, Kiroff G, Game P, et al. Laparoscopic adjustable banding in the treatment of obesity: a systematic literature review. *Surgery*. 2004; 135(3):326-51.

2. Dixon JB, Dixon AF, O'Brien PE. Improvements in insulin sensitivity and beta-cell function (HOMA) with weight loss in the severely obese. Homeostatic model assessment. *Diabet Med*. 2003;20(2):127-34.

3. Dolan K, Bryant R, Fielding G. Treating diabetes in the morbidly obese by laparoscopic gastric banding. *Obes Surg*. 2003;13(3):439-43.

4. Moore LL, Visioni AJ, Wilson PW, D'Agostino RB, Finkle WD, Ellison RC. Can sustained weight loss in overweight individuals reduce the risk of diabetes mellitus? *Epidemiology*. 2000;11(3):269-73.

5. Parikh MS, Laker S, Weiner M, Hajiseyedjavadi O, Ren CJ. Objective comparison of complications resulting from laparoscopic bariatric procedures. *J Am Coll Surg*. 2006; 202(2):252-61.

6. Ren CJ, Horgan S, Ponce J. US experience with the LAP-BAND System. *Am J Surg*. 2002; 184(6B):46S-50S.

7. Ren CJ, Cabrera I, Rajaram K, Fielding GA. Factors influencing patient choice for bariatric operation. *Obes Surg*. 2005;15(2):202-6.

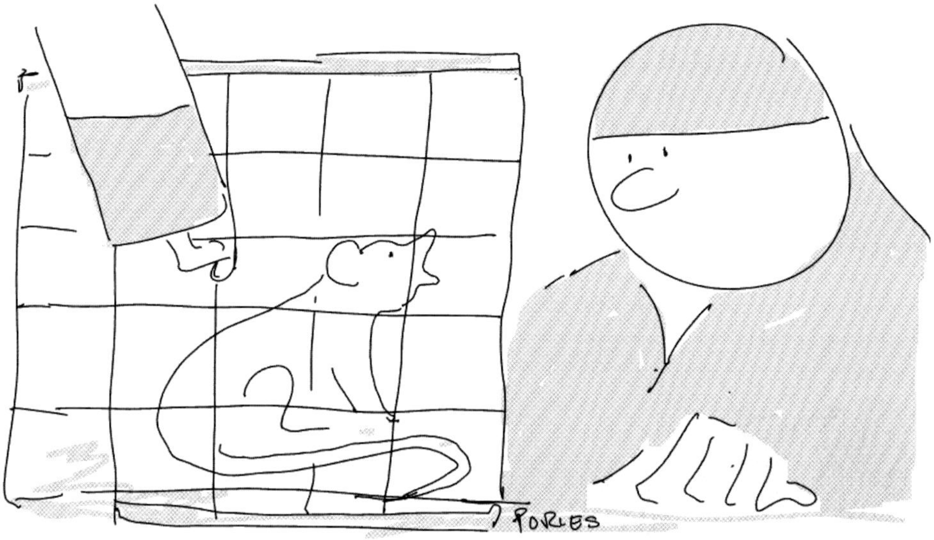


"If you don't mind, I'd rather be randomized to the band instead of the gastric bypass."

# The Biliopancreatic Diversion with Duodenal Switch

Alfons Pomp, MD, FACS
Michel Gagner, MD, FACS

Surgery is the only modality that is proven effective in inducing and maintaining long-term weight loss in the morbidly obese population. Bariatric surgeries are designed to limit the intake of calories. Reduced provision of calories induces the metabolism of stored fuels (adipose tissue) until a new equilibrium is established between caloric consumption and energy expenditure. Surgeries either restrict the amount of food intake, short-circuit the digestive tract to provoke malabsorption, or combine both of these methods to induce weight loss. Given that energy expenditure and weight loss is a complex function of an individual's metabolic rate, genetics, environment, and the interaction of gastrointestinal hormones, it is not realistic to assume that one type of surgery would be the optimal solution for every patient.

The history of malabsoprtion procedures actually predates gastric bypass surgeries. In the early 1950s, Kremen described the first jejunal-ileal bypass procedures. These surgeries and subsequent modifications, while successful as far as weight loss was concerned, were complicated by a high frequency of disabling diarrhea (steatorrhea), vitamin and nutrient deficiency, and a significant rate of liver failure. These surgeries were largely abandoned by the surgical community when Mason introduced the gastric bypass in the mid-1960s. Scopinaro in Italy rekindled interest in the malabsorptive procedures in the late 1970s when he described a partially restrictive gastrectomy with a long-limb–bypass procedure he termed the biliopancreatic diversion (Figure 1).(1)

**Figure 1**
**Scopinaro Procedure-Biliopancreatic Diversion**

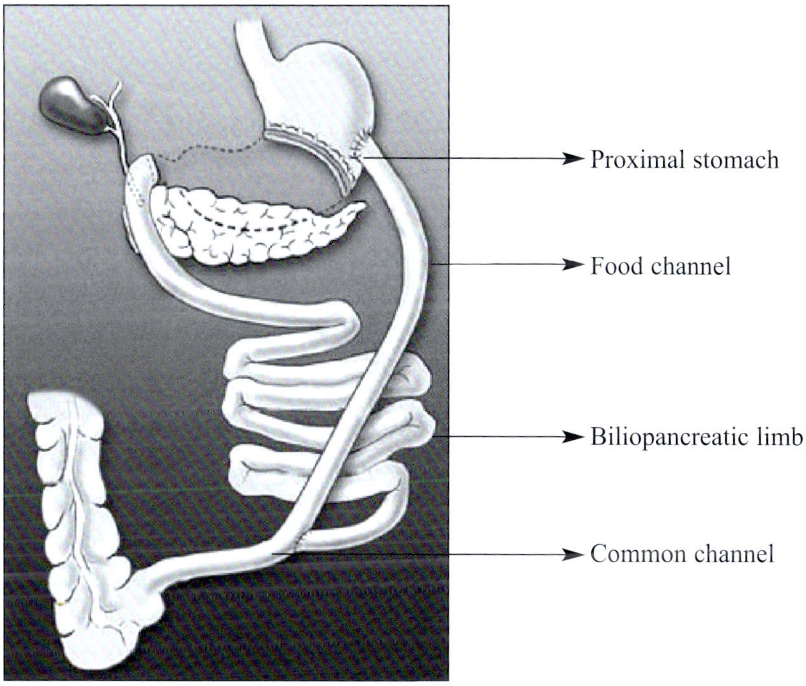

Further modifications by Marceau and then Hess, essentially performing the gastrectomy as a resection of the greater curve (sleeve gastrectomy) and also preserving the pylorus (duodenal switch), gave us the modern biliopancreatic diversion with duodenal switch (BPD/DS) procedure.(2) The current operation consists of a greater curve gastrectomy, leaving a volume of 125 cc to 200 cc and a common channel of 50 to 100 cm in length, depending in part on the patient's weight or the surgeon's preference (Figure 2). Michel Gagner first performed the operation laparoscopically in 1999.(3)

**Figure 2**
**Biliopancreatic Diversion with Duodenal Switch (BPDDS)**

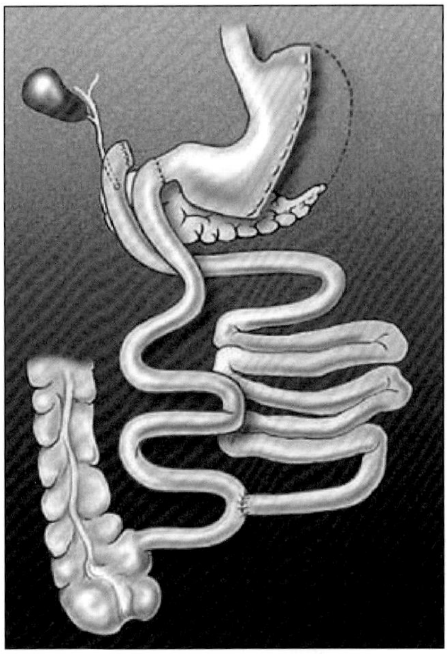

**Patient Selection**

All patients must fulfill National Institutes of Health (NIH) consensus criteria in order to be eligible for surgery.(4) During an initial office visit, specific attention is given to prior surgical history, medical history (comorbidities), and prior weight loss attempts. Patients are evaluated by a dietician/nutritionist and a psychologist or psychiatrist. Upper gastrointestinal endoscopy is performed to evaluate *Helicobacter pylori* status and rule out other incidental findings in the stomach. A cardiologist is usually consulted for patients with a pertinent cardiac history, which may include evidence of coronary artery disease, congestive heart failure, angina or prior myocardial infarction, hypertension, or arrhythmia. Patients with clinical evidence of severe venous stasis disease, prior history of deep venous thrombosis (DVT), or pulmonary embolus (PE) are at increased risk for DVT/PE during the perioperative period of weight loss surgery and are referred for an inferior vena caval filter (temporary or permanent) prior to surgery.

Patients usually present after having obtained information from multiple sources in the popular literature or Web sites, and they often come to the office visit with detailed questions. However all patients still receive a thorough review of all the bariatric surgeries and the potential risks involved. Given the morbidity of weight loss surgery, detailed informed consent is paramount. Every patient must be informed of the potential risk of an anastomotic leak and the possibility of death. Patients should receive the opportunity to discuss their operation with other patients who are either considering or have already undergone the operation in question. Each potential patient completes a questionnaire that demonstrates sufficient knowledge of the surgery and its inherent risks and benefits. Patients should leave the office visit understanding that bariatric surgery is a tool they will use for the rest of their lives to maximize and then maintain weight loss. Specific risks of each type of surgery should be addressed. Patients who undergo BPD/DS have more frequent foul-smelling bowel movements and flatus, which may require lifestyle modifications.

The Roux-en-Y gastric bypass has long been considered the bariatric procedure of choice in North America. Nonetheless, patients who have a body mass index (BMI) that exceeds 50 kg/m$^2$ ("super obese") have less successful results following this operation (5,6). The BPD/DS is our procedure of choice for patients with a BMI in the super-obese range. The necessity for close follow-up of nutritional parameters and mineral and vitamin levels mandate that the patient understand the complexity of a malabsorptive procedure and be diligent about the surgical follow-up. The patient must be compulsive about taking supplements and have the financial resources to be able to afford upwards of $1,000 per year of mineral and vitamin costs that, for the most part, are not covered by insurance polices.

### Technique

A seasoned operating room staff and anesthesiologist familiar with the technique, as well as the instruments and preoperative set-up, are essential. After induction of anesthesia, a urinary catheter is placed. Routine DVT prophylaxis is obtained. Antibiotic prophylaxis (cefazolin and metronidazole) is given to all patients.

The first stage of the procedure begins by performing a sleeve gastrectomy over a 60 Fr bougie (Figure 3) that leaves both the antrum and pylorus intact. The excised stomach is then removed from the abdominal cavity. The duodenal switch begins with a periduodenal dissection that is perhaps the most technically challenging part of the operation. The first 2 to 4 cm of duodenum can usually be dissected free circumferentially and the duodenum can then be transected. To ensure hemostasis, we routinely over-sew the duodenal stump using nonabsorbable suture. The ileocecal valve is identified and the small bowel is run in a distal to proximal direction. While running the bowel, a length of umbilical tape is used to measure out the 100-cm common channel on the antimesenteric border. Several clips are placed in the mesentery to temporarily mark this spot and an additional 150 cm is measured out to become the alimentary (Roux) limb. At this point (now 250 cm from the ileocecal valve), the small bowel is transected.

**Figure 3**
**Sleeve Gastrectomy**

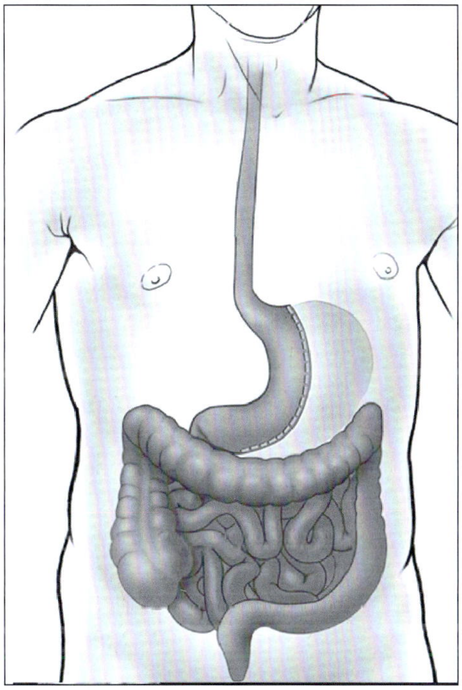

There are a number of ways to perform the duodeno-ileostomy; however, at our institution we use a 21 circular EEA stapler to make this anastomosis. The stapler is placed into the lumen of the ileum and the alimentary limb is brought antecolic toward the anvil, which has been placed in the proximal duodenum. A running nonabsorbable suture is then started at the corner of the duodenum staple line and carried across the anterior duodeno-ileostomy staple line. The open edge of the ileum is then stapled shut and the anastomosis tested using either a gastroscope with air insufflation or with a nasogastric tube and methylene blue dye.

The previously placed 100-cm marking clips are located and the distal end of the biliopancreatic limb is aligned in an isoperistaltic fashion at this point, and the distal anastomosis is created. An enterotomy is made in the end of the biliopancreatic (BP) limb and in the side of the alimentary limb. A linear stapler is then inserted in the two lumens and fired. The remaining enterotomy is closed using a running nonabsorbable 2-0 suture to complete the anastomosis.

Finally, the two mesenteric defects (enteroenterostomy and Petersen's space) are closed using running nonabsorbable sutures. At the end of the case, hemostasis is again ensured and any fluid collections are aspirated.

We no longer leave drains routinely. Incidental cholecystectomy is not performed unless the patient has symptomatic gallstones. Liver biopsies are often indicated to assess the initial severity of obvious macroscopic steatosis. We do not advocate incidental appendectomy.

Routine postoperative care includes close hemodynamic monitoring for 6 hours. During this time, patients are placed on continuous positive airway pressure (CPAP) if they have known sleep apnea. Maintenance intravenous (IV) fluids are continued and urine output is carefully observed. No further antibiotics are given, and we do not use post-op heparin routinely. Early ambulation is essential. If a patient is older than 50 years of age or has a cardiac history, we routinely use perioperative beta-blockers unless contraindicated.

### Postoperative Course and Surgical Follow-up

On the first postoperative day, we begin a bariatric clear liquid diet. This consists of clear liquids low in concentrated sugars given in 30 cc quantities every 20 minutes. If any intraoperative difficulty was observed, an anastomotic repair performed after a positive leak test, or any concern about the patient's clinical exam noted (including hemodynamic instability), an upper-gastrointestinal contrast study is obtained to evaluate the sleeve gastrectomy and duodeno-ileostomy.

When patients tolerate the liquid diet, the urinary catheter is removed. They are also weaned off the IV fluids and patient-controlled analgesic. Oral hydrocodone and IV ketorolac are used routinely for pain control on day 1 and 2. On day 2, patients are advanced to a bariatric puree diet. Our nutritionists extensively review the postoperative diet with patients while they are in the hospital. Most BPD/DS patients are discharged on the third postoperative day and will remain on a puree diet for the next 3 weeks. The only additional medications patients take upon discharge are calcium carbonate (Tums®) and chewable multivitamins.

At about 3 to 4 weeks after surgery, patients return for a first postoperative visit. They are then started on iron supplements, as well as oral bile salts such as ursodeoxycholic acid (if the gallbladder is intact). Vitamin A and D supplements are often prescribed. Patients are transitioned to calcium citrate and continue multivitamins. After this visit, the patient's diet is adjusted to permit small quantities of solid foods. During a follow-up visit with the dietician, the patient is reminded about dietary guidelines (e.g., eat protein first). In addition, many patients schedule routine visits with the psychologist at this time.

Additional follow-up visits are scheduled at 3-month, 6-month, 1-year, 18-month, 2-year, 3-year, and 5-year time points. At each of these visits, patients are again monitored for laboratory values (vitamin and nutrient levels that include A, D, E, and B vitamins, selenium, zinc, calcium, magnesium and iron, and international normalized ratio [INR] and prothrombin time to indirectly measure vitamin K levels). Weight loss is noted and reinforced. Potential complications are screened. The most common deficiencies after BPD/DS include iron (iron-deficiency anemia) and vitamins A and D. Calcium metabolism abnormalities are common and are usually foreshadowed by a high parathyroid hormone (PTH) level. Patients are continuously encouraged to maintain an active lifestyle that includes an appropriate exercise regimen and a healthy diet low in concentrated sweets and fats. In addition, they are encouraged to participate in support groups as participants, as well as mentors for future patients.

### Two-stage Procedures

Surgery in the super obese is technically demanding. The presence of a large bulky omentum, which is often accompanied by significant liver engorgement, makes this procedure intricate, to say the least. When the procedure is performed laparoscopically, the thick abdominal wall increases trocar "torque," which renders difficult the fine-motor control necessary to accomplish the intestinal anastomosis. The situation is further complicated by the limited physiologic reserve of these patients, which makes each significant complication a possible catastrophe.

When we initially reviewed our data, a definite increase in morbidity and mortality rates was apparent in the super, super-obese (BMI >60) patients operated on using open and laparoscopic techniques. A laparoscopic approach in this population has the potential to decrease cardiovascular, pulmonary, and wound-related complications. We hypothesized that separating the restrictive and malabsorptive aspects of the surgery with a laparoscopic sleeve gastrectomy, followed several months later (after significant weight loss) by a laparoscopic duodeno-ileostomy, would reduce the complication and mortality rates. Our initial experience has been very satisfactory—there has been a drastic reduction in morbidity and mortality using this approach, as compared with our historical cohort.(7) In fact, we have now transferred this 2-stage procedure over to our high-risk gastric bypass patients.(8)

Published results of hundreds of patients have demonstrated the efficacy and safety of biliopancreatic diversion with duodenal switch performed laparoscopically. Several groups have now published series on laparoscopic BPD/DS, including hand-sewn techniques, robotically assisted, and hand-assisted modifications.(9,10,11) The effectiveness of this procedure in reducing obesity related comorbidities has been proven using the open approach, and the results should be no different when expert surgeons do the same operation laparoscopically. Further research is needed to examine the long-term efficacy of weight loss surgery, comparing results between different surgical techniques, particularly in patients with BMIs greater than 50 to 60. The combination of modification of techniques based on bariatric data analysis and technical innovation will allow us to continue to improve the surgical treatment of obesity.

**References**

1. Scopinaro N, Marinari G, Camerini G. Laparoscopic standard biliopancreatic diversion: technique and preliminary results. *Obes Surg*. 2002;12(3):362-5.
2. Hess DS, Hess DW. Biliopancreatic diversion with a duodenal switch. *Obes Surg*. 1998; 8(3):267-82.
3. Ren CJ, Patterson E, Gagner M. Early results of laparoscopic biliopancreatic diversion with duodenal switch: a case series of 40 consecutive patients. *Obes Surg*. 2000;10(6):514-23.
4. National Institutes of Health. Gastrointestinal surgery for severe obesity. Consensus statement. NIH Consensus Development Conference, March 25-27, 1991. Public Health Service, National Institutes of Health, Office of Medical Applications of Research.
5. Brolin RE, Kenler HA, Gorman JH, et al Long-limb gastric bypass in the super obese: a prospective randomized study. *Ann Surg*. 1992;215(4):387-95.
6. MacLean LD, Rhode BM, Nohr C. Late outcome of isolated gastric bypass. *Ann Surg*. 2000;231(4):524-8.
7. Kim W, Gagner M , Kini S, et al. Laparoscopic vs open biliopancreatic diversion with duodenal switch: a comparative study. *J Gastrointest Surg*. 2003;7(4):552-7.
8. Regan J, Inabnet W., Gagner M, et al. Early experience with two-stage laparoscopic Roux-en-Y gastric bypass as an alternative in the super-super obese patient. *Obes Surg*. 2003;113(6):861-4.
9. Smith DC, Hendricks K, O'Reilly MJ. Laparoscopic biliopanceatic diversion with duodenal switch, with hand-sewn duodeno-ileostomy. *Obes Surg*. 2002;12:206.
10. Sudan R, Sudan D. Development of a totally intracorporeal robotic assisted biliary pancreatic diversion with duodenal switch. *Obes Surg*. 2002;12:205.
11. Rabkin RA, Savage S. The laparoscopic duodenal switch for the treament of morbid obesity. *Obes Surg*. 2002;12:216.

# Laparoscopic Sleeve Gastrectomy

Ronit Grinbaum, MD
Torsten Olbers, MD, PhD

## The Evolution of Sleeve Gastrectomy

In the United States, Roux-en-Y gastric bypass (RYGB) has emerged as the most popular, as well as the gold standard, of surgical treatments for severe obesity. The procedure is considered to have well-documented, long-term safety, and efficacy.(1)

**Figure 1. Laparoscopic sleeve gastrectomy**

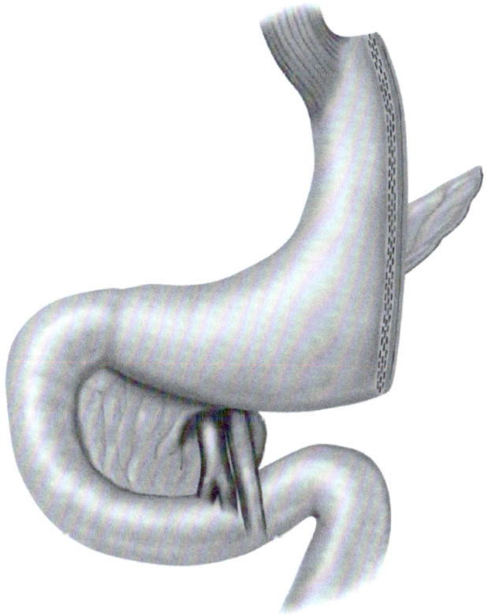

Biliopancreatic diversion (BPD), a procedure devised by Scopinaro more than 20 years ago, has been considered a valuable alternative to gastric bypass in patients with the most severe forms of obesity (e.g., having a body mass index [BMI] >50 kg/m$^2$).(2) Marceau and Hess have modified this procedure to a reconstruction termed the duodenal switch (BPD/DS).(3) This technically complex procedure combines an element of gastric restriction as a result of a longitudinal sleeve gastrectomy (SG) that replaced the distal gastrectomy of the BPD, with a malabsorptive component. The SG maintains the integrity of the antropyloric pump, thus avoiding dumping and reducing ulcerogenicity by lowering parietal cell mass. After this procedure, approximately 250 cm of small bowel remains in contact with the alimentary stream, 50 to 100 cm of which (the "common channel") is available for mixing of ingested food with biliary, pancreatic, and duodenal secretions. Both RYGB and BPD/DS cause a substantial, durable weight loss.

Laparoscopic sleeve gastrectomy (LSG) as a singular operation has recently been gaining popularity as a weight loss procedure. Because of the increased risk inherent in performing complex operations in patients with extremely severe obesity, some surgeons, led by Gagner, have opted to perform the BPD/DS procedure in 2 stages, with an isolated SG used to induce initial weight loss, followed 6 to 12 months later by the bypass reconstruction to create the full BPD/DS.(4-6) In small, uncontrolled series, weight loss after the SG rivaled the effects of gastric bypass. As a result, SG has begun to emerge as a stand-alone weight loss procedure. In 2 series, short-term outcomes appear similar to those of adjustable gastric banding (AGB) or even RYGB.(7, 8) Excess weight loss (EWL) in these small series ranges from 41% to 83% after 1 year.(6, 9) However, clinical experience with this procedure is limited, and its long-term efficacy is unknown.

The mechanism by which SG induces weight loss is unknown. It has been widely considered a restrictive procedure, but the degree of gastric restriction (the resulting gastric volume of SG is approximately 100 to 150 ml) is far less than that produced by RYGB or AGB, and specific mechanisms of action have not yet been studied. Ghrelin is a potent appetite stimulator produced primarily in the body of the stomach. Since SG involves resection of most of the ghrelin-producing mucosa, the reduced ghrelin levels may contribute to weight loss after this procedure.

**Indications**

Surgical treatment of super-obese patients has been challenging due to both weight loss failures (reported in up to 34.9% of RYGB patients) and high perioperative morbidity and mortality.(10) Gagner and colleagues have reported a 38% major complication rate and a 6.25% mortality rate associated with 1-stage laparoscopic BPD/DS in patients with BMI ≥65, compared with 8.3% major complication rate and no mortalities in patients with BMI 40 to 64.(11) Given these results, currently the two main indications for SG are: 1) as a first stage of a 2-stage procedure in super-obese or high-risk patients with BMI >50; and, 2) as an alternative to AGB or RYGB in patients with BMI 35 to 60, since SG provides short-term weight loss similar to the gastric bypass with the option of a later conversion to a RYGB or BPD/DS.

Sleeve gastrectomy has the advantage of being technically easier than RYGB in the previously operated abdomen. This has prompted the use of SG as an alternative to fundoplication and gastropexy for treating complex paraesophageal hernia in obese patients.(12)

Laparoscopic sleeve gastrectomy also has a lower risk profile of long-term failure than laparoscopic gastric banding (LAGB), the most popular restrictive procedure, with the clear advantage of the absence of a foreign body.

**Operative Technique**

The patient is positioned supine, with the surgeon on the patients' right side and the assistant on the patient's left side. We prefer using four (12 mm) working ports, with the camera port inserted about 25 cm to 30 cm below the xiphoid process in the upper midline. After carbon dioxide insufflation to 15 mm Hg pressure, three working ports are inserted as demonstrated in Figure 2. The liver is retracted cephalad with a Nathanson liver retractor. The dissection is performed using either an ultrasound scissor (Harmonic Ace™) or a diathermia-based device (LigaSure™).

**Figure 2**

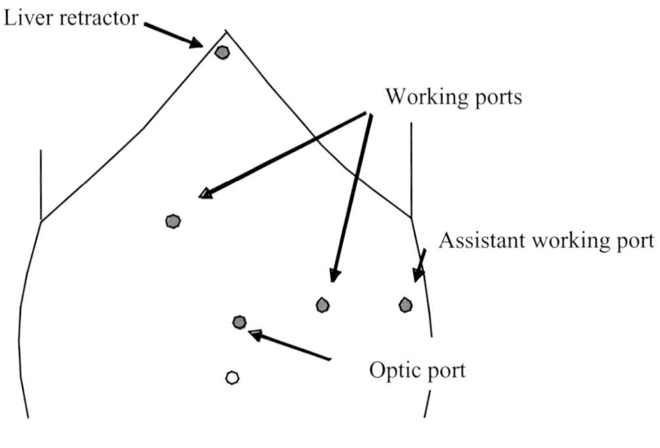


The dissection commences at a vessel-free space close to the stomach along the major curvature. It continues cephalad, staying close to the stomach wall and thus dividing all of the short gastric vessels. Since there are usually two layers of peritoneum, it is advisable to divide them separately. Frequently, there is a very close relationship between the upper fundic part of the stomach and the hilum of the spleen. It is important that all short gastric vessels are taken down, otherwise there will be a substantial portion of fundus spared and bulging dorsally. The dissection should also be through to the back wall of the upper stomach (inside the omental bursa), as there are often some fibrous attachments to the pancreas, etc. It is important to ensure that the stomach is only attached along the minor curvature. The dissection thereafter is performed from the initial start point on the major curvature, but now toward the pylorus. This dissection can end about 6 cm to 8 cm from the pylorus where the staple line will commence.

The resection starts about 6 cm to 8 cm from the pyloric ring on the major curvature, using a linear cutting stapler. The antral part of the stomach is predominantly preserved. A bougie (size 32 to 40 Fr) is inserted transorally and aligned along the lesser curvature to guide the gastric resection. At the angulation of the stomach on the minor curvature, the staple line is fashioned close to the bougie. The gastric tube is thus created with multiple staple firing, going vertically along the minor curvature close to the intraluminal tube and all the way up to the angle of His. We recommend the use of 2 initial 60-mm green cartridges at the lower part of the stomach since the stomach wall here is thick. Thereafter, either yellow or blue cartridges can be used. Applying buttresses on the stapler to increase the strength and decrease the risk of leakage and bleeding from the staple line is optional but should be considered, especially at the lower portion of the stomach (antrum) where the gastric diameter is large. The first two firings are preferably done with the stapler inserted through the right-sided working port. Thereafter, the left-sided working port provides a better angle. The resected stomach portion is inserted into a large specimen bag and is extracted through an extended port incision, usually the upper-right port. A clamp or Babcock is used to grab the specimen inside the bag and subsequently slide it out through the opening that usually does not need to be larger than 20 mm. A closure of at least the extraction port site is recommended, typically with a fascia closure device.

Staple lines should finally be inspected for any signs of insufficiency or bleeding. The estimated volume of the gastric sleeve is in the range of 100 to 150 mL.

**Results**

Gagner, Pomp, and colleagues published the first report of the use of LSG as a first-stage procedure in super-obese patients.(4,13) In their series, from January 2000 to September 2001, 33 patients underwent SG with no major morbidity or mortality. At the 6-month follow-up, the mean BMI declined from 66 ±5 to 53, and EWL was 32±10%. Twenty-three patients proceeded to a second-stage laparoscopic duodenoileostomy/ileoileostomy.(14)

Following these encouraging results, Almogy and colleagues published a series with 21 patients with a mean BMI of 56 who underwent longitudinal gastrectomy.(15) Nine were offered the procedure preoperatively because of their high preoperative risks. In 12 patients, a laparoscopic BPD/DS was planned but intraoperative findings or hemodynamic instability led to SG. Five patients developed complications, but there was no mortality reported. With a median follow-up of 18 months, median EWL at 12 months was 45.1%. Beyond 1 year, 4 of the 10 patients who were followed achieved more than 50% EWL.

For Baltasar and colleagues, the indications for LSG were: 7 patients with very high BMI (mean 65) as first stage of the duodenal switch; 7 with severe medical comorbidities; 16 with BMI 35 to 43; and one patient revised from a prior gastric banding. In the super-obese group, the EWL was 56% (4 to 27 months after SG).(16) The group with lower BMI had EWL of 62%. One patient (3%) with BMI 74 died due to intra-abdominal hemorrhage from a working port; another required explorative laparoscopy for ruptured access-port site with intra-abdominal bleeding.

Mognol and colleagues evaluated outcomes of LSG in 10 patients with a mean BMI of 64.(5) They reported no mortality, no complications, and no conversion to open laparotomy. Average EWL at 1 year was 51%. Based on their outcomes, they support integrating SG as a first-step procedure and as an acceptable singular restrictive procedure if long-term results are good.

In South Korea, Moon Han and colleagues described a series of 130 patients who underwent LSG.(9) They distinguish Asian from Western obesity, hence the growing need to explore this procedure. The LSG was offered as a first stage for all patients with a planned second stage duodenal switch if weight is regained after a year. The mean BMI was 37 (range: BMI 30 to 56). There was one death (1%), which occurred 21 days after surgery; an autopsy revealed peritonitis with no evidence of a leak. One conversion was reported, due to bleeding from a short gastric vessel, and there were 5 (4%) postoperative complications, two of them major—1 leakage and 1 delayed bleeding requiring re-exploration. Excess weight loss was 83% at 1 year. Diabetes resolved in 100% of patients within 6 months of operation; hypertension resolved in 92.9% and improved in 100%; and dyslipidemia resolved in 75% within a year. In 60 patients who were followed for at least 1 year, food intake dropped to 41% of preoperative levels. At 1 year, only one patient failed to achieve satisfactory weight loss (EWL was 21%; BMI from 56 to 51) and consequently underwent a second-stage RYGB. Beyond the first year, another four patients were identified as likely to need a second-stage duedenal switch—most of them had an initial BMI >50.

Langer and colleagues examined the success of LSG as a sole operation, and the incidence of gastric dilatation in 23 patients with mean BMI 48.5±6.9.(17) No morbidities or mortalities were reported. Excess weight loss at 1 year was 56%. Two patients were converted to RYGB—one because of severe gastroesophageal reflux at 15 months postoperatively (EWL of 98%), the other for complete weight regain at 2 years. After 1 year, 14 patients underwent an upper gastrointestinal series to exclude gastric dilatation. One patient met radiological criteria for dilatation but had achieved 59% EWL at 12 months and remained weight stable at 30 months postoperatively. Langer and colleagues concluded that LSG is effective as a sole operation and gastric dilatation may not be a limiting factor. However, patients should be aware of possible dilatation of the SG and the possibility of regained weight requiring a second-stage procedure. Follow-up is necessary to evaluate long-term outcomes.

In another study, Langer and colleagues observed a significant decrease of plasma ghrelin levels at 1 month and 6 months after LSG, while ghrelin levels increased in banding patients postoperatively. Excess weight loss was significantly higher in the LSG group at 6 months when compared with the LAGB group (61% vs 29%). Since ghrelin is predominantly produced in the gastric fundus, they concluded that the reduction in ghrelin levels as a consequence of the gastric resection may contribute to the superior weight loss observed after LSG, compared with after LAGB.

Cottam and colleagues examined the role of LSG within a 2-stage approach for the high-risk, high BMI (>60) patient. One hundred twenty-six patients with a mean BMI of 65.3 were enrolled in the study. Forty-two percent were assessed preoperatively to have American Society of Anesthesiologists (ASA) physicial status III, and 52% were ASA IV. The mean number of comorbid conditions per patients was 9. There was one late death, which occurred in the only conversion to open SG. That patient developed postoperative decubitus ulcers and pulmonary embolus 3 months after surgery. The incidence of major postoperative complications was 14% and included 5 strictures, 2 leaks, 2 pulmonary emboli, 5 patients requiring >24 hours ventilator support and 4 who developed renal insufficiency not requiring dialysis. Mean EWL at 1 year was 45%. Thirty-six patients with a mean BMI of 49 (EWL 38%) underwent a second-stage RYGB after a mean interval of 12 months (range: 4 to 22 months). The mean number of comorbidities in that group decreased to 6 and ASA class was improved prior to stage 2. The authors concluded that the staged approach in these patients is a safer and more effective strategy, with reduced morbidity and mortality rate; however, long-term follow-up is needed.

Silecchia and colleagues in Italy evaluated the effect of LSG on major obesity-related comorbidities as part of 2-stage laparoscopic BPD-DS. Forty-one high-risk patients (mean BMI 57) were enrolled in a prospective study. At surgery, 41.5% were scored ASA IV and 58.5% as ASA III. Ten patients had prior failure of intragastric balloon and four had LAGB failure. No mortality was reported. Major complications were recorded in 5 patients (12%), including a staple-line leak diagnosed 3 weeks after discharge and treated conservatively, staple-line bleeding, and transient acute renal failure. After 12 months, 58% of these patients had resolution of major comorbidities (obstructive sleep apnea syndrome, diabetes, and hypertension) and 31% had only one major comorbid condition. Average BMI after 12 months dropped to 41. Of 41 patients, 14 (34%) completed the second-stage BPD-DS after a mean interval of 16 months, with no mortality. The authors do not advocate LSG as a stand-alone procedure, but rather as a bridge to a second stage, optimizing the patient's condition by weight loss and significant reduction in comorbidities and ASA score.

Roa and colleagues analyzed data from 30 patients out of 62 who had LSG between November 2004 and March 2006.(7) The mean preoperative BMI was 41; mean EWL was 52.8% at 6 months. No mortality was reported. One patient developed a staple-line leak, detected on a Gastrografin study on the first postoperative day, and this was treated surgically. It was concluded that in the short term, LSG is safe and effective for both obese and super-obese patients.

Table 1
**Outcomes of Laparoscopic Sleeve Gastrectomy**

| Author | n | Preop BMI kg/m? | Mortality % | Complications % | Bougie size (Fr) | EWL 12 months % | 2nd stage % |
|---|---|---|---|---|---|---|---|
| **Gagner (2002)** | 33 | 66 | 0 | 3 | 60 | 32 | 70 |
| **Almogy (2004)** | 21 | > 50 | 0 | 24 | - | 44 | 10 |
| **Mognol (2005)** | 10 | 64 (61-80) | 0 | 0 | 32 | 51 | 0 |
| **Baltasar (2005)** | 31 | 35-74 | 3 | 3 | 32 | 46 | 3 |
| **Moon Han (2005)** | 130 | 37 (30-56) | 0 | 1 | 48 | 83 | 1 |
| **Langer (2006)** | 23 | 49 (40-73) | 0 | 0 | 48 | 56 | 9 |
| **Cottam (2006)** | 126 | 65 (45-91) | 0.8 | 14 | 46-50 | 45 | 28 |
| **Silecchia (2006)** | 41 | 57 | 0 | 12 | 48 | NA | 34 |
| **Roa (2006)** | 30 | 41 | 0 | 3 | 52 | 53 ** | 0 |
| **Himpens (2006)** | 40 | 39 (30-53) | 0 | 5 | 34 | 58%, 66%* | 5 |

NA: not available
** %EWL at 6 months
* %EWL at 3 years

The recent study published by Himpens and colleagues compares the outcomes of the most popular restrictive procedure worldwide, the LAGB, with that of the less common, isolated LSG.(8) During 2002, 80 patients were randomly assigned to either LAGB (40 patients) or LSG (40 patients). The LSG had a clear and significant advantage over the LAGB. Median EWL at 1 year was 41% after LAGB and 58% after LSG (*P*=.0004); at 3 years, median EWL was 48% after LGB and 66% after LSG (*P*=.0025). Loss of feelings of hunger after 1 year was recorded in 42.5% of patients with LAGB, and in 75% of patients with LSG (*P*=.003), and decreased after 3 years to 3% and 47% (*P*=.0001), respectively. Complications requiring reoperation postoperatively were recorded in 2 patients after LSG: 1 intraperitoneal bleeding during the first 24 hours, treated by laparoscopy, and 1 ischemia of the sleeve on postoperative day 4, requiring total gastrectomy. In the LAGB group, patients developed late complications requiring surgery: 3 had gastric-pouch dilatation treated by band removal in 2 and, laparoscopic conversion to RYGB in the third patient; 1 patient presented with gastric erosion treated by conversion to RYGB, and 3 had port disconnection treated by reconnection. Each group had 2 patients who had insufficient weight loss, which was treated by conversion to RYGB (from LAGB) or to LDS (after LSG). The authors concluded that weight loss and loss of hunger feelings are better after LSG than LAGB. Despite an important number of reoperations in both groups, complications seemed more severe after LSG.

Consensus regarding the gastric volume size that should be created during the procedure is lacking and ranges from 60 mL to 150 mL. The gastric tube is created using different bougie sizes ranging from 32 Fr to 60 Fr. There is some correlation between bougie size shaping the gastric-tube volume and degree of weight loss, but there is no linear relationship (Table 1).

Moon Han and colleagues demonstrated extraordinary results with a 48 Fr bougie, a result that to some extent may be attributable to the differences between Asians and Western population. Others using 32 Fr had a lesser EWL (41% to 62%), but the use of the largest size bougie (60 Fr) seems to produce the least weight loss (33% to 35%).(4,5,9,16,18)

The success of LSG in achieving weight loss can be partially explained by the mechanical restriction of food intake by the smaller longitudinal gastric pouch. The role of the gastric pouch in weight regulation is complex and involves the neurohormonal gut-brain axis.

Ghrelin, the most potent orexigenic hormone known, is produced primarily by the stomach. Ghrelin powerfully increases food intake, increases gastrointestinal motility and decreases insulin secretion.(19) Langer et al observed a significant decrease of plasma ghrelin 1 month and 6 months after LSG, while ghrelin levels were unchanged in banded patients. SG offers the advantage of decreased ghrelin secretion over other restrictive procedures. Reduced ghrelin levels may contribute to the weight loss, possibly by increasing satiety, as well as by altering gastric emptying. It would be helpful to develop a relevant animal model of SG to explore in more detail the physiological mechanisms by which SG induces weight loss.

Laparoscopic sleeve gastrectomy is an effective primary restrictive procedure with good short-term results and low morbidity rates. It is feasible and better tolerated in high-risk patients because it is relatively technically simpler to perform laparoscopically and hence operative time is shorter. However, long-term follow-up and prospective studies are needed to prove its efficacy as a sole operation. The option of a second-stage procedure in case of weight regain, with minimal anatomic distortion, will promote the acceptance of SG to the bariatric arsenal.

**References:**


1. Buchwald H, Avidor Y, Braunwald E, et al. Bariatric surgery: a systematic review and meta-analysis. *JAMA*. 2004;292(14):1724-37.
2. Scopinaro N, Adami GF, Marinari GM, et al. Biliopancreatic diversion. *World J Surg*. 1998;22(9):936-46.
3. Marceau P, Hould FS, Simard S, et al. Biliopancreatic diversion with duodenal switch. *World J Surg*. 1998;22(9):947-54.
4. Regan JP, Inabnet WB, Gagner M, et al. Early experience with two-stage laparoscopic Roux-en-Y gastric bypass as an alternative in the super-super obese patient. *Obes Surg*. 2003;13(6):861-4.
5. Mognol P, Chosidow D, Marmuse JP. Laparoscopic sleeve gastrectomy as an initial bariatric operation for high-risk patients: initial results in 10 patients. *Obes Surg*. 2005;15(7):1030-3.
6. Cottam D, Qureshi FG, Mattar SG, et al. Laparoscopic sleeve gastrectomy as an initial weight loss procedure for high-risk patients with morbid obesity. *Surg Endosc*. 2006;20(6):859-63.
7. Roa PE, Kaidar-Person O, Pinto D, et al. Laparoscopic sleeve gastrectomy as treatment for morbid obesity: technique and short-term outcome. *Obes Surg*. 2006;16(10):1323-6.
8. Himpens J, Dapri G, Cadiere GB. A prospective randomized study between laparoscopic gastric banding and laparoscopic isolated sleeve gastrectomy: results after 1 and 3 years. *Obes Surg*. 2006;16(11):1450-6.
9. Moon Han S, Kim WW, Oh JH. Results of laparoscopic sleeve gastrectomy (LSG) at 1 year in morbidly obese Korean patients. *Obes Surg*. 2005;15(10):1469-75.
10. Christou NV, Look D, Maclean LD. Weight gain after short- and long-limb gastric bypass in patients followed for longer than 10 years. *Ann Surg*. 2006;244(5):734-40.
11. Ren CJ, Patterson E, Gagner M. Early results of laparoscopic biliopancreatic diversion with duodenal switch: a case series of 40 consecutive patients. *Obes Surg*. 2000;10(6):514-23; discussion 524.
12. Cuenca-Abente F, Parra JD, Oelschlager BK. Laparoscopic sleeve gastrectomy: an alternative for recurrent paraesophageal hernias in obese patients. *JSLS*. 2006;10(1):86-9.

13. Gagner M, Rogula T. Laparoscopic reoperative sleeve gastrectomy for poor weight loss after biliopancreatic diversion with duodenal switch. *Obes Surg*. 2003;13(4):649-54.

14. Gagner M, Boza C. Laparoscopic duodenal switch for morbid obesity. *Expert Rev Med Devices*. 2006;3(1):105-12.

15. Almogy G, Crookes PF, Anthone GJ. Longitudinal gastrectomy as a treatment for the high-risk super-obese patient. *Obes Surg*. 2004;14(4): 492-7.

16. Baltasar A, Serra C, Pérez N, Bou R, Bengochea M, Ferri L. Laparoscopic sleeve gastrectomy: a multi-purpose bariatric operation. *Obes Surg*. 2005;15(8):1124-8.

17. Langer FB, Bohdjalian A, Felberbauer FX, Fleischmann E, et al. Does gastric dilatation limit the success of sleeve gastrectomy as a sole operation for morbid obesity? *Obes Surg*. 2006;16(2):166-71.

18. Milone L, Strong V, Gagner M. Laparoscopic sleeve gastrectomy is superior to endoscopic intragastric balloon as a first stage procedure for super-obese patients (BMI > or −50). *Obes Surg*. 2005;15(5):612-17.

19. Cummings DE, Overduin J. Gastrointestinal regulation of food intake. *J Clin Invest*. 2007;117(1):13-23.

# Intragastric Balloon

Jeffrey Allen, MD

The intragastric balloon is a device that is just beginning to undergo early-stage clinical trials in the United States and I have been fortunate to be working on those. I am not going to write about the trials or patients specifically, because these studies are ongoing. Instead, I will review a history of the device, as well as offer some international data.

The intragastric balloon is a silicone balloon that is endoscopically placed within the body of the stomach. It is designed to induce weight loss by limiting food consumption and should be considered a space-occupying lesion. Internationally, the device is known as the "Bioenterics Intragastric Balloon," shortened to BIB. Bioenterics is a division of Allergan, formerly Inamed Health.

**Advantages of the BIB**

The advantage of such a device is that it is the least invasive surgical treatment to date. In fact, it is not even a surgical treatment, but rather an endoscopic treatment. You have the elimination of a general anesthetic when inserting the BIB, which is a benefit. The BIB can potentially be used as a bridge to a more aggressive surgical therapy such as a gastric bypass or gastric band, or to a ventral hernia repair. Those of us who practice general surgery have all seen patients in the office who have large, complex ventral hernias, and we advise such patients to lose weight. Often they are not able to do so, but we feel if they did just lose weight, a hernia repair would have more chance of being long-lasting.

Another potential advantage of the BIB is that there is no "mutilation" of the stomach. Speak to German surgeons about bariatric surgery and they may point out the archaic German law that prohibits "mutilation" of a normal organ. This is not an issue with the BIB. Once the intragastric balloon is removed, the stomach basically goes back to normal, which can be good or bad as I'll talk about further on. There is a significantly lower out-of-pocket cost with the BIB, as insertion is not likely to be performed in the operating room. We are not in a sterile environment, required to gown and glove and so forth. An anesthesiologist is not required to be present. Thus, the typical out-of-pocket cost, though it varies regionally, is going to be about one fourth of the cost of a LAP-BAND procedure. There are no wounds, so there is virtually no chance for infection or postoperative hernia to occur. In addition it has the potential for being an outpatient procedure. In fact, the majority of intragastric balloons or BIBs that are placed are done so on an outpatient basis.

**Disadvantages**

What are the disadvantages? First, as we know, the stomach has a lot of acid and this acid will attack any kind of material that is in there. The current BIB design does not allow the device to be placed for unlimited periods of time and that's a problem. Furthermore, the BIB can rupture and once it ruptures or deflates, it may then migrate. Peristalsis can cause it to flow through the gastrointestinal tract. There is a planned removal (because of limited durability) of the BIB and subsequent weight gain is certainly a concern, as often happens when we reverse operations such as a gastric bypass or gastric banding. Many patients will gain all their weight back, and then even more. In addition, there are many more primary failures with BIB than with other forms of bariatric surgery. A number of patients simply don't lose any weight at all with the balloon. On the other hand, there are some people who do so well with the BIB that they will avoid presenting to have the balloon removed. When that happens, as noted, the device will likely eventually deflate and migrate.

After one of these balloons is placed, there is some fairly severe postprocedure malaise, for lack of a better word, including nausea, vomiting, abdominal pain, and/or diarrhea. All of the patients in whom I have placed these balloons, and just about every patient whose surgeon I have had discussions with on the topic, have had postprocedure malaise—some of it so severe that the patients demanded to have the device removed.

There are also unusual complications that can occur with this device. Though no longer a problem, I have had patients who have gone overseas, to Mexico or France, for instance, where they had these devices implanted and then came back to the United States with unusual complications. We were not sure how to most effectively take care of them. It's similar to when we first started performing the LAP-BANDs. The physician who saw the first patient with a slipped LAP-BAND who went into a local emergency room 100 miles from Louisville had no idea what to expect, and we have some of those same little quirks and nuances with the intragastric balloon.

There is also a potential for abuse, from physicians and patients alike. As you may know, these are pretty easy things to put in. There is a lot of handholding postoperatively, but if you eliminate that, I can foresee assembly lines where endoscopists will put 20 or 30 of these in per day, then just turn the patients loose. That is clearly not the optimal way in which we want this device to be used. Also, there is abuse by patients—having a balloon put in, taken out, put in, taken out. Or, as previously stated, having it put it in and not coming back for retrieval.

**History**

Let's step back a little and talk about the history of this type of device. A space-occupying lesion as a weight loss modality was first discussed by a gentleman named Davies in the United Kingdom, in 1921. In the 1980s, we began to have different devices at different locations. The Ballobese looks like the electron micrograph of a spermatozoon, but it is simply an intragastric balloon. Two others are important, the Taylor intragastric balloon and the Garren-Edwards Bubble.

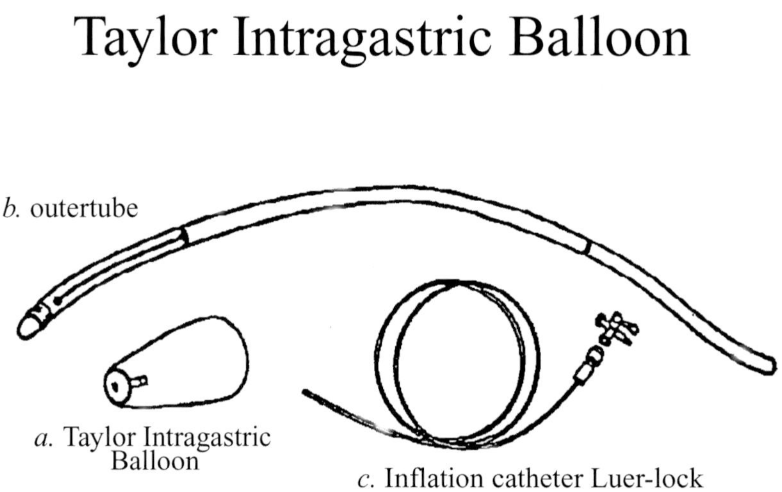


Illustrated here is the Taylor intragastric balloon. All have a similar delivery system with a stalk, and are inflated endoscopically.

**Figure 1**

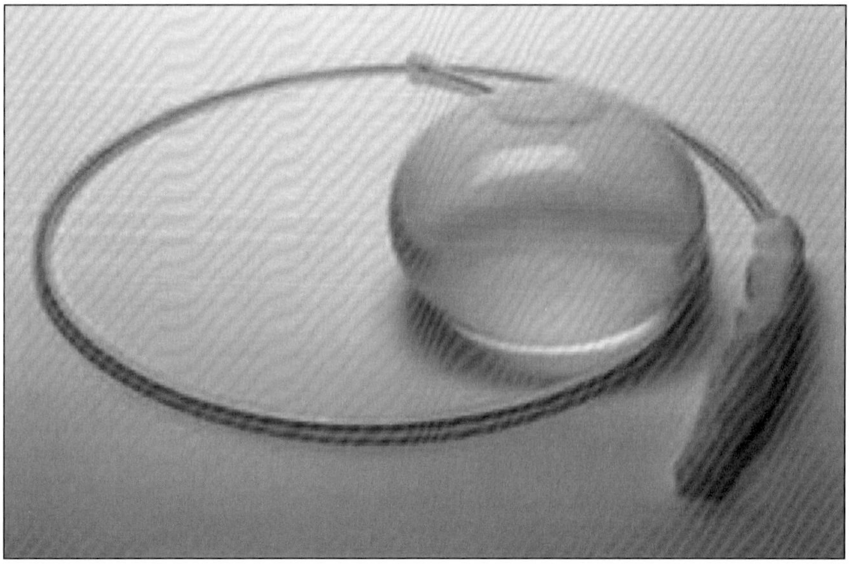

The Garren-Edwards Bubble had something of a space-capsule look to it and was first used in the United States. It had a tin-can shape and was made of an elastomer plastic. The recommended time period for the device to be in place was 3 months, and it was air-filled with 250 cc. It was approved by the FDA in 1985 as a temporary treatment for people who were 20% over their ideal body weight and there were 5 clinical trials. Sales began in 1986, quickly selling 20,000 units. That's an important number to note because, in reality, there were many complications, as the device simply didn't work very well.

In 1988, this lack of efficacy prompted the US Food and Drug Administration (FDA) to restrict the use of the Garren-Edwards Bubble to investigational trials. In May of that year, the company withdrew the product from the market due largely to its high complication rate. It had also prompted a bit of physician abuse, attributed to a "cure-all that can be used by anybody" mentality. There doesn't seem to be any evidence that the device was promoted as part of a comprehensive weight loss program, so the effect was poor results and it was withdrawn from the market.

As a result of this failure and that of the other devices, there was a scientific conference in 1987 in Tarpon Springs, Florida, bringing together 75 experts, including gastrointestinal surgeons and bariatric physicians, for the purpose of developing criteria for the use of an intragastric space-occupying device. The recommendations were:

- The device should work (one thing that the Garren-Edwards Balloon did not do)
- It should be liquid-filled instead of air-filled. That would give it more mass. It would be heavy, pulling down the stomach and activating the stretch receptors
- It should be capable of adjustment to various sizes, as well as have smooth surfaces. They found that the tin-can shape with those sharp edges was very prone to contributing to patients developing gastritis and even ulcers
- It should have a radiopaque marker, so spontaneous deflation and passage could be detected
- It should be made of durable materials that wouldn't leak

The good news is that the BIB currently being used overseas and which we used in our trial meets those criteria. The BIB has no sharp edges, is durable and capable of adjustment, can be tracked, is saline-filled, and has a self-sealing valve.

It is important to note that the BIB is not yet available in the United States. It is being placed in Latin America and Europe now, but clinical trials are in their infancy here in the United States, so the BIB will likely not be available in this country for 3 to 4 years.

The BIB was designed to be part of a comprehensive weight loss program. In the late 1980s, clinical trials began in Arizona on 3 or 4 forerunners of the current device. A second clinical trial was scheduled but never started as money for the project ran out and interest was waning on the part of the investigators involved. So in 1991, the focus shifted to Europe where the clinical trials showed that weight loss could be achieved by the BIB when its use was combined with a restrictive diet. Since that time, the BIB has been sold in limited centers in Europe and Latin America.

**Figure 2**

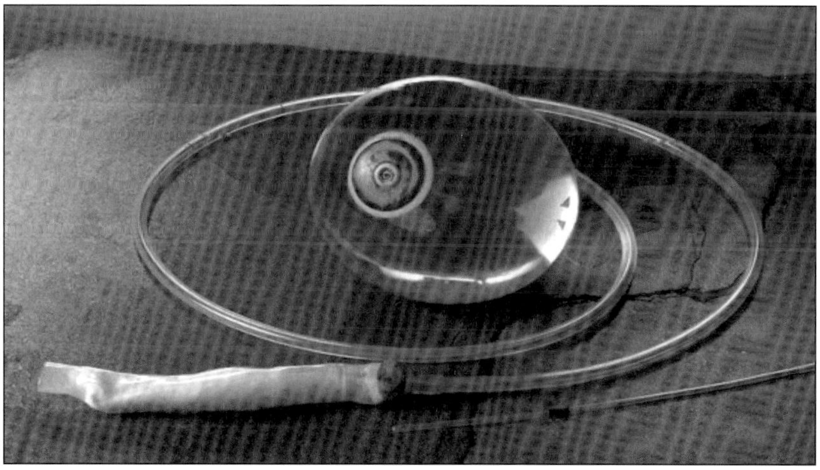

Figure 2 shows what the current device looks like. The tube is passed in to inflate the BIB, and then is snapped off.

**Figure 3**

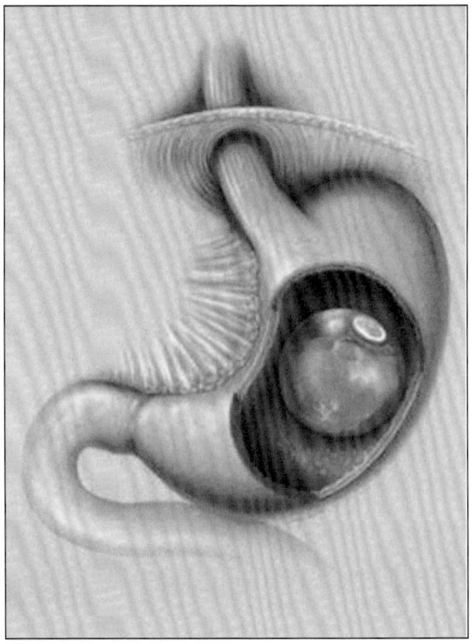

Figure 3 shows the approximate location where the BIB should be placed. If it gets too far down stream, it can go into in the antrum and cause obstruction so that the pylorus works to evict it. If it is too high up in the fundus, it will cause massive gastroesophageal reflux, so careful placement is key.

**Technique of Placement**

First, a diagnostic upper endoscopy is done, carefully checking to make sure that no ulcers, no large hiatal hernia and (especially) no Barrett's or any other kind of intragastric lesions are present. The endoscope is then removed. The stalk and the balloon are lubricated with gel and placement is made just as with an orogastric tube. The device should go down fairly easily. Once it is in, the physician follows its progress with the endoscope, much as with a percutaneous endoscopic gastrostomy (PEG), following the nasogastric tube down into the stomach.

**Figure 4**

X-ray of BIB® in place

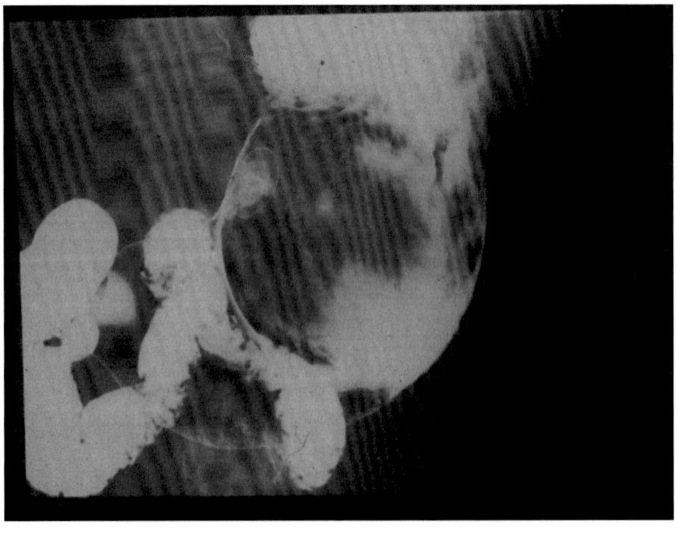

The device is filled with approximately 500 cc of saline under endoscopic vision. It is critical to fill only once it is in the stomach, as filling in the esophagus will perforate the esophagus, which has been reported. Some centers put methylene blue in—a good idea, since, if the BIB ever spontaneously deflates, the patient's urine would immediately turn green, signifying that there had been a deflation. In theory, the deflated BIB could then be retrieved prior to passing through the pylorus.

Having filled the device with saline, the physician then pulls the stalk off. There is a fill valve that automatically seals. The endoscope can then be used to manipulate the BIB into the correct position in the stomach. Once positioned, it works—not unlike the LAP-BAND—with a lot of the food concentrated above it.

After approximately 180 days, the device is removed. This is the most dangerous part of the procedure. Using a gastroscope, the patient is checked to make sure there are not a lot of retained food particles. If there are, the balloon should not be removed at that time, as the patient could aspirate when the balloon is pulled out. Putting the patient on a liquid diet beforehand and giving him/her cathartics should work to clean the stomach. Once all is well, the BIB can be punctured with the "handy dandy" BIB puncture device and then deflated as the fluid is sucked out. Once it is completely deflated, the BIB can be grasped either with an endoscopic snare or the retrieval device that can be provided.

Again, retrieval is potentially extremely dangerous. As the device is pulled through the esophagus, it catches on the sphincters and sphincter-like locations. It catches at the gastroesophageal junction, at the carina and at the upper esophageal sphincter. Thus, it may be wise to perform the retrieval with the patient under general anesthesia. A difficult airway problem or worrying about the device catching or lodging at the carina can be dealt with best by using general anesthesia.

**Complications**

What are the complications of the BIB? Fortunately, we have not seen many of these in our trial. Most patients do have some aspect of severe nausea. Most also have chronic gastroesophageal reflux disease, which requires proton pump inhibitors. Most seriously, esophageal or gastric perforation has been described and results in patient mortality. The rate of death as seen from the company data and what has been reported to Allergan and Bioenterics is probably about one in 10,000.

The balloon deflation and migration problem has been markedly improved based on the new design, although perforation still occasionally does happen. Gastritis and ulcers are also possible due to a deflated intragastric balloon. A patient whose device has deflated must go immediately to the endo suite and have the device retrieved. It is true that once it goes into the small intestine, the balloon often can pass with massive cathartics. Of course, it is going to catch on the ileocecal valve, but once in the colon, it will pass. Clearly, it is best to retrieve the BIB before it can deflate and migrate.

As we all know, and Allergan concurs, the BIB system is not indicated for cosmetic use. A large body of valid, published, clinical evidence of safety and effectiveness could change this. It is likely that the ultimate use of this device will not necessarily be only in the morbidly obese patient, but also in those who have a bit less weight to lose. I would never say that something like this should be implemented for cosmetic reasons, but it certainly could be used to treat the patient who has not reached severe obesity.

**Results**

International studies of note:

- In 126 patients in Belgium, there was 50% excess body weight loss at 6 months. This group had two gastric perforations, neither one of them lethal. These were not associated with the placement of the device. These patients had serious vomiting similar to Boerhaave Syndrome. That is something of which you must be very mindful. A patient with this kind of vomiting needs nutritional counseling and appropriate pharmaceutical care. If these do not work, the patient should probably have the balloon taken out. (It is difficult to gauge how much somebody is vomiting just by talking to them, of course.) The most concerning thing about this study, however, was that 10% of the patients were very unsatisfied, which apparently had no correlation with how much weight they lost. Even the patients who had lost a lot of weight were unhappy. One "take home" message is that the BIB is not necessarily a "walk in the park" for such patients. Unlike many of the bariatric surgery patients that I see (LAP-BAND, gastric bypass, switch patients), these BIB patients were pretty dissatisfied with at least some component of their treatment. These results were published in *Obesity Surgery*.

- One study, which enrolled 326 patients from Italy and was published in 2002, looked at BIB-plus-diet patients versus diet-alone patients and saw that the mean decrease in body mass index (BMI) was 4.8 kg/m$^2$ for the BIB-plus-diet patients—a significant decrease. They also showed real improvement in comorbidities

- In August 2004, a group of 483 patients from Brazil showed a 48% excess body weight loss at 6 months, and the patients had kept 90% of their weight off at 1 year

The obvious question is, "What happens when we remove this balloon? Won't the patient gain all the weight back?" What separates the really successful programs from the unsuccessful ones internationally, at present, appears to be the use of a multidisciplinary treatment approach. In the Belgian study, the patients got dietary therapy. They received nutritional counseling, exercise therapy, and behavior modification, as well as the BIB. In this way, when the balloon came out and they no longer had it to rely on, they had the other three components of the tripod. These patients continued to keep their weight off. Their excess body weight as a group was 39% at BIB removal. One year following BIB removal, the patients were still at 27% excess body weight loss, which is very good. It is important to know that there is some research going on about the basic science of it all.

A French study of 17 patients, published in *Obesity Surgery* in April 2005, showed that when the BIB is in place, there is certainly decreased gastric emptying and there are also significantly decreased ghrelin levels. The weight reduction correlated strongly with decreased ghrelin levels. The "emptying" patients did better compared with the patients who experienced greater retardation of the gastric emptying.

It has been proposed that the intragastric balloon should be a bridge to other weight loss procedures, or even ventral hernias, as I mentioned before. Favretti in Italy and his group looked at putting BIBs in and then doing LAP-BANDs, and what they found was that there were fewer conversions from laparoscopic to open incision in the patients who had lost weight preoperatively with an intragastric balloon. However, there was no increase in total weight loss than in the band alone. So one could argue that it may or may not be a necessary procedure.

It is important when reviewing the literature to use a jaundiced eye because so many of the international centers do not conform to US standards of morbid obesity or agree on who should have bariatric procedures. There are many patients who are in the BMI 30 to 35 range, and it is not appropriate to compare excess body weight loss percentage in those patients with patients who, for instance, have a BMI of 70. So when patients have lost 49% of their excess body weight at 6 months, it seems great, but may not necessarily be as wonderful as it sounds. The truly good results come from centers where patients are offered a good companion program.

Concentrating on the safety aspects of these interventions shows that the intragastric balloon is the safest modality being discussed today, with probably 1 in 10,000 mortality, but it might fail in the morbidly obese patients in an efficacy-to-safety ratio. It is an effective treatment, especially in patients who are not necessarily morbidly obese, and it is very good in some morbidly obese patients. However, I think the likely benefit of this modality is going to be that it will extend the realm of weight loss therapy to patients with lower BMIs.

The bridge theory has not really been proven. The Favretti study was interesting, but there is another study by Michel Gagner that compared sleeve gastrectomy with BIB. Although the statistical power was low, results demonstrated superiority of the sleeve gastrectomy as an initial procedure in super-obese patients.

**Conclusions**

Based on limited experience with the device, as well as review of the international data, the BIB appears to be a safe, reasonably effective therapy and seems especially good for the obese, though not necessarily the morbidly-obese, patient. It is inexpensive and certainly performs best as part of a comprehensive program. In fact, it will fail miserably if limited to assembly-line practices where physicians simply insert the intragastric balloons and later take them out. It is my personal opinion that the best utility of this device will be to bring antiobesity therapy to patients with lower BMIs—such as 30 to 35 or even 25 to 30 in diabetics—or to patients with other comorbidities associated with excess weight.

## Suggested Reading


1. Busetto L, Segato G, De Luca M, et al. Preoperative weight loss by intragastric balloon in super-obese patients treated with laparoscopic gastric banding: a case-control study. *Obes Surg*. 2004;14(5):671-6.
2. Doldi SB, Micheletto G, Perrini MN, Librenti MC, Rella S. Treatment of morbid obesity with intragastric balloon in association with diet. *Obes Surg*. 2002;12(4):583-7.
3. Herve J, Wahlen CH, Schaeken A, et al. What becomes of patients one year after the intragastric balloon has been removed? *Obes Surg*. 2005;15(6):864-70.
4. Milone L, Strong V, Gagner M. Laparoscopic sleeve gastrectomy is superior to endoscopic intragastric balloon as a first stage procedure for super-obese patients (BMI > or =50). *Obes Surg*. 2005;15(5):612-7.
5. Mion F, Napoléon B, Roman S, et al. Effects of intragastric balloon on gastric emptying and plasma ghrelin levels in non-morbid obese patients. *Obes Surg*. 2005;15(4):510-6.
6. Sallet JA, Marchesini JB, Paiva DS, et al. Brazilian multicenter study of the intragastric balloon. *Obes Surg*. 2004;14(7):991-8.
7. Totté E, Hendrickx L, Pauwels M, Van Hee R. Weight reduction by means of intragastric device: experience with the bioenterics intragastric balloon. *Obes Surg*. 2001;11(4):519-23.

# Weight Loss Surgery and Outcomes: Gastric Pacing

Scott Shikora, MD

It has been estimated that there are approximately 16 to 23 million adult Americans who have a body mass index (BMI) greater than or equal to 35 kg/m$^2$. Despite the lack of effective nonsurgical approaches, less than 1% of these patients will undergo bariatric surgery. Why? Many of these patients won't consider surgery because they fear the complications of the procedures, the long-term sequelae that may develop afterwards, or both. This situation creates a tremendous potential for new and less complex procedures to accommodate these patients. One such new technology, the Implantable Gastric Stimulator (IGS), has been shown to be very safe and thus far, in some patients, very effective for weight loss.

The IGS is similar to a pacemaker in that it stimulates the stomach with a small-patterned electrical pulse. The operation is a minimally invasive, laparoscopic procedure, and takes between 30 minutes to an hour to complete. Implantation of the IGS system is a "same day" surgical procedure, as most patients go home from the hospital within a few hours after completion. Like the laparoscopic adjustable gastric band procedure, the IGS is reversible and adjustable.

Unlike cardiac pacing, the IGS does not "pace" the stomach; it merely provides electrical stimulation. The stomach does not function like the heart and the goal is not to "capture its rhythm." In fact, it is currently believed that the resultant weight loss is likely due to factors other than altering gastric peristalsis. Recent research in both animals and humans has demonstrated other mechanisms of action for weight loss, including stimulation or inhibition of the vagus nerve and/or appetite hormones, and even affecting the brain itself.

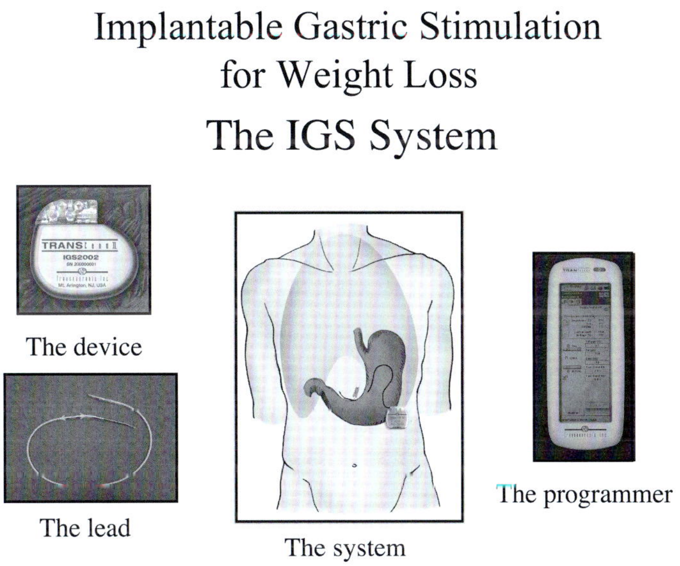


The IGS system consists of an electrical pulse generator, a bipolar lead with a positive and negative electrode, and a programmer. The programmer "communicates" with the IGS generator by external, noninvasive radio frequency via a handheld PDA-like device. The lead or leads are inserted into the wall of the stomach and the generator is implanted into a pocket in the subcutaneous tissues much like the port of a laparoscopic adjustable gastric band.

The operative procedure compares favorably with other bariatric procedures in that it is relatively straightforward and brief. Generally, only 3 or 4 trocars are used. After gaining access to the abdominal cavity and creating a pneumoperitoneum, the liver is retracted and the stomach is visualized. The nerves of Laterge (pes ancerinis) are identified on the lesser curvature of the stomach. Using a tape measure, a 3-cm length is marked with the electrocautery on the stomach just underneath the nerve branches. These marks will be used for the insertion of the lead. The 3 cm mark signifies the entry and exit ports for the lead. Both electrodes must be buried and the 3-cm length is sufficient to accomplish this. In more recent investigations, the IGS system utilized 2 leads consisting of 4 electrodes so the lead insertion procedure was performed twice. Utilizing a 2-lead system dramatically increased the number of stimulation options, as well as the ability to stimulate via 1 or 2 leads.

Lead insertion is not a technically difficult maneuver, but it does require some skill. The lead must be placed sufficiently deep to be in the seromuscular interface of the stomach wall, but not deep enough to penetrate into the lumen of the stomach. After insertion, an endoscopy is performed to confirm proper placement. A lead cannot be left in place after it has penetrated the lumen. If a lead has in fact penetrated the lumen, it can be partially withdrawn and reinserted. Once proper positioning is confirmed both by endoscopic and laparoscopic visualization, the insertion needle is cut off of the lead and removed and the lead is fixed in place by suturing it to the gastric wall. The free ends of the leads are then pulled out of the abdomen and connected to the device. A subcutaneous pocket is created in the abdominal wall on the patient's left side, where the device is implanted. The laparoscopic ports are then closed and the operation completed. Most patients are discharged to home a few hours later.

Implantable Gastric Stimulation
for Weight Loss

Cigaina: Update on 1998 Study

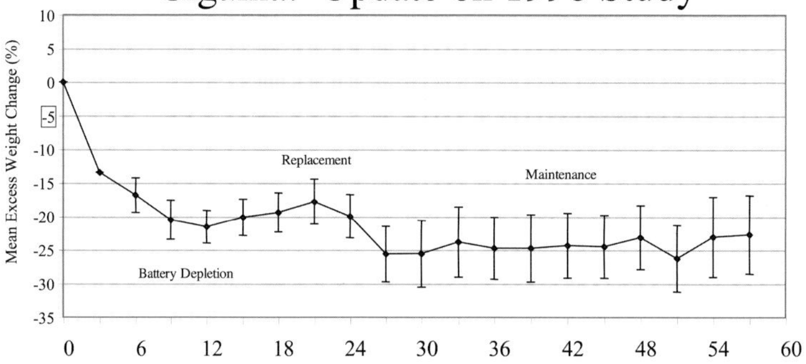


10 Patients

The concept of electric stimulation of the stomach to achieve weight loss was first conceived in the mid-1990s by an Italian surgeon, Valero Cigaina. After preliminary animal trials succeeded in achieving weight loss, he began human trials. His 1998 trial was the first significant research effort. Ten patients were implanted and succeeded in losing more than 20% of their excess weight. Furthermore, patients started to regain weight at approximately 12 months after implant. This corresponded with depletion of the device batteries, as the average battery life of these early devices was only 1 year. Explantation of the depleted devices and replacement with new devices resulted in renewed weight loss. This study and its observations spawned worldwide interest in gastric electrical stimulation for weight loss and set the stage for international investigations.

To date, more than 720 patients worldwide have been implanted and are participating in clinical investigations. For the earliest patients, there is now more than 20 year's follow-up. Thus far, there have been no deaths, and no serious complications, and no long-term consequences have been identified. For those patients who have responded to follow-up, there is more than 35% excess weight loss, and generally speaking, whatever weight loss a patient achieved was maintained as long as the battery was active.

Several trials with the IGS have been conducted in the United States thus far, but the results have been inconsistent. The following is a summary of these trials.

## Implantable Gastric Stimulation for Weight Loss

## US O-01 Study

- 103 patients, 10 centers, PRDBPCT
- Randomization between device ON or device OFF for 6 months
- All devices turned ON 7 months postimplant
- Uniform low output settings
- No behavioral or dietary counseling given
- Results:
  - No statistically significant weight loss between groups
  - Overall weight loss was 20% EWL at 20 months

**The O-01 Trial**

The first US investigation of the IGS for weight loss was initiated in 2000. This was a randomized, double-blind, placebo-controlled trial involving 103 morbidly obese patients. All 103 patients were implanted and, after 1 month, were randomized into "device turned on" and "device left off" groups. As with all double-blind trials, neither patients nor investigators knew which patients had their devices activated and which had devices that were not activated. Patients were then followed for 6 months. Unfortunately, at the end of this 6-month period there was no difference in weight loss between those patients whose devices were on and those whose were off and there was insignificant weight loss overall.

## Implantable Gastric Stimulation for Weight Loss

## US O-01 Trial: Results

- No significant difference in weight loss between the active and control groups
- Overall weight loss was 20% excess wt
- No deaths or major complications
- Study problems
  - Inadequate preoperative screening
  - Lack of patient education and dietary counseling
  - High incidence of electrode dislodgment (20%)
  - Low output (6 mA) - uniform settings

Although the trial results were very disappointing, a number of confounding variables were identified that may have negatively impacted the results. For instance, no behavioral or dietary counseling was provided to either group of patients upon entry into the trial. Few bariatricians would dispute the benefits of both behavioral and dietary counseling for improving the success of any bariatric procedure. There were also very few exclusions for entry into the trial, which meant patients with eating disorders were included. It is now believed that patients with eating disorders are less likely to respond. In addition, midway through the study, it was discovered that the technique for securing the lead to the gastric wall was inadequate, as a number of the patients were found to have lead dislodgments. Like other electrical systems, contact with the gastric wall is essential for having a complete electrical circuit. A dislodged lead breaks the circuit. Lastly, by protocol design, all IGS devices were programmed to uniformly low output settings. In contrast, patients in Europe were programmed to higher settings and achieved better results. Despite these limitations, there appeared to be a subgroup of patients in the trial that did respond to the IGS and succeeded in achieving a 20% or greater excess weight loss.

### The DIGEST Trial

A smaller and less ambitious project, the open-label dual-lead implantable gastric electrical stimulation trial (DIGEST) was conducted at 2 centers with 30 severely obese patients. Compared with O-01 trail, DIGEST had a more selective enrollment. A psychologist screened all patients preoperatively, eliminating patients with personality or eating disorders. The devices were newer, 2-lead electrical generators. All were set to higher outputs and settings were individualized based on the ability to elicit symptoms during device-interrogation in the office. Improved lead security was also employed in this trial.

Implantable Gastric Stimulation
for Weight Loss

DIGEST Results

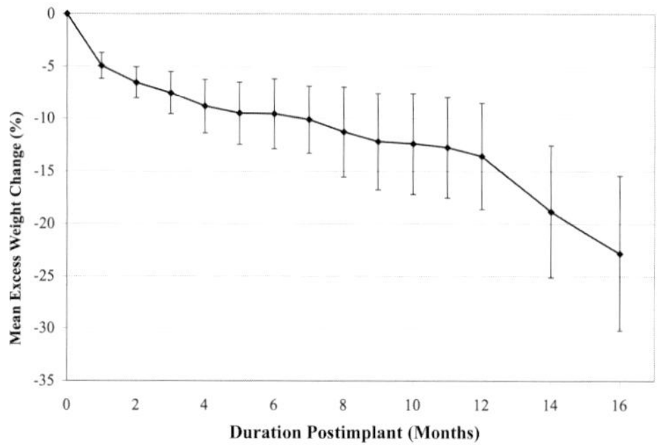


* At 9 months follow up - 65% of patients have lost weight, 41% lost >10% of excess weight, and 18% lost >20% of excess weight.

As a consequence of all of these improvements, the study achieved better weight loss results than the O-01 trial. Thirty percent of patients lost more than 20% of their excess weight. However, like the O-01 trial, there were responders and nonresponders. In addition, in this trial, it was learned that the IGS caused early satiety, based on the responses to satiety questionnaires that patients were required to fill out during their follow-up visits. This led to the hypothesis that successful patients would be those who respond appropriately to satiety while nonresponders would be those who ignore the signals of satiety.

Implantable Gastric Stimulation
for Weight Loss

DIGEST - Satiety and Appetite

Significant improvement seen in:

- ↓ Appetite before meals (15% change)
- ↑ Satiety between meals (60% change)
- ↑ Satiety at the end of a meal (90% change)

Some patients report changes in food choices

The ability to predict whether patients would be likely to respond or not, was considered an important aspect for improving overall success with this technology. The premise was only to implant patients likely to succeed and in this regard, a screening tool was developed by a statistician named Roland Maude-Griffin. Using the data from the first 252 patients implanted with the IGS worldwide, Maude-Griffin constructed a computer-generated statistical model that would predict responsiveness for all patients being considered for implantation. The Baroscreen, as it is named, is a machine-learning, computer-generated algorithm that analyzes information from prospective patients and compares that information with a database of preoperative information gathered from known responders and nonresponders.

## Implantable Gastric Stimulation for Weight Loss

### Effects of screening

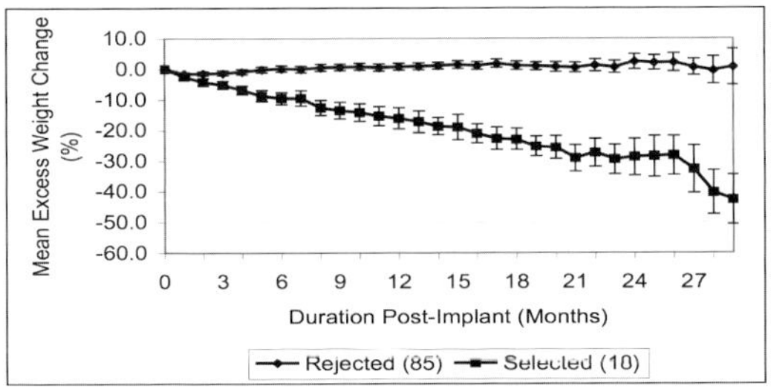


O-01 Trial

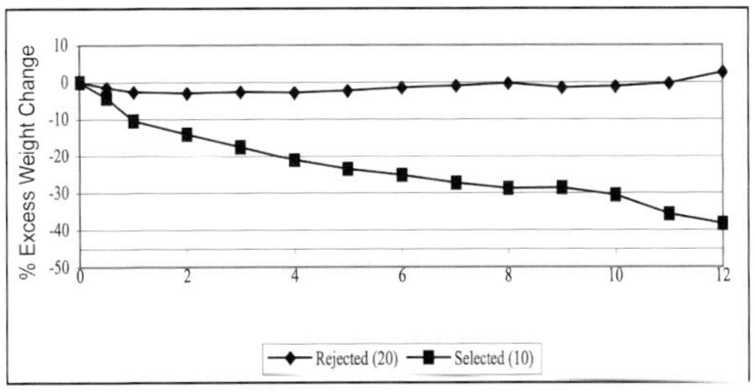


DIGEST Trial

The Baroscreen was validated both retrospectively and prospectively. Retrospectively, it was validated with the data from the O-01 and DIGEST trials. For the 103 patients of the O-01 trial, the Baroscreen suggested that 85 were not good candidates. Those 85 patients, in fact, did not lose weight. Furthermore, it suggested that 18 of the patients would respond and, in fact, those patients lost more than 40% of their excess weight. In the DIGEST trial, the Baroscreen rejected two thirds of the patients entered and these patients indeed failed to lose weight. The remaining one third of patients (who were predicted to be responders) lost nearly 40% of their excess weight.

## Implantable Gastric Stimulation for Weight Loss

### Prospective Screening

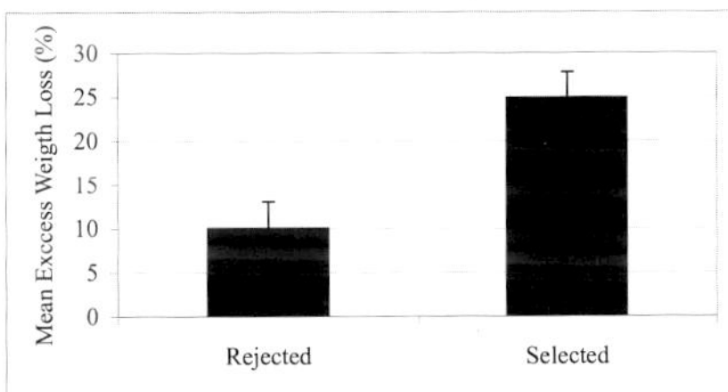


p=.003

11 Rejected with mean follow-up of 10 months, and 13 selected with mean follow-up of 8.2 months.

Similar results were achieved when the Baroscreen was tested prospectively. In a small study, patients were subjected to the Baroscreen, but were implanted regardless of its results. The patients deemed nonresponders by the Baroscreen lost approximately 16% of their excess weight in a 16 month period. However, those patients who were deemed likely responders lost statistically significantly more excess weight—approximately 30%.

**The SHAPE trial**

At the time of this report, the SHAPE trial is well underway.

## ***S***creened ***H***ealth ***A***ssessment & ***P***acer ***E***valuation (***SHAPE***) trial

- Randomized, placebo-controlled, double-blinded trial
- 190 patients at 9 investigative centers
- Patients were only enrolled after passing the screening algorithm
- 11% Excess weight loss thus far

This study enrolled 190 patients at 8 centers across the United States. Prior to acceptance in the trial, all patients had to pass the Baroscreen and of all interested candidates, only approximately 25% passed. These patients were then subjected to standard behavioral screening, which excluded those with behavioral or eating disorders. The remaining candidates were then enrolled in the study. Similar to the O-01 trial, this was a prospective, randomized, placebo-controlled investigation. All patients were implanted with the higher output, 2-lead IGS system. Two weeks after implant, patients were randomized into "device on" and "device off" groups. Data collection would continue for a 12-month period before breaking the blinding. The primary endpoint was a greater than 10% difference in weight loss between the study (device on) and control (device off) groups. At 8-month follow-up, an overall weight loss of 11% of excess weight was observed.

## Possible Mechanisms of Action

Patients eat less due to an enhanced feeling of satiety

- Altered gastric motility
- Fundic expansion
- Change in blood levels of GI hormones
- Direct or indirect vagal stimulation
- Combination of the above

Studies have shown an effect of pacing in all of these factors

One lingering question remains: how does the IGS achieve weight loss? Ongoing basic science research and the results from the many human clinical trials have thus far failed to definitively reveal the mechanism of action; however, several are proposed. Research has shown that with IGS, there are potential changes in gastric motility, fundic tone, and gut hormones, as well as inhibition of the vagus nerves, stimulation of the autonomic nervous system, and even direct effects on the hypothalamus. Whether one or several of these influences are involved with achieving weight loss is still not known.

From a gastric electrophysiologic standpoint, IGS function has been well established. The stomach has a native electrical pacemaker on the proximal greater curvature of the fundus. It fires a small electrical charge at a frequency of 3 cycles per minute. The charge propagates distally toward the antrum and is thought to cause tone and peristalsis. The IGS is placed more distally and fires an electrical impulse at a higher frequency (12 CPM) in a retrograde fashion, which results in inhibition of the natural electrical activity, which may inhibit gastric motility and possibly have other effects such as changing gastric tone, etc.

Given the known safety profile of the IGS, its potential application is very promising. In addition to the severely obese, it may be attractive to consider for patients who suffer from obesity-related health conditions and have a BMI <35, which currently disqualifies them from traditional bariatric surgery. The IGS may have utility as part of a staged approach for extremely high-risk patients—a utility similar to, but safer than, the gastric sleeve. Lastly, the IGS might be appropriate for obese adolescents and even for patients seeking weight loss maintenance after successful medical weight loss.

A very safe and increasingly effective alternative to other bariatric procedures currently being performed to achieve meaningful and sustainable weight loss, the IGS with addition of the screening tool seems promising. Indeed, the IGS may one day assist in offering surgical remedies to the large number of worthy patients who, for a variety of reasons, will not undergo more conventional surgical procedures.

### Suggested Reading

1. Cigaina V. Long-term follow-up of gastric stimulation for obesity: the Mestre 8-year experience. *Obes Surg*. 2004;14(suppl 1):S14-S22.
2. Cigaina V. Gastric pacing as therapy for morbid obesity: preliminary results. *Obes Surg*. 2002;12(suppl 1):12S-16S.
3. Shikora SA. Implantable gastric stimulation for weight loss. *J Gastrointest Surg*. 2004;8(4):408-12.

# The Role of the Endoscopist

James Ellsmere, MD
Ram Chuttani, MD

Endoscopists have an important role in managing problems that may occur following weight loss surgery. This chapter will discuss how we use endoscopy to evaluate symptoms and treat complications, as well as to investigate patients who initially lose, but then regain their weight. Several groups are currently using endoscopic techniques to treat patients who fail to maintain weight loss following bariatric surgery. There is also much interest in performing weight loss procedures using only endoscopic techniques, and we will look at these emerging endoscopic applications and discuss how the role of endoscopy in weight loss surgery may evolve.

## Bariatric Anatomy

The first step for an endoscopist in evaluating a patient who has had weight loss surgery is to understand what operation he/she has had. There have been a number of weight loss operations performed over the last 30 years, both solely restrictive and solely malabsorptive or combinations thereof. The most commonly performed procedures today have been described in this book. Endoscopists looking after bariatric patients must familiarize themselves with these various operations, and the best way for an endoscopist to determine a patient's specific anatomy is to discuss the operation with the patient's surgeon. Alternatively, the endoscopist can review the operative notes. Reviewing the most recent contrast studies will also increase the yield of the endoscopic evaluation.

## Nausea and Vomiting

Nausea and vomiting are the most common complaints after weight loss surgery. Generally this is due to eating too much, too quickly. Most currently performed procedures have some element of gastric restriction. Learning to eat smaller meals and chew food adequately is an important lifestyle change that patients need to adopt to achieve their weight loss goals. If correcting eating habits does not address the patient's complaints, then it is appropriate to perform an upper endoscopy to assess the distal esophagus, gastric pouch, and both gastric remnant and duodenum in solely restrictive procedures, or the jejunum in the case of a gastric bypass.

## Obstruction

Stenosis at the gastric pouch outlet is common and easily treated endoscopically with balloon dilation. The incidence of this stenosis depends heavily on the surgical technique used and ranges from 2% to 30%. In our experience, anastomoses created with circular staplers have a higher rate of stenosis than those that are hand sewn.

**Figure 1**
**A stenotic gastrojejunostomy seen 3 months post-Roux-en-Y gastric bypass**

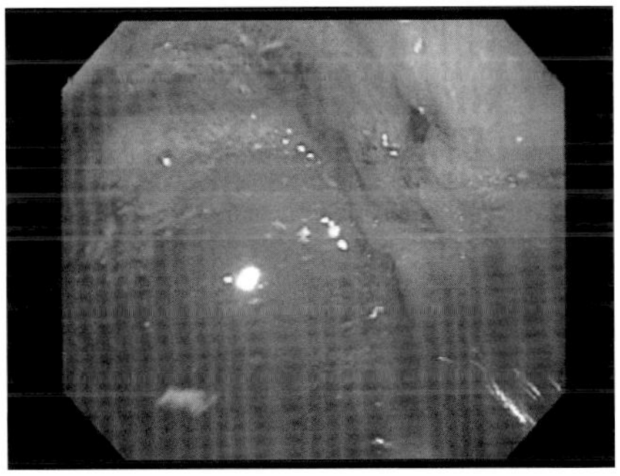

Figure 1 shows a gastrojejunal stenosis at 3 months after a gastric bypass. Endoscopic balloon dilation is successful in most subjects, although 2 to 3 sessions may be required to achieve long-term results. Balloon dilation can be performed with hydrostatic balloons of fixed or graded diameters.

**Figure 2**

**Dilating a gastrojejunostomy stenosis with a balloon dilator under direct vision**

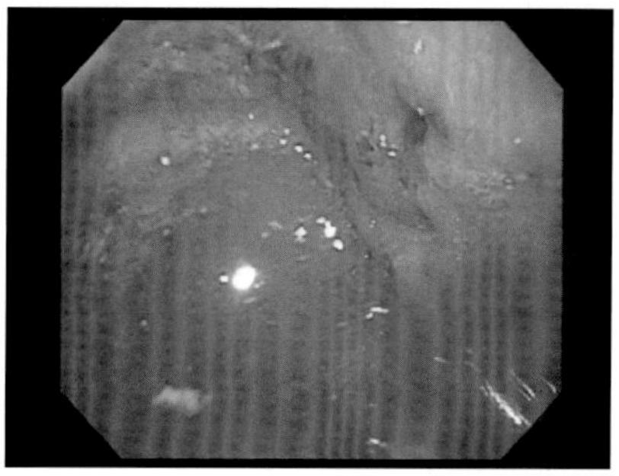

Figure 2 shows a stenotic gastric outlet being dilated with a balloon. We have found gradual dilation using the controlled radial expansion (CRE) balloon (Boston Scientific, Natick, MA) to be very effective. We dilate to a diameter of 15 mm and generally not beyond in order to avoid losing gastric restriction.

Obstruction from causes other than gastric outlet stenosis can occur. These potential causes include a slipped gastric band, a constricting mesocolon, a narrowed jejunojejunal anastomosis, adhesions, or volvulus. Much less common than stenosis, these are important to recognize as they can lead to life-threatening complications. There are limited endoscopic options for these patients. It may be beneficial to dilate a constricting mesocolon or a narrowed jejunojejunal anastomosis, but this should only be done in consultation with the patient's surgeon.

### Epigastric or Retrosternal Pain

New onset epigastric or retrosternal visceral-like pain following weight loss surgery can occur and is typically secondary to gastroesophageal reflux. Obese patients can have several risk factors for coronary artery disease so this needs to be excluded as the cause. Gastroesophageal reflux usually can be treated with acid suppression and lifestyle changes, including avoiding large meals and eating before bed. As all patients have some degree of gastric outlet restriction, liquid or orally dissolvable acid-suppression formulation should be prescribed. If acid suppression is not effective, endoscopy should be performed to evaluate for other possible causes, such as obstruction or ulceration, which need to be managed differently.

### Anastomotic Ulcers

Anastomotic ulcers, as shown in Figure 3, can occur following weight loss surgery, although the incidence is less than that of other gastric surgery because the cardia does not secrete acid like the rest of the stomach. The incidence of symptomatic ulceration is less than 15%. The exact etiology is unclear; however, many factors are thought to be associated with development of these ulcers. The usual causes, such as *Helicobacter pylori*, smoking, and non steroidal anti-inflammatory drugs (NSAIDs), should be sought out and treated appropriately. Ischemia from devascularized tissue is always a concern with surgical anastomoses and can lead to ulcers that are difficult to heal. A high level of acid in the pouch should raise suspicion that either the pouch encompassing the gastric fundus is too large or that there may be a fistula between the gastric pouch and gastric remnant. Treatment with acid suppression alone is generally effective. Sulcrafate may be added for patients with persistent ulcers but obstruction must first be excluded to avoid creating a sulcrafate bezoar.

**Figure 3**

**Anastomotic ulcers typically occur just beyond the gastrojejunostomy**

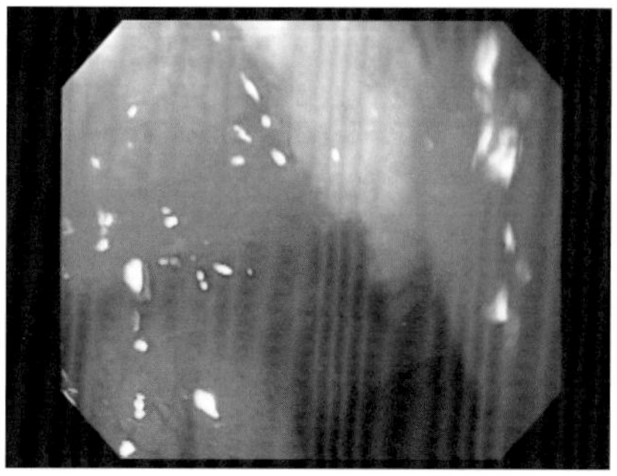

### Gastro-gastric Fistula

In the past, one third of gastric bypass patients developed gastro-gastric fistula because the stomach was partitioned, but not divided, using noncutting staplers. Today, fistulas are much less common because the gastric pouch is actually divided from the remnant using cutting staplers. Failure to lose weight and marginal ulcers should increase suspicion for a gastro-gastric fistula. Both contrast studies and endoscopy are helpful in making the diagnosis. An endoscopic image of a fistula is shown in Figure 4. If problems secondary to the fistula persist despite optimizing medical management, endoscopic or surgical attempts to close the fistula should be considered.

**Figure 4**
**The fistula between the gastric pouch and the gastric remnant can be seen above the gastrojejunostomy**

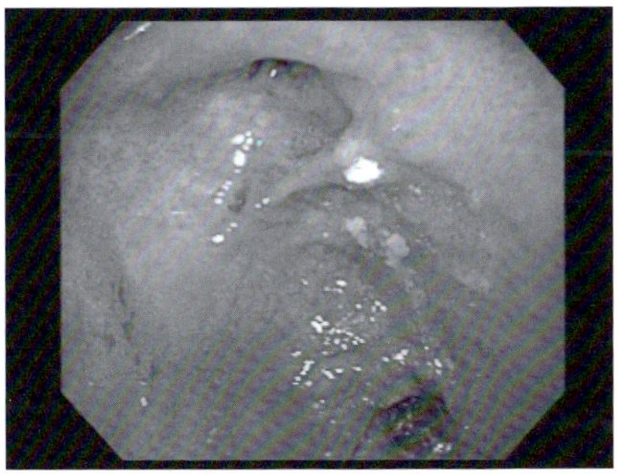

### Bile-duct Stones

Managing bile-duct stones endoscopically is more complicated following weight loss surgery. In patients with gastric bands, the band needs to be emptied in order to permit a 12-cm duodenoscope to pass through. Similarly, patients with vertical banded gastroplasties may need to have their stomas dilated to accommodate the duodenoscope. In our experience, bariatric patients with long-limb Roux-en-Y gastric bypasses are not amenable to duodenoscopy using retrograde techniques that can be used in patients with Bilroth II and short-limb Roux-en-Y reconstructions. In the past, we have recommended either transhepatic or surgical bile-duct exploration. More recently, we have been successful passing a duodenoscope through a laparoscopic gastrostomy in the gastric remnant. Figure 5 is an x-ray showing an endoscopic cholangiogram being performed during a laparoscopic procedure.

**Figure 5**
**The bile duct being cannulated using a duodenoscope passed through the wall of the gastric remnant**

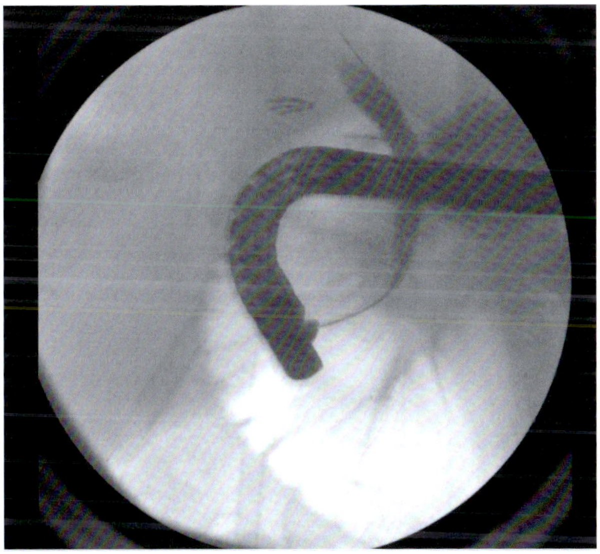

### Anemia

Anemia is another problem seen in patients undergoing weight loss surgery that endoscopists are asked to evaluate. All gastric bypass patients have some degree of iron malabsorption, and thus supplementary iron is recommended, particularly for female patients. Postoperative iron-deficiency anemia in patients who do not respond to iron supplementation needs to be evaluated endoscopically. Upper endoscopy should be performed to evaluate for erosions and ulcerations. Colonoscopy should also be considered to exclude polyps and malignancies. Bariatric patients generally prefer low-volume colonic preparations because of the small size of their gastric pouch.

**Failure to Lose Weight**

Failure to lose weight, or weight regain is sometime seen following bariatric surgery. The most common cause is poor eating habits; however, there are several important anatomical problems that need to be evaluated, including gastric fistula and stomal or gastric-pouch dilatation. The best way to evaluate for these changes is a contrast study. Endoscopy has a role in further evaluating any ambiguous radiographic findings and quantifying the degree of dilatation. Because of the morbidity of reoperative surgery, surgical repair is generally reserved for those with documented fistula. There are a number of groups that are using endoscopic techniques to treat both fistula and stoma dilatation with promising early results.

**Endoscopic Techniques**

Endoscopic techniques have been used to effectively reduce the size of the gastric outlet in bariatric patients. The first group to report the experience injected a sclerosing agent circumferentially around the gastric outlet. The group reported that sclerotherapy was safe and effective in reducing the gastric outlet diameter and it was associated with a trend toward weight loss over a 6-month period. A more recent report described using the EndoCinch Suturing System (Davol Inc., Cranston, RI) to plicate the gastric outlet. This device was originally designed to plicate the gastroesophageal junction in patients with gastroesophageal reflux. They successfully narrowed dilated anastomosis in 8 participants. Six of the 8 patients showed an average weight loss of 10 kg at 4 months. Though both of these results are promising, the likelihood of long-term success with either technique is low. Our group is currently investigating the use of a full-thickness gastric suturing system to improve durability. More durable techniques are likely to emerge, and so it seems endoscopy will have an increasing role in revisional bariatric surgery.

**Endoscopic Weight Loss Procedures**

Endoscopy may also have a role in the primary treatment of obesity. Currently, intragastric balloons and endoscopic suturing devices are being used in human trials. The intragastric balloon is unlikely to achieve good long-term results because the stomach simply distends to accommodate balloon volume increases. It may have a role as a bridge to surgery in patients at high surgical risk for bariatric or general surgical procedures. It seems that with the improvements in endoluminal suturing devices, endoscopic gastroplasty techniques will assume a more prominent role.

The rationale for an endoscopic gastroplasty is to provide a weight loss solution that does not require incisions, thereby avoiding incision-related complications. Providing surgical exposure to the target organ often results in much of the morbidity. Common incision-related complications such as wound infections, incisional hernias, and adhesions can be eliminated, or at least minimized, using an endoscopic approach. The major benefits of gastrointestinal procedures without abdominal wall incisions include the need for less anesthesia and lowering patient apprehension to elective surgeries. Pain related to external incisions is also eliminated. Less pain should translate into shorter recovery times, reduced hospitalization rates, and, consequently, less inpatient complications such as nosocomial infection, deep venous thrombosis, and pulmonary embolism.

There have been two groups to date who have reported their experience with endoscopic restrictive gastroplasty. One group from Brazil enrolled 10 subjects with body mass index (BMI) ranging from 28 to 43 kg/m$^2$, and plicated the anterior and posterior walls along the lesser curvature in the proximal stomach using the EndoCinch Suturing System. All subjects lost weight, with total weight loss ranging from 15 to 49 kg at 9 months postprocedure. Another international group enrolled 21 patients (9 patients in Brussels and 12 in Mexico). The BMI ranged from 35 to 53. Using the TransOral Gastroplasty System (Satiety Inc., Palo Alto, CA), the anterior and posterior wall of the proximal stomach were approximated and stapled. A second row of staples was placed to narrow the gastric outlet. At 3-month follow-up, all 21 patients had lost an average of 12 kg.

Thus, these preliminary data suggest that endoluminal techniques are safe and effective in producing short-term weight loss. Given this data, we suspect that more device manufacturers will pursue this application, and it is likely that endoscopic therapy will have an increasing role in the primary treatment of obesity.

## Suggested reading


1. Stellato TA, Crouse C, Hallowell PT. Bariatric surgery: creating new challenges for the endoscopist. *Gastrointest Endosc*. 2003;57(1):86-94.

2. Brethauer SA, Nfonsam V, Sherman V, Udomsawaengsup S, Schauer PR, Chand B. Endoscopy and upper gastrointestinal contrast studies are complementary in evaluation of weight regain after bariatric surgery. *Surg Obes Relat Dis*. 2006;2(6):643-8; Discussion 649-50.

3. Thompson C, Slattery J, Bundga M, Lautz D. Peroral endoscopic reduction of dilated gastrojejunal anastomosis after Roux-en-Y gastric bypass: a possible new option for patients with weight regain. *Surg Endosc*. 2006;20(11):1744-8.

4. Ellsmere J, Jones D, Pleskow D, Chuttani R. Endoluminal instrumentation is changing gastrointestinal surgery. *Surg Innov*. 2006;13(2):145-51.

# Body Contouring

Loren J. Borud, MD

Until recently, it was extraordinary for an individual to lose more than 100 lbs. Over the past decade, the explosion in bariatric surgery in the United States has created an unprecedented population of massive weight loss (MWL) patients. Although the postbariatric patient has achieved the major primary medical goal of MWL in most cases—with its attendant reduction in comorbid conditions and associated risk factors—the journey is not over for many. The skin and subcutaneous tissues of the formerly obese patient, for years, have been stretched beyond their elastic ability to contract. After MWL, some degree of skin contraction does occur. However, it is inevitable that significant areas of residual skin excess will be present.

Prior to bariatric surgery, most of the patient's attention is appropriately focused on the weight loss procedure, patient education, and nutritional counseling. In general, there is little or no discussion of postbariatric, body contouring surgery. Even in the media, stories of MWL focus on the surgery or diet program, with before and after photos, omitting mention of the body contouring surgery that was clearly part of the featured cases. Prior to deciding on the surgery, many patients and their families are under the false impression that with sufficient exercise or muscle "toning," the patient's skin excess will resolve.

Although the psychological impact of MWL has not been rigorously characterized, it is readily apparent that MWL is only part of the goal for many patients. Most of these patients have a lifelong history of obesity, with all its attendant personal, social, and even potentially economic consequences. The massive residual skin excess in MWL patients prevents them from reaping the aesthetic rewards of the process. They may have trouble fitting into garments due to excess thigh or arm skin. The waistline, even when thin, is marred by excessive skin folds that must be concealed in oversize clothing. Large, full breasts before weight loss have deflated into pancake-thin ptotic breasts that fill out a bra by virtue of creating the illusion of volume based on skin excess. Many of our patients view the postbariatric body contouring process as an essential final step in their journey to achieve a healthier, more balanced, happier, and psychologically sound and aesthetically appealing lifestyle.

### Evaluation of the Postbariatric Surgery Patient

Evaluation begins with a detailed history and physical examination. History should focus on health before and after weight loss. The surgeon must carefully review prior surgical history, especially with respect to any anesthesia, bleeding, or clotting complications. After the history is evaluated, a detailed physical examination of the entire body should ensue (Figure 1). Photographs, which do not capture the patient's face, are taken in standard positions with a blue background to establish the preoperative baseline appearance. A nurse or medical assistant should be present in the examination room for the entirety of the physical examination and photographing to assist the patient during what can be a difficult encounter. The physical examination should make note of jowling, excess skin in the submental area; breast and nipple ptosis with measurement of notch-to-nipple distance; and should include pinch-test examination of the vertical skin excess in the upper body, which extends circumferentially around the upper trunk at approximately the level of the bra line. The upper arm skin excess is examined and note is made of the degree of excess extending down onto the chest wall itself.

**Figure 1**

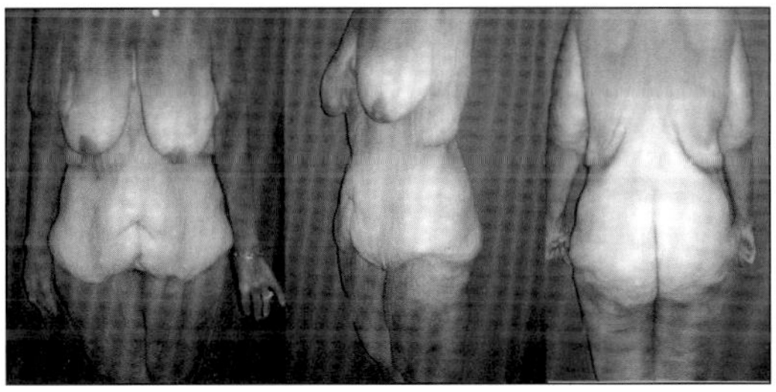

Typical deformity in the MWL patient: this patient went from a BMI of 61 to a BMI of 26. Note skin-excess patterns in upper arm, breast ptosis and flattening; pannus, circumferential-skin excess, buttock and lateral-thigh ptosis, and medial-thigh skin excess extending down to the knee areas.

The lower trunk is generally the area of greatest concern for the MWL patient. Anteriorly, the pannus (which consists of vertically oriented skin excess) should be noted, but the anterior skin also should be examined for a component of transverse skin excess. Lateral hip ptosis and buttock ptosis should be examined in planning for a circumferential lower-body lift. The medial thighs should be examined separately to evaluate the degree of medial skin excess. In younger patients with less weight loss, the skin excess is generally a horizontal crescent at the proximal-most inner thigh. In older patients or those with more substantial weight loss, there is a significant transverse dimension of skin excess that extends all the way inferiorly down to or below the knee. These patterns have an important role in determining surgical approach, prognosis, and staging options.

The most important prerequisite to body contouring surgery is that the patient's health is reasonable for the risks of anesthesia and surgery. Body contouring surgery can be a much greater physiological stress than the patient's prior surgery, which in many cases consisted of a brief, minimally invasive, laparoscopic procedure. All body contouring procedures are designed to remove and tighten skin, and this cannot be accomplished without large incisions, and large excisions of tissue, with substantial fluid loss, blood loss, and operative time expended.(1)

If the patient is an adequate medical risk for body contouring surgery, has achieved a plateau in weight loss (generally 12 to 24 months after the bariatric surgery), and is in good nutritional health, the next step is to develop a priority list of areas to be treated (Table 1). Each anatomical region is then discussed in turn and an extensive informed consent process must take place. The key element of this process is to (as accurately as possible) provide a realistic outline of what is achievable, as well as to present the overall risks and benefits of the procedures. We emphasize that the common element of all body contouring procedures is to "exchange skin for scar." All procedures involve resecting large areas of skin, and thus lengthy scars are inevitable. Although we are able to camouflage most scars in anatomically favorable areas, that is not always the case, and some patients have unpredictably poor scarring that occurs beyond the control of the plastic surgeon. Risks specific to each body contouring procedure are discussed in more detail below.

### Face and Neck Lifts

Sagging jowls and neck skin can be more apparent in the MWL patient than in other age-matched patients and can mimic the appearance of premature aging. Paradoxically, due to poorly understood fat distribution patterns, the MWL patient sometimes loses more than the expected or desired fat from the cheek and orbital areas, resulting in a malnourished or cachectic look. At the time of facelift and necklift, which are the only viable options for the sagging jowl and neck areas, autologous fat transfer from the abdomen or other part of the body to the cheek and orbit areas can restore the youthful, normal contour in these areas.

### Arm Lift

Although extremely variable from patient to patient, most MWL patients have some degree of excess hanging skin in the arm areas. Sometimes referred to as "bat wings" by patients, these extend from the axilla down to the elbow. On closer inspection, the skin excess in fact extends well onto and down the chest wall itself. Any procedure designed to remedy the skin excess must take into account the predominance of skin excess in the circumferential dimension, by extending the incision near or below the elbow. This scar cannot be well hidden, and is often a bit hypertrophic in places, especially in the distal forearm. Other potential complications include wound dehiscence and lymphocele. A lymphocele is a small fluid collection resulting from injury to a lymphatic duct. These can be troublesome, but usually resolve with local measures. Wound dehiscence is a partial separation of the wound, which can require local wound care until the wounds close spontaneously over a few weeks. Lymphedema is a devastating and fortunately unusual complication that results from significant impairment of lymphatic drainage from the extremity. There are a number of surgical techniques for brachioplasty, but we prefer the L brachioplasty design described by Hurwitz (Figure 2).(2)

**Figure 2**

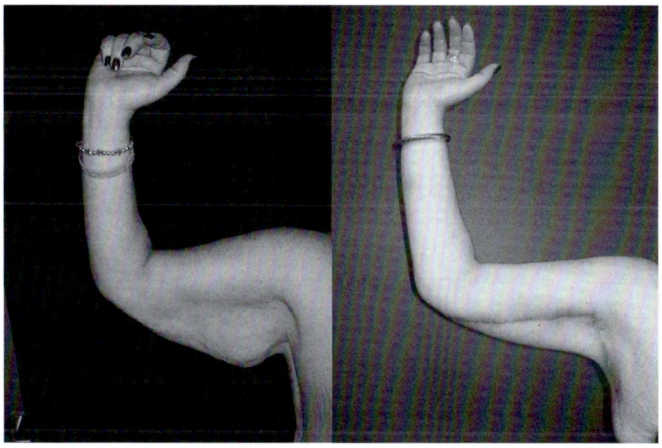

Brachioplasty. This patient underwent brachioplasty at the same time as lower-body lift. Her maximum BMI was 76, down to her current BMI of 31, 3 years after bariatric surgery. The scar lies in the inner arm along the bicipital groove and is not evident with the arms down. This early scar fades up until about 1 year after the surgery.

### Breast and Upper Body Procedures

All breast procedures in the MWL patient involve a mastopexy (breast lift), with resection of excess skin and elevation of the nipple. Since the vertical skin excess of the lateral breast extends circumferentially (causing the upper body "rolls"), patients with significant upper body rolls undergo an extended mastopexy, or upper body lift, in which the skin excision extends circumferentially around the upper body along the posterior bra line. The posterior skin can either be discarded or it can be used, based on the intercostals artery perforator (ICAP) to provide autologous tissue for breast augmentation for the lateral or central breast.(3) In the rare MWL with residual excess breast volume, breast reduction can be performed at the time of mastopexy (breast reduction). Patients with ideal breast mass need only a simple mastopexy. Patients who need additional augmentation to achieve adequate breast volume generally have sufficient tissue for augmentation from an ICAP flap and usually do not need breast augmentation with an implant (Figure 3). Some patients require implant augmentation with or without a simultaneous ICAP flap. Risks of these operations include substantial scars; loss of nipple sensation; inability to lactate; numbness; hypertrophic scarring; right/left asymmetry in nipple position and/or size; hematoma; wound infection; and/or need for reoperation. If implants are used, capsular contracture, rupture, and other problems can occur. Despite these risks, most patients are very happy with their results.

**Figure 3**

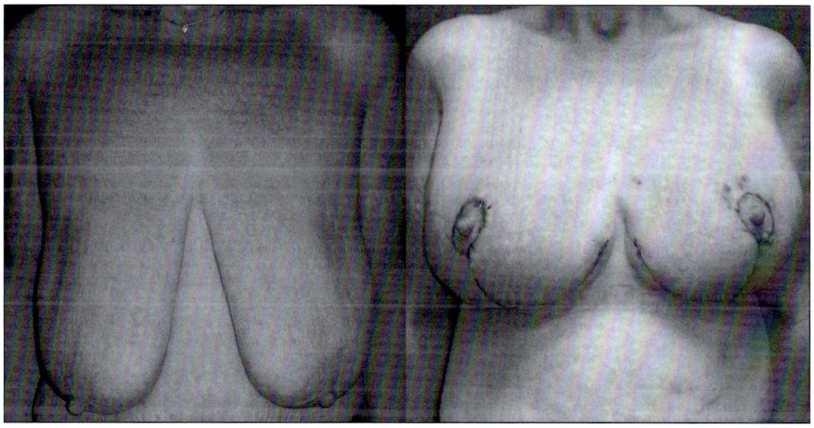

ICAP breast augmentation: following gastric bypass, this patient's BMI dropped from 53 to 28. Her second stage of body contouring consisted of an upper-body lift and medial-thigh lift. After lifting the breast, it was noted that there was insufficient volume. The tissue from the back harvested for the upper-body lift was moved using ICAP vessels to allow it to act as breast-augmentation tissue. With this technique, we were able to avoid use of a breast implant and still achieve full breast volume.

**Panniculectomy and Abdominoplasty**

The most common procedure for removal of skin from the anterior abdomen is the panniculectomy. This operation is designed simply to remove the "pannus," or overhanging skin below the umbilicus. No undermining of the superior flap is performed, the upper skin is not stretched inferiorly, the umbilicus is not translocated, and there is no abdominal wall plication. It is an operation designed to remedy a medical problem such as chronic intertrigo from a skin fold, but it is not designed to achieve a positive aesthetic outcome.

In the abdominoplasty, a panniculectomy is performed first, the skin above the umbilicus is mobilized so it may be stretched taught, and a new site is chosen to bring the umbilicus through. In addition, substantial tightening of the abdominal wall itself is performed by plicating the abdominal wall from the xiphoid to the pubis. Sometimes, in order to treat the transverse dimension of abdominal skin excess, a modified abdominoplasty with a vertically oriented triangular skin excision can be performed, although the wound complication risks are higher and this should not be done in patients with high residual body mass index (BMI) >32 kg/m$^2$ (Figure 4).(4)

**Figure 4**

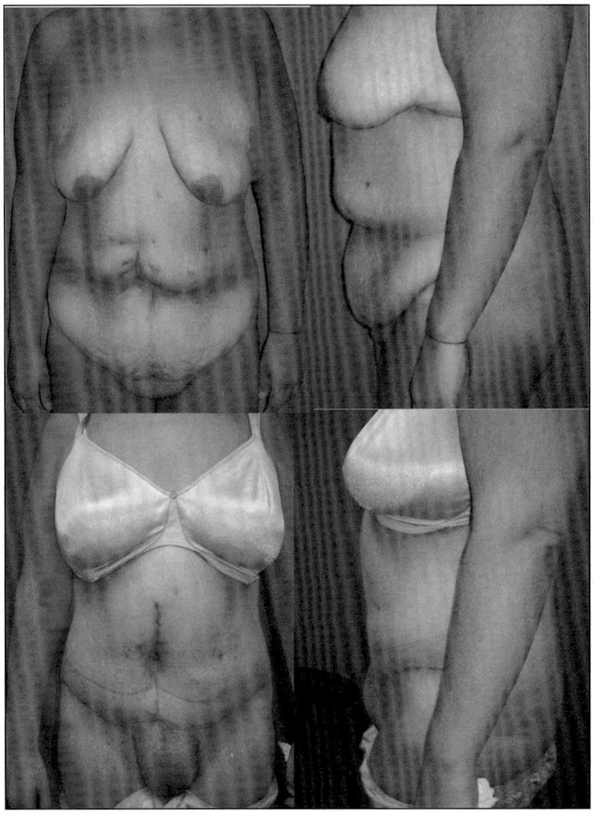

Abdominoplasty: this patient had an initial BMI of 49, which pleateaued at 30 at 1 year after gastric bypass. Knowing the limitations of the front-only procedures, this patient elected to have the abdominoplasty only, rather than the more extensive lower-body lift. Although much improved, the lateral thigh and buttock remain unchanged by this operation. In addition, there is still transverse-skin excess in the mons, which could be corrected with a medial-thigh lift.

In either case, a long transverse scar results. Major potential complications are bleeding, hematoma, need for reoperation, seroma requiring reoperation or multiple drainage attempts, and wound dehiscence. In addition, there is a poorly understood phenomenon of skin relaxation. The stretched skin of the MWL patient seems to have different viscoelastic properties than "normal" skin. Even when pulled very tight in the operating room, skin in some patients can stretch out in the first few weeks after surgery, resulting in the appearance of residual skin excess that would need to be revised in a later procedure.

In the MWL patient, the truncal skin excess extends circumferentially around the body. Attempting to address this cosmetic deformity with a front-only procedure (such as abdominoplasty) alone is bound to be limited in its result. Wherever the incision ends laterally, there is a "dog ear" of skin excess, followed posteriorly by unaltered regions of excess sagging skin involving the buttock and lateral thighs. The next section discusses the remedy for this problem.

### Lower body lift

To address the lateral thigh and buttock, abdominoplasty must be complemented by a lateral thigh lift and buttock lift. Together, these three procedures constitute a lower body lift, which involves a circumferential incision around the lower torso.(5) The greatest skin excess and thus the greatest skin excision, actually occurs along the lateral midline.(6) This region of skin is least adherent to underlying fascia and, thus, skin tends to descend more here than in any other area.(7)

In the past 2 years, significant progress has been made in the analysis of and the optimization of buttock aesthetics. The buttock is another area where there is excess loss of volume in the MWL patient. Simply resecting and lifting tissue improves the contour, but can leave the buttock appearing remarkably flat. Several new techniques have been developed to use otherwise discarded tissue to augment the buttock.(8) Our favored technique makes use of blood supply from the superior gluteal artery perforators (SGAP) so that the block of lateral tissue can be moved medially and inferiorly, where it is needed to restore aesthetic contour to the buttock area (Figure 5).

**Figure 5**

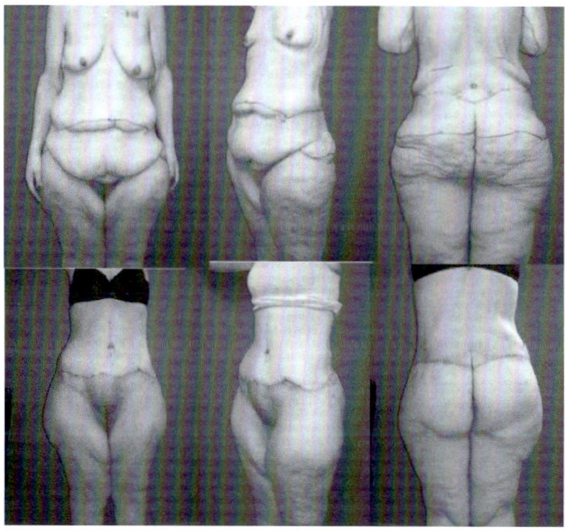

Lower-body lift: this 38-year-old patient had a maximum BMI of 68, down to a current BMI of 30. She demonstrated a low residual BMI and good quality skin, and was a good candidate for multiple simultaneous procedures. She underwent lower-body lift and brachioplasty. Her second stage will consist of a medial-thigh lift and upper-body/breast lift.

The lower body lift is an extensive procedure that requires 4 to 7 hours of surgery and at least one intraoperative position change. Risks are the same as those for abdominoplasty. Seroma and wound dehiscence seem to be more common than with abdominoplasty alone.

### Medial thigh lift

While the lateral thigh component of the lower body lift marginally improves the medial thigh area, the medial thighs need to be addressed separately in order to achieve an adequate cosmetic outcome. In the young patient with average weight loss and good skin elasticity, a simple crescentic excision of the vertical skin excess is possible, with scars extending posteriorly along the inferior gluteal crease and anteriorly along the groin crease. In the older patient, the patient with poor skin elasticity or with massive skin excess, the crescentic excision is insufficient and must be augmented with a vertical skin excision that extends down the medial thigh all the way to the knee. This medial thigh scar is unfavorable and patients should be counseled about this if they are considering the vertical medial thigh lift. Risks include scars, lymphocele, and lymphedema as in the brachioplasty; prolonged swelling, wound dehiscence, and wound infection are additional risks.

### Combining and staging strategies

The simultaneous treatment of multiple regions of the body can result in prolonged operations with significant anesthesia time and blood loss. Combined procedures should only be done by surgeons with extensive experience in each component body contouring procedure. They should only be performed in a setting where adequate technical assistance is available in the operating room and where inpatient care is available and intensive care is accessible. Apart from these personnel and institutional criteria, there are patient criteria to consider when embarking on major combined procedures. Patients undergoing multiple, concurrent, body contouring operations should be good risks for general anesthesia and should be willing to accept the possible need for blood transfusion and prolonged recovery time.(9)

One of the most feared complications of any surgical procedure is the deep venous thrombosis (DVT), which can lead to a potentially life-threatening pulmonary embolus (PE). These can seem even more daunting in the setting of an aesthetic procedure such as body contouring, than for life- or limb-saving procedures which are not as elective. There is no consensus on DVT prophylaxis in major body contouring procedures. In fact, there is no evidence that total operative time (say 10 hours vs. 4 hours) is a major factor in DVT risk in body contouring procedures. Our prophylactic regimen includes the routine use of pulsatile antithromboembolism stockings in the operating room and in the postoperative period, as well as early postoperative ambulation on the night of surgery or the first postoperative day. We do not routinely use heparin or other anticoagulants because these procedures create large raw surfaces and are high risk in terms of bleeding complications. In the patient with a history of prior DVT, we would be more aggressive about splitting the procedure into multiple stages, obtaining hematological consultation, using anticoagulants, or avoiding body contouring procedures altogether.

**Insurance**

The issue of insurance coverage inevitably arises in the setting of postbariatric body contouring. There are significant regional differences in the benefits covered by insurance across the country. No insurance company will cover "cosmetic" surgery. The criteria for "medical necessity" are different for each insurance carrier. The most commonly covered procedure is the panniculectomy. The criteria for medical necessity in this case generally rely on the presence of intertrigo, possibly refractory to a certain period of prescription remedies, and possibly requiring photographic documentation. Other criteria in use by some companies involve photographic landmarks such as coverage of the groin by the pannus on a frontal view or contact between the pannus and the thigh skin on lateral view. The presence of a hernia has, in our experience, not been beneficial in terms of obtaining coverage for the panniculectomy. Most insurance companies consider the panniculectomy and the hernia to be two separate problems requiring two separate operations. In cases of simultaneous hernia, our experience is that the insurers will approve the hernia repair but deny coverage of the panniculectomy.

Other common, postbariatric, body contouring procedures, such as mastopexy, upper-body lift, medial-thigh lift, buttock lift, and lower-body lift (exclusive of the panniculectomy component), are generally considered aesthetic procedures and are rarely, if ever, covered by insurers. The surgeon's role is to act as an advocate for the patient by taking photographs and, if there are genuine criteria for medical necessity, submitting a letter to the insurance company appealing for coverage for the panniculectomy on behalf of the patient.

Body contouring surgery is becoming a routine final step in the MWL transformation. Candidates must be in reasonable health and have reasonable expectations to benefit from these procedures. The most important principle of body contouring in MWL is the "exchange of skin for scar." Major complications are rare, but minor complications are very common. In recent years, significant advances have been made in the treatment of each body region in the setting of MWL. In selected patients, procedures can be combined to save on total recovery time and total financial cost.

Table 1

# Indications for Body Contouring Surgery in MWL

### *Common Indications for Surgery*

- Massive weight loss with substantial skin excess
- Intereference with ability to fit clothing
- Interference with optimum aesthetic appearance
- Presence of rash or other medical condition associated with skin

### *Preoperative Requirements for Surgery*

- Achievement of stable weight loss plateau
- Adequate nutritional status, espeically protein intake
- Adequate overall health for prolonged elective anesthestic
- Psychologically stable
- Able to understand risks and beneifits ot procedures
- Willling to accept risks of minor and major complications
- Willing to accept possibility of need for more than one operation
- Willing to accept possibility of DVT and PE
- Willing to accept lengthy and permanent scars
- Low residual BMI (<32) if multiple simultaneous procedures are considered
- Willing to accept blood transfusion if mulitple simultaneous procedures are planned

**References**


1. Borud LJ, Warren AG. Body contouring in the post-bariatric surgery patient. *J Am Coll Surg*. 2006;203(1):82-93.
2. Hurwitz DJ, Holland SW. The L brachioplasty: an innovative approach to correct excess tissue of the upper arm, axilla, and lateral chest. *Plast Reconstr Surg*. 2006;117(2):403-11; discussion 412-3.
3. Kwei S, Borud LJ, Lee BT. Mastopexy with autologous augmentation after massive weight loss: the intercostal artery perforator (ICAP) flap. *Ann Plast Surg*. 2006;57(4):361-5.
4. Borud LJ, Warren AG. Modified vertical abdominoplasty in the massive weight- loss patient. *Plast Reconstr Surg*. 2007;119(6): 1911-21; discussion 1922-3.
5. Nemerofsky RB, Oliak DA, Capella JF. Body lift: an account of 200 consecutive cases in the massive weight loss patient. *Plast Reconstr Surg*. 2006;117(2):414-30.
6. Lockwood TE. Superficial fascial system (SFS) of the trunk and extremities: a new concept. *Plast Reconstr Surg*. 1991;87(6):1009-18.
7. Aly AS, Cram AE, Chao M, Pang J, McKeon M. Belt lipectomy for circumferential truncal excess: the University of Iowa experience. *Plast Reconstr Surg*. 2003;111(1):398-413.
8. Pascal JF, Le Louarn C. Remodeling body lift with high lateral tension. *Aesthetic Plast Surg*. 2002;26(3):223-30.
9. Borud LJ. *Combined Procedures and Staging: Aesthetic Surgery in the Massive Weight Loss Patient*. Rubin JP, Matarasso A, eds. 2006: Elsevier, in press.
10. Borud LJ, Jones DB, Slavin S, Rezak KM. *Atlas of Body Contouring After Weight Loss*. Woodbury, CT: Ciné-Med, Inc., in press.

# LABS Next Steps

Bruce M. Wolfe, MD

The manner by which the National Institutes of Health (NIH) funds research has evolved in recent years. The NIH scientists themselves are more proactive in determining exactly which research is to be done, and in providing input and guidance to the conduct of the research itself. In response to the great interest in obesity, specifically bariatric surgery, a decision was made at the National Institute of Diabetes and Digestive and Kidney Diseases (NIDDK) to fund a bariatric surgery consortium. It was funded for 5 years and is known as the Longitudinal Assessment of Bariatric Surgery, or LABS.

The evolution of LABS began in 1991, when the NIH held a consensus conference on obesity surgery. That conference was a seminal event in defining the role of bariatric surgery and, to some extent, indications and specific procedures. It became clear in recent years, however, that this document needed updating, but NIDDK scientists felt that there was insufficient new evidence available to support another consensus conference. Instead, an NIDDK/NIH working group was convened in May 2002 and research questions were discussed and outlined, with recommendations made to guide research in the field. The NIH, with input from Walter Pories and others, moved forward with its plan for the consortium and released its request for applications (RFA) in November 2002. The centers were selected and funding initially began in September 2003.

The consortium has been molded by the NIH to include not only bariatric surgeons, but also investigators from internal medicine research and treatment, as well as endocrinology and hepatology. There has also been considerable input from behavioral science and outcomes research. Epidemiologists and scientists from various other disciplines have been brought together to compose the steering committee of this consortium. Six university centers (Table 1) comprise the clinical centers. There is also a data coordinating center, which consists of statisticians, epidemiologists, and coordinators, that functions as the organizational center of the project at the University of Pittsburgh. Multiple scientists from NIH/NIDDK participate actively in all meetings of the consortium.

**Table 1**

**LABS**

- Clinical Centers
  - Cornell/Columbia (NY), Paul Berk
  - East Carolina University, Walter Pories
  - Neuropsychiatric Research Institute (ND), Jim Mitchell
  - Oregon Health & Science University, Bruce Wolfe
  - University of Pittsburgh, Anita Courcoulas
  - University of Washington, David Flum
- Data Coordinating Center (DCC)
  - University of Pittsburgh, Steve Belle
- National Institute of Diabetes and Digestive and Kidney Diseases (NIDDK)
  - Carolyn Miles, Project Scientist

Over the next year and a half, extensive discussions were held as to how to formulate and guide the research plan. Three basic projects were identified: LABS 1, 2, and 3.(1) LABS 1 is intended to evaluate the short-term safety of bariatric surgery. LABS 2 will evaluate longer-term efficacy and safety of bariatric surgery. LABS 3 will involve smaller numbers of patients and will study mechanisms and conduct more detailed studies of comorbidities.

A decision made after considerable discussion was that LABS would be an observational study. A randomized, controlled trial to compare medical treatment or nonsurgical treatment with surgical outcomes was neither practical nor necessary (Table 2). The reasons for this decision are many, including that a nonoperative comparative group is not immediately available to the surgeons and surgical centers that comprise the LABS consortium. Given the present lack of long-term effectiveness of nonsurgical therapy in achieving weight loss, it is thought that comparison of the outcomes to the patient's status at baseline is a reasonable substitute.(2)

**Table 2**

# Rationale for an Observational Study

- Randomized controlled trial
  - Not seeking surgery—risk
  - Seeking surgery—consent
  - No access to surgery—coercion
  - Not necessary at this time

Some more specific problems with conduct of a prospective randomized trial comparing medical with surgical therapy in this setting include multiple logistic problems. First, a proper randomized trial would not just randomize patients who present to a surgical program for consideration of surgery. This is clearly a subgroup of the patients with body mass index (BMI) ≥ 35 kg/m$^2$. These patients have in their own minds determined that further efforts at medical therapy are futile; they are ready to proceed with surgery. Therefore, a bias would be introduced if only those patients who sought surgery were randomized. To randomize patients to surgery who do not seek surgery would require access to that patient population and getting the subjects to consent to a procedure with definite risk, which was rejected by the Swedish obese subjects (SOS) trial. The Swedish system, however, facilitates better access to a medical comparator group than our system affords. There are few obesity treatment clinics at US centers that follow patients for 10 years and maintain such follow-up so that this could practically be done. Long-term follow-up is crucial to any outcome study in the treatment of obesity, and we believe that the follow-up conducted by the surgeons of the nonsurgical patients would be quite difficult.

The issue of patient safety in bariatric surgery is of importance. Obesity is a life-threatening disease and is associated with multiple comorbidities. It is reasonable to assume that significant weight loss is beneficial among patients with morbid obesity and(3) bariatric surgery produces superior short- and long-term weight loss. Dr. Pories has indicated that about 1% of the population in the United States with a BMI >40, and an even lesser percentage with a BMI >35, actually undergoes bariatric surgery in a given year. The disease is life threatening and surgery is the most effective treatment.

Why does only 1% of the population undergo the treatment in a given year? A patient will present with an obviously life-threatening disease associated with obesity and comorbidities. Bariatric surgery is recommended, but somebody involved—the primary care physician, a family member, or another patient in the chat room—is hesitant because of concerns regarding safety. Patient safety concerns, I believe, are the most significant and perhaps appropriate deterrent to widespread application of bariatric surgery among this very large patient population.

Consequently, LABS made it a first priority to further progress in the area of safety in bariatric surgery (Table 3). LABS 1 is designed to determine the frequency of events associated with temporal trends and bariatric surgery. We intend to compare the frequency of events between groups (Table 4), such as patient subtypes and different providers, and establish benchmarks. We also hope to provide a basis for risk stratification to the extent this would be possible. Thus, having a large number of subjects is an important goal. To date, the surgery database established by the Society of Thoracic Surgeons has entered 2.4 million subjects. The mortality rate in bariatric surgery overall is less than 1%, lower than the 3% reported for cardiac surgery. For this reason, we need a very large number of subjects in order to accurately and definitively establish risk stratification. Without risk stratification, it is difficult to characterize the risk of a patient who has a combination of risk factors.

We will include all of the cases done by all of the surgeons at each of the participating centers during the 3-year acquisition of patients involved. In total, we estimate 3,000 to 4,000 patients will be entered, far short of the cardiac surgery pool of 2.4 million, but a larger series than has been accumulated to date. Again, we need as large a sample as possible to define infrequent events and to establish the risk adjustment for several outcomes—not only death, but also specific complications.

**Table 3**

## 3 Phases of LABS

- LABS 1: short-term safety
- LABS 2: longer-term safety and efficacy
- LABS 3: mechanisms, greater detail

**Table 4**

## LABS 1 Parameters

- Patient characteristics
- 30-day outcomes
  - Wound complication
  - Requirement for anticoagulation
  - Percutanous or operative reintervention
  - Death
- Risk stratification

There are many parameters that could conceivably impact this risk adjustment, such as height, weight, BMI, percent body fat, age, gender, and smoking history. In addition, revisions may increase risk. All of this demographic information will be reported and we also will assess specific comorbidities associated with obesity, and objective measures so that these can be quantitatively analyzed. Laboratory values are useable in some situations, but not others because treatment, as for diabetes, dyslipidemia, and hypertension, influences these laboratory values. Thus, a system needs to take into account the impact of treatment, which is particularly pertinent, because surgeons are obligated to control medical comorbidities as much as possible preoperatively.(4) One clearly cannot measure the blood sugar, the A1C, or any of those types of parameters in order to quantitate the severity of the comorbidities.

The specific comorbidities that we will assess are the usual multiple comorbidities associated with obesity: diabetes, hypertension, dyslipidemia, sleep apnea, hepatic disease, cardiac dysfunction, and ambulatory status. Description of the operative procedure will be done, including such possible impacting events as duration, blood loss, and intraoperative events. We will measure the outcomes at 30 days. Although a longer interval was considered, it was felt that 30 days would be optimal to make maximum use of limited resources. In order to establish the definitions of complications, which are so variable among various surgical reports, we decided to focus on rehospitalizations or postoperative reinterventions (procedures). If the patient is rehospitalized within 30 days, it will be reported as a complication and the cause for the rehospitalization will be logged in as that complication. Similarly, interventions such as endoscopic dilation of a stricture will be recorded.

The fidelity of the data is a major concern in any research project. Objective observers will be recording the data and objective measures will be used to every extent possible, with audits performed for accuracy. The data coordinating center will site-visit each center at regular intervals to audit the data. An adjudication committee will review all deaths and major complications in which the diagnosis is uncertain.

There are, of course, limitations to all studies and LABS is no exception. A decision was made to not influence the type of operation that is done. The operations that will be studied by LABS will consist of those operations performed by the surgeons at the participating sites, so the procedure selection is not standardized. The number of patients will be too small to fully characterize infrequent events. For example, we would like to know as much as possible about the risk factors and the role of prophylaxis in fatal postoperative pulmonary embolism. If the incidence is just 0.2% in 4,000 cases, that would give us only 8 such patients to analyze. It would be difficult to fully characterize that event with so few patients. Hopefully, we can set the stage for standard data collection, which will net the program much more data, permitting us to characterize these very infrequent, but still major events.

In LABS 2, we will sample 1,000 to 1,200 of the patients from the total cohort. In this study, we will obtain considerably more detail regarding preoperative comorbidity assessment and postoperative complications, and it will be a longitudinal follow-up for the duration of the project. In order to focus on priorities and instruments of measure, workgroups were established in many areas and reports and recommendations were made to the steering committee. These included workgroups in diet behavior. We have come up with several psychological instruments that will be used to define behavioral health, eating disorders, and other issues that may be pertinent to the obese population, as well as to their outcomes. Diabetes, liver disease, cardiovascular function, musculoskeletal function, health economics, and other comorbidities will be studied. All of these areas will be assessed to the extent possible. As there is not a comparative group, we will be comparing longitudinal status with baseline, which will be extensively evaluated. We do have resource limitations, yet there is a lot of expectation in the bariatric community. The NIH-funded consortium will not be able to resolve all the important problems, but should provide definitive answers to a number of questions.

We have spent a great deal of time at our meetings weighing the relative or expected benefit of one study or one parameter or instrument and weighing how much personnel time and resources will be consumed. There is also a patient burden, which limits how much can be done. For example, we estimate that it will take patients at least 2 hours to complete the questionnaires that we have selected for their preoperative and postoperative assessments. We are optimistic that patients will indeed give us this effort. Finally, a limitation to all such research is the challenge of long-term follow-up. We have a retention and follow-up committee that investigates methods to enhance follow-up participation.

The gastric bypass and banding patients are excellent models for the study of obesity and the responses to intervention. The fact that there is such a variable response to a single intervention, such as gastric bypass, is ideal for studying the effectiveness of the intervention. Mechanisms of action of bariatric surgery are of substantial interest due to the superior weight loss that is achieved, and may have implications for future directions in the development of nonsurgical treatments for obesity.

LABS 3 will pursue these issues with carefully selected substudies, using smaller numbers of subjects. Three specific substudies have been identified. Intravenous and oral glucose tolerance tests with appropriate endocrine studies will be done before and after gastric bypass to assess the early response of diabetes that is seen following gastric bypass. Further details regarding behavioral issues of bariatric surgery will be studied with investigator-conducted interviews. Finally, a detailed study of resource consumption and related health economics in bariatric surgery will be done.

Ancillary research to the basic LABS 2 protocol will also be conducted. A total of 7 research projects have been funded by NIDDK/NIH to date (Table 5). These studies will take advantage of the primary or basic database that will be established from LABS 2 patients. They will then expand on the specific issue that is the subject of the ancillary research. The study of nonalcoholic fatty liver disease seeks to establish the relationship between free fatty acid metabolism as defined by adipose tissue biology in the causation of liver disease. The body composition study will do detailed studies of the components of body composition in the bariatric surgical population. An effort to relate the variations in body composition to a pattern of comorbid conditions, as well as responses to surgical intervention will be done, and longitudinal changes of body composition associated with postoperative weight loss will be identified.

**Table 5**

**LABS Ancillary Studies**
**NIH-Funded**

- Adipose tissue biology, NAFLD
- Body composition
- Cognitive effects
- Energy balance
- MC4R mutations
- Sexual function
- Teen LABS

Preliminary data regarding identification of cognitive impairment associated with morbid obesity have been published. This study will involve a comprehensive battery of cognitive tests to define the severity and nature of the cognitive impairment associated with obesity and its response to weight loss. DNA from all of the LABS 2 patients will be analyzed for mutations of the melanocortin-4 receptor (MC4R) gene. These possible mutations or variations will be correlated with the severity of the obesity and its comorbidities, as well as the response to weight loss.

A subset of the bariatric surgical patients will also undergo detailed assessment of the components of energy expenditure, both before and after surgery. Total energy expenditure, as well as nonexercise activity thermogenesis will be defined. The impairment in sexual functioning associated with morbid obesity will be characterized in detail and the response to bariatric surgery determined. Finally, an ancillary program to study bariatric surgery in adolescent patients has been established. An adult comparator group whose obesity dates to their adolescent years will be included.

All of the data from LABS, as well as frozen plasma, serum, and DNA will be maintained in an NIH repository. In the future, investigators will be able to request access to both the data and specimens for future research of this well-characterized surgical population.

In summary, the consortium for the longitudinal assessment of bariatric surgery has been funded by NIDDK/NIH in order to establish a comprehensive, core database derived from bariatric surgical patients, and to standardize definitions and data collection procedures for this and future databases. It will determine predictive factors for positive and negative outcomes that will assist in the selection of appropriate patients and procedures. In addition, studies regarding the mechanisms of action of surgical procedures as they might be applied to medical therapies will be done.

**References**

1. Belle SH, Berk PD, Courcoulas AP, et al. Safety and efficacy of bariatric surgery: Longitudinal Assessment of Bariatric Surgery. *Surg Obes Relat Dis*. 2007;3(2):116-26.

2. Shekelle PG, Morton SC, Maglione M, et al. Pharmacological and surgical treatment of obesity. *Evid Rep Technol Assess*. 2004;(103):1-6.

3. Dixon J. Survival advantage with bariatric surgery: report from the 10th International Congress on Obesity. *Surg Obes Relat Dis*. 2006;2(6):585-6.

4. Ali MR, Maguire MB, Wolfe BM. Assessment of obesity-related comorbidities: a novel scheme for evaluating bariatric surgical patients. *J Am Coll Surg*. 2006;202(1):70-7.

# Staple-Line Buttress Materials

Ninh T. Nguyen, MD

Laparoscopic gastric bypass is gaining popularity as an acceptable option for the treatment of morbid obesity. With the growing number of bariatric procedures being performed in the United States, it is important for surgeons to continue to evaluate methods to improve the outcomes of patients undergoing laparoscopic gastric bypass.

One potentially life-threatening complication after laparoscopic gastric bypass is postoperative gastrointestinal hemorrhage. The incidence of intra-abdominal and gastrointestinal hemorrhage after laparoscopic gastric bypass ranges from as low as 0.8% to as high as 9.4%.(1-5) We previously reported a 3.2% incidence of gastrointestinal bleeding after laparoscopic gastric bypass(4) and this postoperative gastrointestinal bleeding can be life threatening, particularly if it occurs within a short time after the index operation.

Until proven otherwise, the cause for gastrointestinal hemorrhage after laparoscopic gastric bypass is bleeding somewhere along the rows of the staple line within the gastrointestinal tract. There are four potential sites for gastrointestinal hemorrhage: staple lines along the gastrojejunostomy, the gastric pouch, the jejunojejunostomy, and the gastric remnant.(6) A variety of intraoperative methods have been implemented to prevent staple-line bleeding, including the use of staplers with shorter staple height and over-sewing of staple lines. For example, we now utilize the blue stapler load (3.5 mm staple height) for construction of the gastric pouch instead of the green stapler load (4.8 mm staple height). The shorter height provides more compression on the transected tissues and hence provides better hemostasis. Over-sewing of the staple lines is an effective maneuver to enhance hemostasis, but can be time consuming during laparoscopic gastric bypass. More recently, staple-line reinforcement products have been introduced to be used as an adjunct in minimizing postoperative gastrointestinal hemorrhage and leaks

Staple-line reinforcement has been recognized as an effective adjunct for decreasing the occurrence of air leaks following pulmonary wedge resection.(7-9) Recently, the concept of buttressing the staple line was applied to patients undergoing gastrointestinal surgery in an effort to improve the integrity of the staple lines and reduce staple-line bleeding.(10-11) Staple-line reinforcement consists of sleeves of absorbable or nonabsorbable material placed onto the linear stapler prior to firing. Upon firing, the staple-line–reinforcement material is incorporated into both sides of the transected tissue. For use in the gastrointestinal tract, absorbable staple-line–reinforcement product is preferred, as there is the risk for erosion of the staple line when using nonabsorbable material.(12)

**Figure 1**

Staple-line reinforcement sleeves fit onto a linear stapler

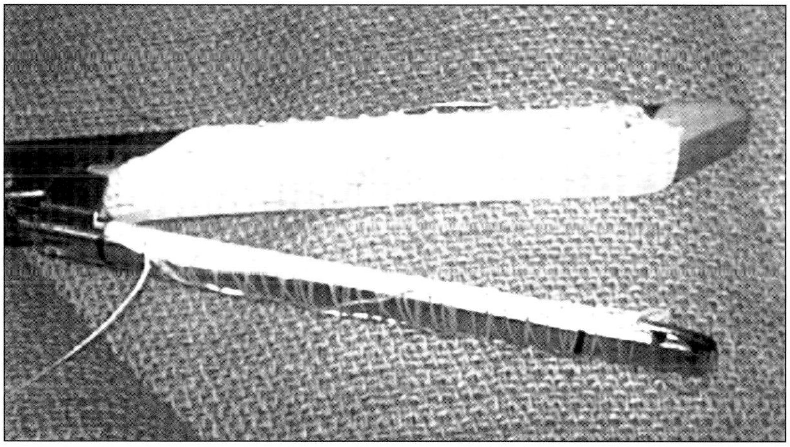

Staple-line–reinforcement sleeves are supplied in pairs. One sleeve fits onto the cartridge jaw of the stapler and the other sleeve onto the anvil jaw of the stapler.

Once the linear stapler is passed through the trocar and positioned onto the tissue, the suture attached to the staple-line–reinforcement sleeves is removed (prior to firing). The stapler is released after firing, leaving the reinforcement material remaining along the staple line on both sides. There are two types of staple-line–reinforcement materials available on the market: bioabsorbable Seamguard® (W.L. Gore & Associates, Inc., Flagstaff, AZ) and Peri-Strips Dry® with Veritas® collagen matrix (Synovis Surgical Innovations, St. Paul, MN). The bioabsorbable Seamguard® is composed of a glycolide copolymer that retains measurable strength for up to 6 weeks postoperatively. The Peri-Strips Dry® is composed of bovine pericardium and the Veritas® technology introduces a remodelable and biocompatible characteristic.

**Mechanisms of Hemorrhage**

Bleeding of the staple lines occurs either at the transected staple-line edge or at the mucosal layer where the staple penetrates the mucosa. Bleeding at the staple-line edge during laparoscopic gastric bypass can be easily visualized; however, intraluminal bleeding can be difficult to detect. Intraluminal bleeding occurs at the mucosa layer as a result of the staple penetrating through the mucosa, or as the result of laceration of the mucosal layer during mechanical closure of the staple.

Staple-line–reinforcement materials are used as buttressing material on both sides of the staple line to enhance integrity and provide additional compression of the tissue. The mechanism for hemostasis with the use of staple-line–reinforcement material is the compressive effect of the buttress material on the staple lines, which results in redistribution of pressure exerted upon individual staples over a wider tissue-surface area. In addition, the presence of the staple-line–reinforcement material enhances the integrity of the staple line by preventing laceration of the mucosal layer during formation of the individual staples.

**Clinical Studies**

Intraoperative staple-line bleeding and postoperative gastrointestinal hemorrhage are well known complications of laparoscopic gastric bypass.(1-4) Intraoperative staple-line hemorrhage is a common occurrence during laparoscopic gastric bypass, whereas the incidence of gastrointestinal hemorrhage postoperatively is less common.(1-5) Clinically, the most common sites for gastrointestinal hemorrhage are the gastrojejunostomy or the staple lines of the gastric pouch or gastric remnant. Bleeding at the jejunojejunostomy is uncommon.

Intraoperative staple-line bleeding can be a nuisance, requiring control by over-sewing the staple-line edges or the use of clips and/or electrocautery. Champion and Williams(13) reported that the mean number of clips applied to staple lines during laparoscopic gastric bypass for control of staple-line bleeding ranged from 21 to 30 clips. Staple-line bleeding is also a reflection of potential intraluminal bleeding. In a randomized clinical trial examining the efficacy of staple-line–reinforcement product in reducing intraoperative staple-line bleeding and gastrointestinal hemorrhage, Nguyen and colleagues(14) reported that patients receiving staple-line–reinforcement sleeves had lower numbers of staple-line-bleeding sites, lower blood loss, and less time was required to obtain hemostasis of the staple lines. The rate of gastrointestinal hemorrhage in this small trial (N=34) was 5.9% for the control group (no staple-line reinforcement) and 0% for the treatment group (with staple-line reinforcement). A single patient in the control group developed postoperative gastrointestinal hemorrhage requiring blood transfusions and operative intervention for control of the hemorrhage.

Another benefit in the use of staple-line–reinforcement is the possible reduction in staple-line leak. Shikora and colleagues reported no acute leaks in 250 consecutive patients who underwent laparoscopic gastric bypass with bovine pericardial staple-line–reinforcement strips.(10) One reason for development of anastomotic leak is the presence of either linear or radial tension acting upon the staple lines. For example, increased intraluminal pressure acting upon the gastric pouch and gastrojejunostomy staple lines can lead to staple-line disruption. In a swine model, Arnold and colleagues(15) reported that staple lines buttressed with Peri-Strips Dry® sustained significantly higher mean burst pressures than nonbuttressed staple lines. Their study demonstrated that buttressed staple lines can maintain seam integrity at a significantly higher intraluminal pressure when compared with nonbuttressed staple lines.

Gastrointestinal bleeding is a potentially life-threatening postoperative complication. Efforts to improve outcomes for patients undergoing bariatric surgery include evaluating studies that review the effectiveness of products purported to make surgeries safer. The use of staple-line–reinforcement products during laparoscopic gastric bypass is clearly proving itself to be safe and effective in reducing intraoperative staple-line bleeding and possibly lowering the risk for postoperative gastrointestinal hemorrhage.

**References**


1. Mehran A, Szomstein S, Zundel N, Rosenthal R. Management of acute bleeding after laparoscopic Roux-en-Y gastric bypass. *Obes Surg*. 2003;13(6):842-7.
2. Higa KD, Ho T, Boone KB. Laparoscopic Roux-en-Y gastric bypass: technique and 3-year follow-up. *J Laparoendosc Adv Surg Tech A*. 2001;11(6):377-82.
3. Schauer PR, Ikramuddin S, Gourash W, et al. Outcomes after laparoscopic Roux-en-Y gastric bypass for morbid obesity. *Ann Surg*. 2000;232(4):515-29.
4. Nguyen NT, Rivers R, Wolfe BM. Early gastrointestinal hemorrhage after laparoscopic gastric bypass. *Obes Surg*. 2003;13(1):62-5.
5. Luján JA, Frutos MD, Hernández Q, et al. Laparoscopic versus open gastric bypass in the treatment of morbid obesity: a randomized prospective study. *Ann Surg*. 2004;239(4):433-7.
6. Nguyen NT, Longoria M, Chalifoux, Wilson SE. Gastrointestinal hemorrhage after laparoscopic gastric bypass. *Obes Surg*. 2004;14:1308-12.
7. Murray KD, Ho CH, Hsia JY, Little AG. The influence of pulmonary staple-line reinforcement on air leaks. *Chest*. 2002;122(6):2146-9.
8. Vaughn CC, Wolner E, Dahan M, et al. Prevention of air leaks after pulmonary wedge resection. *Ann Thorac Surg*. 1997;63(3):864-6.
9. Miller JI, Landreneau RJ, Wright CE, et al. A comparative study of buttressed versus nonbuttressed staple line in pulmonary resections. *Ann Thorac Surg*. 2001;71(1):319-32; discussion 323.
10. Shikora SA, Kim JJ, Tarnoff ME. Reinforcing gastric staple lines with bovine pericardial strips may decrease the likelihood of gastric leak after laparoscopic Roux-en-Y gastric bypass. *Obes Surg*. 2003;13(1):37-44.
11. Consten EC, Gagner M, Pomp A, Inabnet WB. Decreased bleeding after laparoscopic sleeve gastrectomy with or without duodenal switch for morbid obesity using a stapled buttressed absorbable polymer membrane. *Obes Surg*. 2004;14(10):1360-6.
12. Consten EC, Dakin GF, Gagner M. Intraluminal migration of bovine pericardial strips used to reinforce the gastric staple-line in laparoscopic bariatric surgery. *Obes Surg*. 2004;14(4):549-54.
13. Champion JK, Williams MD. Prospective randomized comparison of linear staplers during laparoscopic Roux-en-Y gastric bypass. *Obes Surg*. 2003(6);13:855-9; discussion 860.
14. Nguyen NT, Longoria M, Welbourne S, Sabio A, Wilson SE. Glycolide copolymer staple-line reinforcement reduces staple site bleeding during laparoscopic gastric bypass: a prospective randomized trial. *Arch Surg*. 2005;140(8):773-8.
15. Arnold W, Shikora SA. A comparison of burst pressure between buttressed versus non-buttressed staple-lines in an animal model. *Obes Surg*. 2005;15(2):164-71.

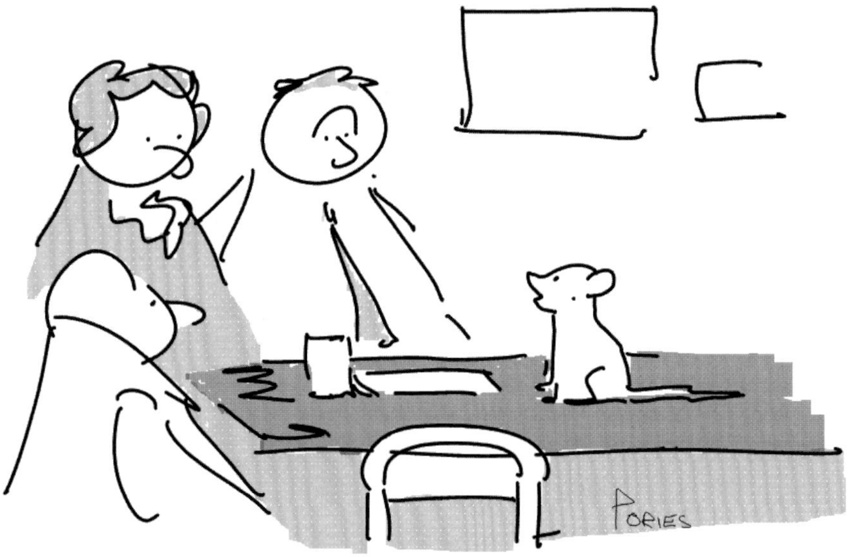


"So tell me this. How does the Institutional Review Board have the right to decide what happens to me?"

# Fibrin Sealants

Meng-G Martin Lee, MD

Since 1916 fibrin sealant has been used as a fibrin patch to stop bleeding in intra-abdominal surgery. In 1940, Young and Medawar reported using fibrin sealant in nerve anastomosis. In the 1960s, the advancing technology led to highly concentrated fibrinogen-sealing preparation by fractionation. The US Food and Drug Administration (FDA) approved the first commercially available fibrin sealant, called Tisseel® in 1988.

**Figure 1**

Fibrin sealant contains fibronectin, Factor XIII, thrombin, ionized calcium, and fibrinogen.

## Mechanism of Action

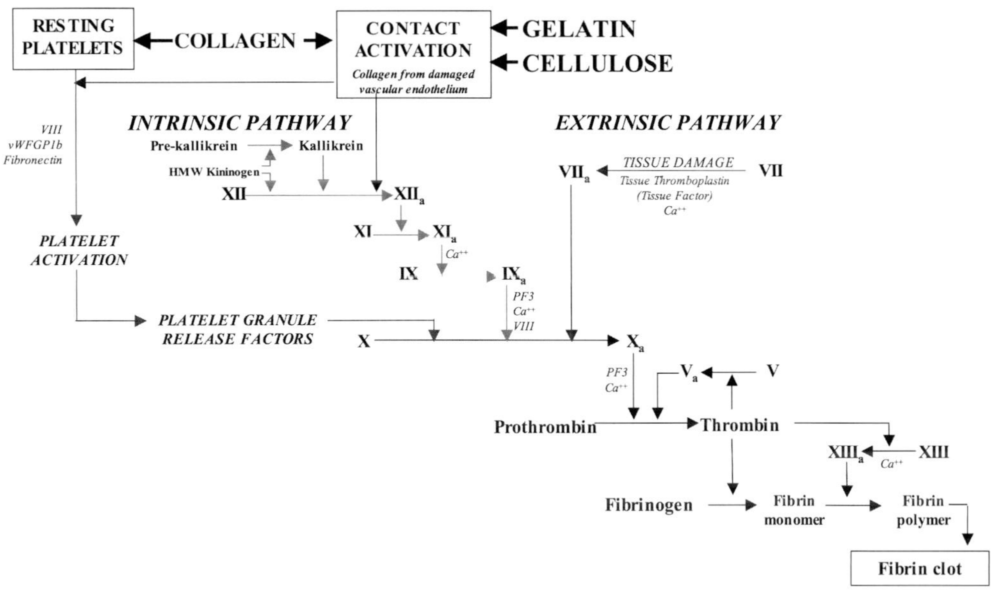


The wound-healing coagulation cascade includes the intrinsic pathway, the extrinsic pathway, and the common pathway on which the fibrin sealant acts. Thrombin contained in the fibrin sealant breaks the fibrinogen down to fibrin monomers; the Factor XIII, along with calcium, causes those fibrin monomers to form into clots. The fibrin sealant solidifies into a firm, wide material with a rubbery appearance and very strong adhesive properties. It is biodegradable and can be broken down to about 20% of its original mass over 72 hours in the wound. By adding proteins such as aprotinin to the mixture, the lifespan of the clot is prolonged.

**Figure 2**

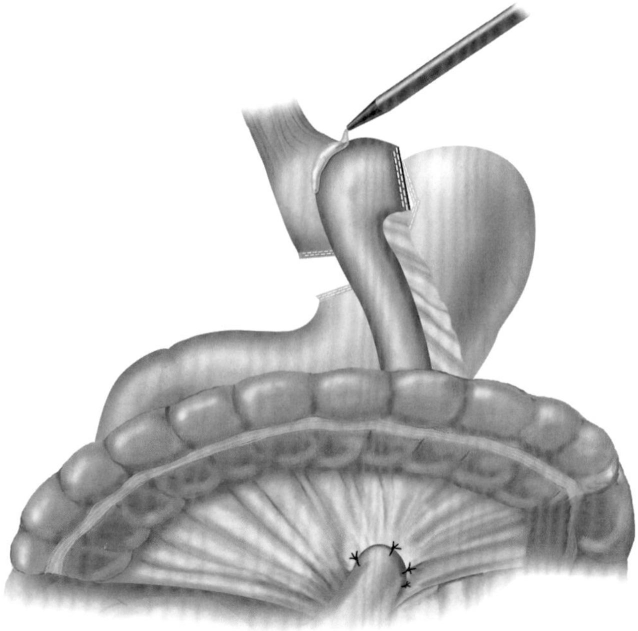

When applied onto the collagen of damaged tissue surface, the fibrin-sealant material usually reabsorbs within 7 to 14 days. There are several different applicators, usually in the form of a 2-syringe system. One syringe will contain thrombin and the other fibrinogen. The two materials are mixed in the common Y-limb and by the time the material reaches the tissue it will be activated. The fibrin sealant is extremely safe. In more than 1 million applications, there were no documented cases of hepatitis or HIV transmission.

Tisseel®, which is the older generation fibrin sealant, contains a bovine protein and there have been case reports of anaphylactic reactions to the bovine protein. Newer generations of fibrin sealant, such as COSEAL® or Hemaseel®, contain only human protein, which reduces the risk of adverse reaction.

In terms of clinical application, fibrin sealant has been used in reinforcing gastrointestinal anastomosis; in the management of perforated peptic ulcer disease; in the management of hepatic and splenic trauma; and as part of laparoscopic inguinal hernia repairs. In terms of constructing a sound gastrointestinal anastomosis, some of the technical factors, such as adequate blood supply, tension free anastomosis, and hemostasis of the suture line, are irreplaceable. But fibrin sealant can enhance the anastomosis by achieving better hemostasis at a suture line and preventing microscopic leaks, as well as by confining the bacteria intraluminally.

Fibrin sealant may be used in constructing anastomoses. In a study by Morales, silk, polyglycolic acid, and fibrin sealant were used to construct anastomoses in a rat model. Silk lasted the longest and fibrin sealant the shortest, but fibrin sealant generates the lowest amount of inflammation and edema around the anastomosis.

Another study, by Zilling, looked at stapled anastomoses, hand-sewn anastomoses and fibrin-sealant–constructed anastomoses. Leakage rate was the same with different kinds of anastomoses. Fibrin-sealant anastomoses were weakest in terms of tensile strength. On the other hand, a Harvard study found that fibrin-sealant anastomosis showed the least amount of inflammation. So, it appears that using fibrin sealant to construct anastomoses by itself may be contraindicated, as it has the lowest tensile strength. However, it has been looked at by some as a useful reinforcement agent at the staple line to decrease the rate of leakage.

A study by Kanellos and his colleagues looked at using fibrin sealant to reinforce the suture in anastomoses in a rat model. Although there was no leakage rate in different groups, the fibrin-sealant–reinforced anastomosis had a higher bursting pressure.

In Roux-en-Y gastric bypass, one major complication is leak at the gastrojejunal anastomosis. This can lead to sepsis, stricture, and fistula formation.

**Figure 3**

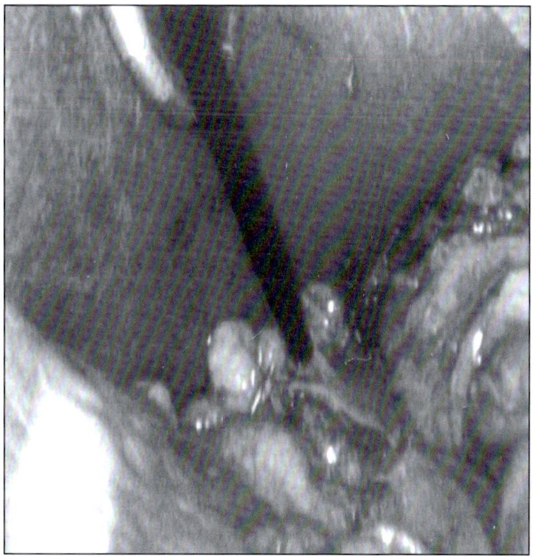

In applying fibrin sealant to a staple line at the gastric pouch, the goal is to decrease any leak at the gastrojejunal anastomosis.

A study by Liu and colleagues looked at using fibrin-sealant–reinforced anastomosis compared with nonreinforced anastomosis. One surgeon used fibrin sealant to reinforce 120 of his patients and the other two surgeons in the same practice served as controls and did not use fibrin sealant for their anastomoses. They found that in the fibrin sealant group, there was no leak. Of the other two surgeons, each of whom had 120 patients, 5 leaks occurred in one group and 2 leaks in the other.

In another study published by Sapala, 738 patients who had undergone Roux-en-Y gastric bypass were included. Fibrin sealant was used to reinforce the gastrojejunal anastomosis in these patients. Two patients developed a leak requiring a laparotomy for re-exploration; however, neither of them was from the reinforced gastrojejunal anastomosis. This is an improvement over the historic leakage rate of 0.9%. These studies, though obviously not randomized controlled trials, do indicate that fibrin sealants decrease anastomotic leaks in high-risk anastomosis and the data can certainly be extrapolated to other laparoscopic procedures.

Fibrin sealant has other potential applications, such as is in the laparoscopic repair of perforated peptic ulcer disease. The advantage here is that the site of perforation can be easily identified without making a large incision. This technique is easy to learn and use and results in shorter operative time, as well as shorter lengths of hospital stay for patients. A gelatin sponge is rolled into a cone shape and pulled into the perforation site. Fibrin sealant is injected around the site to seal it.

In Hong Kong, Lau reported a study of 100 consecutive patients with stomach perforation who were treated with fibrin-sealant repair. No difference was observed in terms of mortality and morbidity in patients who underwent laparoscopic fibrin-glue repair versus suture repair and open repair. The same group, in a study published later on, reported randomizing 93 patients into different groups, including laparoscopic fibrin-glue repair. In that study, 1 patient in the laparoscopic fibrin-sealant group developed a leak, as did 1 in the open group.

Lee and colleagues looked at 374 patients who had perforated peptic ulcer disease, with 109 having repair done by laparoscopic fibrin-sealant repair. In this study, there was a significantly higher leakage rate after repair in the laparoscopic fibrin-glue–repair group (16% compared with 2% with open repair.). After they stratified all their patients, it was concluded that laparoscopic fibrin-sealant repair can be achieved with low risk in select patients. The criteria that should be used for the fibrin-sealant repair is small ulcer size (<5 mm), and that the patient should not be significantly ill, with an Acute Physiology and Chronic Health Evaluation (APACHE) score of less than 5.

Fibrin sealant has very good hemostatic abilities and surgeons have been taking advantage of that in the management of hepatic and splenic injuries. It has been shown to be safe and efficacious in animal studies; however, as of this writing, there are no large clinical trials in the literature. In an interesting report by Chen and colleagues, management of blunt hepatic trauma using laparoscopy and fibrin sealant was studied. Patients underwent laparotomy if they presented as hemodynamically unstable, and in 61 patients who were managed conservatively, 6 failed conservative management and underwent laparoscopy. All 6 were repaired by injecting fibrin sealant at the area of hemorrhage, avoiding laparotomy. Thus, although using a laparoscope to manage a trauma patient is certainly controversial, laparoscopic evaluation of a trauma patient can allow better characterization of the injury and more accurate assessment of the anatomic injury grade and rate of ongoing hemorrhage. It can also provide additional diagnostic information while at the same time decreasing the rate of nontherapeutic laparotomies.

As we know, intra-abdominal adhesions are the major cause of small bowel obstruction following surgery. Some researchers have been reporting that fibrin sealant can actually reduce the density and the severity of the intra-abdominal adhesions in animal models following surgery. Researchers have found that fibrin sealant actually alters the mRNA expression of the factors regulating plasminogen activator activity. They postulate this might be the reason why fibrin sealant can potentially decrease intra-abdominal adhesions.

Several groups have been looking at using fibrin sealant as a plug such as in the closure of the choledochotomy site in laparoscopic common bile duct exploration. A stent is placed across the choledochotomy and then fibrin sealant is injected on top in order to seal the opening. Others have been looking at using fibrin sealant in pancreatic resection. By injecting the sealant into the pancreatic duct, you aim to seal the duct and decrease post-op pancreatic leaks. Another application is treating an anal fistula by injecting the sealant into the fistula tract in order to seal it. In addition, case reports have injected intralumenal fibrin sealant to manage leaks at circular stapled gastrojunostomy after gastric bypass. Finally, the US Army has been looking at using a dry fibrin-sealant dressing to control bleeding in a traumatic wound. Thus, the ongoing advances in tissue sealants appear likely to make laparoscopic surgery safer in the future.

**Suggested Reading**

1. Chen RJ, Fang JF, Lin BC, Hsu YB, Kao JL, Kao YC, Chen MF. Selective application of laparoscopy and fibrin glue in the failure of nonoperative management of blunt hepatic trauma. *J Trauma.* 1998;44(4):691-5.
2. Kanellos I, Mantzoros I, Goulimaris I, Zacharakis E, Zavitsanakis A, Betsis D. Effects of the use of fibrin glue around the colonic anastomosis of the rat. *Tech Coloproctol.* 2003;7(2):82-4.
3. Lee MG, Provost DA, Jones DB. Use of fibrin sealant in laparoscopic gastric bypass for the morbidly obese. *Obes Surg.* 2004;14(10):1321-6.
4. Liu CD, Glantz GJ, Livingston EH. Fibrin glue as a sealant for high-risk anastomosis in surgery for morbid obesity. *Obes Surg.* 2003;13(1):45-8.
5. Sapala JA, Wood MH, Schuhknecht MP. Anastomotic leak prophylaxis using a vapor-heated fibrin sealant: report on 738 gastric bypass patients. *Obes Surg.* 2004;14(1):35-42.
6. Zilling TL, Jansson O, Walther BS, Ottosson A. Sutureless small bowel anastomoses: experimental study in pigs. *Eur J Surg.* 1999;165(1):61-8.

# Surgical Device Industry

Dean J. Geraci, MSc

**It is All About Patient Safety**

Patient safety is paramount for any medical device manufacturer. Proper training on use of surgical devices is necessary for successful outcomes in surgery. Therefore, manufacturers use continuous quality assurance programs to reduce complications that may arise when their instruments are used in surgery. In weight loss surgery, however, most complications that affect patient safety manifest themselves outside the operating room. Therefore, these manufacturers are actively involved in improving patient safety across the continuum of care for the bariatric patient.

Because of the physical, nutritional, and psychosocial characteristics of extreme weight loss that accompany bariatric surgery, patient safety for manufacturers of the primary devices used in such procedures often goes beyond the operating room.

Patient safety goes hand-in-hand with patient outcomes. If the surgery is unsuccessful due to postoperative complications, there can be dire consequences for the patient. In some cases, patient safety and outcomes are dependent upon factors that arise prior to surgery—i.e., proper patient selection. In this case, a manufacturer may provide services to those professionals who interact with patients before they are considered for surgery, in order to ensure that the right patients undergo the appropriate procedures.

We can place device manufacturers' interaction with healthcare providers regarding patient safety into the following categories:

- Technology that primarily focuses on providing devices that conform to their intended use
- Training of healthcare providers so that the devices are properly used
- Support activities that augment the above technology and training so that patients can safely achieve their weight loss goals

Serious consequences, ranging from commercial failure to litigation to potential felony violations, await manufacturers who produce unsafe medical products.(1,2,3) The Federal Drug and Cosmetic Act(4) specifically established laws that control the introduction of medical devices manufactured and offered on the market, which are determined by the US Food and Drug Administration (FDA) to be "safe and effective."(5) For a device manufacturer to offer a product in Europe, it must obtain a CE mark that establishes that the device improves the safety and health of patients exposed to its use.(6)

When products fail in use, the FDA relies on patients and the healthcare industry to identify and report these adverse events, including rare serious failures. In fact, approximately 95% of the more than 100,000 device-related, adverse event reports sent to the FDA are from manufacturers. Product recalls (i.e., removal from the market) occur when a reasonable probability of serious harm exists. Recalls may be initiated by the manufacturer or the FDA.(7) Violations in the regulations regarding devices can be misdemeanors or felonies, resulting not only in possible incarceration, but also in fines up to $500,000 for each offense.(8)

In bariatric surgery, the responsibility for patient safety rests not only with the manufacturer who employs the device, but also with the surgeon who uses it in procedures, as well as other healthcare professionals who encounter the patient. As with all medical devices, a healthcare professional is responsible for employing the device; the manufacturer is responsible for providing adequate instructions for use. While a surgical stapler or adjustable band may work exactly as designed, the surgery may not be as successful because of other factors inherent in treating bariatric patients.

Overall, patient safety initiatives are more successful when patient safety and outcomes are not the responsibility of any single person, but of all caregivers as a system. This latter concept is the progenitor of Centers of Excellence programs,(9,10) which have proven themselves in the cardiac and transplant fields and are being adopted in bariatric surgery.(11)

### Technology and Procedures are Linked

The development and introduction of open and laparoscopic stapling devices was one of the key aspects in developing procedures for morbid obesity. For this reason, the surgical/medical device industry was involved directly and indirectly in patient safety as the procedures were developed, adapted, and adopted.(12)

Surgical staplers, whether used in open or laparoscopic cases, are the primary devices employed in several bariatric procedures. In the Roux-en-Y gastric bypass, several firings of a linear stapler transect the stomach, forming the pouch. When a linear stapler is fired, several rows (4 or 6 in total) are formed in parallel. An internal knife is then passed down the center of the rows, dividing the sections. The linear stapler is used in this fashion to divide the jejunum, forming the biliopancreatic and Roux limbs. The linear stapler is also used to form a functional side-to-side anastomosis between the Roux and biliopancreatic limb. Further, a linear stapler can be used to form the posterior layer of the gastrojejunosotomy.(13,14) A circular stapler can also be used to form the gastrojejunostomy.(15,16) In other iterations of the Roux-en-Y, the gastrojejunostomy is hand sewn and no staplers are used.(17)

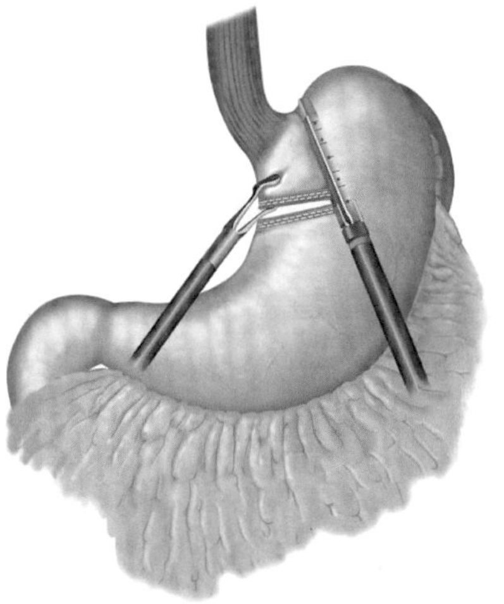

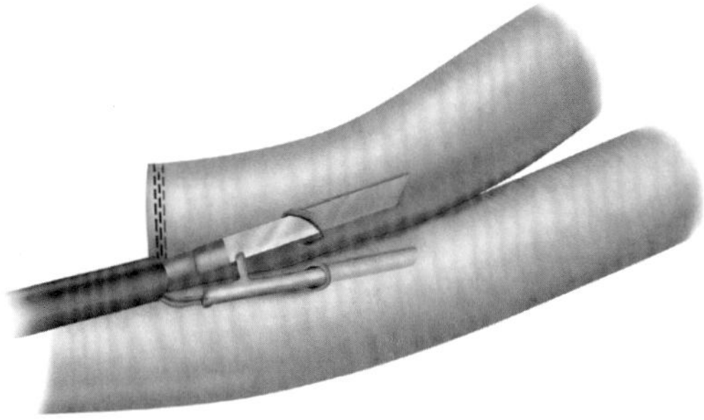

**Roux-en-Y Gastric Bypass**

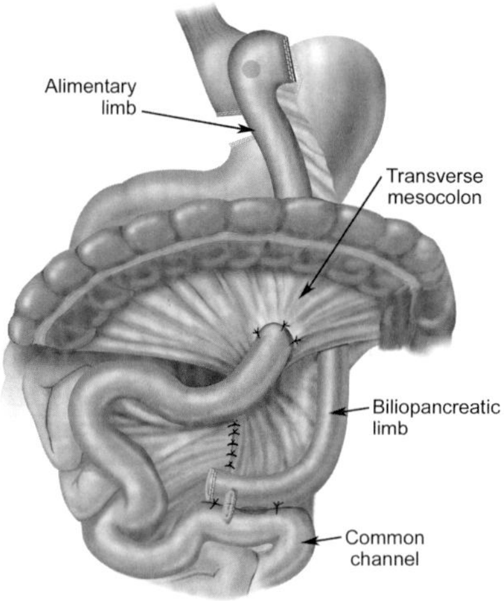


Devices specifically designed for open surgery have a longer history than those designed for laparoscopic surgery.(18) The surgical steps are very similar to the laparoscopic approach; however, the technique is very different.(19) One of the primary reasons for the move to laparoscopic procedures is the direct impact on patient safety in reducing the complications associated with the laparotomy in the open approach—reduction of hernias, infection, and dehiscence.(20,21)

In contrast, no staplers are used in performing a laparoscopic adjustable band procedure. In this case, the device is specifically designed for the procedure, whereas in gastric bypass procedures, staplers and other ancillary instruments are used. Most band procedures are performed through a laparoscopic approach.

**Figure 1**

Risk-benefit relationship of several bariatric procedures.

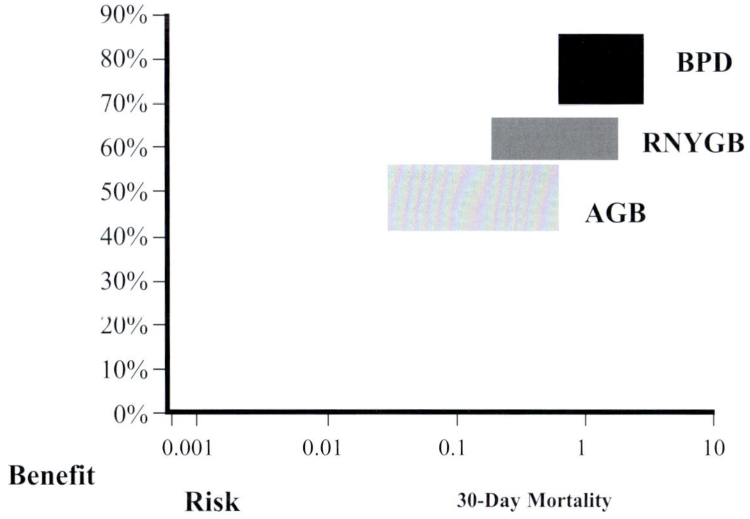


Adapted from Buchwald et al, (20) and Maggard et al(21).

## Know the Technology, Know the Procedure

All device manufacturers provide instructions for use of their products. However, in procedures where the device has a significant impact on patient safety, many manufacturers provide additional training in the form of workshops, animate model exposure, or cadaver model exposure. Some workshops may concentrate on instrumentation, while others may concentrate on procedural aspects—i.e., learning the steps of the procedure. In other instances, the workshop may be aimed at increasing surgical skills such as intracorporeal suturing. In many cases, the FDA will require the manufacturer to offer specific training programs to potential users prior to selling the device to them.(22)

In bariatric surgery, manufacturers of staplers, as well as adjustable bands, offer an array of training programs, ranging from introductory courses to full-year, postgraduate fellowships, which they sponsor at leading institutions.

Several reports have shown that a surgeon's level of experience is directly related to patient mortality and morbidity.(23,24,25) Few studies have shown the effect of the training path on patient safety in bariatric surgery, although reports suggest that an extensive fellowship program provides the best training for complex surgical procedures.(26,27)

**Figure 2**

Training pathway for surgical teams for bariatric surgery.

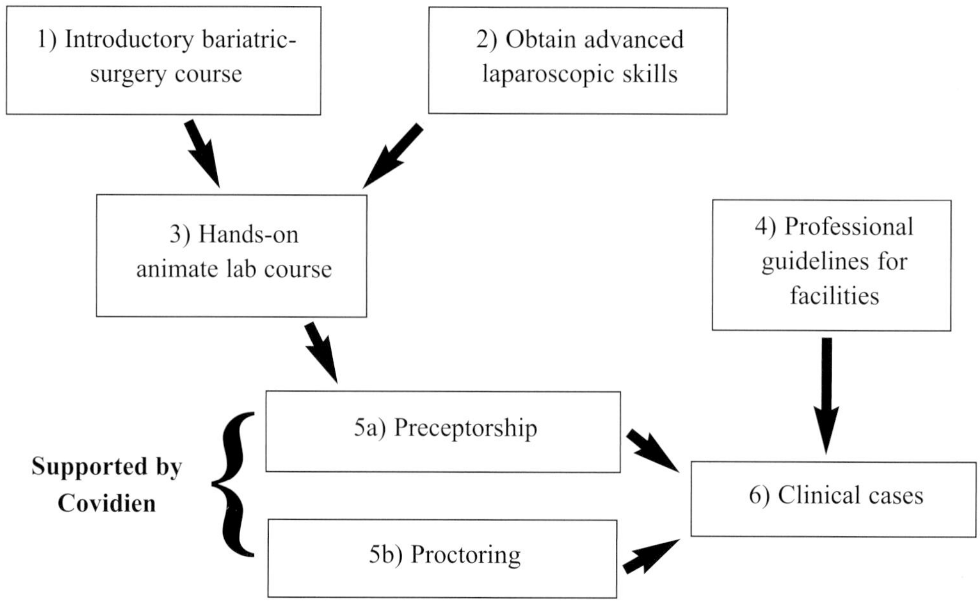


Manufacturers participate in professional medical education for both physicians and nurses by providing resources for postgraduate education. In some instances, the education is broad-based, as with an introductory course for bariatric surgery, or very specific, as when issues regarding clinical pathway steps are explored.

Many professional societies offer postgraduate programs for both surgeons and allied healthcare personnel. These programs are often supported by the medical device manufacturers in the form of educational grants, faculty support, or in-kind equipment donation.

**Patient Safety Does Not Stop at the Operating Room Door**

Patient education is a prime example of industry efforts to positively impact patient safety. Almost all of the major manufacturers have provided information aimed directly at the patient, especially through the Internet, as to various aspects of procedures.(28,29,30) They have been providing generalized patient education via pamphlets, journals, syllabi, posters, educational videos, and slide presentations. Because many surgical practices adopt these educational tools, *de facto* standards in patient education have been established. Furthermore, manufacturers provide substantial information to patients at a more technical level through other means—again, particularly through the Internet, where any patient can access the information.

As with surgical education, allied health education is also supported by industry. Allied health education addresses patient care, from post-op training of the hospital allied health team, to creating comprehensive care plans, to sensitivity training of the entire staff. Since clinically severe obesity is associated with higher perioperative risks and many comorbidities, allied health education becomes imperative in ensuring positive outcomes for the patient.

Continued medical education for hospital staff members is often provided or supported by device manufacturers, either through in-hospital education programs, professional societies, or industry-sponsored programs. Training on concepts such as early ambulation to prevent thromboembolic complications, or early recognition of band obstructions are pertinent to positive outcomes for patients.

Hospital staff can be considered the front line of patient safety, particularly for postoperative issues. In many instances, timely intervention by allied healthcare personnel prevents minor problems from becoming major complications or catastrophic failures. For example, if a hospital staff member is properly trained to recognize a staple-line leak in a gastric bypass patient, serious complications can be avoided by following a predetermined patient-care path.

Establishing standards of care and clear patient-care pathways encompasses a large area of allied health training. The bariatric patient tends to be more complex than most postoperative patients and requires a specialized team that can recognize the often-masked symptoms of complications and understand the special care needs of this population. Thus, hospital staff education becomes a crucial part of patient safety.

Hospital staff can be resistant to a new bariatric program, not only because of the worry over not being able to manage perioperative complications, but also because of mobility issues the patient might have and the concern the staff members have for the patient's safety. Hospital staff must be given support and instruction on how to care for and mobilize bariatric patients, as well as education on their own body mechanics and physical limitations.

Even though the industry is obviously concerned about the technical/surgical aspect of bariatric surgery, patient safety and outcomes go beyond this. It is well understood that multidisciplinary teams have a positive impact on the short- and long-term success of bariatric procedures.(9,10,31) A sound standard of care for patient safety, with exceptional outcomes as a primary focus, requires clinical, physical, psychological, and educational concentration to directly impact the effectiveness of a bariatric surgery program.

Furthermore, recognizing that safety and optimal outcomes are a result of continuous managment and improvement of healthcare delivery, oversight organizations(32,33) and professional societies(9,10) have developed guidelines that focus on patient-safety indicators specific to the bariatric surgery patient, including the continuous need for allied health education.(9)

Because the comorbidities associated with obesity are so wide-ranging, many multidisciplinary functions are involved in the care of the patient. Still, many caregivers are biased against the obese,(34) and medical care prior to surgery may be lacking, to the point of being nonexistent. Continuing medical education also focuses on adjacent healthcare professionals such as the family physician, cardiologists, or endocrinologists that would usually treat the comorbidities associated with clinically severe obesity.

**Good Outcomes are Good Business**

Reducing complications in the operating theater and postsurgery is a continued effort and requires collaboration between all the stakeholders involved in the care of bariatric surgery patients—surgeons, allied health professionals, device manufacturers, professional medical societies, and even the patients themselves. While defects do occur in the manufacture of medical devices, as with any production process, they are quite rare when taken in context of the number of uses. Product improvement and development efforts are constantly underway to improve the performance of bariatric devices.

When complications do occur, the outcome can be catastrophic. Manufacturers of bariatric medical devices stress continued education for healthcare professionals in recognizing and resolving patient issues. Early intervention in resolving the complications is stressed in continued medical education programs sponsored or provided by the industry.

Patient safety and overall outcomes of bariatric surgery are closely tied together; complications reduce the effectiveness of the procedures. Obviously, companies that manufacture devices used in bariatric surgery are in business to make a profit. At the end of the day, it is recognized that delivering products and services that result in good outcomes is good business.

## References

1. Simons J. Not for the faint of heart: Boston Scientific's stent recall is a blow to earnings—but an opportunity for investors. *Fortune*. 2004; 150(3):164-166.
2. Henkel J. Device maker receives five-year sentence in fraud case. FDA Consumer. 1995. Available at: http://www.fda.gov/FDAC/departs/695_irs.html. Accessed January 2007.
3. Maisel WH. Safety issues involving medical devices; implications of recent implantable cardioverter-defibrillator malfunctions. *JAMA*. 2005;294(8):955–8.
4. US Food and Drug Administration. Food, Drug, and Cosmetic Act. Code of Federal Regulations, United States Code (USC) Title 21, Chapter 9.
5. US Food and Drug Administration. Food, Drug, and Cosmetic Act, 21CFR860.7, Determination of Safety and Effectiveness.
6. Council of the European Communities; Council Directive 93/42/EEC, Article 2; June 14, 1993.
7. Maisel WH. Medical device regulation: an introduction for the practicing physician *Ann Intern Med.* 2004;140(4):296-302.
8. Monsein LH. Primer on medical device regulation: part III. Regulatory mechanisms and import/export regulation. *Radiology*. 1997;205(1):19-25.
9. American Society for Metabolic and Bariatric Surgery Centers of Excellence Program; Mission Statement, Surgical Review Corporation. Available at: http://www.surgicalreview.org/about_us.aspx. Accessed January 2007.
10. American College of Surgeons, Bariatric Surgery Center Network Accreditation Program: Overview. Available at: http://www.facs.org/cqi/bscn/overview.html. Accessed January 2007.
11. Birkmeyer JD, Dimick JB, Birkmeyer NJ. Measuring the quality of surgical care: structure, process, or outcomes? *J Am Coll Surg*. 2004;198(4):626-32.
12. Buchwald H. Overview of bariatric surgery. *J Am Coll Surg*. 2002;194(3):367-75.
13. Schauer PR, Ikramuddin S, Gourash W, Ramanathan R, Luketich J. Outcomes after laparoscopic Roux-en-Y gastric bypass for morbid obesity. *Ann Surg*. 2000;232(4):515–29.
14. Champion JK, Williams MD. Prospective randomized comparison of linear staplers during laparoscopic Roux-en-Y gastric bypass. *Obes Surg*. 2003;13(6):855-9; discussion 860.
15. de la Torre RA, Scott JS. Laparoscopic Roux-en-Y gastric bypass: a totally intra-abdominal approach—technique and preliminary report. *Obes Surg*. 1999;9(5):492-8.
16. Jones DB. The circular stapler for the gastrojejunostomy in laparoscopic gastric bypass. *Obes Surg*. 2005;15(8):1102-3.
17. Higa KD, Boone KB, Ho T, Davies OG. Laparoscopic Roux-en-Y gastric bypass for morbid obesity: technique and preliminary results of our first 400 patients. *Arch Surg*. 2000;135(9):1029-33; discussion 1033-4.
18. Willbanks OL. Long-term results of silicone elastomer ring vertical gastroplasty for the treatment of morbid obesity. *Surgery*.1987;101(5):606-10.
19. Nguyen NT, Goldman C, Rosenquist CJ, Arango A, et al. Laparoscopic versus open gastric bypass: a randomized study of outcomes, quality of life, and costs. *Ann Surg*. 2001;234(3):279-89; discussion 289-91.
20. Buchwald H, Avidorf Y, Braunwald E, et al. Bariatric surgery, a systematic review and meta-analysis, *JAMA*. 2004;292(14):1724-37.

21. Maggard M, Shugarman LR, Suttrop M, Maglione M, et al, Meta-Analysis: surgical treatment of obesity. *Ann Intern Med*. 2005;142(7):547-59.

22. US Food and Drug Administration. LAP-BAND® Adjustable Gastric Banding (LAGB®) System.–[P000008, FDA June 2001] Available at: http://www.fda.gov/cdrh/pdf/p000008.html. Accessed December 2006.

23. Flum DR, Dellinger EP. Impact of gastric bypass operation on survival: a population-based analysis. *J Am Coll Surg*. 2004;199(4):543-51.

24. Christou NV, Sampalis JS, Liberman M, Look D, Auger S, et al. Surgery decreases long-term mortality, morbidity, and health care use in morbidly obese patients. *Ann Surg*. 2004;240(3):416-23; Discussion 423-4.

25. Nguyen NT, Paya M, Stevens CM, Mavandadi S, et al. The relationship between hospital volume and outcome in bariatric surgery at academic medical centers. *Ann Surg*. 2004;240(4):586-93; Discussion 593-4.

26. Kothari SN, Boyd WC, Larson CA, et al. Training of a minimally invasive bariatric surgeon: are laparoscopic fellowships the answer? *Obes Surg*. 2005;15(3):323-9.

27. Ballantyne GH, Ewing D, Capella RF, et al. The learning curve measured by operating times for laparoscopic and open gastric bypass: roles of surgeon's experience, institutional experience, body mass index and fellowship training. *Obes Surg*. 2005;15(2):172-82.

28. http://www.autosuturebariatrics.com. Accessed January 2007.

29. http://www.lapband.com Accessed January 2007.

30. http://www.bariatricedge.com Accessed January 2007.

31. McMahon MM, Sarr MG, Clark MM, et al. Clinical management after bariatric surgery: value of a multidisciplinary approach. *Mayo Clin Proc*. 2006;81(10 suppl):S34-S45.

32. Agency for Healthcare Research and Quality. Quality Indicators. Available at: http://www.qualityindicators.ahrq.gov/documentation.htm.Accessed January 2007.

33. Joint Commission. Disease Specific Care, Certification. Available at: http://www.jointcommission.org/HTBAC/DSC/dsc_eligibility.htm. Accessed January 2007.

34. Schwartz M, et al. Weight bias among health professionals specializing in obesity. *Obes Res*. 2003;11:1033–1039.

# Corporate America's Role

Kevin Lobo

We live in a world where too many Americans—adults and children—are overweight, obese, or morbidly obese. Too many people have heart disease. Too many suffer from type 2 diabetes, have cancer, or are dying from obesity and the 35 major diseases that have been linked to obesity, and the economic costs are huge. The obesity epidemic costs this nation more than $100 billion each year in medical services and lost productivity alone.

The statistics are frightening; the real life consequences are devastating. Obesity is not a matter of personal choice but a complex disease requiring innovative solutions and our collective commitment to find them. Finding these innovative solutions is not only good for business—it's the right thing to do.

The good news is that with a long-term and responsible multifaceted approach, corporate America along with medical professionals and the institutions they represent have the power to help millions of people prevent, or obtain treatment for obesity. But we need to do more. Fundamentally and profoundly, people must know and understand that obesity is not healthy. They must understand that it is a progressive disease with predictable outcomes, which include high blood pressure, heart disease, type 2 diabetes, and, in many cases, premature death. We must stop the progression of this disease for ourselves, our families, our friends, our society, and for our companies. We must disrupt the family tree of obesity in this country so that our children and future workforces are healthier and free from obesity-related diseases.

But what can corporate America do? Where do we begin? How do we address this enormous problem and make a difference? Here below are 5 guiding principles that I believe can make an impact.

**1. Understand the impact of obesity on our organizations, recognize the true threat it is, and commit to developing and articulating a strategy to combat it**

A report by the health advocacy group Trust for America's Health, which is supported by the Robert Wood Johnson Foundation, concluded that America lacks a comprehensive strategy for dealing with obesity, and we need to change that. The first place to do that is in our own organizations. We must ask ourselves, do we know how much obesity costs us? How pervasive it is in our organization? How many people in our organization are overweight, obese, or morbidly obese? Do we know precisely what our insurance policy covers and what it doesn't? Are we clear on the rationales behind those coverage decisions? Do they make sense to our organization?

Each organization needs to fully understand the impact of obesity on its business and its employees. Only then can the process for developing a comprehensive obesity strategy begin. This is done in business all the time. A need is identified in the marketplace and a business plan is developed to include objectives, strategies, strengths, and weaknesses. Products and services are developed that seize upon a business opportunity or reduce or pre-empt threats to the health of the business.

Obesity is one of the biggest threats facing business today. A greater percentage of revenues are going to pay for healthcare costs associated with obesity than ever before. According to a national survey by the Kaiser Family Foundation, healthcare premiums of employers and their workers have climbed twice as fast as wages and inflation. Part of the problem is that we seem more willing to pay for the treatment of the complications of obesity than we are willing to pay for treatments that address obesity itself. This has to change.

Bottom line: we must use the same critical thinking and apply the same analyses that we do for our products and services in order to specifically and effectively address the issue of obesity. Each company and organization must put its best thinkers to work on the problem, developing long-term strategies, programs, and incentives that will solve it in a realistic way.

**2. Increase education and patient access to proven preventative measures, as well as to treatments for obesity**

Insurance policies must reflect what truly works, what doesn't, and for whom, and corporate America must make obesity a top priority with insurers. As a progressive disease, obesity brings with it a higher risk of developing related conditions, including type 2 diabetes and heart disease, the longer an individual suffers from it. We must, therefore, direct our own insurance companies—those that cover our employees and their families—to fully address the issue of this disease from its early onset to its late stages, and to do so in a comprehensive and cost-effective way. Prevention isn't enough. Policies must adequately address and recognize proven treatments along the entire disease continuum.

Decisions should be made on evidence-based medicine and what is good for the patient and, therefore, the system in the long term—not simply on short-term economic concerns. This is not just an issue for insurance companies. Corporate America must step up and provide leadership on this issue. We are, after all, the payers. We need to make obesity a priority, not simply a problem for insurers to solve alone without consultation and direction.

By becoming partners with insurers on the issue of obesity, we will encourage them to look at the disease in the context of all the other diseases that are associated with it. In addition, we must support the research that shows the impact of prevention and treatment of obesity.

Employers can insist on having active dialogue with their insurance companies to develop policies that reflect the priority that obesity must command, insisting that addressing obesity as the source will have positive impact on related diseases and therefore substantially reduce overall health expenditures. Thus, it is important to have solid rationales for the decisions made in this context, for the challenge will be in prioritizing resources to ensure that there is sufficient funding for both short- and long-term initiatives. This is both a business and societal imperative.

**3. Promote the diagnosis and treatment of obesity responsibly**

For those in the healthcare industry, providing fair, balanced information about the risks and benefits of any procedure or intervention is a key responsibility. Obesity is a serious disease with serious consequences and people cannot be set up for failure. Instead, they must be provided with reasonable expectations without overstated or understated risks or benefits. Claims about treatments should only be made when supported by strong clinical evidence. We must commit to educating patients suffering from obesity so that they are the best informed consumers of health care.

The goal should be to foster an informed conversation between patient and physician, and to educate the consumer not only about the treatment, but also about the disease or condition itself. Appropriate time should be spent educating health professionals about new treatments before beginning an educational campaign to consumers. Of key importance is to remember that, in terms of obesity, it's not about the method of weight loss; it's about the right procedure, treatment, or intervention for the right patient, delivered by a highly skilled and sensitive health professional at the right time.

**4. Pay special attention to the impact of obesity on minority populations**

Only 13% of the US population is African American, yet 33% of our *entire* type 2 diabetes population is African American. There are great disparities. Obesity and its related diseases cut across all racial lines, economic backgrounds, and age, but many individuals carry a heavier burden than others because of circumstance, culture, awareness, knowledge, and access to care.

To address this unacceptable situation, programs must be created that focus on the special needs of minority populations. Tearing down the societal, cultural, and economic barriers that interfere with the prevention and treatment of obesity must be a priority in the overall campaign to promote the positive lifestyles that lead to wellness among our citizens.

**5. Recognize that we are in this together**

No one group can solve the obesity epidemic alone. No one procedure, no one medicine, no one diet plan, no one insurer, no one hospital or company can make this disease—which has so many disparate facets—disappear from the fabric of today's society.

Partnerships should be fostered with academia, healthcare professionals, local communities, government agencies, hospitals, insurers, schools, the healthcare industry, the food industry, and the people with obesity themselves and their families. We are all affected and therefore we all need to be part of the solution. It is our responsibility to "take on" this disease in order to prevent more people from getting it and to do more for those who already have it.

**Ethicon Endo-Surgery, Inc.**

Ethicon Endo-Surgery is most involved with those who have morbid obesity and those who treat them. In 2004, the company established BariatricEdge as a therapeutic franchise dedicated to the concerns of morbid obesity and bariatric surgery. It's a way of doing business that goes beyond the procedure. It organizes us globally so that we can identify and address needs in the community, whatever they are, wherever they occur. Ethicon Endo-Surgery recognizes that as a company it must be more than a manufacturer and marketer of products. It must consist of experts who provide services, solutions, and support from pre-op to post-op for all stakeholders, including doctors, hospitals, allied health professionals, patients, government, and insurers.

Investments must be made in research, education, and training to improve patient outcomes and find new solutions to old problems. In addition, we must continue to support evidence-based medicine and initiatives. In this regard, the data supporting the use of bariatric surgery in combating morbid obesity are overwhelming. Bariatric surgery has been shown to have the unique ability to improve or resolve several diseases at once in appropriate patients. The effect on diabetes is truly profound. Patients who for years had type 2 diabetes have in many cases left the hospital no longer experiencing symptoms of the disease. Others are significantly improved within months and well before the weight has come off. What other procedure or treatment has that power? People not only get their lives back, they get new lives.

Bariatric surgery, however, is not a magic pill or a quick fix; rather, it is a lifelong commitment to good health. Ethicon Endo-Surgery believes it has a responsibility not only to provide quality products to support this commitment, but also to provide quality information about these products and procedures so that the best healthcare decisions can be made. Doing right by customers is right for business, and the company takes a long-term view on obesity. Ethicon Endo-Surgery continues to develop its strategy on the disease for business, but believes more needs to be done. Defeating this complex disease will require a multifaceted solution from all stakeholders. No one group can do it alone.

# Safer Surgery Through Simulation

Kinga A. Powers, MD, PhD
Scott T. Rehrig, MD
Daniel B. Jones, MD, MS

The literature on patient safety is beginning to recognize partial-task training and medical simulation as a methodology to improve the quality of health care. In the era of work-hour restrictions, rising costs of operating room time, and patient/insurer intolerance of complications, surgical simulation and skills training offer safe alternatives outside of the operating room for improving the quality and efficiency of teaching and learning new procedures.

## Simulator-based training

Minimally invasive surgery has created new challenges for the surgeon as new technology gets introduced to the operating room. Operating in a 3-dimensional field with 2-dimensional visualization demands far different psychomotor skills. Haptics, tactility, and instrument ergonomics, as well as how the operating room (OR) is set up, may challenge the novice in the field, as these components of minimally invasive surgery require a steep learning curve for proficiency. Patient safety concerns have reduced trainees' opportunity to acquire surgical skills by "practicing" on patients in the OR; therefore, simulator training has emerged and offers surgeons a safe alternative for mastering laparoscopic skills.

Advances in simulators offer a variety of tools to help hone laparoscopic skills. The visual realism and overall scope of partial task trainers is rapidly expanding. Simulation tools may be labeled as *physical-reality* systems that include box trainers and animal models; *virtual reality* (VR) systems that are software-based; and *mixed-reality* trainers offering a combination of video equipment and electronic sensors that activate when instruments touch physical objects. (Figure 1). The simulators can be used for part-task training of basic-to-complex skills required during surgical procedures (e.g., suturing or dissection). Full procedural simulators enable the user/learner to practice integrating different skills into a continuous procedure. The latest emerging technology integrates part-task training and procedural-simulator training with team training in simulated ORs where trainees have opportunities to rehearse skillful handling of emergency situations.

**Figure 1**

An example of a physical reality box trainer (A) and a virtual reality system (B).

A B

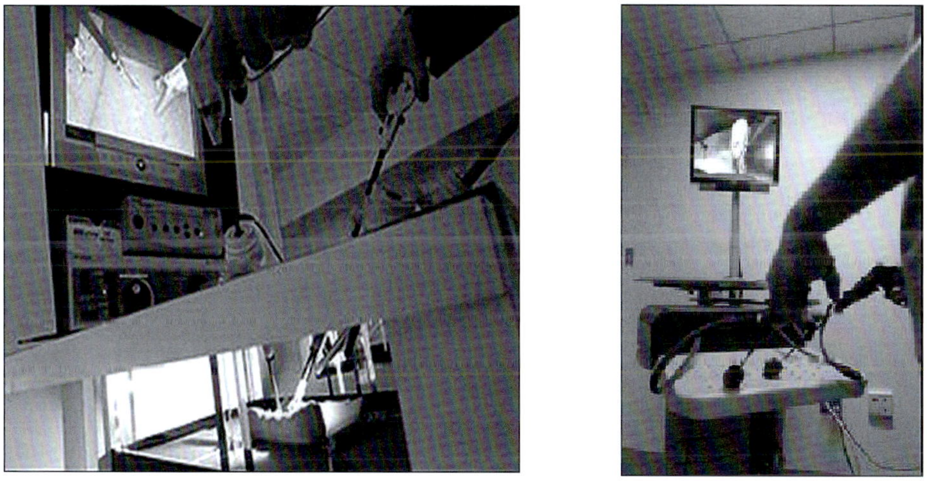

Box trainers are relatively inexpensive and widely available to most surgeons. Box trainers offer a number of drills that can be practiced using real instruments, however, the face validity of these models is poor and their application—specifically toward bariatric procedures—is still in development. The Society of American Gastrointestinal and Endoscopic Surgeons (SAGES) uses the box trainer for certification in fundamentals of laparoscopic skills (FLS). Fundamentals of laparoscopic skills certification is recommended by SAGES for all senior residents in general surgery and may represent a benchmark for surgeons performing laparoscopic bariatric procedures (Figure 2). Industry grants make FLS testing available to all senior residents and MIS Fellows.

**Figure 2**

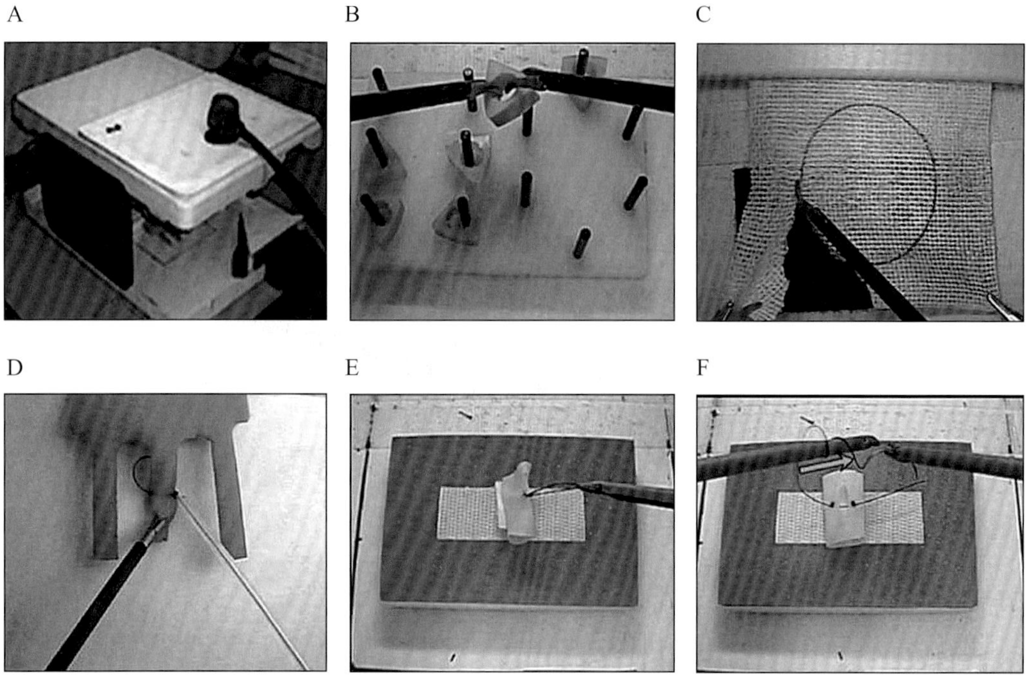

Fundamentals of laparoscopic skills certification is a 2-part process, testing cognitive knowledge through a multiple-choice examination and testing manual skills through a hands-on skills examination administered via the FLS Laparoscopic Trainer Box (A). Five standardized exercises are evaluated both for precision and speed: peg transfer (B), pattern cutting (C), placement of a ligating loop (D), intracorporeal knot (E), and extracorporeal knot (F).

Animal models, as well as cadaveric models are used for laparoscopic surgery training courses, including bariatric procedure training. Much of the porcine foregut anatomy is similar to the human anatomy and, therefore, this model provides high fidelity. In addition, animal lab operating suites offer the opportunity for trainees to work in teams, more closely approximating procedures on humans. Ethical restraints, as well as costs are limiting the use of animal models for wide-scale procedure training.

Virtual reality (VR) represents a computer-based avenue for laparoscopic surgery training. Although sophisticated simulators are available commercially and provide higher face validity than box trainers, they are still in relatively early stages of development. virtual reality provides an opportunity to practice tasks and entire procedures in ways that trainees not only learn technical skills, but also the key steps of procedures. However, one major limitation of VR simulators is their lack of haptic, or touch, recognition (haptics). Force-feedback mechanisms are currently being integrated into newer simulators. Some of the endoscopic procedure simulators have a better-developed haptics feedback mechanism. These simulators are based on a common platform with real endoscopes introduced into an elongated box, in which the travel of the end-piece activates progressive views of anatomy or specific haptic responses. One criticism of VR simulation is that graphics remain "cartoonish"; however, these graphics are also likely to improve with time. The VR simulators currently available for laparoscopic surgery are the following: Procedicus MIST, Haptica ProMIS, METI SurgicalSIM, Simbionix Lap-Mentor and Surgical Science LapSim.

The LAP Mentor™ by Simbionix has a library of modules that contain part-task and procedure-specific VR training cases. One of the modules currently under development offers training in the laparoscopic Roux-en-Y gastric bypass procedure (RYGB). The surgeon can perform and perfect the different steps of RYGB. All cases have several trocar configurations for convenience. General features of the module allow the surgeon to choose an "assisting tool" from the tool menu, to be used only with the right trocar. The surgeon can also use virtual linear staplers for creating the anastomosis. Each part of the procedure is broken down into several critical steps that are described, and the surgeon can perform these using the virtual tools (Figure 3).

**Figure 3**

**A**

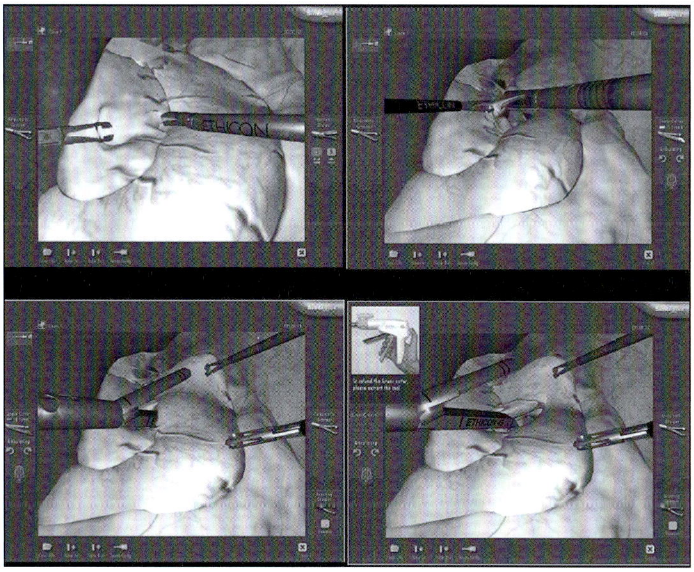


**B**

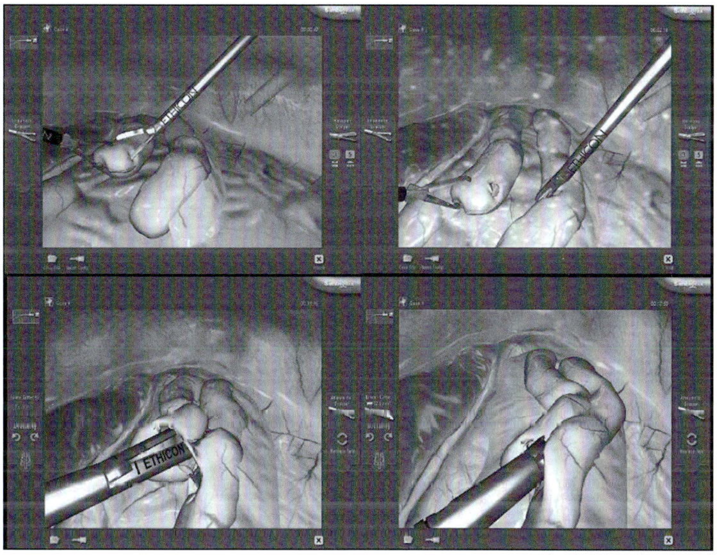


Simbionix Gastric Bypass Virtual Reality module: creating the gastric pouch.

(A) Enteroenterostomy anastomosis (B) Gastrojejunal anastomosis

C

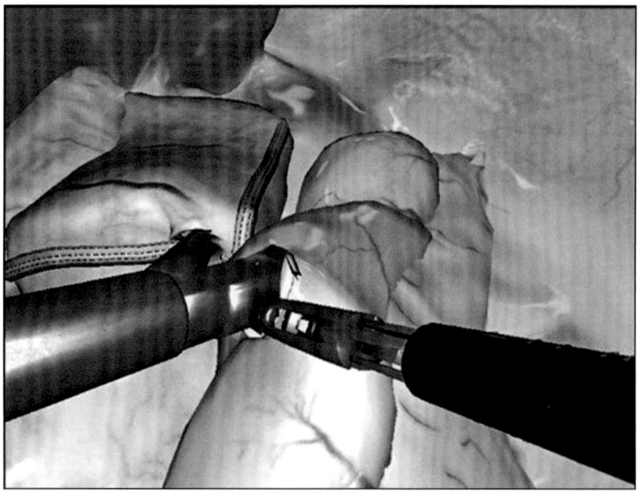

### Operating-room Team Training

Beyond part-task trainers and VR procedure simulators, team training in virtual operating theaters is being developed to enable the user/learner to practice within more comprehensive laparoscopic surgery scenarios. Virtual ORs target the higher level of skills that enable the surgeon to not only perform a surgical task, but also to interact in a healthcare team environment that simulates an actual OR. Traditionally, quality patient care was believed to result from healthcare teams and surgeons being well trained in particular sets of individual skills. Unfortunately, even skilled, experienced providers will make mistakes that are often viewed as personal failures, with the predictable result that these events are minimized and not openly discussed. Human-factors research suggests that surgical outcomes are not only a result of an individual's skill, but also a result of complex interactions of healthcare personnel working as a team, with each team member influenced by the working environment. A report from The Joint Commission revealed that in more than 70% of 2,455 sentinel events reported, the primary cause of medical error was communication failure. The seriousness of these occurrences is immeasurable; indeed, approximately 75% of the patients involved died. In aviation and other industries, the propensity for human error was recognized long ago and steps to circumvent error were implemented as part of mandatory team training. Simulator-based training with the Crew Resource Management (CRM) system has been used to train flight crews in crisis management. Anesthesiologists have developed a number of simulation models, including Anesthesia Crisis Resource Management courses. The repeated practice of scenario-based training models gives participants the knowledge and skill to manage routine and crisis situations as they occur in real life.

Crisis-simulation team training in surgery using a simulated operating theater was first described in the United Kingdom by Sir Ara Darzi. That scenario assessed the trainee's technical ability to control femoral arterial bleeding, and also assessed team/human-factors skills such as communication, situational awareness, and team and leadership skills during a crisis.

Virtual endosuites are a novel concept and one of the first of these used for laparoscopic skills training was established at Beth Israel Deaconess Medical Center. The Carl J. Shapiro Simulation and Skills Center (SASC) (www.BIDMC.Harvard.edu\SASC) is accredited as a level 1 education institute by the American College of Surgeons (ACS). As one of only 6 inaugural certified centers in the United States, SASC provides simulation-based skills training to healthcare students and professionals from all medical and surgical disciplines. A mock endosuite replicates a real operating theater. All standard laparoscopic surgical equipment, as well as an anesthetic simulator, are present and allow manipulation of the mannequin's hemodynamic parameters through a software program. An adjacent room serves as control room (Figure 4). A variety of video and audio recording equipment allows the researchers or trainers to view the simulation in real time, as well as in playback on a DVD disc to evaluate or use for debriefing. A synthetic model of the abdomen is fixed to the anesthetic simulator which simulates the abdominal wall skin as well as intra-abdominal organs and fat. The model is draped with surgical drapes and simulated laparoscopic procedures can be performed with simulated blood loss initiated, controlled, and monitored.

Figure 4

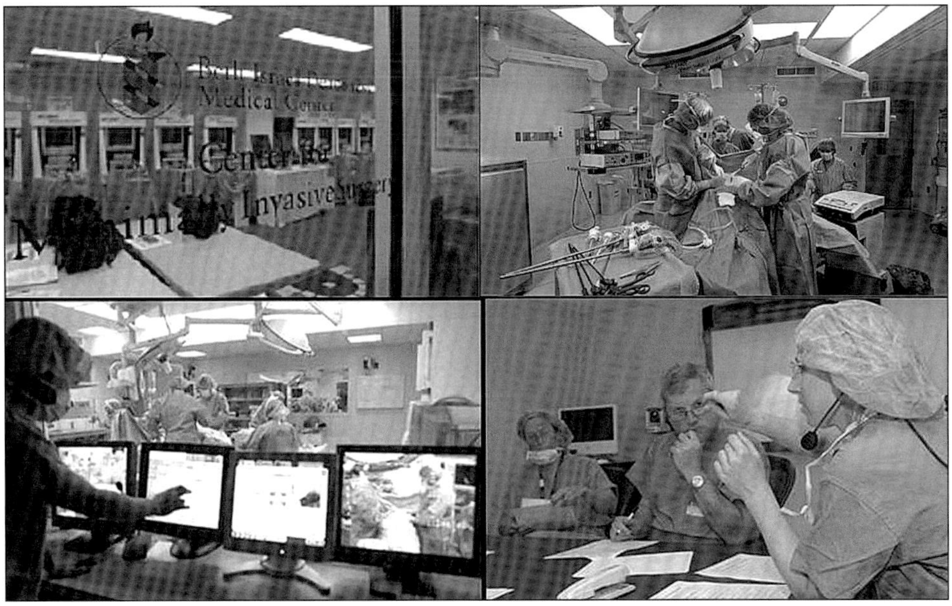

Mock endosuite for simulated surgical crisis-management training at the Carl J. Shapiro Simulation and Skills Center (www.BIDMC.Harvard.Edu\SACS), Beth Israel Deaconess Medical Center, Boston, MA.

### Future Outlook

We predict that team training courses specifically for bariatric procedures will one day provide a basis for credentialing bariatric surgeons. Task trainers will instruct trainees in the newest techniques and instrumentation in minimally invasive bariatric surgery, as well as allow for practice of the steps of laparoscopic gastric banding, gastric bypass, and other bariatric procedures in a safe environment. The use of a cadaver or animal lab will likely be replaced with VR simulators within a mock endosuite. Surgeons will thus be able to practice procedures, reduce operative time, and decrease complications.

Although there are limitations to surgical simulation, it is a field undergoing growth and transformation. Simulators, even in their current form, have clearly improved laparoscopic surgical skills. In an era of increased patient demands for safety and for change in the healthcare culture from an individual expert physician to collaborative team environments, surgical simulators have enormous potential to be developed into standardized training programs for laparoscopic and other surgical procedures. Simulation—even with its limitations—should prove to be among this century's most powerful surgical training and planning tools.

### Suggested Reading

1. Thomas EJ, Brennan T. Errors and adverse events in medicine: an overview. In: Vincent CA, ed. *Clinical Risk Management. Enhancing Patient Safety*. London. BMJ Publications; 2001:31-44.
2. Carter D. The surgeon as a risk factor. *BMJ*. 2003;326(7394):832-3.
3. Reznick RK. Surgical simulation: a vital part of our future. *Ann Surg*. 2005;242(5):640-1.
4. Sutherland LM, Middleton PF, Anthony A, Hamdorf J, Cregan P, et al. Surgical simulation: a systematic review. *Ann Surg*. 2006;243(3):291-300.
5. Dutta S, Gaba D, Krummel TM. To simulate or not to simulate: what is the question? *Ann Surg*. 2006;243(3):301-3.
6. Reznick RK, MacRae H. Teaching surgical skills—changes in the wind. *N Engl J Med*. 2006;355(25):2664-9.
7. Rehrig ST, Powers KA, Jones DB. Simulation and simulators. In: *Mastery of Endoscopic and Laparoscopic Surgery*. Lippincott Williams & Wilkins; 2008. In press.

8. Powers KA, Rehrig ST, Irias N, Albano HA, Malinbnow A, Jones SB, et al. Simulated laparoscopic operating room crisis: An approach to enhance the surgical team performance. *Surg Endosc*. 2008; 22(4):885-900.

9. Helmreich RL, Merritt AC, Wilhelm JA. The evolution of Crew Resource Management training in commercial aviation. *Int J Aviat Psychol*. 1999;9(1):19-32.

10. Helmreich RL, Schaefer H. Team performance in the operating room. In: Bogner MS, ed. *Human Error in Medicine*. Hillsdale, NJ: Lawrence Erlbaum; 1994.

11. Moorthy K, Munz Y, Forrest D, et al. Surgical crisis management skills training and assessment: a stimulation-based approach to enhancing operating room performance. *Ann Surg*. 2006;244(1):139-47.

12. Moorthy K, Munz Y, Adams S, Pandey V, Darzi A. A human factors analysis of technical and team skills among surgical trainees during procedural simulations in a simulated operating theatre. *Ann Surg*. 2005;242(5):631-9.

# Gastric Bypass Controversies: Implications for Patient Safety

Daniel J. Scott, MD
Farid J. Kehdy, MD

Since the introduction of the gastric bypass operation in the 1960s and 1970s, many issues have been explored relating to optimal methods for performing the operation and for patient-care strategies. From the era of open gastric bypass surgery, long-term follow-up data are available that document the safety and efficacy of this procedure, with remarkable benefit to patients.(1,2) With the advent of laparoscopic techniques in the 1990s, further benefits were established(3-6).

Even though this operation has been in use for more than 30 years, controversies still remain with direct implications for patient safety and cost-effectiveness. With the establishment of accredited Centers of Excellence for bariatric surgery, however, investigators are now well positioned to perform high-quality research in a networked fashion, with studies involving large numbers of patients, in order to answer many of these questions.

**Preoperative Endoscopy: Should it Become Mandatory in Asymptomatic Patients?**

Upper endoscopy is often performed on patients undergoing bariatric procedures, especially for gastric bypass patients, since the operation excludes the distal stomach and makes future endoscopic access very difficult. Many surgeons voice concern over the potential presence of upper gastrointestinal (GI) pathology that may alter the preoperative or operative course of treatment. In a study by Madan et al(7), it was found that 90% of gastric bypass patients had some type of pathology detected on routine preoperative endoscopy. Pathologies included erosive esophagitis, gastritis, duodenitis, hiatal hernia, and the presence of *Helicobacter pylori*. Madan recommended screening all patients with preoperative endoscopy. It was also recommended that all hiatal hernias be repaired before the gastric bypass, despite the fact that a gastric bypass is an excellent antireflux procedure, where the gastrojejunostomy will also tether the neo-stomach underneath the diaphragm. Notwithstanding the increased rate of positive findings, some authors argue that the proportion of patients who had a change in surgical management remained small.

In a study by Azagury, 47% of patients had positive findings on routine upper endoscopy prior to a bariatric procedure.(8) These findings were similar to Madan's study and pathology included gastric and duodenal ulcers, gastric polyps, and Barrett's esophagus. Out of 319 patients, only 13 patients (4%) needed definitive therapy other than eradication of *Helicobacter pylori*. This group did not fix hiatal hernias. Two of the 13 patients underwent a subtotal gastrectomy for gastric polyp. Even though the risk of developing cancer is slim, the difficulty in accessing the stomach after the bypass was the incentive to perform a partial gastrectomy on these patients. Because of the cost of upper endoscopy and the dangers of airway management in this patient population, as well as the presence of *Helicobacter pylori* as the most frequent abnormality on routine upper endoscopy, Azagury and his colleagues recommended noninvasive screening for *Helicobacter pylori* and treatment with proton inhibitors accordingly.

In most studies, esophagitis and esophageal pathology account for the majority of endoscopic abnormalities; since the esophagus remains accessible, many surgeons feel that routine endoscopy or radiographic screening is unnecessary in the absence of dysphagia or other concerning symptoms. On the other hand, it is well established that the absence of symptoms cannot be relied upon to predict the absence of upper GI pathology. However, given the weak clinical relevance, most of the detected pathology raises the question of the cost benefit of upper endoscopy before bariatric procedures.

**Are Routine Upper GI Studies Necessary After Gastric Bypass?**

An anastomotic leak is the most feared complication of a gastric bypass procedure. There can be catastrophic consequences that may end in the demise of the patient. It is, therefore, understandable that surgeons would do their utmost to avoid this complication. Many surgeons routinely perform upper GI studies on all postoperative patients; some surgeons follow selective protocols, while others obtain no imaging studies.

In a study by Hamilton where routine postoperative upper GI studies were used, only 22% of leaks were detected on radiographic imaging. Despite this low yield, these authors argue that the consequences of leaks may be so disastrous that even the early detection of one leak is worth the cost.(9) If a patient succumbs to sepsis and has a prolonged hospital course, the cost may be astronomical—certainly much higher than the cost of routinely performing postoperative imaging studies. The limits of upper GI series in this setting, however, are significant: x-ray penetration may be poor in severely obese individuals, resulting in poor quality imaging and in nondetection of some gastrojejunostomy leaks. Due to the gastric bypass configuration and relatively long Roux limb, most upper GI studies are not able to detect leaks at the gastric remnant or jejunojejunostomy. Fortunately, leaks at the latter two locations are more rare than gastrojejunostomy leaks, giving credence to the utility of postoperative upper GI studies.

Other investigators have proposed a more selective strategy for postoperative upper GI studies. Katasani and colleagues reported on a series of 553 patients who underwent imaging on a selective basis. This group performed upper GI studies on 120 patients who demonstrated clinical signs of leaks—signs that included at least one of the following: tachycardia (pulse more than 120 beats/min), respiratory distress, fever, and significant abdominal pain. Using this protocol, four anastomotic leaks were detected and no leaks were missed. All disruptions were in areas where soluble contrast could easily identify the abnormality.(10)

From a patient safety standpoint, it is critical to correlate the clinical picture with the radiologic picture, as indicators such as tachycardia greater than a rate of 120 and respiratory distress may be the most sensitive indicators.(9) The fact remains that there is no single test that can reliably and accurately diagnose all anastomotic leaks in a gastric bypass. Surgeons must remain extremely vigilant and must employ a constellation of available data to accurately and promptly identify this terrible complication.

**To Drain or Not to Drain...**

The utility of closed drains in gastric bypass procedures is another controversial issue. Drain placement is thought to facilitate the diagnosis of either an anastomotic leak or an intra-abdominal bleed in a gastric bypass. Both complications are rare, but the former is a formidable complication. Placement of drains around the gastrojejunal anastomosis is thought to identify leaks earlier in a patient population that makes physical exam notoriously unreliable; such drains may also facilitate nonoperative management in stable patients with small, contained leaks. In an era where managed care mandates the shortest possible hospital stay, early feeding is a prerequisite. In a study by Serafini et al, 100 patients underwent a gastric bypass, after which the region around the gastrojejunostomy was drained. These investigators inspected the drain fluid in order to recognize oral contents in the drain output. Three out of 100 patients were identified with leaks on upper GI studies performed 36 hours after surgery. Clinically, the anastomotic leaks declared with purulent drainage after the upper GI studies. None of these patients required an operation. Management was conservative. Repeat upper GI studies studies after 5 to 7 days were normal, after which oral intake was initiated.(11)

Another study by Chousleb investigated drains in 593 patients. In this study, 24 patients (4.4%) were diagnosed with a postoperative bleed. Eight of these patients had an increased serosanguinous effluent from the drains placed around the anastomoses. However, 16 were intraluminal, manifested by melena and not detectable by drain output. Of these 24 patients, 75% required transfusions, and 4 required reoperation. On the other hand, 10 patients (1.68%) were diagnosed with leaks. Half of these patients (0.84%) had evidence of a leak in the character of their drain output, and this group was managed conservatively. The other group required reoperation for control of the leak.(12)

It seems that placement of drains next to the anastomoses in patients' status following gastric bypass may decrease the incidence of returning to the operating room for control of a leak. This may generate a false sense of security in a patient population that requires surgeons to be extremely attentive. Drains are not 100% foolproof and there are incidents where leaks are not drained. This will cause a delay in diagnosis with the dire consequences of unrecognized abdominal sepsis and a very prolonged and morbid hospital course. On the other hand, drain placement for the detection of bleeds in a gastric bypass is much more controversial. In the Chousleb study, the percentage of intraluminal bleeds was higher than extraluminal bleeding. The patients in whom reoperation was necessary all had intraluminal bleeds. Drains will not detect intraluminal bleeds and will definitely not detect a remnant-stomach bleed, which in many instances will lead to remnant blowout and intra-abdominal sepsis. In addition, no matter how large drains are, the literature is replete with reports describing the failure of drains to demonstrate bleeding secondary to clogged lumens.

**Is a Routine Cholecystectomy Necessary During a Gastric Bypass?**

There is continued controversy regarding prophylactic cholecystectomy during gastric bypass procedures. It is well documented that obesity constitutes a risk factor for cholelithiasis, as does rapid weight loss, with gallstone formation in up to 32% of patients after surgery.(13) In the 1980s, routine removal of the gallbladder was performed by many surgeons during open gastric bypass procedures, since open abdominal access afforded suitable exposure to the gallbladder. Thus, the gallbladder was commonly removed for patients with gallstones as a therapeutic intervention and for patients without gallstones as a prophylactic strategy.

This universal cholecystectomy approach was supported by a study reported by Guadalajara in which 100 patients undergoing an open gastric bypass had a cholecystectomy and 93% of the patients had a pathologically documented gallbladder abnormality.(14) Pathology included cholelithiasis, cholecystitis, and granulomatous cholecystitis. There were no operative complications related to simultaneous cholecystectomy and it was concluded that this practice is safe and appropriate. Despite these findings, many surgeons questioned the clinical significance of gallbladder pathology noted at the time of gastric bypass.

Sugerman explored a different approach through several studies and documented that administration of ursodiol, a synthetic bile salt, postoperatively might be a suitable alternative to routine (prophylactic) cholecystectomy. With a 6-month course of 300 mg of ursodiol twice daily, Sugerman documented a 2% gallstone formation rate compared with a 32% rate for patients randomized to the placebo-controlled group. This was a high-quality, multicenter trial with a very high rate of compliance, ensured by weekly pill counts conducted by the investigators.

Compared to an open gastric bypass approach, the laparoscopic technique poses greater challenges to safely performing simultaneous cholecystectomy. Namely, fixed trocar positions limit range of motion and often necessitate additional trocar placement for adequate access. Even with additional trocars and angled laparoscopes, abundant portal and omental fat often obscure complete visualization, making cholecystectomy a challenging procedure in severely obese patients, with concerns of inadvertent injury. Because of these difficulties, investigators at UT Southwestern Medical Center studied the use of ursodiol for laparoscopic gastric bypass patients.(15) In 151 patients, the gallstone formation rate was 22% over 12 months of follow-up. The study investigators explained their findings of decreased efficacy compared with the Sugerman studies as due to poor compliance (64%). Known medication side effects include nausea, emesis, and skin rashes, which significantly hinder full compliance in actual clinical practice, and render this treatment only partially effective. Of note, very few patients (7%) developed gallstones associated with symptoms, and even fewer (3%) developed complications of acute cholecystitis, cholangitis, or pancreatitis.

In a study by Taylor, 535 patients who underwent a laparoscopic gastric bypass were studied over a 5.5-year period. Of these patients, 15% had documented cholelithiasis, for which a cholecystectomy was performed. Following gastric bypass, only 3% of this population needed an operation for symptomatic cholelithiasis. These operations were successfully performed as needed in the period following gastric bypass, with no complications; as expected, patients had lost significant weight by the time of their cholecystectomy, making the operation much easier and presumably safer. It was concluded that symptomatic cholelithiasis following gastric bypass is infrequent and routine cholecystectomy is not necessary.(16)

Additional data concerning simultaneous cholecystectomy at the time of laparoscopic gastric bypass were reported by Hamad et al. This group documented that patients who underwent simultaneous cholecystectomy had a prolonged hospital stay (increased by 1.6 days) compared with patients who underwent gastric bypass alone. The investigators offered the explanation that cholecystectomy adds significantly to the operative time and hence prolongs recovery.(17)

Thus, the optimal strategy for screening, preventing, and treating gallstones related to gastric bypass operations is still in evolution and additional long-term, multicenter trials are warranted. Given the current information about the paucity of patients who develop serious complications from gallstones after gastric bypass, a routine cholecystectomy approach is likely not warranted. In asymptomatic patients with gallstones at the time of gastric bypass, there is still no consensus.

Other issues related to biliary disease after gastric bypass are related to the inaccessibility of the biliary system by conventional endoscopic routes. Should choledocholithiasis, cholangitis, a cystic stump leak, a common bile duct stricture, or severe pancreatitis occur, endoscopic retrograde cholangiopancreatography (ERCP) is often not a therapeutic option. This does not apply to specialized centers that may be able to perform endoscopic procedures using long endoscopes passed transorally or conventional scopes passed transgastrically via access achieved in the operating room. These constraints underscore the importance of having surgeons skilled in open and laparoscopic biliary procedures, including common bile duct exploration, and of further optimizing protocols for optimal patient care.

### Creation of the Gastrojejunostomy

While not a debated issue in the era of open gastric bypass, with the technical demands of a laparoscopic approach, considerable debate over the optimal anastomotic technique for gastrojejunostomy (GJ) creation now exist. The main concerns are over leak and stricture rates and, to a lesser extent, marginal ulcer formation. Whereas leaks occur early and have potentially devastating consequences, GJ stenosis is a late complication with favorable outcomes, in most cases, after endoscopic balloon dilation. Laparoscopic GJ creation can be done in a number of ways and is currently dictated by surgeon preference rather than objective data from large trials. Techniques include: circular stapler, linear stapler, hand-sewn, and robotically assisted hand-sewn anastomoses. There are enough reports in the literature to both encourage and discourage each of the above techniques except the last, which is still fairly novel. Large controlled trials are still lacking.

The circular stapler was one of the earliest laparoscopic techniques to create the GJ and was introduced in 1994 by Wittgrove and Clark.(3) Introduction of the anvil by this group was via a transoral route and the technique was used and reported to have good success at other institutions.(18) However, other groups cited safety concerns with lodging of the anvil in the pharynx or esophagus, with inadvertent injury reported.(19,20) An alternative approach evolved, using the distal stomach as a route for transgastric anvil passage, obviating the potential for injuries outside the abdominal cavity.(19)

Early reports using the circular stapler technique documented acceptable leak rates but relatively high rates of stenosis. This complication was attributed to different factors, including small subclinical leaks, tension at the anastomosis, ischemia, and submucosal hematoma formation. However, the most objective cause was found to be the diameter of the stapler itself. In a trial that included 261 patients, Gould(21) demonstrated that using a 25-mm circular stapler, with an internal diameter of about 16 mm (varies according to the manufacturer), resulted in a lower rate of stenosis of the GJ when compared with using a 21-mm circular stapler (8.8% vs 26.8%, respectively). The leak rate in this series was 0% and weight loss was comparable in both groups, which is important given the clinical concern that a stoma that is too large will provide rapid emptying of pouch contents and impede weight loss. Proponents of the circular stapler anastomosis suggest that this technique creates a uniform stoma size reproducibly and with relative simplicity. From a technical standpoint, circular staplers are not designed for laparoscopic use; insertion of the stapler through the abdominal wall and maintenance of the pneumoperitoneum can be troublesome. In addition, the port site used for insertion becomes significantly dilated, necessitating fascial closure to prevent port-site hernia formation, and patients routinely complain of increased pain at this location.

Using the linear stapler to create an end-to-side GJ is another popular technique. Schweitzer (22) reported a zero leak rate in a study that included 251 patients, in which 30 mm of a 45-mm linear stapler was used. The defect used for stapler insertion was then closed using a hand-sewn technique, with posterior reinforcement of the staple line. The rate of stomal stenosis in this series was 4%, which is similar to other reports for this technique. Using the linear stapler is advantageous since insertion of the stapler is accomplished using conventional trocars with maintenance of the pneumoperitoneum. The technique can be technically challenging from calibration and defect-closure standpoints. Most surgeons use a bougie to stent the anastomosis open as the defect is closed, in an effort to achieve a uniform anastomotic diameter. While good results may be achieved, there may be a more prolonged learning curve with this approach compared with using a circular stapler, which automatically calibrates the stoma. In addition, suturing the defect closed may be technically challenging and/or time consuming in severely obese patients or patients with severe hepatomegaly, with limited exposure to the subdiaphragmatic area.

The completely hand-sewn technique is probably the least popular of the techniques, given its technical challenges. Suturing the entire anastomosis requires additional operative time for most surgeons (except for a few select virtuosos), and is associated with a steep learning curve. Surgeons who do not have outstanding intracorporeal suturing skills will not perform this technique. Given the fact that very few surgeons in practice possess the necessary skills, the hand-sewn technique will likely remain the operative strategy for only a few groups.(23) From a technical standpoint, the anastomosis is usually performed over a bougie to calibrate the stoma size. In the hands of extremely skilled surgeons, the technique can result in very good outcomes, with no leaks and a stenosis rate of 4.9%.(24)

Robotically assisted surgery has made great strides in recent years in urology, with many groups using these systems for minimally invasive prostatectomies, but few groups have adopted this technology for intestinal surgery. Nonetheless, some data are available for robotic gastric bypass. Yu reported the use of the da Vinci robot to perform a laparoscopic gastric bypass in 100 patients, with a leak rate of zero and a stricture rate of 2%.(25) These data are encouraging and robotic assistance may be quite helpful for complex procedures. These systems potentially make surgery easier, with increased range of motion via instrument-wrist articulation, scaling of motion, tremor filtration, and 3-dimensional imaging. These attributes may help surgeons with nonexpert laparoscopic skills to perform a hand-sewn anastomosis. However, there are numerous constraints associated with this equipment that impede widespread adoption. Current systems cost about $1.4 million and cost is a serious factor. Operative times tend to be longer due to robot "docking," additional instrument set-up requirements, and a new learning curve for the surgeon, nurses, and technicians, which must be overcome. Many laparoscopists believe that using the robot is an expensive and time-consuming extra step, unnecessary for surgeons who possess adequate skills to perform an operation without it.

**Antecolic or Retrocolic Roux Limb?**

The Roux-en-Y gastric bypass may be performed using either an antecolic or a retrocolic approach. Anatomically, the major difference between these two techniques is the number of potential internal hernia defects that are generated. The retrocolic technique creates a mesenteric defect, a mesocolic defect, and a Peterson defect, whereas the antecolic approach generates only the mesenteric and Peterson defects. The concern over internal hernia formation is well founded; since early in the evolution of laparoscopic techniques, such hernias were reported with increased frequency compared with past open-approach reports. Decreased adhesion formation following laparoscopic surgery is likely the culprit, but a clear understanding of the anatomy and potential spaces, along with meticulous closure of all defects is critical to achieving good outcomes.

Several series have been reported that favor the antecolic route.(24,26,27) Proponents cite the ease of this approach from a technical standpoint, with faster operative times and a decreased rate of internal hernia formation. Debate continues as to whether the Petersen hernia defect created by this approach requires closure. With the antecolic approach, the Petersen hernia defect is quite large, which many surgeons feel obviates the possibility of clinically significant hernia formation given a low likelihood of intestinal obstruction. Early reports supported this concept, but reports with longer follow-up have documented internal hernias at the Petersen defect requiring reoperation as late as 3 years following gastric bypass.(27)

On the other hand, the retrocolic approach has seen an evolution of outcomes over time. Early reports documented relatively high rates of internal hernia formation using this technique. Anecdotally, some surgeons reported changing to permanent (as opposed to absorbable) suture for performing defect closure, with improved results.(24,28) Using meticulous closure techniques, data now support acceptably low rates (0.55%) of internal hernia formation following a retrocolic approach.(29) Proponents of this approach suggest that the retrocolic approach is a shorter route to the gastric pouch and provides less tension on the GJ anastomosis.

**Length of Roux limb**

Increasing the length of the Roux limb in the super obese patient (body mass index [BMI] >50) effectively increases weight loss in this patient population, at least in the early postoperative course. Brolin documented superior weight loss with no increase in micronutrient deficiencies or watery stools at 2-year follow-up for super-obese patients who had a 150-cm Roux limb compared with a 75-cm limb.(2)

However, for nonsuper-obese (BMI <50) patients, the optimal length of the Roux limb has not been established. In a study by Feng, there was no difference in weight loss in patients with BMI <50 and Roux limbs either 100 or 150 cm in length after 1-year follow-up.(30) A study by Inabnet arrived at a similar conclusion for the same patient population using similar limb lengths.(31) In addition, the results demonstrated a higher rate of internal hernias in patients with the 150-cm Roux limb over a 1-year period, presumably related to the increased mobility of the longer limb.

Lee reported superior weight loss for patients with a BMI ≥40 or more who received a longer Roux limb. In a cohort of 165 patients who underwent laparoscopic Roux-en-Y gastric bypass, 97 were evaluated at 1 year. Limb lengths of 100 to 150 cm were constructed, and a linear relationship between limb length and weight loss was established. The investigators concluded that patients with Roux limbs >100 cm had a faster weight loss than those patients with limbs <100 cm in a 1-year time frame.(32)

Bariatric surgery has proven itself as a tremendously beneficial process for patients, and this includes the well-established gastric bypass procedure. Nonetheless, significant debate exists on how best to perform various aspects of the operation, as well as to screen for and prevent adverse patient outcomes.

Given the national focus on patient safety and the elective nature of these procedures, which are designed to improve health and quality of life, the bariatric surgical community will continue to receive external pressure to improve outcomes. Fortunately, internal motivation amongst surgeons is equally strong and, when coupled with the powerful alliance of centers specializing in bariatric surgery (as organized by the Centers of Excellence programs now in existence), ensures that participants in the field have an important opportunity to collaborate in a networked fashion, design and implement large, high-quality studies, and answer many of the questions highlighted in this chapter. Ultimately, such efforts will improve outcomes further and have a positive impact on patient safety, as well as on achieving cost-effectiveness.

**References**


1. Pories WJ, Swanson MS, MacDonald KG, Long SB, Morris PG, Brown BM, et al. Who would have thought it? An operation proves to be the most effective therapy for adult-onset diabetes mellitus. *Ann Surg*. 1995;222(3):339-50; discussion 350-2.
2. Brolin RE, Kenler HA, Gorman JH, Cody RP. Long-limb gastric bypass in the superobese: a prospective randomized study. *Ann Surg*. 1992;215(4):387-95.
3. Wittgrove AC, Clark GW, Tremblay LJ. Laparoscopic gastric bypass, Roux-en-Y: preliminary report of five cases. *Obes Surg*. 1994;4(4):353-7.
4. Nguyen NT, Lee SL, Goldman C, et al. Comparison of pulmonary function and postoperative pain after laparoscopic versus open gastric bypass: a randomized trial. *J Am Coll Surg*. 2001;192(4):469-76; discussion 476-7.
5. Puzziferri N, Austrheim-Smith IT, Wolfe BM, Wilson SE, Nguyen NT. Three-year follow-up of a prospective randomized trial comparing laparoscopic versus open gastric bypass. *Ann Surg*. 2006;243(2):181-8.
6. Schauer PR, Ikramuddin S, Gourash W, Ramanathan R, Luketich J. Outcomes after laparoscopic Roux-en-Y gastric bypass for morbid obesity. *Ann Surg*. 2000;232(4):515-29.
7. Madan AK, Speck KE, Hiler ML. Routine preoperative upper endoscopy for laparoscopic gastric bypass: is it necessary? *Am Surg*. 2004;70(8):684-6.
8. Azagury D, Dumonceau JM, Morel P, Chassot G, Huber O. Preoperative work-up in asymptomatic patients undergoing Roux-en-Y gastric bypass: is endoscopy mandatory? *Obes Surg*. 2006;16(10):1304-11.
9. Hamilton EC, Sims TL, Hamilton TT, Mullican MA, Jones DB, Provost DA. Clinical predictors of leak after laparoscopic Roux-en-Y gastric bypass for morbid obesity. *Surg Endosc*. 2003;17(5):679-84.
10. Katasani VG, Leeth RR, Tishler DS, et al. Water-soluble upper GI based on clinical findings is reliable to detect anastomotic leaks after laparoscopic gastric bypass. *Am Surg*. 2005;71(11):916-8; discussion 918-9.
11. Serafini F, Anderson W, Ghassemi P, Poklepovic J, Murr MM. The utility of contrast studies and drains in the management of patients after Roux-en-Y gastric bypass. *Obes Surg*. 2002;12(1):34-8.
12. Chousleb E, Szomstein S, Podkameni D, et al. Routine abdominal drains after laparoscopic Roux-en-Y gastric bypass: a retrospective review of 593 patients. *Obes Surg*. 2004;14(9):1203-7.
13. Sugerman HJ, Brewer WH, Shiffman ML, et al. A multicenter, placebo-controlled, randomized, double-blind, prospective trial of prophylactic ursodiol for the prevention of gallstone formation following gastric-bypass-induced rapid weight loss. *Am J Surg*. 1995;169(1):91-6; discussion 96-7.
14. Guadalajara H, Sanz Baro R, Pascual I, et al. Is prophylactic cholecystectomy useful in obese patients undergoing gastric bypass? *Obes Surg*. 2006;16(7):883-5.
15. Villegas L, Schneider B, Provost D, et al. Is routine cholecystectomy required during laparoscopic gastric bypass? *Obes Surg*. 2004;14(2):206-11.
16. Taylor J, Leitman IM, Horowitz M. Is routine cholecystectomy necessary at the time of Roux-en-Y gastric bypass? *Obes Surg*. 2006;16(6):759-61.
17. Hamad GG, Ikramuddin S, Gourash WF, Schauer PR. Elective cholecystectomy during laparoscopic Roux-en-Y gastric bypass: is it worth the wait? *Obes Surg*. 2003;13(1):76-81.
18. Biertho L, Steffen R, Ricklin T, et al. Laparoscopic gastric bypass versus laparoscopic adjustable gastric banding: a comparative study of 1,200 cases. *J Am Coll Surg*. 2003;197(4):536-44; discussion 544-5.
19. Scott DJ, Provost DA, Jones DB. Laparoscopic Roux-en-Y gastric bypass: transoral or transgastric anvil placement? *Obes Surg*. 2000;10(4):361-5.

20. Nguyen NT, Wolfe BM. Hypopharyngeal perforation during laparoscopic Roux-en-Y gastric bypass. *Obes Surg*. 2000;10(1):64-7.

21. Gould JC, Garren M, Boll V, Starling J. The impact of circular stapler diameter on the incidence of gastrojejunostomy stenosis and weight loss following laparoscopic Roux-en-Y gastric bypass. *Surg Endosc*. 2006;20(7):1017-20.

22. Schweitzer MA, Lidor A, Magnuson TH. A zero leak rate in 251 consecutive laparoscopic gastric bypass operations using a two-layer gastrojejunostomy technique. *J Laparoendosc Adv Surg Tech*. 2006;16(2):83-7.

23. Stefanidis D, Sierra R, Korndorffer JR Jr, et al. Intensive continuing medical education course training on simulators results in proficiency for laparoscopic suturing. *Am J Surg*. 2006;191(1):23-7.

24. Comeau E, Gagner M, Inabnet WB, Herron DM, Quinn TM, Pomp A. Symptomatic internal hernias after laparoscopic bariatric surgery. *Surg Endosc*. 2005;19(1):34-9.

25. Yu SC, Clapp BL, Lee MJ, Albrecht WC, Scarborough TK, Wilson EB. Robotic assistance provides excellent outcomes during the learning curve for laparoscopic Roux-en-Y gastric bypass: results from 100 robotic-assisted gastric bypasses. *Am J Surg*. 2006;192(6):746-9.

26. Champion JK, Williams M. Small-bowel obstruction and internal hernias after laparoscopic Roux-en-Y gastric bypass. *Obes Surg*. 2003;13(4):596-600.

27. Hwang RF, Swartz DE, Felix EL. Causes of small-bowel obstruction after laparoscopic gastric bypass. *Surg Endosc*. 2004;18(11):1631-5.

28. Higa KD, Boone KB, Ho T. Complications of the laparoscopic Roux-en-Y gastric bypass: 1,040 patients—what have we learned? *Obes Surg*. 2000;10(6):509-13.

29. Carmody B, DeMaria EJ, Jamal M, et al. Internal hernia after laparoscopic Roux-en-Y gastric bypass. *Surg Obes Relat Dis*. 2005;1(6):543-8.

30. Feng JJ, Gagner M, Pomp A, et al. Effect of standard vs extended Roux limb length on weight loss outcomes after laparoscopic Roux-en-Y gastric bypass. *Surg Endosc*. 2003;17(7):1055-60.

31. Inabnet WB, Quinn T, Gagner M, Urban M, Pomp A. Laparoscopic Roux-en-Y gastric bypass in patients with BMI <50: a prospective randomized trial comparing short and long limb lengths. *Obes Surg*. 2005;15(1):51-7.

32. Lee S, Sahagian KG, Schriver JP. Relationship between varying Roux limb lengths and weight loss in gastric bypass. *Curr Surg*. 2006;63(4):259-63.

# Acceptable Comorbidity

Scott Shikora, MD

Bariatric surgery is performed not for cosmetic reasons, but because severe obesity is a major health concern. Most morbidly obese patients have poor health and consume a significant proportion of healthcare resources. It's been well documented that for adult patients, bariatric operations improve and even cure a vast majority of these comorbidities. Despite this well-publicized data, bariatric surgeons must often still debate with the health insurance industry as to what constitutes an "acceptable" comorbidity in order to proceed with surgery.

## Obesity Associated Medical Conditions

- Coronary artery disease
- Cardiomyopathy
- Diabetes mellitus
- Infertility
- Depression
- Degenerative joint disease
- Respiratory abnormalities
- Pseudotumor cerebri
- Hypertension
- Stroke
- Endocrine abnormalities
- Hepatobiliary disease
- Malignancies
- Chronic back pain
- Gastroesophageal reflux
- Sudden death

Above is just a partial list of obesity-related conditions. Heart disease, diabetes mellitus, hypertension, and sleep apnea are the most recognized. These patients are also at risk for premature death, compromised quality of life, and a host of behavioral difficulties. Current guidelines for surgery, at least for adults, suggest that to be considered candidates for surgery, patients must have a body mass index (BMI) $\geq 35$ kg/m$^2$ and suffer from comorbid conditions, or have a BMI $\geq 40$ kg/m$^2$ with or without associated comorbid conditions. Incidentally, as BMI goes up, comorbidities generally are more severe and patients often have more than one.

As stated above, there is ample evidence in the literature demonstrating improvement in comorbidities with bariatric surgery. To paraphrase Dr. Harvey Sugerman, there is no other single modality in all of medicine that can cure or improve so many different conditions with one intervention.

## Outcomes after Bariatric Surgery

| Comorbidity | % Improved | % Resolved |
|---|---|---|
| OA/DJD | 47 | 41 |
| Hyperlipidemia | 33 | 63 |
| GERD | 24 | 72 |
| HTN | 18 | 70 |
| OSA | 19 | 74 |
| Depression | 47 | 8 |
| Peripheral edema | 55 | 41 |
| Urinary incontinence | 39 | 44 |
| Asthma | 69 | 13 |
| Diabetes | 18 | 82 |
| CAD | 75 | 25 |

Schauer et al. *Ann Surg*. 2002.

Schauer et al in a study published in a 2002 issue of *Annals of Surgery* demonstrated dramatic improvement in, or resolution of, the majority of these comorbid conditions 12 months after Roux-en-Y gastric bypass surgery. In fact, their data showed that for nearly all of these conditions, the sum of the percent improved and percent resolved was consistently 90% or greater. There are many published articles that have reached similar conclusions, yet none seem to have emerged reporting any worsening of these comorbidities due to bariatric surgery.

## Surgery is *NOT* Without Risk

Meta-analysis of 136 studies and 22,094 patients (1990-2003)

| Procedure | Op mortality (%) |
|---|---|
| Gastric banding | 0.1 |
| Gastric bypass | 0.5 |
| Gastroplasty | 0.1 |
| BPD+/-DS | 1.1 |

Buchwald et al, *JAMA* 2004

It must be stated that none of these surgeries are without risk. Buchwald et al, in a 2004 issue of *JAMA*, published a meta-analysis of the world literature on bariatric surgery. Included were data on 22,000 patients who had undergone this surgery. Outcomes demonstrated an operative mortality variance from 0.1% for gastric banding to 1.1% for biliopancreatic diversion procedures. While these numbers are respectably low, they do emphasize that the surgical procedures are not without risk.

When considering patients for surgery, all surgeons must determine their own strengths and limitations. This decision-making process will vary based on a number of interrelated factors such as the surgeon's own experience, hospital size and type, and available resources. Surgeons who work out of small community hospitals or in small programs, or have limited experience, may want to be more selective and refer the higher-risk and more complex patient to a larger medical center and/or bariatric surgical program.

## Unacceptable Comorbidity

- Severe comorbid diseases that would create unacceptably high operative risk
- Incurable or end stage diseases (cancer, AIDS, cirrhosis)
- Unstable diseases (CHF, COPD, unstable angina, thyroid disease)
- Gastrointestinal diseases (dysmotilities)
- Conditions that would not be expected to improve with weight loss

When discussing "acceptable" comorbidities, one must first discuss the "unacceptable" conditions. The serious health issues would likely be less disputable. They comprise those conditions that are so severe that the risk of surgery is great and may, in fact, outweigh the benefits of the surgery. These include incurable or end-stage diseases (advanced cancer, AIDS, cirrhosis), unstable or deteriorating conditions (congestive heart failure, chronic obstructive pulmonary disease, angina), certain gastrointestinal disorders (inflammatory bowel disease, motility disorders, abdominal radiation), or previous abdominal surgeries that might significantly complicate the surgery or make it unlikely to result in a good outcome.

## What are Acceptable Comorbidities?

- Comorbid conditions that would qualify a patient for surgery
- Whose interpretation?
  - Insurance industry?
  - Clinicians?
  - Patient?
- Minor conditions now are likely to become more severe over time

What then are "acceptable" comorbidities? We would like to say that they are health conditions that would justify surgery for these patients, because the risk-to-benefit ratio favors proceeding with surgery. Unfortunately, there is no universal consensus and the interpretation is highly variable. In addition, it should be of no surprise that interpretation differs greatly between the bariatric surgical community and the health insurance industry. Making matters worse is the likely probability that many conditions may currently be minor in nature, but would become more severe over time. Should these conditions be considered "acceptable" when they are minor or should the patient wait until they become more severe? Waiting would likely increase the perioperative risks for the patient and possibly have a negative impact on the overall outcome of the surgery when it is ultimately performed.

The 1991 National Institutes of Health (NIH) Consensus Conference on Obesity is the foundation for the current guidelines for surgery. Of significance is the fact that the conference was more than 15 years ago. There has been nothing new in these guidelines since then, though the evidence considered by the panel is long outdated. For example, in 1991, there were essentially only 2 bariatric operations performed: open gastric bypass and open vertical banded gastroplasty. Bariatric laparoscopy didn't exist, nor did the adjustable gastric band. The biliopancreatic diversion was done in only a few programs and not commonly accepted in the United States. There also have been significant improvements, since 1991, in areas such as intensive care, anesthesia management, perioperative care, patient selection and preparation, and postoperative management. Clearly the 1991 NIH guidelines were based in part on the technology at the time and, therefore, the panel's decision to use a BMI of 40 without comorbidity, or 35 with major comorbidity reflected the intersection of the risk-benefit curves appropriate to 1991. It would be interesting to see what the guidelines would be if the risk-benefit curves were calculated based on the data coming out of the practice of bariatric surgery today.

Controversy continues to surround the definition of "acceptable" comorbid conditions, which often pits the health insurance industry against the clinicians. The industry strives to establish guidelines that, in its view, are fair, able to be standardized across its domain, and are fiscally sound. On the other hand, the clinician responds only to the health and well-being of his/her patients. While clinicians adhere to the 1991 NIH standards, the insurance industry establishes standards of its own. In doing so, it often requires that the comorbid conditions be defined as "severe" or "life threatening," as, for instance, in severe obstructive sleep apnea, Pickwickian syndrome, obesity-related cardiomyopathy, severe diabetes, unmanageable hypertension, etc. The NIH in 1991 did not include such language. Unfortunately for the patient, these additional modifiers are vague and too often used to deny access to surgery. For instance, what defines the term "life threatening?" Is it a condition so severe that death is imminent? What is meant by "severe"? And how does one determine that a health condition is truly obesity-related or clinically unmanageable?

Let's look at a sampling of comorbid conditions whose "acceptability for surgery" is currently being debated.

### Cardiovascular Disease

Many insurance policies allow obesity-related cardiovascular disease as an "acceptable" comorbid condition for approving surgery. Cardiovascular disease is commonly seen with obesity and includes hypertension, hyperlipidemia, coronary artery disease, arteriosclerosis, congestive heart failure, and pulmonary hypertension. Congestive failure in this population is thought to be due to the expanded blood volume that results in a greater amount of left-ventricular work expended in order to propel the blood. In the setting of hypertension, left-ventricular dilatation and ultimately congestive heart failure are common sequelae. Many severely obese patients may have premature heart disease, but may not be diagnosed, because they are not sufficiently ambulatory to elicit symptoms. Should the patient be required to delay surgery until the heart disease is more advanced?

There is ample evidence in the literature to suggest that heart disease improves after bariatric surgery. Alpert et al, in an article published in a 1985 issue of the *American Journal of Cardiology*, studied 62 patients preoperatively with extensive cardiac evaluations. They reported a high incidence of severe heart disease, including left-ventricular dysfunction and chamber enlargement. Postoperatively, after weight loss, the patients were re-evaluated and found to have improvements in ejection fraction, chamber size, and wall thickness.

### Respiratory Insufficiency

There is a strong association between respiratory deficiencies and obesity. Obstructive sleep apnea is very common, but dramatically under-diagnosed in these patients. Many patients have never been evaluated. One study suggested that the majority of patients who present to bariatric programs for surgery have evidence of it. Yet, sleep apnea itself does not seem to closely correlate with BMI. Sleep apnea can be found in patients with lower BMIs and be absent in patients with extremely high BMIs. Sleep apnea can cause sudden death and also can increase perioperative risks. A related condition is the obesity-hypoventilation syndrome associated with baseline hypoxia and hypercapnea. This syndrome can also lead to heart failure and/or death.

Sleep apnea can vary in severity and it is likely that the severity of a patient's symptoms will increase over time and with increasing weight. Therefore, even mild sleep apnea must be considered life threatening in obese individuals. Delaying surgery until a patient has severe disease will only place that patient at greater risk for both death and surgical complications.

Sugerman et al authored several papers on sleep apnea and hypoventilation syndrome in the morbidly obese, which were published in the *American Journal of Clinical Nutrition* in 1992. In these writings, they consistently demonstrated improvements in both conditions after bariatric surgery.

### Glucose Intolerance

It is highly unlikely that patients with BMIs 35 to 39, as well as glucose intolerance (or "prediabetes"), would get approval for bariatric surgery from many of the health insurance carriers. Most plans require the patient to have actual diabetes. It has been demonstrated, however, that the majority of obese patients with glucose intolerance will proceed to develop diabetes over time.

Long et al, as published in a 1994 issue of *Diabetes Care*, followed 61 patients who had glucose intolerance. Of these, 11 did not have bariatric surgery and over an 8-year period, 55% of them became diabetic. Of the 50 patients who had surgery, none went on to develop diabetes. Since diabetes increases the risk of surgery and decreases the overall health of these patients, why should there be a delay in providing them with a procedure that is highly likely to cure their glucose intolerance and prevent the deterioration that will lead to diabetes? As an additional cautionary note, several studies have found that the longer a patient suffers from diabetes, the less likely he/she is to benefit from surgery.

### Pseudotumor Cerebri

This condition is rarely, if ever, considered an "acceptable" comorbidity for surgery by the health insurance industry. Its symptoms include severe headaches and blurred vision. However, the disease can also result in blindness, neuralgia, and Bell's palsy.

Sugerman et al, in a 1999 article in *Annals of Surgery*, demonstrated that the weight loss achieved with bariatric surgery would improve and often cure pseudotumor cerebri.

**Hyperlipidemia**

While there are currently several prescription medications that can decrease serum hyperlipidemia, this condition should still be viewed as a serious health concern because it can result in heart attack or stroke. The NIH has found that patients with elevated triglyceride levels have a two-fold excess risk of cardiovascular disease. Yet, it too is rarely considered an "acceptable" comorbid condition. Consistent with the previously addressed conditions, dramatic improvements in serum lipids, cholesterol, and triglycerides have been reported after bariatric surgery.

Brolin et al, in a 2000 issue of the *Journal of Gastrointestinal Surgery*, documented a 50% reduction in triglycerides, 15% reduction in cholesterol, and an improvement in "good" cholesterol (i.e., high-density lipoprotein) after surgery.

**Hypertension**

Hypertension is commonly seen in this population. There are no published standards defining mild, moderate, severe, manageable, or unmanageable hypertension. All levels must be considered a risk factor for heart attack or stroke.

## What About Hypertension?

- Surgery can cure and even prevent the development of hypertension
- 1025 patients (51% HTN) had GBP
- Results
  - 1 year post-op - 69% cured
  - 5-7 years post-op - 66% resolution of HTN
  - Resolution of HTN less likely in older patients

Sugerman et al. *Ann Surg.* 2003.

Several studies have reported cure rates as high as 90% with bariatric surgery. Of course, there are also data to suggest that if you wait too long or if the condition progresses too far, the likelihood of resolution drops (i.e., Sugerman et al, in a 2003 issue of *Annals of Surgery*). As with diabetes, the likelihood for resolution is reduced the longer the patient must wait for bariatric surgery.

**Gastroesophageal Reflux Disease (GERD)**

Gastroesophageal reflux disease is commonly associated with obesity. While many cases can be adequately treated with medications, GERD can, on occasion, result in serious consequences such as Barrett's esophagus, cancer, esophageal ulcers, tooth decay, chronic pneumonitis, chronic laryngitis, and hoarseness. How many health insurance plans will approve fundoplication surgery for severe GERD as a condition for bariatric surgery? Weight loss surgery has been shown to be more beneficial in this population.

Frezza et al, in an issue of *Surgical Endoscopy* in 2002, looked at 238 morbidly obese patients with GERD who underwent laparoscopic gastric bypass surgery. The study concluded that dramatic improvements were seen in heartburn, wheezing, laryngitis, aspiration, and use of medications to relieve GERD.

**Venous Stasis Disease**

Venous stasis disease can cause serious problems in this population, including pitting edema, poorly healing ulcers, chronic infections, and persistent breakdown. These can lead to impaired ambulation and even complete immobility. Severe infections can even result in limb amputations.

Venous stasis disease and its complications will improve dramatically in the majority of patients after bariatric surgery, as was noted by Sugerman et al in a 2001 issue of *Annals of Surgery*, whereas other modalities of treatment are generally ineffective.

**Stress Urinary Incontinence**

Stress urinary incontinence can be a serious problem in this population and can result in chronic skin irritation and breakdown. In morbidly obese and severely obese patients with this condition, most medical therapies, medications, and even urologic surgical procedures are generally ineffective.

In the *Journal of Obstetrics and Gynecology* in 1992, Bump et al demonstrated that after bariatric surgery, a relatively good cure rate and even a physiological improvement was observed in bladder pressure. Most symptoms dramatically improved and patients reported decreased pad usage and episodes of incontinence.

Thus, we recognize that the majority of obese, severely obese, and morbidly obese individuals are afflicted with significant comorbid conditions that are associated with their obesity. Weight loss surgery has been shown, in most cases, to improve or cure these conditions. Therefore, the definition of what is "acceptable" in order to qualify for surgery should be expanded to include these less severe conditions, as well as those that are viewed by some to be mild and/or early stage. Since these early or mild conditions will likely progress over time, waiting for deterioration to take place may move the patient into a very high complication risk group, or they may not be able to benefit from the surgery. Ultimately, "acceptable" comorbidities may turn into "unacceptable" ones.

**Suggested Reading**

1. Alpert MA, Terry BE, Kelly DL. Effect of weight loss on cardiac chamber size, wall thickness and left ventricular function in morbid obesity. *Am J Cardiol.* 1985;55(6):783-6.
2. Buchwald H, Avidor Y, Braunwald E, Jensen MD, et al. Bariatric surgery: a systematic review and meta-analysis. *JAMA*. 2004;292(14):1724-37.
3. Brolin RE, Bradley LJ, Wilson AC, Cody RP. Lipid risk profile and weight stability after gastric restrictive operations for morbid obesity. *J Gastrointest Surg*. 2000;4(5):464-9.
4. Bump RC, Sugerman HJ, Fantl JA, McClish DK. Obesity and lower urinary tract function in women: effect of surgically induced weight loss. *Am J Obstet Gynecol.* 1992;167(2):392-7.
5. Frezza EE, Ikramuddin S, Gourash W, Rakitt T, Kingston A, Luketich J, Schauer P. Symptomatic improvement in gastroesophageal reflux disease (GERD) following laparoscopic Roux-en-Y gastric bypass. *Surg Endosc.* 2002;16(7):1027-31.
6. Long SD, O'Brien K, MacDonald KG Jr, Leggett-Frazier N, et al. Weight loss in severely obese subjects prevents the progression of impaired glucose tolerance to type II diabetes. A longitudinal interventional study. *Diabetes Care.* 1994;17(5):372-5.
7. O'Keeffe T, Patterson EJ. Evidence supporting routine polysomnography before bariatric surgery. *Obes Surg.* 2004;14(1):23-6.
8. Sugerman HJ, Fairman RP, Sood RK, Engle K, Wolfe L, Kellum JM. Long-term effects of gastric surgery for treating respiratory insufficiency of obesity. *Am J Clin Nutr*. 1992;55(2 suppl):597S-601S.
9. Sugerman HJ, Felton WL 3rd, Sismanis A, Kellum JM, DeMaria EJ, Sugerman EL. Gastric surgery for pseudotumor cerebri associated with severe obesity. *Ann Surg*. 1999;229(5):634-40; Discussion 640-2.
10. Sugerman HJ, Sugerman EL, Wolfe L, Kellum JM Jr, Schweitzer MA, DeMaria EJ. Risks and benefits of gastric bypass in morbidly obese patients with severe venous stasis disease. *Ann Surg*. 2001;234(1):41-6.
11. Sugerman HJ, Wolfe LG, Sica DA, Clore JN. Diabetes and hypertension in severe obesity and effects of gastric bypass-induced weight loss. *Ann Surg*. 2003;237(6):751-6; Discussion 757-8.

# Weight Gain and Reoperative Surgery

Aurora D. Pryor, MD
Eric J. DeMaria, MD

As the number of bariatric cases continues to increase and the number of surgeons grows, we will also see an increase in the number of patients with "failed" bariatric procedures presenting for possible revisional surgery. Revisional surgery is, in general, higher risk than the initial procedure with potentially lower benefit.(1) The key to addressing these patients is to identify the reason for failure. Patients can fail for reasons relating to anatomic, as well as behavioral problems; all patients should undergo a thorough evaluation to identify the cause. Patients with behavioral issues may benefit from additional counseling, whereas anatomic problems can be addressed surgically.

One issue when deciding to revise a bariatric surgery patient is that we don't know exactly why the surgical procedures work in the first place. Some surgeons focus on restriction and consider outlet/stoma size (or caliber band) and pouch volume as the key. Others focus on malabsorption and address the bypass or Roux limb length. Abnormalities in any of these may be a reason for failure. As with initial bariatric surgery procedures, surgeons will have personal preferences for revisional procedures. There are data to support a variety of approaches.(2-5) This chapter will focus on anatomic reasons for failure and technical issues involved with revising these patients.

There are several major anatomic reasons why bariatric procedures can fail, including breakdown of previous restriction, such as staple-line disruption or anastomotic dilation, as well as complications such as band erosion, pouch dilation, or esophageal dilation. Patients may also seek revision for intolerance of existing anatomy, such as for reflux or obstruction symptoms. We will try to focus on reasons that may lead to inadequate weight loss, or weight regain.

Any discussion of inadequate weight loss needs to first define what it is. For the purpose of our discussion, we will consider excess weight loss of 50% at least 1 year postoperatively, as the cut-off for adequate weight loss. Patients who lose less than this should be evaluated for possible reasons of failure. They should undergo a thorough nutritional assessment, including a calorie count for both quantity and quality. A contrast upper gastrointestinal (upper GI) series is the most helpful test, as it can delineate normal or abnormal anatomy. This is essential if the patient underwent surgery somewhere else. Endoscopy can also be helpful to evaluate stoma size and assess for erosion of a band, if present. We will discuss some of the pathology that may be encountered during this work-up.

## Gastric Pouch Evaluation by Upper GI Contrast Study

We really don't have data to prove what the ideal pouch size needs to be to have successful weight loss and maintenance of that weight loss. Many people put it around the 60-mL size for a pouch, but some will claim it needs to be in the 15 to 30-mL range. Either way, that is not something that is strongly proven in the surgical literature. Figure 1 depicts normal Roux-en-Y gastric bypass (RYGB) anatomy.

**Figure 1**

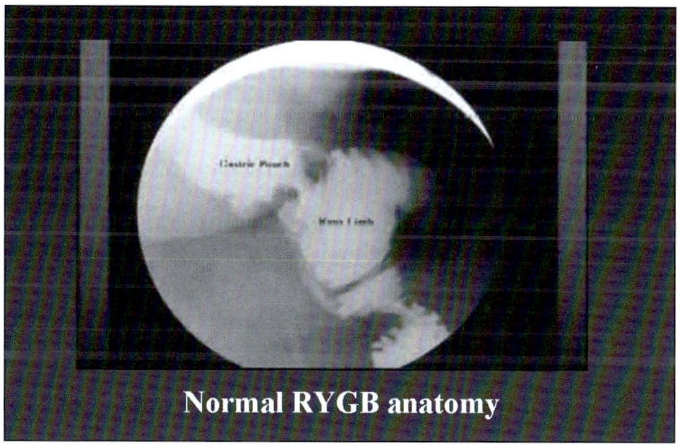


This demonstrates an upper GI contrast study of normal postoperative gastric bypass anatomy.
Note the very small gastric pouch and small gastrojejunostomy orifice between that and the roux limb.

**Gastro-gastric fistula**

**Figure 2a**

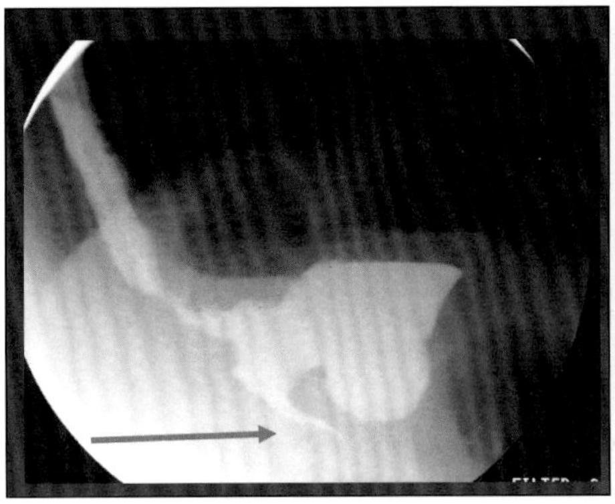

**Figure 2b**

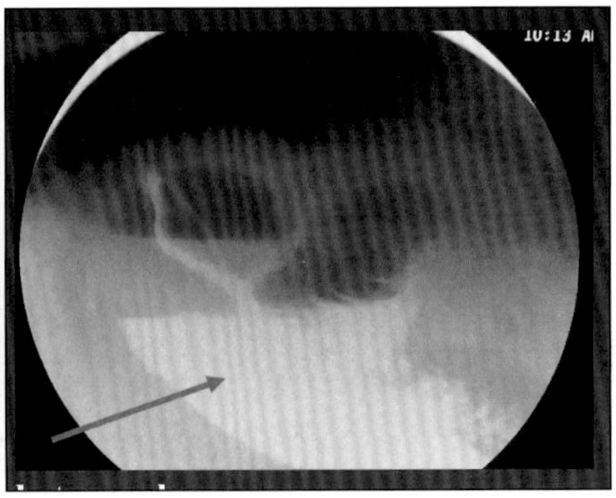

**Figure 2a**

This is an upper GI series of a patient with a gastro-gastric fistula. The tongue off the pouch is the fistula tract.

**Figure 2b**

This is a delayed image of the same patient. The contrast was followed from the tongue by the pouch in Figure 2a into the distal stomach. This ultimately proved to be a connection to the distal stomach.

In a nondivided stomach, you'd call it a staple-line disruption. Although it is logical that a patient with a gastro-gastric fistula (GGF) can overeat the size of his/her pouch, it's not always a reason for failure.(6) Nevertheless, if a patient with failure presents with a fistula, he/she should be revised. In this situation, when revisional surgery is undertaken, we believe there's a need to retransect the pouch, and that it's important to try to do this so that you do not leave an isolated portion of gastric pouch or stomach. If you leave isolated stomach you can get a phenomenon called sequestrum of the stomach, where that isolated piece of stomach can secrete and actually become dilated over time. We have seen a patient like this in our practice; it is very difficult to manage over a long period of time.

**Revisional Procedures and Controversies**

For an evidence-based discussion of revisional surgery after gastric bypass, the state-of-the-art, we must go fairly far back in the literature to a series by Schwartz's group(1). This involved 900 initial cases and 42 revisions over a 10-year period. Some of the reasons for revision included: dilated stoma in 16 cases, 10 patients who had inadequate weight loss but anatomy intact, 6 staple-line disruptions, 4 obstructions, 4 anastomosic leaks, and 2 enlarged pouches—all at nearly 2 years of follow-up after the original procedure. If you go back to this cohort of information, initial surgery complications were very common in the 61% of patients who needed revision. Outlet obstructions, staple-line disruptions, leaks and bowel obstruction were particularly frequent causes of ultimate revisional surgery. In 20 cases, the procedure was completely redone. In 17 redos of the gastrojejunal anastomosis alone, the stomach was restapled in 4 cases and an intraoperative dilatation of a resistant stricture was done in one. A 50% major complication rate was shown. Although this was a different era, there's significant room for improvement. Ten ultimate obstructions, 4 anastomotic leaks out of 42 (10%)—that's not far off from what we know happens today. Further, there were two subsequent staple-line disruptions and a death from a pulmonary embolus. Nine of the 42 patients needed more than one reoperation to correct problems. Here's the really bad news—when they looked at weight loss beyond 6 months after the revision, the initial weight loss from the original procedure was 49% vs. 51% at 2 years. Revision in this group did not provide subsequent weight loss(1), again, a real caution. What is the benefit, what is the risk? Conclusions that still hold today are that there is a high rate of major complication with revisional surgery and inadequate subsequent weight loss for many patients. This is why it's key to select the right patient and the right revisional operation.

**Conversion to a Distal Gastric Bypass**

So, what should you do with intact anatomy after a gastric bypass? In Schwartz's study they actually did a revision of the gastric bypass itself.(1) To us, that did not seem like the optimal approach when the anatomy is intact. We have used conversion to distal gastric bypass, which is based on a biliary pancreatic diversion procedure.(7) Again, this depends on compliance of the patient. We want a documented history of the patient's compliance with treatment. We are motivated in making the decision for surgery by the persistence of serious comorbidity. In other words, these are not the patients who come in and say, "You know, I just can't lose that extra 20 pounds and I don't look good in a bathing suit." This is a bad choice for patients like that. So, we're motivated by comorbidity and are aware that distal gastric bypass conversion carries a significant risk of malnutrition.(8)

**Figure 3**

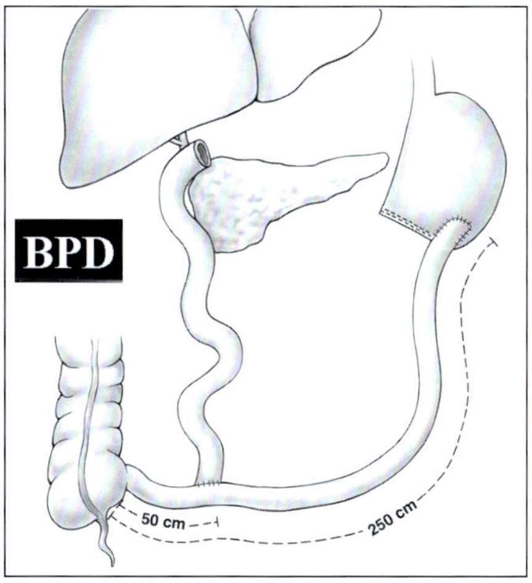


Biliopancreatic diversion (BPD) anatomy: a large gastric pouch is left and the remainder of the stomach removed. The small bowel is dived 250 cm proximal to the ileocecal valve and anastomosed to the stomach. The biliopancreatic limb is then anastomosed to the distal small bowel 50 cm proximal to the ileocecal valve to create a short common channel.

Here is the basis for the concept of distal gastric bypass: Figure 3 depicts biliopancreatic diversion (BPD) anatomy. This has a much larger pouch than after a gastric bypass and we do not recreate a pouch when we perform a distal gastric bypass conversion. Considering that a RYGB pouch is much smaller than a BPD pouch, we think it's important to lengthen the common channel with the revision operation to avoid nutritional problems. In other words, do not create very restrictive, proximal anatomy with very malabsorptive distal anatomy because, in our experience, the risk of protein-calorie malnutrition is prohibitively high. When this operation is used selectively, we have demonstrated good results.

### Vertical Banded Gastroplasty to RYGB

We also have experience with 58 conversions of failed vertical banded gastroplasty (VBG) to gastric bypass.(9) Fifteen of these were for weight loss failures and 43 were for other complications of VBG, such as leaks, band erosions, staple-line disruptions, and resistant stenoses with obstruction. The operative technique for revising a VBG to a gastric bypass initially involves encircling the esophagus to get exposure to the pouch. Then it becomes a matter of strategy as to what the anatomy is at the time of the revisional procedure. When we're faced with a small pouch that's intact and associated with band erosion, it's important to do the dissection and reopen the end-to-end anastomosis (EEA) window from the VBG. Then you remove the band and staple and transect the stoma. The small pouch is then used for subsequent anastomosis. It is important to confirm that it is isolated by multiple staple firings. In the case of a large dilated VBG pouch, or no pouch at all (which is very common when patients have had a previous horizontal gastroplasty which tends to just fall apart completely over time), we open the lesser curve and restaple the stomach. (Figures 4 and 5)

Figure 4

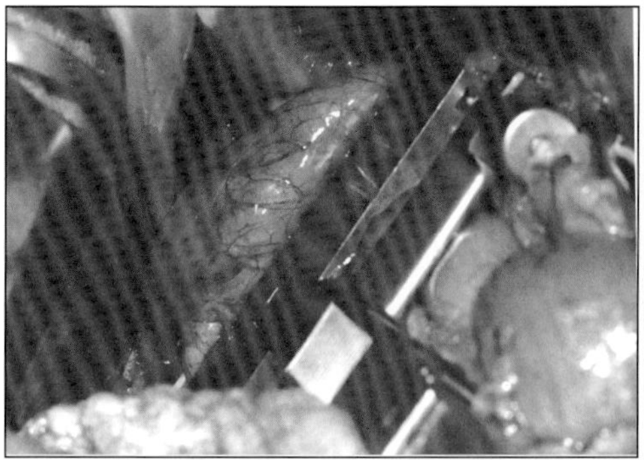

Figure 5

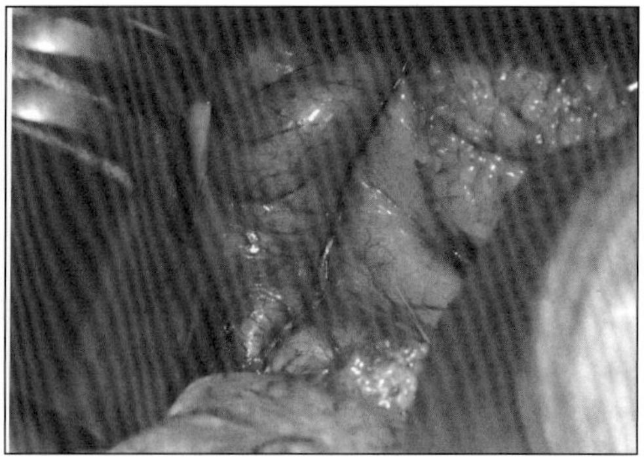

**Figure 4**

Schematic depicting the transaction line when converting a VBG to Roux-en-Y gastric bypass

**Figure 5**

Neo-pouch formed in converting a VBG to RYGB

This leaves a small pouch with the remainder of the stomach intact. In this situation, it is not necessary to remove the band. If the band is intact, we believe in disruption of the band if it's technically feasible (Figure 6).

**Figure 6**

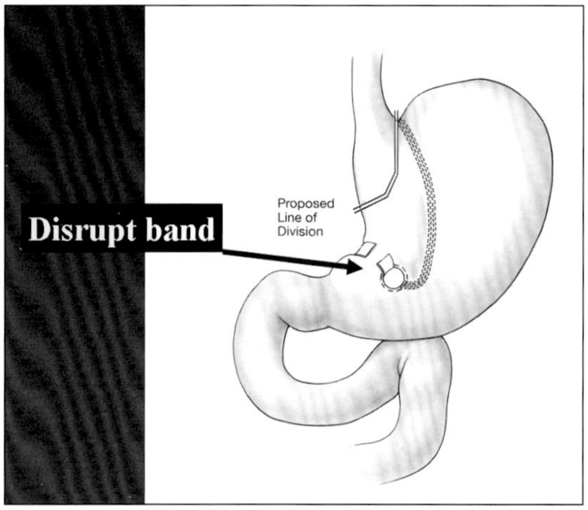


If the band is intact following a VBG, it must be disrupted or removed at the time of conversion to prevent a gastric sequestrum.

To do that, we restaple the stomach and transect to confirm the disruption. The distal stomach will then drain appropriately, and we do the RYGB anastomosis to this neo-pouch (Figure 7).

**Figure 7**

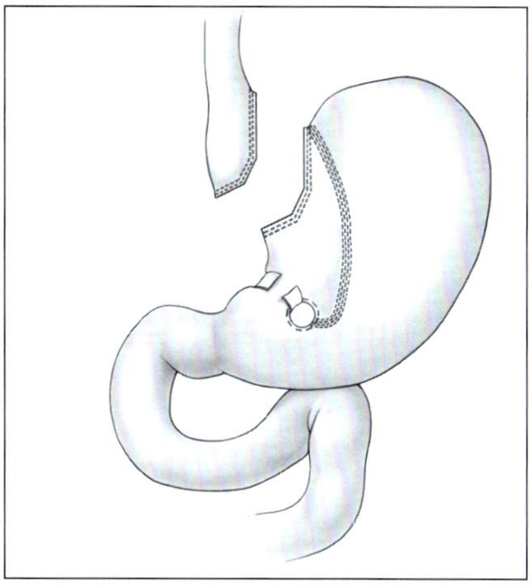

Anatomy following revision of a VBG to RYGB

If you are dissecting out staple lines, you need to try to superimpose your staple lines to avoid a gastric sequestrum. We recommend intraoperative endoscopy, or at least a methylene blue leak test due to a much higher instance of anastomotic leak in revisional cases. Patients will do better if you pick up leaks intraoperatively. In difficult or open revisions, we often place a gastrostomy tube, particularly when there is significant lysis of adhesions, to help prevent distal gastric blowout from ileus or obstruction.

In our experience with these 58 patients, we fortunately had no mortality, but we did have complications in nearly half of our patients. We had a leak from the bypassed stomach, we had 3 disruptions of the vertical staple line, and we had 20 stomal stenoses, and 3 bowel obstructions. As compared with Schwartz's weight loss,(1) when you do take the patient through the risky procedure of going from vertical-banded-gastroplasty failure to gastric bypass, you do see additional weight loss. This was confirmed by others, as well.(10-13) Our patients had only one third of excess weight loss after the VBG and, after a gastric bypass conversion, lost the fairly typical amount of two thirds excess body weight in up to 8 years following the procedure. Particularly rewarding was our cohort of sweets eaters who, obviously, didn't do well with the VBG restrictive procedure, but lost weight just like any gastric bypass patient would be expected to lose weight.

### Laparoscopic Revisional Surgery

There are varieties of laparoscopic revisional procedures that are reported in the literature (14-20) and that we have experience with. We've repaired internal hernias, transected gastro-gastric fistulas and had the opportunity to convert many loop gastric bypasses to RYGBs. We've done LAP-BAND removal procedures and converted bands to gastric bypasses. In many ways, we consider the lap band to be the new VBG. The benefit of the LAP-BAND is that it's a lot easier to technically convert.

### LAP-BAND to Gastric Bypass

In our experience with converting LAP-BAND to gastric bypass, we've seen complications at the rate we would have predicted with any revisional surgery. In other words, higher than the original procedure's complication rate. Out of 19 conversions, we had 3 intraoperative gastrojejunal leaks, 1 postoperative leak, and 1 reoperation for bleeding from a torn liver capsule; and, when we had to do open conversion, 3 of 5 patients had incisional hernias. So again, a spectrum of complications and incidence of complications that is not unusual for patients who are having revisional surgery. But again, some positive information: when we had the LAP-BAND in place for an average of 34 months, the patients that were converted lost 19% of their excess weight; but when they had their gastric bypass conversion, they lost more weight and ended up losing about 61% of their total preoperative excess weight. So, there was a benefit to the conversion—it just came at a later time, after the gastric bypass. Figure 8 depicts an example of a LAP-BAND in place.

**Figure 8**

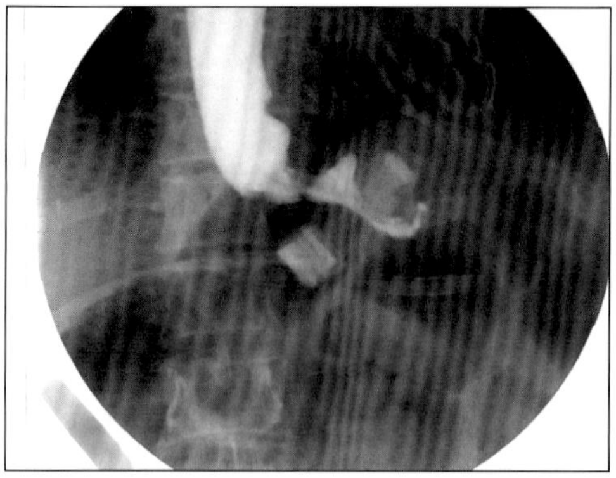

Appropriately positioned Lap Band

There is a unique issue with the LAP-BAND of dilated esophagus.

**Figure 9**

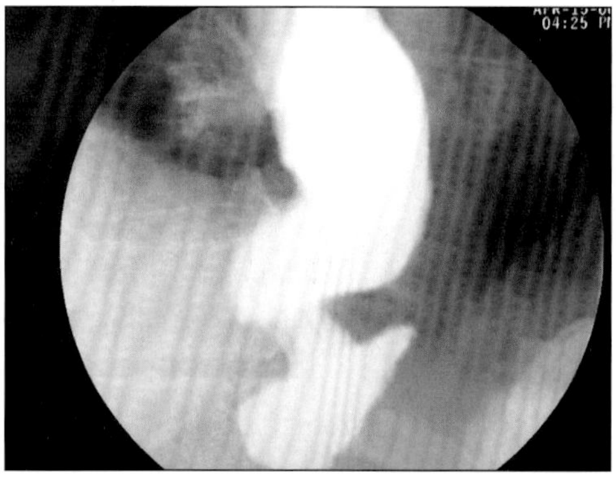

Dilated esophagus following Lap Band placement

In this case, we remove the band and perform gastric bypass with a fairly generous anastomosis. However, in the long-term follow-up, the esophageal dilatation does not always resolve (Figure 10), so the story is still unclear as to what will happen to these patients.

**Figure 10**

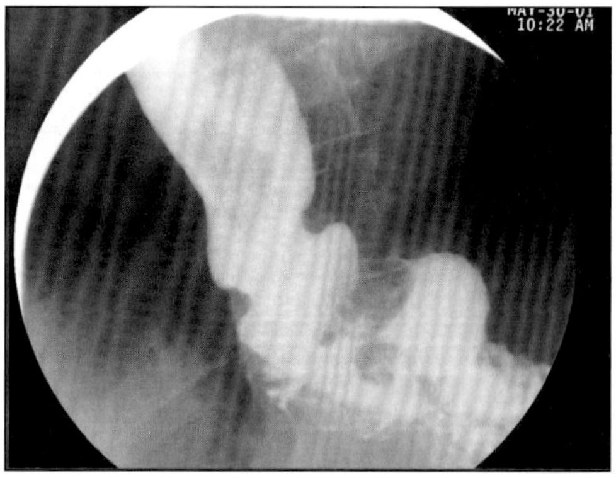


The same patient as in Figure 9 with dilated esophagus following LAP-BAND after conversion of the band to a RYGB

## Management of a Dilated Anastomosis

Dilated anastomosis is something that we really don't know what to do with and that a number of groups around the country are beginning to address through various mechanisms. There are people banding the gastric pouch.(3,21) We have sclerosing interventions that utilize the gastroscope aimed at sclerosing the gastrojejunal anastomosis. There are even methods of endoluminal plication of the anastomosis, which seem to be very promising.(22,23) There are a tremendous number of patients who are in this situation. When we've hinted to our support groups (which was a mistake) that we might be able to deal with dilated anastomosis using some newer techniques, we were flooded with e-mails and phone calls. Since nearly 10% of gastric bypass patients have potential failure, and we follow a population of 4,000 patients, that adds up to a lot of phone calls about this problem. Patients intuitively believe it's the loss of restriction that causes their problems in the long term. "I can eat whatever I want now…I can eat as much as I want now." That's what they say over and over again. So, it may be an overly simplistic solution to recreate the restriction of the procedure, but the fact is that patients easily buy into its value.

Let's discuss a case with a dilated pouch (Figure 11).

**Figure 11**

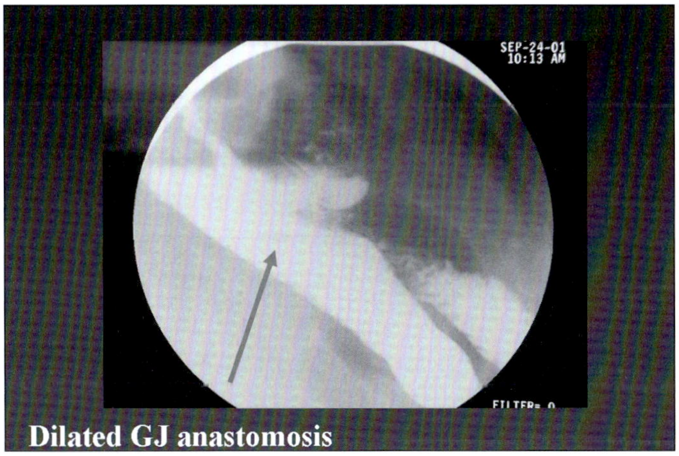


Dilated gastrojejunostomy: the lumen size remains constant from the gastric pouch and into the small bowel

You can almost not see where the anastomosis is. It's in the 2.0 to 2.5-cm range on this upper GI series. The concept has been vetted to "reconstrict" or "rerestrict" these patients, and we've actually done one case where we've banded the pouch using the laparoscopic adjustable gastric band.

**Figure 12**

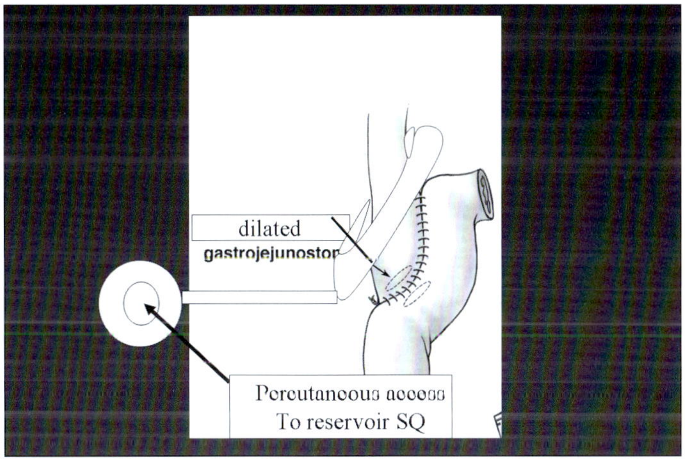


Banding the pouch and gastrojejunostomy: an adjustable gastric band can provide added restriction to a dilated pouch or stoma.

Figure 12 depicts a schematic for banding the pouch. There are many unanswered questions for banding in this situation. How do you secure the band? How do you prevent slippage of the pouch or even Roux limb through the band? In our case, we chose to ignore all those questions and just put a band around the pouch in a gentleman who had lost 150 lbs from a super-obese baseline. He weighed more than 500 lbs. This is a gentleman who's been very compliant all the way down the line with eating behavior, follow-up appointments, and even had a pool installed in his backyard so he could exercise. So, 18 months ago when we did his revisional operation, he was still about 400 lbs. Since then, he's lost another 70 lbs with banding his pouch. There are others who have more experience in this area, but it does appear to be a lower-risk form of revisional surgery.(3,21)

### Gastric Bypass Reversal

We should also mention reversal of gastric bypass. In general, this is a problem with poor patient selection rather than technical failure. In a cohort of patients that number more than 5,000 between Medical College of Virginia and Duke over the course of 20 years, I am aware of four reversals in our hands. I can't say what has happened to patients who have gone to other providers, but this is something that, unfortunately, we hear about fairly often these days. "The patient didn't tolerate the procedure and insisted on a reversal." This is something that I would urge great caution in deciding to do as a surgeon. I think this should be a very rare intervention. The reason for this is that, although we do encounter patients who have intolerances to the procedure, particularly during the first months or year after the procedure, almost invariably they can be counseled through this period. We have put patients on intravenous nutrition and we have used enteral nutrition during this period of time. But, it is a risky proposal to reverse the procedure, particularly following transection of the stomach, which is much more difficult to reverse than a nontransected, nondivided gastric pouch. Therefore, we really lean in the direction of counseling the eating behavior, with a lot of handholding, frequent contacts with the patient, and a lot of instruction.

From personal experience, we can provide insight into three of these cases. The first case is a patient who had a major small-bowel infarction from an internal hernia. She simply could not overcome the restriction of her small gastric pouch to eat enough to absorb adequate nutrition; we had to reverse her procedure. The other two were psychologically unable to cope with gastric bypass and should never have undergone the initial operation. Unfortunately, that is something that you will identify in a busy practice of bariatric surgery. This again illustrates the importance of careful patient selection. Unfortunately, one of these conversion patients died from complications of a postoperative leak. Reversals are not benign.

In summary, when we talk about revisional bariatric surgery, it's hard to give an evidence-based presentation, because there really aren't many large series out there. Yet it's something to never underestimate. Always be cautious in the patient selection. During the informed-consent discussion, make sure that you're very clear about the dramatically higher risks for revisional procedures. It's important to understand what failed or how the patient failed before you offer the intervention. Again, many times when you see patients who aren't doing well, it has nothing to do with the anatomy of the operation, but rather the behavior of the patient. Know your patients; know their compliance; know their comorbidity. Be motivated, I think, to offer this surgery by the comorbidity rather than any other issues, such as cosmesis. Again, beware the informed consent process. If you think that you've offered detailed informed consent to a routine bariatric surgery patient, multiply that process two- or threefold. Make it a repeat-visit scenario with the revisional patients so that you're sure and very clear with the risk-profile information.

### References:

1. Schwartz RW, Strodel WE, Simpson WS, Griffen WO Jr. Gastric bypass revision: lessons learned from 920 cases. *Surgery*. 1988;104(4):806-12.
2. Slater GH, Fielding GA. Combining laparoscopic adjustable gastric banding and biliopancreatic diversion after failed bariatric surgery. *Obes Surg*. 2004;14(5):677-82.
3. Bessler M, Daud A, DiGiorgi MF, Olivero-Rivera L, Davis D. Adjustable gastric banding as a revisional bariatric procedure after failed gastric bypass. *Obes Surg*. 2005;15(10):1443-8.
4. Keshishian A, Zahriya K, Hartoonian T, Ayagian C. Duodenal switch is a safe operation for patients who have failed other bariatric operations. *Obes Surg*. 2004;14(9):1187-92.
5. Martin MJ, Mullenix PS, Steele SR, See CS, et al. A case-matched analysis of failed prior bariatric procedures converted to resectional gastric bypass. *Am J Surg*. 2004;187(5):666-70; discussion 670-1.
6. Stanczyk M, Deveney CW, Traxler SA, et al. Gastro-gastric fistula in the era of divided Roux-en-Y gastric bypass: strategies for prevention, diagnosis and management. *Obes Surg*. 2006; 16(3):359-64.
7. Sugerman HJ, Kellum JM, DeMaria EJ. Conversion of proximal to distal gastric bypass for failed gastric bypass for superobesity. *J Gastrointest Surg*. 1997;1(6):517-24; discussion 524-6.

8. Fobi MA, Lee H, Igwe D Jr, et al. Revision of failed gastric bypass to distal Roux-en-Y gastric bypass: a review of 65 cases. *Obes Surg*. 2001;11(2):190-5.

9. Sugerman J, Kellum JM, DeMaria E. Conversion of failed or complicated vertical banded gastroplasty to gastric bypass in morbid obesity. *Am J Surg*. 1996;171(2):263-9.

10. Roller J, Provost DA. Revision of failed gastric restrictive operations to Roux-en-Y gastric bypass: Impact of multiple prior bariatric operations on outcome. *Obes Surg*. 2006;16:865-9.

11. Buckwalter JA, Herbst CA Jr, Khouri RK. Morbid obesity. Second gastric operations for poor weight loss. *Am Surg*. 1985;51(4):208-11.

12. Gonzalez R, Gallagher SF, Haines K, Murr MM. Operative technique for converting a failed vertical banded gastroplasty to Roux-en-Y gastric bypass. *J Am Coll Surg*. 2005;201(3):366-74.

13. van Gemert WG, van Wersch MM, Greve JW, Soeters PB. Revisional surgery after failed vertical banded gastroplasty: restoration of vertical banded gastroplasty or conversion to gastric bypass. *Obes Surg*. 1998;8(1):21-8.

14. Calmes JM, Giusti V, Suter M. Reoperative laparoscopic Roux-en-Y gastric bypass: an experience with 49 cases. *Obes Surg*. 2005;15(3):316-22.

15. Cohen R, Pinheiro JS, Correa JL, Schiavon C. Laparoscopic revisional bariatric surgery: myths and facts. *Surg Endosc*. 2005;19(6):822-5.

16. de Csepel J, Nahouraii R, Gagner M. Laparoscopic gastric bypass as a reoperative bariatric surgery for failed open restrictive procedures. *Surg Endosc*. 2001;15(4):393-7.

17. Gagner M, Gentileschi P, deCsepel J, et al. Laparoscopic reoperative bariatric surgery: experience from 27 consecutive patients. *Obes Surg*. 2002;12(2):254-60.

18. Khaitan L, Van Sickle K, Gonzalez R, Lin E, et al. Laparoscopic revision of bariatric procedures: is it feasible? *Am Surg*. 2005;71(1):6-10; discussion 10-2.

19. McCormick JT, Papasavas PK, Caushaj PF, Gagné DJ. Laparoscopic revision of failed open bariatric procedures. *Surg Endosc*. 2003;17(3):413-5.

20. Müller MK, Wildi S, Scholz T, Clavien PA, Weber M. Laparoscopic pouch resizing and redo of gastro-jejunal anastomosis for pouch dilatation following gastric bypass. *Obes Surg*. 2005;15(8):1089-95.

21. Kyzer S, Raziel A, Landau O, Matz A, Charuzi I. Use of adjustable silicone gastric banding for revision of failed gastric bariatric operations. *Obes Surg*. 2001;11(1):66-9.

22. Schweitzer M. Endoscopic intraluminal suture plication of the gastric pouch and stoma in postoperative Roux-en-Y gastric bypass patients. *J Laparoendosc Adv Surg Tech A*. 2004;14(4):223-6.

23. Thompson CC, Slattery J, Bundga ME, Lautz DB. Peroral endoscopic reduction of dilated gastrojejunal anastomosis after Roux-en-Y gastric bypass: a possible new option for patients with weight regain. *Surg Endosc*. 2006;20(11):1744-8.

# Weight Loss Surgery and Pregnancy

Giselle Hamad, MD

The issue of pregnancy following bariatric surgery is important because the vast majority of patients who undergo bariatric surgery are women of childbearing age. Among the issues that will be discussed in this chapter include pregnancy-related complications seen in obesity, the effect of weight loss on fertility, the safety and optimal timing of pregnancy after bariatric surgery, and possible complications of concern in pregnant bariatric surgical patients.

The morbidly obese are prone to pregnancy-related comorbidities.(1) Some of these risks negatively impact gravid females in the antepartum period, such as gestational diabetes,(2) macrosomia, preeclampsia,(3) pregnancy-related venous thromboembolism,(4) stillbirth,(5) and hypertension, while others have an adverse effect on labor and delivery itself,(6) including the need for labor induction, meconium staining, cesarean delivery,(7) and wound complications.

Obesity is a common feature of polycystic ovary syndrome (PCOS). Associated menstrual irregularities and infertility are common. With surgically induced weight loss, fertility has been shown to improve. In a retrospective study by Eid et al, 24 women with PCOS who underwent gastric bypass were studied, and 81% had regulation of their menstrual cycle after 3 months.(8) One out of 4 who were previously infertile became pregnant 2-years postoperatively. Therefore, postoperative bariatric patients of reproductive age are at increased risk of becoming pregnant and must adhere to birth control practices during the period of rapid weight loss. In addition, the drastic weight loss resulting from bariatric surgery may exert harmful effects on the fetus. It is critical for the bariatric surgeon to discuss the importance of birth control for 18 to 24 months. A pregnancy test should be obtained preoperatively and on the day of surgery, in women of reproductive age.

There are data to support delaying pregnancy until after the period of rapid weight loss following gastric bypass. In a study of pregnancy after gastric bypass by Printen and Scott, 54 pregnancies were observed;(9) forty-six delivered, most within 2 years after the gastric bypass. There was a 4% incidence of spontaneous abortion and other severe complications, including premature delivery, microcephaly, and elective termination.

Weight loss may ameliorate some of the complications of pregnancy. Richards et al compared 57 pregnancies in gastric bypass patients with pregnancies in morbidly obese controls.(10) There was a lower incidence of hypertension and large-for-gestational-age infants in the mothers who had undergone bariatric surgery. The authors found no significant difference in the rate of pregnancy-related complications. In a study by Wittgrove et al, there was a lower incidence of pregnancy-related complications, including gestational diabetes and macrosomia, and a lower prevalence of cesarean sections compared with previous pregnancies from the preoperative period in the same patients.(11)

Pregnancy has been shown to be safe after restrictive procedures. In a study of patients undergoing vertical banded gastroplasty (VBG), there were 14 pregnancies in 9 patients.(12) Preoperatively, 7 out of 18 pregnancies ended in miscarriage prior to VBG, with 1 miscarriage from toxemia after VBG. Prior to VBG, 5 out of 6 women had pregnancy-related complications compared with one third who had complications after VBG.

In the setting of laparoscopic adjustable gastric banding (LAGB), the band may be deflated for patients having severe nausea or vomiting, or to avoid weight loss in the antepartum period. In a study of 20 women with 23 pregnancies who had undergone LAGB, there was 1 ectopic pregnancy, 2 elective abortions, and 2 spontaneous abortions.(13) Three of the patients required band deflation for nausea and vomiting. Two of those patients were observed to gain weight during their pregnancies. In another study of 7 unexpected pregnancies in LAGB patients, 2 women miscarried.(14) All bands were decompressed in order to manage nausea and vomiting. Two patients required reoperations during this period for either band erosion or a defect in the band. In a study from Australia of patients having LAGB, 79 postbanding pregnancies were compared with the patients' previous pregnancies, matched obese subjects, and community outcomes. Stillbirths, preterm deliveries, and abnormal birth weights were comparable with the community outcomes.

There are two large studies of pregnancy after malabsorptive procedures. In one study, 239 pregnancies were observed in more than 1,000 women with a mean weight gain of 6.2 kg.(15) Twenty-one percent of the patients required total parenteral nutrition (TPN), but the vast majority delivered full term, and about one third of them were small for gestational age. However, given that there were 73 abortions, 2 severe birth malformations, and 3 fetal deaths, these patients must be observed closely. In a study of 783 biliopancreatic diversion (BPD) patients by Marceau et al, nearly half had an improvement in fertility.(16) While there was a reduction in macrosomia and a normalization of birth weight, miscarriage occurred in 26%. These data provide further support of delaying pregnancy until weight stabilizes.

Sheiner et al reported on a population-based study comparing all pregnancies with and without previous bariatric surgery.(17) Out of a database of 159,000 pregnancies, there were 298 deliveries in bariatric surgery patients with a significant association between cesarean section and previous bariatric surgery, but overall, there was not an association with adverse outcome.

Bariatric surgery may result in nutritional deficiencies that can be deleterious to the developing fetus. Both obesity and bariatric surgery are risk factors for folate deficiency.(18,19) Folate deficiency can lead to neural tube defects, which can result in spina bifida and brain malformations such as anencephaly. In one case report, 3 out of 110 pregnancies or a sixfold risk increase in neural tube defects was observed after gastric bypass.(20) One woman had 2 miscarriages and 2 others had anencephalic fetuses. All of these women were noncompliant with their vitamin supplementation. Therefore, a patient considering pregnancy after bariatric surgery must be screened for folate deficiency and must be counseled about the importance of vitamin supplementation.

Following gastric bypass, premenopausal women are vulnerable to anemia, which may be exacerbated by pregnancy. Therefore, routine monitoring for vitamin $B_{12}$ and iron deficiency should be performed. Oral or parenteral supplementation may be indicated.

More recently, there have been reports of catastrophic consequences of internal herniation in pregnant patients.(21-23) Internal herniation is a complication that may elude diagnosis because of nonspecific signs and symptoms. Imaging studies such as CT and upper GI are often nondiagnostic. In the pregnant bariatric patient, abdominal pain may be erroneously dismissed as a common sequela of pregnancy. Unfortunately, internal herniation left unrecognized may result in intestinal ischemia and ultimately intestinal perforation, and may lead to the demise of the mother and/or fetus. Unexplained abdominal pain and persistent nausea and vomiting should raise the suspicion for internal herniation. CT scanning and exploratory laparotomy should be pursued aggressively.

In conclusion, there is a higher risk of becoming pregnant after bariatric surgery because of the improvement in fertility that accompanies weight loss. Patients should be counseled to use birth control during the period of rapid weight loss. Pregnant bariatric patients should be monitored very closely, especially for vitamin and mineral deficiencies. Finally, one must consider internal herniation in the differential diagnosis of a pregnant bariatric patient with abdominal pain.

**References**

1. Johnson JW, Longmate JA, Frentzen B. Excessive maternal weight and pregnancy outcome. *Am J Obstet Gynecol.* 1992;167(2):353-70; discussion 370-2.

2. Anderson JL, Waller DK, Canfield MA, Shaw GM, Watkins ML, Werler MM. Maternal obesity, gestational diabetes, and central nervous system birth defects. *Epidemiology*. 2005;16(1):87-92.

3. Bodnar LM, Ness RB, Markovic N, Roberts JM. The risk of preeclampsia rises with increasing prepregnancy body mass index. *Ann Epidemiol.* 2005;15(7):475-82.

4. James AH, Jamison MG, Brancazio LR, Myers ER. Venous thromboembolism during pregnancy and the postpartum period: incidence, risk factors, and mortality. *Am J Obstet Gynecol.* 2006;194(5):1311-5.

5. Kristensen J, Vestergaard M, Wisborg K, Kesmodel U, Secher NJ. Pre-pregnancy weight and the risk of stillbirth and neonatal death. *BJOG*. 2005;112(4):403-8.

6. Robinson HE, O'Connell CM, Joseph KS, McLeod NL. Maternal outcomes in pregnancies complicated by obesity. *Obstet Gynecol*. 2005;106(6):1357-64.

7. Dempsey JC, Ashiny Z, Qiu CF, Miller RS, Sorensen TK, Williams MA. Maternal pre-pregnancy overweight status and obesity as risk factors for cesarean delivery. *J Matern Fetal Neonatal Med*. 2005;17(3):179-85.

8. Eid GM, Cottam DR, Velcu LM, et al. Effective treatment of polycystic ovarian syndrome with Roux-en-Y gastric bypass. *Surg Obes Relat Dis*. 2005;1(2):77-80.

9. Printen KJ, Scott D. Pregnancy following gastric bypass for the treatment of morbid obesity. *Am Surg*. 1982;48(8):363-5.

10. Richards DS, Miller DK, Goodman GN. Pregnancy after gastric bypass for morbid obesity. *J Reprod Med*. 1987;32(3):172-6.

11. Wittgrove AC, Jester L, Wittgrove P, Clark GW. Pregnancy following gastric bypass for morbid obesity. *Obes Surg*. 1998;8(4):461-4; discussion 465-6.

12. Bilenka B, Ben-Shlomo I, Cozacov C, Gold CH, Zohar S. Fertility, miscarriage and pregnancy after vertical banded gastroplasty operation for morbid obesity. *Acta Obstet Gynecol Scand*. 1995;74(1):42-4.

13. Martin LF, Finigan KM, Nolan TE. Pregnancy after adjustable gastric banding. *Obstet Gynecol*. 2000;95(6 Pt 1):927-30.

14. Weiss HG, Nehoda H, Labeck B, Hourmont K, Marth C, Aigner F. Pregnancies after adjustable gastric banding. *Obes Surg*. 2001;11(3):303-6.

15. Friedman D, Cuneo S, Valenzano M, et al. Pregnancies in an 18-year follow-up after Biliopancreatic Diversion. *Obes Surg*. 1995;5(3):308-13.

16. Marceau P, Kaufman D, Biron S, et al. Outcome of pregnancies after biliopancreatic diversion. *Obes Surg*. 2004;14(3):318-24.

17. Sheiner E, Levy A, Silverberg D, et al. Pregnancy after bariatric surgery is not associated with adverse perinatal outcome. *Am J Obstet Gynecol*. 2004;190(5):1335-40.

18. Haddow JE, Hill LE, Kloza EM, Thanhauser D. Neural tube defects after gastric bypass. *Lancet*. 1986;1(8493):1330.

19. Werler MM, Louik C, Shapiro S, Mitchell AA. Prepregnant weight in relation to risk of neural tube defects. *JAMA*. 1996;275(14):1089-92.

20. Martin L, Chavez GF, Adams MJ Jr., et al. Gastric bypass surgery as maternal risk factor for neural tube defects. *Lancet*. 1988;1(8586):640-1.

21. Charles A, Domingo S, Goldfadden A, Fader J, Lampmann R, Mazzeo R. Small bowel ischemia after Roux-en-Y gastric bypass complicated by pregnancy: a case report. *Am Surg*. 2005;71(3):231-4.

22. Kakarla N, Dailey C, Marino T, Shikora SA, Chelmow D. Pregnancy after gastric bypass surgery and internal hernia formation. *Obstet Gynecol*. 2005;105(5 Pt 2):1195-8.

23. Moore KA, Ouyang DW, Whang EE. Maternal and fetal deaths after gastric bypass surgery for morbid obesity. *N Engl J Med*. 2004;351(7):721-2.

# Adolescent Bariatric Surgery Debate

Victor Garcia, MD

The central issue in the debate regarding bariatric surgery for adolescent patients is not so much whether the surgery should be performed on obese adolescents, but when, in the life course of the disease, it should be done. The closely related question is: what is the appropriate body mass index (BMI)/weight threshold for the adolescent, given the available treatment options and the relative ability to achieve and sustain a healthy weight? Adolescent obesity is arguably the most significant public health crisis, and the most serious nutritional disorder in children. It is my contention that, by postponing to a BMI of 50 kg/m$^2$ the application of what the available studies suggest is the most effective help for sustained weight loss, we are denying treatment and—for some with type 2 diabetes—inviting a crisis.

The available literature suggests that the BMI threshold proposed in guidelines developed by the panel of pediatric specialists, with interest in childhood obesity, increases the risk of procedure-related death and complications. Furthermore, at this higher BMI, we also increase the likelihood of a poor outcome in terms of achieved weight and increase the likelihood of weight regain, as well as the need for revisional surgery.

What is the context in which we should consider the aforementioned? Obesity, in its extreme, is chronic, progressive, and intractable. A longitudinal comparison of birth cohorts demonstrated that there is a progressive increase in BMI and that even among adolescents, this increase in BMI results in immediate, as well as long-term, health consequences. There was an association with premature mortality among those with higher BMIs, particularly minorities. Furthermore, it is well appreciated that children are the fastest growing segment of the obese population in the United States. An emerging body of evidence suggests that obesity-related metabolic disorders in adolescents have a shorter latency period compared with adults, and a younger age of onset. A group at Yale published, in the *New England Journal of Medicine*, their findings among a cohort of severely obese adolescents that 50% already have metabolic syndrome. The Bogalusa Heart Study demonstrated that a severely obese adolescent already has evidence of cardiovascular disease. Other investigators have suggested that the development and progression of metabolic syndrome may be a process more virulent than the course in adults. One study of Asian Americans noted evidence of retinopathy among patients newly diagnosed with type 2 diabetes related to obesity. Some would argue that the metabolic consequences of extreme obesity pale in comparison to the psychosocial and emotional consequences of being severely overweight—consequences that defy treatment and may leave an indelible mark on the adolescent.

With that as background, we now must examine the available treatment options, critically considering their relative efficacy and durability. Again, there is a robust body of literature that argues that there is no effective behavioral or pharmacological treatment for extreme obesity among adolescents. We often quote the work of Epstein et al that would suggest that children are more amenable to behavioral therapy. This indeed is the case with two notable exceptions: 1) there are very few, if any, adolescents in Epstein's cohort of patients, and 2) according to a personal communication from one of Epstein's coinvestigators, Holly Raynor, there were no adolescents who had more than 100 lbs excess weight over their ideal body weight. These two notable exceptions significantly limit the generalization of Epstein's findings with respect to the population of extremely obese adolescents.

We increasingly recognize that surgical weight loss achieves amelioration, if not a resolution of, most obesity-related comorbidities. What bears emphasis, however, are the studies demonstrating that for some conditions, particularly the metabolic disorders that have an earlier age of onset, the ability of surgical weight loss to ameliorate and resolve these comorbidities is dependent on the duration and the severity of the disease. The work of O'Brien, Dixon, and Schauer has demonstrated this, as far as diabetes is concerned.

As a result, in recognition of escalation and the severity of these health consequences, there has been a clamoring to perform bariatric surgery on children, as well as adolescents. Indeed, what served as a wake-up call for me was a comment that "guidelines were necessary," made at a recent meeting of the American College of Surgeons, where adult and pediatric surgeons were suggesting the merits of weight loss surgery for a morbidly obese 8-year-old child. This convinced me of the need for guidelines based on the best available evidence. Despite the absence of long-term data on the outcomes of weight loss surgery among adolescents, there must be an algorithm to inform the practitioner of who the appropriate candidates are and at what point in the life course of the disease the most effective way to achieve sustained weight loss should be considered.

Now, with regard to guidelines, a word should be mentioned about the need to conservatively restrict the application of this as-yet-unproven entity to those who really require the surgery and stand to benefit the most. The panel, of which I was a member, *arbitrarily* chose a BMI of 40 and 50. It could have been 40 and 45. The choice was not informed by a critical review of the existing bariatric surgical literature. Nor did we solicit or ultimately have input from experienced bariatric surgeons. In my role as a panel member, the clinical/surgical significance of a higher BMI was not evident—that a super-obese patient undergoing surgery had a significantly higher procedure-related mortality and risk of procedure-related complications.

In my view, conservative guidelines would have particular attributes. First, they would provide a complex procedure with a defined, procedure-related risk at a point in the life course of disease, when the risk of procedure-related complications is lowest; and second, they would suggest that procedure only when it is clear that medical therapy is either ineffective or its continuation is detrimental.

I think it's important to interject here that the adolescents that I would suggest we operate on are those who have significant comorbidities and, of their own volition, say that they want this operation. One comorbidity that is under-appreciated is the psychosocial consequences of being severely overweight. Some would argue that the psychosocial consequence is the most significant comorbidity of severe obesity in adolescents.

Second, with regard to guidelines, they should offer this procedure when the BMI/weight-related outcomes are likely to be the best possible; that is to say, when the endpoints of weight, resolution of symptoms, functional outcomes, and psychosocial quality of life have the best likelihood of being achieved and sustained. An additional interpretation of final BMI is that the endpoint BMI would be one associated with an improved actuarial risk, not one that would result in a persistent increase in actuarial risk of early or premature death. Furthermore, surgery would be performed when the likelihood of recidivism is lowest and there is little likelihood that subsequent Reoperative surgery would be required.

A word of caution, as far as guidelines are concerned! Healthcare payers look at guidelines as mandates, regardless of the intent of the developers of the guidelines. Per Bob Scalettar, corporate medical director of Anthem Blue Cross and Blue Shield, "We payers will employ guidelines as mandates and *not be receptive to independent inventions*." That is to say, even though the guidelines may suggest latitude in interpretation of a BMI threshold for surgery, the healthcare payer is not going to look very favorably upon paying for the operation for an obese adolescent presenting with a BMI of less than 40, regardless of accompanying comorbidities, and will contest the issue to no end. Guidelines from the healthcare payer's standpoint are different than guidelines from a clinician's standpoint.

In hindsight, the consensus panel guideline of a BMI of 50, in fact, defines a super-obese population; a population that the literature regards at increased risk of weight loss procedure-related death and complications. I contend that for the adolescent who must wait to reach that level of obesity to have bariatric surgery, we are unnecessarily exposing that child to increased risks. This is not opinion, but rather the inescapable conclusion drawn from the best available evidence. Higher BMI equates to poorer intermediate and long-term outcomes, increasing the need for revisional surgery to achieve a healthier weight/BMI and to deal with recidivism.

What does available evidence show? I've outlined here only a sample of the studies that have demonstrated that increasing BMI is not only a predictor, but also an independent risk factor, for operative mortality and morbidity, as well as a longer duration of operation and higher conversion rate. Dr. Shikora's report from his high-volume program found that for increasing BMI, more intestinal segments were required to be bypassed to achieve weight loss. This corroborates what I stated earlier. Pediatric healthcare specialists must be sensitive to this observation and to the implications for postponing weight loss surgery until a threshold of super obesity. By increasing the segments of intestine bypassed, you're increasing both the likelihood and consequences of postgastric bypass malnutrition. Furthermore, I also found it of interest that, for the first 100 cases in his practice, the mean BMI was 47. At our own institution, the mean BMI is 58. As an experienced bariatric surgeon, Dr. Shikora did not perform any laparoscopic bypass procedures in his early experience on patients with BMI of 55 or greater. In his discussion, he states that patient size contributes to the complexity of the operation. On a scale of 1 to 10, laparoscopic gastric bypass is viewed as a 9.5. It's an extraordinarily complex operation, and we should try to perform it only at a point in time when we can minimize the risk of complications, particularly for the adolescent population.

Also of note, is that the average age of adolescents undergoing bariatric surgery is 17 years. Given that the National Institutes of Health (NIH) consensus development conference panel's guidelines address patients 18 years and older, the adolescent desiring weight loss surgery could simply wait another year and have the operation at a lower BMI. I suggest that this probably prompts adolescents to gain weight so they can actually meet the arbitrary BMI criteria at an earlier age, rather than endure another year of stigmatization.

So, what do I conclude from this discussion? What does the best available evidence say about ultimate weight loss? What is again clearly shown by a number of studies is that the heavier the patient is at the time of surgery, the less the degree of total weight loss. Furthermore, the higher BMI lowers the likelihood that some of the obesity-related conditions will be ameliorated or resolved, and of particular concern is the likelihood of recidivism. That is, the chance of weight regain is significantly greater at the higher BMIs, particularly for patients with a BMI of 50. Bob Brolin's prospective study of patients with BMI 50 demonstrated that at 4 to 5 years after surgery, recidivism was common.

The super-obesity concept is nothing new; but patients who are super obese are a unique entity. It was Ed Mason, back in the 1980s, who actually defined super obesity. Since then, it has been demonstrated that these patients, because of their increased weight, lose a significantly lesser percentage of their excess weight after conventional Roux-en-Y gastric bypass and the likelihood of successfully maintaining that weight loss is significantly reduced. The point that's embedded in this statement is that in order to achieve ideal weight loss or increased weight loss, a more aggressive, more malabsorptive operation is required. Perhaps the reason the biliopancreatic duodenal switch operation came into vogue is because of this poor weight-response after standard Roux-en-Y gastric bypass.

What are the implications, then, considering this persistent actuarial risk? As a pediatric surgeon, you want to perform an operation that offers your patient the best likelihood of cure, because what you do will echo throughout your patient's life. Studies suggest that surgical weight loss improves survival. Fontaine's work has recently demonstrated that excessive weight, obesity, results in almost a 22% reduction in survival. That's of particular concern for minorities. We have also learned that this reduction in survival is something that affects a much younger group than we had presumed earlier. Add to that the fact that adolescents have an earlier age of onset and perhaps a more virulent disease process with a shorter latency period. We also recognize that surgery may improve their survival. So, what about the adolescent who is denied bariatric surgery until he/she is super obese? I submit that in all likelihood he/she will experience, as the data would suggest, suboptimal weight loss. In fact, we may be denying adolescents, as a result of pushing their surgery back to the BMI of 40 to 50, the survival benefits that bariatric surgery would promise.

The consequence of these more conservative guidelines is that we increase the risk for procedure-related complications and death. I think the literature is almost incontrovertible in that regard, showing that there is an increased risk of weight regain and ultimately of an even higher BMI. At that higher final BMI, the likelihood of recidivism is increased. Thus, we may in fact, be denying adolescents the survival advantages that bariatric surgery can offer.

Therefore, I would conclude that the best available evidence that we have, and we cannot wait for the best possible evidence, points to a crisis in adolescent obesity that represents a clear and present danger, arguing against a higher BMI threshold for adolescent bariatric surgery. The studies referenced in this volume suggest that, as a result of the complexity of the operation, a regionalization and evidence-based referral of adolescent patients should be the norm. In addition, I would enthusiastically support the use of Dr. David Flum's paradigm for capturing all patient information so that we have a national database. In this way, all adolescents undergoing bariatric surgery would be tracked; we will be able to accelerate our understanding of outcomes of this procedure that is so desperately needed by these patients.

**Suggested Reading**

1. Brolin RE. Bariatric surgery and long-term control of morbid obesity. *JAMA*. 2002;288(22):2793-6.
2. Christou NV, MacLean LD. Effect of bariatric surgery on long-term mortality. *Adv Surg*. 2005;39:165-79.
3. Flum DR, Dellinger EP. Impact of gastric bypass operation on survival: a population-based analysis. *J Am Coll Surg*. 2004;199(4):543-51.
4. Fontaine KR, Redden DT, Wang C, Westfall AO, Allison DB. Years of life lost due to obesity. *JAMA*. 2003;289(2):187-93.
5. Inge TH, Krebs NF, Garcia VF, et al. Bariatric surgery for severely overweight adolescents: concerns and recommendations. *Pediatrics*. 2004;114(1):217-23.
6. Mason EE, Doherty C, Maher JW, Scott DH, Rodriguez EM, Blommers TJ. Super obesity and gastric reduction procedures. *Gastroenterol Clin North Am*. 1987;16(3):495-502.
7. National Heart, Lung and Blood Institute. Bogalusa Heart Study. Tulane University; June 1972 – July 2002. New Orleans, La.
8. Shikora SA, Kim JJ, Tarnoff ME, Raskin E, Shore R. Laparoscopic Roux-en-Y Gastric Bypass: results and learning curve of a high-volume academic program. *Arch Surg*. 2005; 140(4): 362-7.
9. Weiss R, Dziura J, Burger TS, et al. Obesity and the metabolic syndrome in children and adolescents. *N Engl J Med*. 2004;350(23):2362-74.

# More Conservative Indications for Bariatric Surgery for Adolescent Patients

Thomas H. Inge, MD, PhD, FACS, FAAP

As the myriad benefits of surgical weight loss for morbidly obese adults have become evident, the need for similarly effective and durable weight loss options for morbidly obese adolescents has emerged. Although bariatric surgery offers undisputed benefits for severely obese adults, including resolution or amelioration of many health complications of long-standing obesity,(1) these benefits do not come without risks. The rationale for the operative criteria established by the 1991 National Institutes of Health (NIH) Consensus Development Conference specifically for adults(2) is based primarily upon the serious and significant short- and long-term health risks of morbid obesity. Use of surgery in adolescents was not addressed in the Conference, primarily due to the lack of information about the safety, effectiveness and need for such treatment options in adolescents over a decade ago. Since that time, however, the United States and much of the world has witnessed a progressive increase in the prevalence of obesity in all age groups, including adolescents.(3)

Adolescence is defined as the period of physical and psychological development from the onset of puberty to maturity, and typically encompasses ages 12 to 19. There is a growing recognition and concern about the short- and long-term complications of severe obesity in youth, including decreased longevity.(4) Due to the medical necessity for durable weight loss in severely affected adolescents, the medical community is faced with the need to define appropriate guidelines for implementing bariatric procedures in pediatric patients, as there is still only limited evidence to draw on for appropriate decision-making regarding weight loss surgery (WLS) in teens. In adults, bariatric surgery is commonly performed in those with a body mass index (BMI) $\geq$35 kg/m$^2$ with comorbidities of obesity, or a BMI $\geq$40 without comorbidities.(5) However, a more conservative approach, using higher BMI thresholds and the presence of comorbidities is justifiable for teenagers, as the risk-to-benefit ratio may be different than for adults, and adolescents will present with unique age-related metabolic, developmental, and psychological needs.

A number of valid concerns support the current use of more conservative patient selection criteria in adolescents. In contrast to adults, severely obese adolescents have, most commonly, not developed comorbidities of obesity that would justify surgery. When typical comorbidities of obesity *are* documented in severely obese adolescents, the lower severity of these comorbidities may not warrant surgical intervention, as other nonsurgical treatment interventions may be more appropriate. Compared with adults, BMI in pediatric patients less accurately predicts adiposity and, thus, obesity health risks, making it difficult to justify selection criteria for adolescents based solely on BMI thresholds. In addition, behavioral therapy approaches to weight management have been shown to be more effective in some children compared with adults(6), and a proportion (20% to 30%) of obese adolescents may not be destined to become obese adults.(7) The long-term outcomes of currently available surgical techniques for obesity in adolescents are unknown and surgical techniques for obesity treatment are rapidly evolving with less-risky and less-invasive surgical interventions expected in the near future.(8,9) Add to this the fact that adolescents may have different susceptibility to nutritional effects of gastric bypass surgery(10) and may be less apt to comply with important, life-long postoperative nutritional guidelines and medical visits after surgery,(11) which could increase the lifetime risk of significant nutritional disorders. Finally, there are few data in adults and no data in adolescents suggesting that surgical weight loss improves the early mortality suffered by those with severe obesity.

A group of pediatric specialists convened in January 2003 to consider how to safely introduce bariatric care to qualifying adolescents. That group consisted of 8 pediatric obesity treatment experts, 7 pediatric surgeons, a pediatric healthcare policy expert, and 4 obesity experts from federal agencies, including the NIH, the Centers for Disease Control and Prevention (CDC), and the Health Resources and Services Administration (HRSA). Also included were a representative from the American Pediatric Surgery Association and members of the American Academy of Pediatrics. The recommendations that were ultimately formed after this meeting were published in *Pediatrics*(12) and have been recognized and utilized by a number of groups, including the International Pediatric Endosurgical Group, the American Pediatric Surgery Association,(13) American Academy of Pediatrics, the American Heart Association,(14) the Agency for Healthcare Research and Quality (www.ahrq.gov), and the Betsy Lehman Center.(15) These expert recommendations were based on adult bariatric experience, as well as an understanding of the complexities of, and emerging problems associated with pediatric severe obesity. The recommendations confirm that bariatric surgery should be an option for carefully selected adolescents and they discuss the importance of thoughtful patient selection and both BMI- and comorbidity-based surgical indications. Morbidly obese teenagers (BMI ≥40) with comorbidities of obesity, who have completed linear growth, should be considered candidates for surgical weight loss (Figure 1). Based in part on the variability in physical and neurocognitive maturity level seen in adolescents, it was proposed that a multidisciplinary team, including pediatric, dietary, psychology, bariatric surgery, and exercise physiology expertise should evaluate each potential pediatric WLS candidate.

**Figure 1**

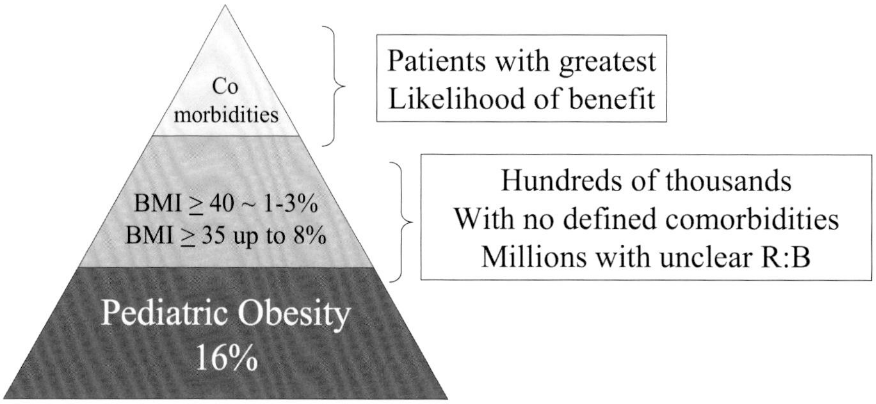


This group also recommended that there be failure of previous organized weight loss attempts before considering surgery. This is a difficult requirement, as it presumes that: 1) that effective, nonsurgical weight loss options exist for severely obese teenagers; and 2) patients have access to such services. In practice, neither is completely true for the vast majority of adolescents with severe obesity. However, because *some* severely obese patients can achieve weight loss with behavioral, dietary, and physical activity programs, it is both practical and necessary to recommend that surgical weight loss not be a first choice for the teen suffering from severe obesity, but that surgery be considered only after reasonable nonsurgical attempts at weight management have been exhausted.

If we were to adopt adult bariatric treatment guidelines for use in teenagers, a large number of pediatric patients without a defined health problem related to obesity may undergo bariatric procedures before risks and benefits are elucidated with clinical studies. Why is this issue an important consideration? When the 1991 NIH consensus development conference(5) proposed that adults with a BMI ≥ 40 should be eligible for WLS, it was done with the understanding that few, if any, adults with this degree of obesity have no comorbidities. On the other hand, it is not at all clear that the same obesity comorbidity burden is borne by adolescents who have achieved a BMI of 40. Thus, if we use adult guidelines and propose that adolescents with BMI ≥40 without comorbidities should be eligible for WLS, we may find that the great majority of teenagers who undergo WLS do not have medical necessity for this intervention. Indeed, there may be hundreds of thousands of adolescents with no, or only minor, comorbidities who might undergo surgical therapy before optimal patient management algorithms are developed and outcomes are completely understood (Figure 2). Stated another way, there may be millions with an unclear risk-to-benefit ratio for bariatric interventions. While surgical weight loss may well be justified based on poor self-image, poor quality of life, and/or depression or social stigmatization, we must also recognize that for adolescents, there are as yet no data to support efficacy of WLS for these psychosocial comorbidities.

Until comparisons of adult and adolescent outcomes of bariatric surgery can be made, substantial caution must be used when extrapolating adult guidelines and outcomes data to teenagers. Use of less stringent adult operative criteria (e.g., lower

BMI thresholds, no requirement for obesity-related comorbidity) as proposed by some(16,17) instead of the more conservative criteria proposed for adolescents,(12-15,18) could result in far greater numbers of adolescents potentially undergoing surgical procedures for weight loss before appropriately designed, prospective studies are conducted to better define best operative procedure, postoperative management (including managing difficult problems with adherence to nutritional supplements), benefits, and risks. Plans to investigate these important surgical outcomes questions now exist. A multicenter, NIH-sponsored, clinical research initiative to document longitudinal outcomes for adolescents undergoing bariatric surgery (Teen-LABS), launched in fall of 2006, will collect data until 2011. The goal of this project (led by the pediatric-bariatric research group at Cincinnati Children's Hospital) is to begin to understand differences between adults and teenagers undergoing bariatric surgery, as well as to define benefits and risks for adolescents. The research is conducted in parallel with the NIH adult bariatric consortium's project entitled Longitudinal Assessment of Bariatric Surgery (LABS). Adolescent outcomes stratified by preoperative BMI is one important aspect of the study, which should bring solid data to bear on BMI-based indications for WLS in teenagers.

Finally, the use of general recommendations for treatment of patients suffering from any disease should be viewed only as a starting point for decision-making. The myriad benefits of bariatric surgery should not be denied to an individual (adult or teenager) in whom benefits of the intervention are judged to outweigh risks. Indeed, there will be adolescent patients who do not fit guideline criteria for surgery and others who *do* meet the guidelines and yet, should not undergo surgery. A multidisciplinary team (including pediatric and bariatric experts) should thoughtfully weigh the pros and cons of keeping the individual adolescent's best interests in mind before offering a surgical procedure. If our supposition that offering bariatric surgery to adolescents has net benefits, this should become readily evident through outcomes research in the near future, and guidelines will likely change based on such scientific evidence.

**Figure 2**

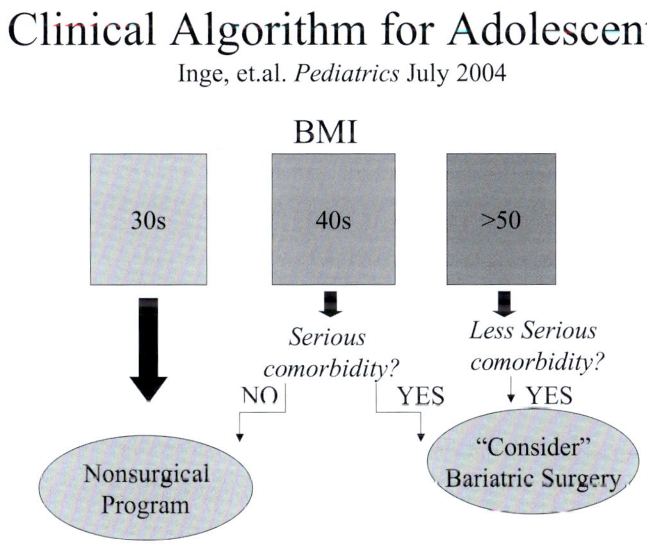

## References


1. Buchwald H, Avidor Y, Braunwald E, Jensen MD, Pories W, Fahrbach K, et al. Bariatric surgery: a systematic review and meta-analysis. *JAMA*. 2004;292(14):1724-37.
2. Gastrointestinal surgery for severe obesity: National Institutes of Health Consensus Development Conference Statement. *Am J Clin Nutr*. 1992;55(2 suppl):S615-S619.
3. Troiano RP, Flegal KM. Overweight children and adolescents: description, epidemiology, and demographics. *Pediatrics*. 1998;101(3 Pt 2):497-504.
4. Engeland A, Bjorge T, Sogaard AJ, Tverdal A. Body mass index in adolescence in relation to total mortality: 32-year follow-up of 227,000 Norwegian boys and girls. *Am J Epidemiol*. 2003;157(6):517-23.
5. Gastrointestinal surgery for severe obesity. Proceedings of a National Institutes of Health Consensus Development Conference. March 25-27, 1991, Bethesda, MD. *Am J Clin Nutr*. 1992;55(2 suppl):S487-S619.
6. Epstein LH, Valoski A, Wing RR, McCurley J. Ten-year follow-up of behavioral, family-based treatment for obese children. *JAMA*. 1990;264(19):2519-23.
7. Whitaker RC, Wright JA, Pepe MS, Seidel KD, Dietz WH. Predicting obesity in young adulthood from childhood and parental obesity. *N Engl J Med*. 1997;337(13):869-73.
8. Shikora SA. Implantable gastric stimulation for weight loss. *J Gastrointest Surg*. 2004;8(4):408-12.
9. Dolan K, Creighton L, Hopkins G, Fielding G. Laparoscopic gastric banding in morbidly obese adolescents. *Obes Surg*. 2003;13(1):101-4.
10. Towbin A, Inge TH, Garcia VF, Roehrig HR, Clements RH, et al. Beriberi after gastric bypass surgery in adolescence. *J Pediatr*. 2004;145(2):263-7.
11. Rand CS, Macgregor AM. Adolescents having obesity surgery: a 6-year follow-up. *South Med J*. 1994;87(12):1208-13.
12. Inge TH, Krebs NF, Garcia VF, et al. Bariatric surgery for severely overweight adolescents: concerns and recommendations. *Pediatrics*. 2004;114(1):217-23.
13. Rodgers BM. Bariatric surgery for adolescents: a view from the American Pediatric Surgical Association. *Pediatrics*. 2004;114(1):255-6.
14. Daniels SR, Arnett DK, Eckel RH, et al. Overweight in children and adolescents: pathophysiology, consequences, prevention, and treatment. *Circulation*. 2005;111(15):1999-2012.
15. Apovian CM, Baker C, Ludwig DS, et al. Best practice guidelines in pediatric/adolescent weight loss surgery. *Obes Res*. 2005;13(2):274-82.
16. Wittgrove AC, Buchwald H, Sugerman H, Pories W. Surgery for severely obese adolescents: further insight from the American Society for Bariatric Surgery. *Pediatrics*. 2004;114(1):253-4.
17. Garcia VF, DeMaria EJ. Adolescent bariatric surgery: treatment delayed, treatment denied, a crisis invited. *Obes Surg*. 2006;16(1):1-4.
18. Inge TH, Garcia V, Daniels S, et al. A multidisciplinary approach to the adolescent bariatric surgical patient. *J Pediatr Surg*. 2004;39(3):442-7;discussion 446-7.

# Patient Outcomes: Collecting Data

Matthew M. Hutter, MD, MPH

Medical speakers often allude to the importance of data. Phrases such as, "The data show this," or "Data will be collected," or "The data will determine who will be accredited" express the impact that study numbers and measurements have on the medical sector. This chapter will focus on data collection itself—not what the outcomes specifically are, but how important data collection is, how it should be used to assess and improve quality and how it is going to be even more important for pay-for-performance or pay-for-participation initiatives and for accreditation.

**Why Data Should be Collected**

The primary reason to collect data is to measure and improve quality. However, another compelling reason is that you will have to collect it—due to regulations by the state or other regulating bodies and in order to comply with requests by insurers and payers for pay-for-performance contracts.

In the Commonwealth of Massachusetts, the Patient Care Assessment (PCA) arm of the Board of Registration in Medicine (BORM) requires the reporting of all major complications and deaths and the statistical collection of these reports, specifically for weight loss surgery (WLS). Regulatory bodies like the Department of Public Health request similar data. Insurance companies and payers have their own specific requests with regard to the reporting of surgical outcomes following WLS. Unfortunately, these multiple requests require filling out numerous different forms asking for similar information. As accreditation, pay-for-performance, and pay-for-participation initiatives come to play a greater role in coverage and reimbursement decisions, data collection and reporting will take on even more importance.

Assessing quality of care is imperative for continuous quality improvement. If you don't know how well you are doing, then you don't know where to focus your efforts and you don't know if your quality improvement initiatives are having an impact. Even in the absence of specific quality improvement initiatives, the simple act of looking at data leads to improvements over time—an observation that has come to be known as the Hawthorne Effect.

**Figure 1**

How do you measure the quality of surgical care? First you assess outcomes, then you analyze the data with risk adjustment, benchmarking and statistical analysis in order to ultimately determine the quality of surgical care.

| Surgical Outcomes = | Accounted for with: |
|---|---|
| Patient factors | *Risk adjustment* |
| + | |
| Treatment effectiveness | *Benchmarking* |
| + | |
| Quality of care | |
| + | |
| Random chance | *Statistical analysis* |

The key question remains: how do you measure quality and how is quality related to outcomes? Figure 1 outlines how surgical outcomes are impacted by a combination of factors, which include patient factors, treatment effectiveness, random chance, and the quality of care. Therefore, in order to isolate and evaluate quality of care, you have to accurately assess and record your outcomes and account for these factors. Patient factors can be accounted for with proper risk adjustment, which can take into account the fact that patients with certain characteristics (i.e., advanced age or comorbid conditions such as heart disease and diabetes) are more likely to have a complication or to die following a surgical operation. Treatment effectiveness can best be accounted for with benchmarking. If the outcome you are measuring is mortality rate, then knowing the national average for the death rate for that procedure is an important determinant of an expected mortality rate. For example, if the death rate was 1%, you would not know if that is high or low unless you had something to compare it with. Thus, benchmarking is critical.

Random chance can be accounted for with appropriate statistical analysis, which includes the evaluation for type I and type II errors. Appropriate statistical analysis is important, but even more important is the task of drawing responsible conclusions from the analysis of these data. Statistically significant findings and clinically significant findings can be two different things and many factors—especially the sample size—must be taken into consideration when deciding what constitutes a meaningful finding. Differentiating a real finding from random variation or noise is crucial in the determination of what constitutes an outlier. Therefore, by assessing surgical outcomes with appropriate risk adjustment, benchmarking, and statistical analyses, one can begin to measure the quality of care.

What is the evidence that data collection would improve the quality for weight loss surgery? The Patient Safety in Obesity Surgery: Defining Best Practices conference produced numerous reports about what the data actually are. Studies include both single-institution and multi-institution studies.(1-3) Studies from the International Bariatric Surgery Registry, the Swedish Obese Subjects Study Group, and the National Surgical Quality Improvement Program (NSQIP) have been reported, and currently the National Institutes of Health Longitudinal Assessment of Bariatric Surgery (NIH LABS) consortium is collecting results.(4-7) Administrative data sets, claims data, and population-based studies have been reported, including results from the National Inpatient Sample, the Office of Statewide Health Planning Database in California, Washington State discharge abstracts, the University Health Consortium, Canadian Health, Medicare and MarketScan, and meta-analyses of these studies.(8-15) But do these studies actually assess whether data collection will make a difference or not? No. There's no evidence specific to WLS proving that collecting data is going to make a difference.

Why, then, should we do it? Well, in addition to the fact that theoretically it makes sense, there is actually very good evidence from fields other than bariatric surgery that confirms this. In the area of cardiac surgery, data have been collected since the 1980s through statewide, regional, and national reporting. For cancer, there is the National Cancer Database and for thoracic surgery, the Society of Thoracic Surgeons (STS) database. Trauma has the National Trauma Databank, and for general and vascular surgery, the NSQIP, which was first started within the Veteran's Administration (VA), is being expanded to the private sector as a program with the American College of Surgeons (ACS), yielding an ACS NSQIP database.

The common result of all these multi-institutional, standardized data collection programs was a decrease in morbidity and mortality over time, after data collection was instituted. For example, in the 12 years following the collection of data at the VA with the NSQIP, there was a 34% reduction in mortality and 41% reduction in morbidity.(16) Similar findings have been seen in cardiac surgery in New York State and northern New England and in basically any large-scale, comprehensive, risk-adjusted surgical outcomes reporting system that has been developed.(17,18) Not only is there a decrease in morbidity and mortality, but over time there have been fewer high-outlier institutions with bad results. So, even though there are no data specifically from the field of bariatric surgery that assess whether data collection is helpful, there is good evidence from other surgical fields that it can improve quality.

**Determining the Data to be Collected**

Once it has been decided that data should be collected, the next step is to decide which data to collect. From the onset, one must decide on what the goal is—specifically, whether the data are to be used for research, quality improvement, public health considerations, or potentially for a combination of all the above. An integral part of the decision of what to collect must be the recognition of what realistically *can* be collected, and the availability of the resources required to actually collect the data.

For bariatric surgery, data points should include preoperative factors, intraoperative factors, and postoperative occurrences, as well as long-term results, including efficacy of the procedure with regard to weight loss and reduction of comorbidities. Preoperative variables are necessary for risk adjustment and to get a baseline to track comorbidities over time. Risk adjustment is critical. Without risk adjustment, any discussion of the results is going to be limited by the comment, "But *my* patients are sicker!" Risk adjustment is crucial to allow surgeons to accept some of the more challenging cases without being penalized, and to provide access of care to the people who most need it. Comorbid conditions in bariatric surgery include obstructive sleep apnea, diabetes, cardiovascular disease, reflux disease, hypertension, gallstone disease, arthritis, stress incontinence, and many more. Intraoperative variables include the type of operation performed, the level of training of the assistant, and process measures of what happens in the operating room. Outcomes must include not only 30-day complication rates and mortality, but also bariatric-specific complications like anastomotic leaks, internal hernias, stomal stenoses, marginal ulcers or band slippage. A reliable way to assess postoperative occurrences might be to document specific interventions or reoperations. Readmissions to the hospital or admission to the intensive care unit from the floor could also be markers of untoward events. Long-term endpoints, including late complications like hernias, bowel obstruction, or need for revisional surgery, as well as documented weight loss and reduction of comorbidities must be tracked as well. Follow-up is critical. If the patient isn't following up with the surgeon, then attempts to reach the patient must be documented, and whether the patient is following up with another weight loss physician must be ascertained.

**Data Collection**

It is critical that good data be used in order to arrive at accurate conclusions. The phrase "garbage in—garbage out" is quite applicable to the collection of data. If you collect bad data, you're going to have imprecise or erroneous conclusions, which can shut down good programs, limit access to care, and wrongly tarnish programs and surgeons. Erroneous conclusions can also fail to identify bad programs and patients could be harmed.

But what are good data? Good data are prospective. It is risk adjusted to take into account case mix and patient factors. Good data are based on standardized definitions that can be accurately and reliably assessed across different institutions. For example, the definition of a urinary tract infection must be the same whether it is diagnosed in an academic teaching hospital in Massachusetts, a clinic in rural North Dakota, or a VA hospital in San Francisco. That's very important.

Another key issue is who is going to collect the data? Will the surgeon self-report or will the data be collected by the resident or fellow who happens to be on the service at the time? Will it be collected by an administrator with no clinical background or by a trained, clinical nurse reviewer? How will the person be trained, deemed competent, and audited to verify the quality of the data being entered?

One critical factor is having a third, otherwise uninvolved person assess and document complications and occurrences. The surgeon, or the person involved in the patient's care, has a biased view and cannot be as objective because there may be too much inherent self-interest at stake. Having another person, who is not directly involved with the patient, determine whether a complication has occurred makes the data more reliable and reproducible. Other questions include:

- To what extent should the data collector look for occurrences in order to document results?
- Is documentation in the hospital chart enough?
- Should the records in the physician's office be reviewed?
- Should the patient be contacted, by phone, mail, or e-mail, in order to document whether or not there was a postoperative occurrence?
- How long should the patient be followed-up? Is 30 days enough or is longer-term follow-up important?

All these considerations must be decided upon a priori and implemented homogeneously across institutions if aggregated data are to be compared in a meaningful way. Once good data are collected, they must be analyzed with sound statistics and conclusions must be decided upon and reported in a thoughtful and responsible manner. However, the process of obtaining good data is expensive. The resources needed to collect, audit, analyze, and report are significant, and this may be the biggest factor limiting rollout across the country.

**Bariatric Surgery Data Collection Methods**

Theoretically, there are many ways to collect data following bariatric surgery, from using a simple Excel' spreadsheet or Access' database, to purchasing a data-collection/patient-management service or developing a semi-automated collection system on an SQL server. The advent of accreditation for the field of WLS, however, means that for the near future there are only two foundations upon which a data collection system may be developed: the American College of Surgeons (ACS) Bariatric Surgery Center Network Data Collection system or the system noted in the American Society of Metabolic and Bariatric Surgery (ASMBS)/Surgical Review Corporation Centers of Excellence program.(19,20) When the Center of Medicare and Medicaid Services (CMS) made a national-coverage decision in February 2006 to reimburse bariatric surgery only if it is performed by surgeons or institutions accredited by one or the other of these organizations, it ushered in a policy of general surgeons being required to have specific accreditation to perform specific operations.(21) The fact that many other payers and insurers usually follow the lead of the CMS with regard to coverage decisions means that for most providers, if a surgeon or institution wishes to perform bariatric surgery in the United States in the future, accreditation by one or the other of these organizations will be required. Ideally, these two accreditation bodies would come together as one, or at least agree to collect the same data points, in order to simplify the process for providers and payers, as well as for the patients. However, as of now they have not.

**What to Do With the Data After Collecting It**

To get the greatest benefit from a given set of data requires examining, understanding, and acting upon it as it is collected. Sure, improvements have occurred simply by individuals realizing that their actions are being monitored; but more pronounced gains can and should be achieved by delving deeper into the data itself. It should be monitored regularly, with trend analyses made and benchmarking used. The data should be cut several different ways to discover specific areas that can be improved upon. Subanalyses by provider, procedure, type of complications, and patient characteristics (such as BMI),\ should be made with regard to complications and efficacy (which might include weight loss and reduction of comorbidities). Short- and longer-term results should be evaluated.

The results should be evaluated by all caregivers involved. Results do little good if they are locked up in the office of the chief of service; they must be distributed widely. It is amazing how different people have different perceptions of the same data. Ultimately, all collected data should be shared across institutions with consortiums set up to benchmark and analyze results and to share best practices regarding systems and processes of care. The goal is quality improvement. Though data analysis is helpful in identifying problems or areas that need improvement, there must be a mechanism to actually do something about these findings. Quality improvement (QI) initiatives must be undertaken and, once implemented, the impact should be assessed and monitored in an ongoing manner, again using the data collection system.

**The WLS Data Collection Imperative**

Data collection of 100% of all weight loss procedures performed, using bariatric-specific preoperative, intraoperative, and postoperative data points, is critical. Short- and long-term results must be analyzed. Not only is this the right thing to do for quality improvement, but it is also going to be mandated by almost every health- or medical-governing body, whether it's the Board of Registration of Medicine, the Department of Public Health, payers like CMS, insurers, or professional societies like the ASMBS or the ACS. If we, the healthcare professionals who care for these patients, do not determine the data points and collect this vital information ourselves, then any or all of these other regulating bodies will. If external bodies were to rely on administrative or bad data or data points, then quality of care would not be assessed in a meaningful or fair way for our patients.

The data that are captured must be high quality, assessed by a third person with a clinical background, and backed up by rigorous documentation and follow-up and regular auditing to verify accuracy. The data must be prospective, risk-adjusted, based on standardized definitions, and benchmarked to multi-institutional results. In addition, it must be evaluated with sound statistics. With these parameters observed, the new data collection systems for WLS developed by both the ASMBS and the ACS will lead to substantial advances in quality and patient safety across the country.

**References:**

1. Wittgrove AC, Clark GW, Tremblay LJ. Laparoscopic gastric bypass, Roux-en-Y: preliminary report of five cases. *Obes Surg*. 1994;4:(4):353-7.
2. Higa KD, Boone KB, Ho T, Davies OG. Laparoscopic Roux-en-Y gastric bypass for morbid obesity: technique and preliminary results of our first 400 patients. *Arch Surg*. 2000;135(9):1029-33;discussion 1033-4.

3. Schauer PR, Ikramuddin S, Gourash W, Ramanathan R, Luketich J. Outcomes after laparoscopic Roux-en-Y gastric bypass for morbid obesity. *Ann Surg*. 2000;232(4):515-29.

4. Nguyen NT, Goldman C, Rosenquist J, et al. Laparoscopic versus open gastric bypass: a randomized study of outcomes, quality of life, and costs. *Ann Surg*. 2001;234:279-91.

5. Mason EE, Tang S, Renquist KE, et al. A decade of change in obesity surgery. National Bariatric Surgery Registry (NBSR) contrib. *Obes Surg*. 1997;7(3):189-97.

6. Sjostrom L, Lindroos A, Peltonen M, et al. Lifestyle, diabetes, and cardiovascular risk factors 10 years after bariatric surgery. *N Engl J Med*. 2004;2683-93.

7. Hutter MM, Randall S, Khuri SF, Henderson WG, Abbott WM, Warshaw AL. Laparoscopic versus open gastric bypass for morbid obesity: a multicenter, prospective, risk-adjusted analysis from the National Surgical Quality Improvement Program. *Ann Surg*. 2006;243(5):657-62;discussion 662-6.

8. Santry HP, Gillen DL, Lauderdale DS. Trends in bariatric surgical procedures. *JAMA*. 2005;294(15):1909-17.

9. Zingmond DS, McGory ML, Ko CY. Hospitalization before and after gastric bypass surgery. *JAMA*. 2005;294(15):1918-24.

10. Flum DR, Dellinger EP. Impact of gastric bypass operation on survival: a population-based analysis. *J Am Coll Surg*. 2004;199(4)543-51.

11. Nguyen NT, Paya M, Stevens CM, Mavandadi S, Zainabadi K, Wilson SE. The relationship between hospital volume and outcome in bariatric surgery at academic medical centers. *Ann Surg*. 2004;240(4):586-93; discussion 593-94.

12. Christou NV, Sampalis JS, Liberman M, et al. Surgery decreases long-term mortality, morbidity, and health-care use in morbidly obese patients. *Ann Surg*. 2004;240:416-23.

13. Flum DR, Salem L, Elrod JA, Dellinger EP, Cheadle A, Chan L. Early mortality among Medicare beneficiaries undergoing bariatric surgical procedures. *JAMA*. 2005;294(15):1903-08.

14. Encinosa WE, Bernard DE, Chen CC, et al. Healthcare utilization and outcomes after bariatric surgery. *Med Care*. 2006;44(8):706-12.

15. Buchwald H, Avidor Y, Braunwald E, et al. Bariatric surgery: a systematic review and meta-analysis. *JAMA*. 2004;292:1724-37.

16. Henderson WG, Khuri SF, Mosca C, et al. Comparison of risk-adjusted 30-day postoperative mortality and morbidity in Department of Veterans Affairs hospitals and selected university medical centers: general surgical operations in men. *J Am Coll Surg*. 2007; 204(6):1103-14.

17. Hannan EL, Kilburn H Jr, O'Donnell JF, et al. Adult open-heart surgery in New York State. An analysis of risk factors and hospital mortality rates. *JAMA*. 1990;264(21):2768-74.

18. O'Connor GT, Plume SK, Olmstead EM, et al. A regional prospective study of in-hospital mortality associated with coronary artery bypass grafting. The Northern New England Cardiovascular Disease Study Group. *JAMA*. 1991;266(6):803-9.

19. The American College of Surgeons Bariatric Surgery Center Network. Available at: http://www.facs.org/cqi/bscn/. Accessed December 27, 2006.

20. The American Society for Metabolic and Bariatric Surgery/ Surgical Review Corporation Centers of Excellence Program. Available at: http://www.surgicalreview.org/. Accessed December 27, 2006.

21. CMS. Decision memo for bariatric surgery for the treatment of morbid obesity (CAG-00250R). Available at: http://www.cms.hhs.gov/mcd/viewdecisionmemo.asp?id=160. Accessed December 27, 2006.

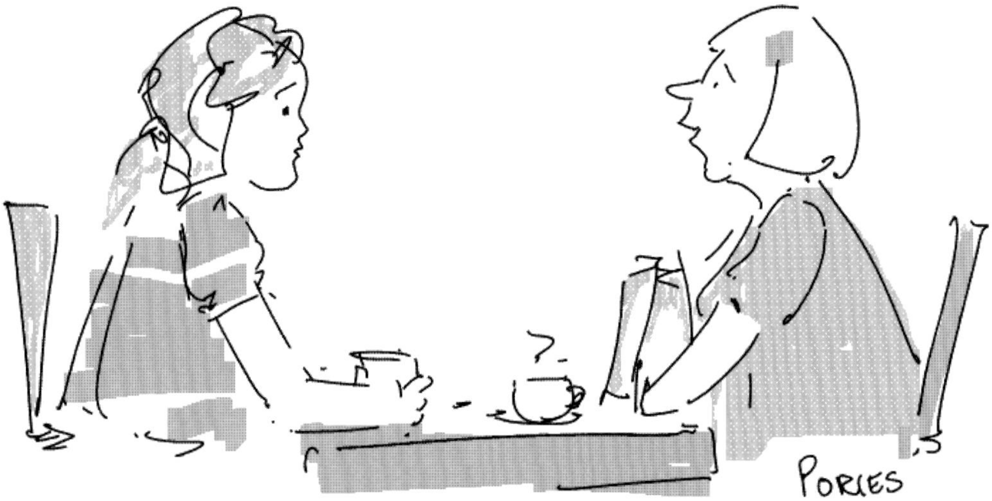


"I just lost 185 pounds of worthless fat.
The divorce became final today."

# Quality of Life

Ninh T. Nguyen, MD
Marcelo Hinojosa, MD
Samuel E. Wilson, MD

Obesity in adults is a chronic disease commonly associated with significant health-related comorbidities, which together can severely degrade the quality of life and limit longevity. The reduction in quality of life of morbidly obese persons has been estimated to be of the same degree as other major debilitating illnesses such as stroke, heart attack, and congestive heart failure.(1) In a study by Rand et al,(2) obese individuals were found to prefer a normal weight even at the cost of a severe disability such as deafness, heart disease, or amputation. The comparison of severe obesity with debilitating illnesses expresses poignantly the negative impact of obesity on an individual's quality of life. One can see why impairment in quality of life is a major reason why morbidly obese patients seek bariatric surgery. Indeed, the most important benefit of bariatric surgery, often under-emphasized, may be the improvement of one's quality of life.

To properly assess the efficacy of an intervention such as bariatric surgery, one must determine which measures of outcome accurately represent improvement in lifestyle. From the patient's perspective, satisfaction with quality of life involves multiple components of physical, mental, emotional, social, and spiritual aspects of life.(1) In surgical treatment of obesity, health-related quality-of-life issues have received less attention from the medical community than measurement of postoperative morbidity and mortality. Quality of life, however, is an essential parameter in measuring the effectiveness of bariatric surgery and should be assessed objectively as a valid outcome measure of any clinical trial. Objective measurement of quality of life requires the use of appropriate instruments that have been tested for reliability and validity.

**Quality-of-life instruments**

Quality of life cannot be measured directly, but is often estimated indirectly by using a measurement scale constructed in the form of questionnaire. Important properties of quality-of-life measurement scales are reliability, validity, responsiveness, and sensitivity. Quality of life can be measured by either generic or obesity-specific instruments. The generic instruments provide a global assessment of the patient's overall health. Examples of generic quality-of-life instruments that have been used to assess the outcome of diverse operations, such as surgery for peptic ulcer disease or aortic aneurysm repair, include the Medical Outcomes Study 36-Item Short Form (SF-36),(3) the Nottingham Health Profile (38 questions),(4) the Sickness-Impact Profile (136 items), the Gastrointestinal Quality-of-Life Index (GIQLI, 36 questions), and the Health-related Quality-of-Life questionnaire (55 items). Obesity-specific, quality-of-life instruments focus on obesity health conditions and are useful for detecting changes caused by bariatric surgery. These instruments include the Moorehead-Ardelt questionnaire (5 questions),(5) the Obesity-Specific Quality-of-Life questionnaire (11 questions),(6) the Quality-of-Well-Being Scale (50 questions), and the Impact of Weight on QOL questionnaire (IWQOL, 74 items).

The SF-36 health survey is the most widely used and validated quality-of-life instrument. The scores are standardized from 0 for poor health to 100 for good health. Scores from the SF-36 survey can be compared with established scores of healthy persons in the United States (US norms). There are 8 health domains within the SF-36: physical functioning (measures limitation in performance of physical activities); role physical (measures limitation in daily activities as a result of physical health); role-emotional (measures limitation in daily activities as a result of emotional problems); bodily pain (measures pain-related functional limitations); vitality (measures energy level); mental health (measures the presence and degree of depression and anxiety); social functioning (measures limitations in social functioning); and general health (measures an individual's perception of his/her health). The GIQLI is a validated instrument, developed specifically for patients with gastrointestinal disease.(7) The GIQLI consists of a one-page questionnaire consisting of 36 questions, each with 5 response categories focusing on 5 dimensions of quality of life: symptoms, emotions, physical function, social function, and medical treatment. The responses are totaled to give a numerical score.

The Moorehead-Ardelt instrument is a simple bariatric-specific questionnaire, used effectively as part of the bariatric analysis and reporting outcome system (BAROS). The Moorehead-Ardelt questionnaire assesses self-esteem, physical activity, social life, work conditions, and sexual activity/interest. Points are added for positive changes and subtracted for negative changes. The BAROS defines 5 outcome groups (failure, fair, good, very good, and excellent) based on a scoring table that adds or subtracts points in three main areas: percentage of excess weight loss, changes in medical conditions, and quality of life as measured by the Moorehead-Ardelt questionnaire.(5)

**Changes in Quality of Life Following Gastric Bypass**

Changes in quality of life after gastric bypass reported from selected series are listed in Table 1. In a randomized trial comparing the outcome of laparoscopic vs. open gastric bypass, Nguyen et al(8) administered both the SF-36 health survey and the Moorehead-Ardelt quality-of-life questionnaire preoperatively and at frequent intervals postoperatively. At baseline, the quality-of-life scores of morbidly obese patients were significantly suppressed in 7 of 8 health domains of the SF-36, compared with the scores of US norms. By 1- month postsurgery, there was improvement in all health domains except for "role-physical," demonstrating that these patients are still limited in their daily activities as a result of the operation. By 3 months postsurgery, the SF-36 quality-of-life scores improved markedly and were comparable to those of the US norms. In addition, all 5 categories of the Moorhead-Ardelt quality-of-life questionnaire had improved compared with baseline at 3 and 6 months postsurgery.(8) Similarly, Dymek and colleagues(9) reported a remarkable improvement in all domains of the SF-36 health survey in patients who underwent open and laparoscopic gastric bypass at 6 months postsurgery. Improvement in quality of life after Roux-en-Y gastric bypass is ongoing at long-term follow-up. Choban et al(10) found that upon reaching the plateau period of weight loss after gastric bypass (18 months postoperatively), patients improved scores in all health domains and were the same as the national "normal" population. At long-term follow-up after a mean time period of 13.8 years after gastric bypass, Zwaan et al(11) reported persistent improvement of both physical and mental composite scores of the SF-36. Scores of 7 of 8 health domains were similar to the scores of the US norm values. Interestingly, scores for bodily pain were lower than that of the US norm.

**Table 1**
**Changes in Quality of Life (QOL) After Gastric Bypass (Selected Series)**

| Authors (year) | QOL measures | No. patients | Main effect |
|---|---|---|---|
| Choban et al(10) (1999) | SF-36 | 107 | Significant improvement at 18 months |
| Velcu et al(12) (2001) | SF-36 | 41 | Significant improvement at 5 years |
| Nguyen et al(8) (2001) | SF-36 | 155 | Significant improvement at 6 months |
| Dymek et al(9) (2001) | SF-36 | 20 | Significant improvement at 6 months |
| de Zwaan et al(11) (2002) | SF-36 | 78 | Significant improvement at 13 years |
| Sanchez et al(13) (2006) | Heath-related QOL | 50 | At 5 years<br>Excellent 22%,<br>Very good 56%<br>Good 18%<br>Fair 2%<br>Failure 2% |
| Puzziferri et al(14) (2006) | Moorehead-Ardelt | 155 | Significant improvement at 3 years |

**Changes in Quality of Life Following Gastric Banding**

Changes in quality of life after gastric banding noted in selected series are listed in Table 2. Using the Bariatric Analysis and Reporting Outcome System, Favretti et al(15) reported that of 180 patients who underwent laparoscopic gastric banding, 4% reported excellent; 44% reported good; 42% reported fair; and only 10% reported failure with follow-up >18 months postoperatively. Similar to changes in quality of life observed after gastric bypass, Freys et al(17) reported immediate improvement of the GIQLI score as early as 3 months after laparoscopic adjustable gastric banding. In their study, all patients had a subnormal GIQLI score before surgery and improved to the level of healthy volunteers by 3 months postoperatively. The GIQLI total score improved significantly from 95 points at baseline to 116 points at 3 months and 112 points at 18 months.(17)

**Table 2**
**Changes in Quality of Life (QOL) After Gastric Banding (Selected Series)**

| Authors (year) | QOL measures | No. of patients | Main effect |
|---|---|---|---|
| Favretti et al(15) (1998) | BAROS | 170 | At 2 years<br>Excellent 5%<br>Good 46%<br>Fair 45%<br>failure 4% |
| Horchner et al(16) (1999) | SF-36 | 39 | Significant improvement at 1 year |
| Freys et al(17) (2001) | GIQLI | 188 | Preoperative score = 95<br>score increased to 112 at 18 months |
| Victorzon et al(18) (2001) | BAROS | 60 | At ≥ 17 months<br>Very good 12%<br>Good 38%<br>Fair 29%<br>Failure 21% |
| Martikainen et al(19) (2004) | BAROS | 123 | At mean 55 months<br>Very good or Good 10%<br>Fair 40%<br>Failure 50% |
| Mathus et al(20) (2004) | Heath-related QOL | 50 | Significant improvement at 1 year |
| Ahroni et al(21) (2005) | SF-36 | 195 | Significant improvement at 1 year |
| Champault et al(22) (2006) | GIQLI | 152 | Preoperative score = 95<br>Score increased to 119 at 2 years |
| Lee et al(23) (2006) | GIQLI | 107 | Preoperative score = 110<br>Score unchanged at 107 at 2 years |

BAROS: bariatric analysis and reporting outcome system; GIQLI: gastrointestinal quality-of-life index

**Summary**

Morbid obesity results in severe impairment of one's quality of life. After bariatric surgery, improvement in quality of life is observed as early as 3 months. Long-term successful weight loss results in a durable improvement in the quality of life, often reaching scores equal to those of the national population. Benefits of weight loss after bariatric surgery include not only reduction in associated comorbidities, but also improvement in an individual's quality of life.

**References**


1. Livingston EH, Fink AS. Quality of life: cost and future of bariatric surgery. *Arch Surg*. 2003;138(4):383-8.
2. Rand CS, Macgregor AM. Successful weight loss following obesity surgery and the perceived liability of morbid obesity. *Int J Obes*. 1991;15(9):577-9.
3. Ware JE, Sherbourne CD. The MOS 36-item short-form health survey (SF-36): Conceptual framework and item selection. *Med Care*. 1992;30(6):473-83.
4. McKenna SP, Hunt SM, Tennant A. The development of a patient-completed index of distress from the Nottingham Health Profile: a new measure for use in cost-utility studies. *Br J Med Econ*. 1993;6:13-24.
5. Oria HE, Moorehead MK. Bariatric analysis and reporting outcome system (BAROS). *Obes Surg*. 1998;8(5):487-99.
6. Le Pen C, Levy E, Loos F, Banzet MN, Basdevant Al. "Specific" scale compared with "generic" scale: a double measurement of the quality of life in a French community sample of obese subjects. *J Epidemiol Community Health*. 1998;52(7):445-50.
7. Eypasch E, Williams JI, Wood-Dauphinee S, et al. Gastrointestinal Quality of Life Index: development, validation, and application of a new instrument. *Br J Surg*. 1995;82(2):216-22.
8. Nguyen NT, Goldman C, Rosenquist CJ, Arango A, Cole CJ, et al: Laparoscopic versus open gastric bypass: a randomized study of outcomes, quality of life, and costs. *Ann Surg*. 2001;234(3):279-89.
9. Dymek MP, le Grange D, Neven K, Alverdy J. Quality of life and psychosocial adjustment in patients after Roux-en-Y gastric bypass: a brief report. *Obes Surg*. 2001;11(1):32-9.
10. Choban PS, Onyejekwe J, Burge JC, Flancbaum L. A health status assessment of the impact of weight loss following Roux-en-Y gastric bypass for clinically severe obesity. *J Am Coll Surg*. 1999;188(5):491-7.
11. de Zwaan M, Lancaster KL, Mitchell JE, et al. Health-related quality of life in morbidly obese patients: effect of gastric bypass surgery. *Obes Surg*. 2002;12(6):773-80.
12. Velcu LM, Adolphine R, Mourelo R, Cottam DR, Angus LD. Weight loss, quality of life and employment status after Roux-en-Y gastric bypass: 5-year analysis. *Surg Obes Relat Dis*. 2005;1(4):413-6.
13. Sanchez-Santos R, Del Barrio MJ, Gonzalez C, et al. Long-term health-related quality of life following gastric bypass: influence of depression. *Obes Surg*. 2006;16(5):580-5.
14. Puzziferri N, Austrheim-Smith IT, Wolfe BM, et al. Three-year follow-up of a prospective randomized trial comparing laparoscopic versus open gastric bypass. *Ann Surg*. 2006;243(2):181-8.
15. Favretti F, Cadiere GB, Segato G, et al. Bariatric analysis and reporting outcome system (BAROS) applied to laparoscopic gastric banding patients. *Obes Surg*. 1998;8(5):500-4.
16. Horchner R, Tuinebreijer W. Improvement of physical functioning of morbidly obese patients who have undergone a LAP-BAND operation: one-year study. *Obes Surg*. 1999;9(4):399-402.
17. Freys SM, Tigges H, Heimbucher J, et al. Quality of life following laparoscopic gastric banding in patients with morbid obesity. *J Gastrointest Surg*. 2001;5(4):401-7.
18. Victorzon M, Tolonen P. Bariatric Analysis and Reporting Outcome System (BAROS) following laparoscopic adjustable gastric banding in Finland. *Obes Surg*. 2001;11(6):740-3.
19. Martikainen T, Pirinen E, Alhava E, et al. Long-term results, late complications and quality of life in a series of adjustable gastric banding. *Obes Surg*. 2004;14(5):648-54.
20. Mathus-Vliegen EM, de Weerd S, de Wit LT. Health-related quality-of-life in patients with morbid obesity after gastric banding for surgically induced weight loss. *Surgery*. 2004;135(5):489-97.

21. Ahroni JH, Montgomery KF, Watkins BM. Laparoscopic adjustable gastric banding: weight loss, co-morbidities, medication usage and quality of life at one year. *Obes Surg*. 2005;15(5):641-7.

22. Champault A, Duwat O, Polliand C, et al. Quality of life after laparoscopic gastric banding: prospective study (152 cases) with a follow-up of 2 years. *Surg Laparosc Endosc Percutan Tech*. 2006;16(3):131-6.

23. Lee WJ, Wang W, Yu PJ, et al. Gastrointestinal quality of life following laparoscopic adjustable gastric banding in Asia. *Obes Surg*. 2006;16(5):586-91.

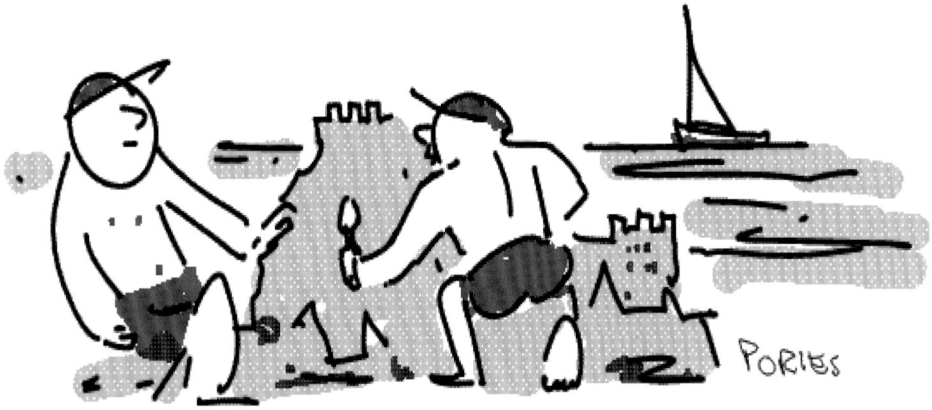


"My daddy is a doctor and he treats diabetes."

"My daddy is a surgeon and he cures it."

# Patients With Type 2 Diabetes

Osama Hamdy, MD, PhD
Ebaa Al-Ozairi, BMSc, MD, MRCP

The growing prevalence of diabetes and cardiovascular disease (CVD) parallels the increased prevalence of obesity. According to the National Health and Nutrition Examination Survey (NHANES), the estimated prevalence of obesity among US adults reached 30.5% in the year 2000, while the prevalence of combined overweight and obesity increased to 64.5%. This percentage is even higher among patients with type 2 diabetes—80% are overweight, obese, or severely obese. During the 10-year period between 1991 and 2001, the prevalence of obesity among the US population increased by 74%. In 1991, the Center for Disease Control and Prevention (CDC) reported that 19 states had a prevalence of obesity between 15% and 19%, with no single state above 20%. Eleven years later in 2002, 20 states had a prevalence of obesity between 15% and 19%, 29 states had a prevalence between 20% and 24%, and 1 state exceeded 25%.

Obesity is strongly associated with several medical problems. Some of these problems are considered direct complications of longstanding obesity. These problems include increased risk for cardiovascular morbidity and mortality, hypertension, cholethiasis, sleep apnea, and endometrial and colon cancers. Table 1 enumerates the most common obesity-related medical problems. Among them, the strongest link is found between obesity and type 2 diabetes. It has been projected that each 1 kg increase in body weight above the estimated ideal weight increases the risk for developing type 2 diabetes by almost 9%.

**Table 1. Common obesity related medical problems**

| |
|---|
| Type 2 diabetes |
| Cardiovascular disease (CVD) |
| Hypertension |
| Sleep apnea |
| Breast, colon and uterine cancer |
| Gall-bladder disease |
| Nonalcoholic steatohepatitis (NASH) |
| Orthopedic dysfunction |
| Depression |

Numerous human studies show increased mortality with increased body mass index (BMI). It has been repeatedly demonstrated that weight reduction, even modest loss, reduces the incidence of most obesity complications and improves the overall sense of well-being. Although lifestyle modifications have been the traditional clinical recommendation for overweight and obese, prediabetic and diabetic individuals, bariatric surgery recently became another valid and effective option for weight control among those high-risk individuals, considering that diabetes is a major comorbid condition. It has been generally accepted for physicians to recommend bariatric intervention for diabetic patients with a BMI >35kg/m$^2$ (class II obesity). For prediabetic individuals and patients diagnosed with impaired glucose tolerance (IGT) or impaired fasting glucose (IFG), bariatric surgery is generally recommended for those with BMI ≥40 (class III obesity) if they do not have any other comorbid conditions.

### Effect of Weight Reduction in Type 2 Diabetes and Prediabetes

Several landmark studies have shown that modest weight loss of approximately 6% to 10% has a remarkable effect on diabetes control in patients with type 2 diabetes, and a profound effect in preventing natural progression of glucose intolerance from IGT to type 2 diabetes. Recently, the Diabetes Prevention Program (DPP) in the United States showed that an approximate 7% weight reduction achieved by lifestyle modification, which was sustained for an average duration of 2.8 years, reduced the risk for developing type 2 diabetes by almost 58% among individuals diagnosed with IGT, compared with the control group.

Similar findings were observed in other large preventive trials in Finland (the Finnish Diabetes Prevention study) and China (the Da Qing IGT and Diabetes study).

Published results from our group demonstrated that 7% weight reduction over a 6-month period, through calorie restriction and moderate-intensity physical exercise, significantly improved endothelial function (EF) in obese subjects with insulin resistance. This significant and profound improvement in EF was similar regardless of the degree of glucose tolerance (normal glucose tolerance, IGT, and type 2 diabetes). Trials were also conducted using pharmacotherapy. The Xenical in the prevention of diabetes in obese subjects (XENDOS) study, showed that weight reduction in prediabetic IGT individuals through lifestyle modification, in addition to orlistat treatment, reduced the incidence of diabetes by 37% compared with lifestyle placebo. Table 2 shows the landmark trials for weight reduction in both prediabetic and diabetic individuals.

**Table 2**

**Landmark Trials for Weight Reduction in Prediabetes and Type 2 Diabetes**

| | **Lifestyle** | **Pharmacotherapy (Orlistat)** | **Bariatric Surgery** |
|---|---|---|---|
| **Trial name** | DPP<br>FINISH,<br>Da Qing | XENDOS | SOS |
| Efficacy<br>(% weight reduction) | 5-7% | 9.6% at 1 year<br>5.2% at 4 years | 21-38% at one year<br>13.2-25% at 10 years |
| Long-term effectiveness | 3-6 years | 4 years | 10 years |
| Side events | Minimal | Moderate | Moderate to severe |

DPP: Diabetes Prevention Program
FINISH: The Finnish diabetes prevention study
Da Qing: The Da Qing IGT and diabetes Study
XENDOS: XENical in the prevention of Diabetes in Obese Subjects (XENDOS) study: Swedish Obese Subjects study (SOS)

Maintenance of weight loss after nonsurgical interventions has been the greatest challenge. Meta-analysis of 16 different studies showed that among people who successfully lost weight through nonsurgical interventions, 60% regained the lost weight by 1 year and 100% by 5 years.

**Effect of Bariatric Surgery in Type 2 Diabetes**

Currently, bariatric surgery is the only interventional method proven to induce significant long-term weight reduction. The number of bariatric surgeries per year in the United States increased dramatically from approximately 16,000 in the early 1990s, to 100,000 in 2003. Despite this significant increase, published long-term results among patients with type 2 diabetes are still scarce, although two large studies provide some evidence of long-term benefits of bariatric surgery in these patients.

**The Swedish Obese Subjects (SOS) study**

The SOS study evaluated the long-term effects of three different bariatric surgery procedures (vertical banded gastroplasty, gastric banding, gastric bypass) compared with nonsurgical intervention at 2 and 10 years postoperatively. Of the 4,047 obese subjects included in this study, the authors were able to evaluate 86.6% at 2 years and 74.5% at 10 years. Of those, 156 patients were diagnosed with type 2 diabetes. The average weight loss at 2 years was 23.4% in the surgical groups vs. 0.1% in the control group. At 10 years, the surgical group continued to maintain an average weight loss of 16.1% of their initial body weight, while the control group gained an average 1.6% in the same period. The amount of weight reduction varied according to procedure used, with the highest following gastric bypass surgery (-38% and -25% at 1 year and 10 years, respectively) and the lowest following gastric banding (-21% and -13.2% at 1 year and 10 years, respectively). Percentage changes in anthropometric and metabolic changes in this study are shown in Table 3.

**Table 3**

Percentage change in anthropometric and metabolic parameters from baseline (adapted from the Swedish Obese Subjects study)

| Percentage Change | Control Group | Gastric Banding | Vertical- Banded Gastroplasty | Gastric Bypass |
|---|---|---|---|---|
| Body weight at 2 years | +0.1% | -23.4% | | |
| Body weight at 10 years | +1.6% | -13.2% | -16.5% | -25% |
| Waist at 10 years | +2.8% | -7.6% | -10.2% | -19.3% |
| BMI at 10 years | +2.3% | -12.8% | -16.0% | -23.8% |
| Fasting plasma glucose at 10 years | +18.7% | -0.8% | -2.5% | -10.0% |
| Fasting serum insulin at 10 years | +12.3% | -25.3% | -27.2% | -54% |
| HDL-C at 10 years | +10.8% | +20.4% | +23.5% | +47.5% |

Prevalence of diabetes mellitus (DM) in the control group increased from 7.8% at baseline to 24.9% at 10 years. In contrast, prevalence of diabetes in the surgical group remained the same (10.8% at baseline vs. 10.5 %) at 10 years after surgery. These changes reflect the overall outcome of the newly diagnosed cases with diabetes in the nondiabetic subjects and the recovery from diabetes in the diabetic subjects. More specifically, among nondiabetic patients, 22% and 27% developed diabetes at 2 years and 10 years respectively, in contrast with 8% and 17% at 2 years and 10 years, respectively, in the surgical intervention group. Among people diagnosed with diabetes at baseline, 72% and 36% recovered from diabetes in the surgical group at 2 years and 10 years respectively, in contrast with 21% and 13% at 2 years and 10 years, respectively, in the control group (Figure 1a and 1b).

**Figure 1a**

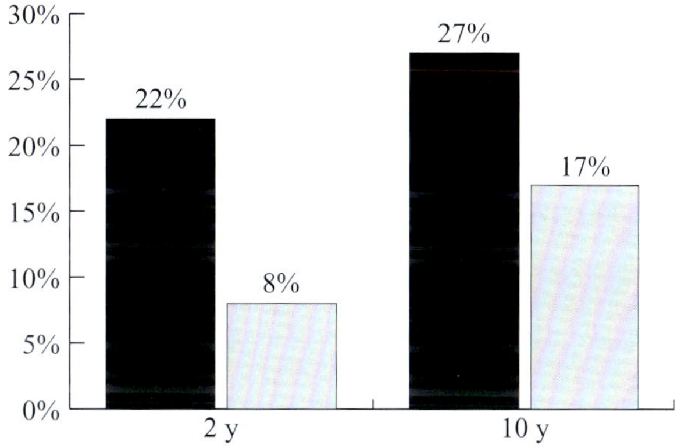


**Figure 1b**

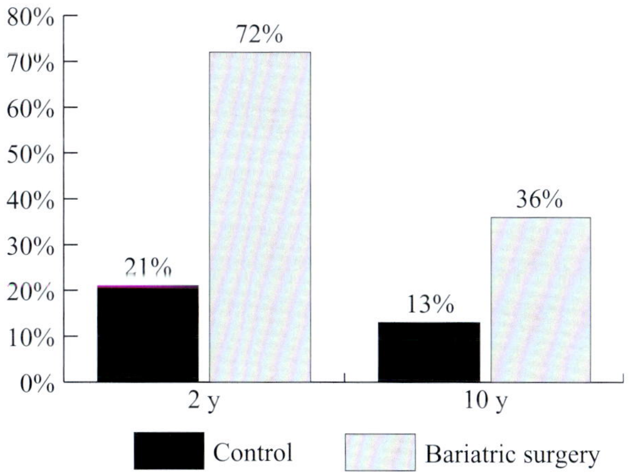


(A) Incidence of diabetes in obese nondiabetic subjects after 2 and 10 years; (B) rate of recovery from diabetes after 2 and 10 years (adapted from Sjöström et al. *NEJM*, 2004.

### Systematic Review and Meta-analysis of Bariatric Surgery

A recently published meta-analysis reviewed 136 bariatric intervention studies that included 22,094 obese patients (5 randomized control trials [RCTs], 28 non-RCTs, and 101 uncontrolled case series). The amount of weight reduction was comparable with that seen in the SOS study: -20% after gastric banding, -25% after vertical banded gastroplasty, and -35% after gastric bypass surgery. Such considerable weight loss was associated with significant reduction in overall obesity complications. Type 2 diabetes was completely resolved in 76.8% of the diabetic subjects included in these trials, with full normalization of fasting blood glucose and A1C. The recovery from diabetes depends on the procedure used: 47.9% recovered after gastric banding, 71.6% after vertical banded gastroplasty, 83.7% after gastric bypass surgery, and 98.9% after the more aggressive malabsorpative procedures.

The study also showed that major improvement in diabetes control was observed in 85% of the included patients. Similar results were also seen in two other studies—the first showed major improvement in diabetes control in 83% of included diabetic patients, and the second demonstrated similar results in 81% of included diabetic patients.

Of particular interest is that the improvement in diabetic control starts within days after bariatric intervention, before a significant weight reduction is achieved. It has been noticed in nonsurgical weight reduction studies that most of the fat reduction that occurs in the first 2 weeks is derived from visceral fat. This visceral fat reduction is associated with significant changes in the gene expression of lipoprotein lipase, PPARγ, and hormone-sensitive lipase. This may explain the quick improvement in diabetes control within the first few postoperative days, while patients are just on a liquid diet with low caloric intake. It is important to note that not all diabetic patients achieve treatment withdrawal postoperatively. It also seems that the success of bariatric surgery in resolving diabetes is not only dependent on the magnitude of weight loss, but also on the duration of diabetes. It is most effective in diabetic patients with shorter duration of the disease, before significant and permanent beta-cell damage has occurred.

### Risk of Bariatric Surgery in Diabetic Patients

The benefits of weight reduction through bariatric surgery intervention in diabetic patients should be weighed against the operative risk in this population. In the previously mentioned meta-analysis, the mortality rate was low: 0.1% in gastric banding, 0.5% in gastric bypass, and 1.1% in malabsorpative procedures. It is worth mentioning that most of the included studies in this meta-analysis were conducted in highly specialized centers and by experienced bariatric surgeons. It might be expected that mortality would be higher in less-experienced centers.

However, none of these studies looked specifically at mortality among a diabetic population. In our opinion, what is more relevant is a comparison between mortality among severely obese diabetic patients treated by bariatric surgery vs. those who chose to continue with combined severe obesity and diabetes. In a retrospective study, overall mortality was compared between a group of 154 obese, diabetic patients who underwent Roux-en-Y gastric bypass operations and a group of 78 diabetic patients who did not go for surgical intervention and served as control group. The results found significant reduction in mortality in the surgically treated group (1% per year) compared with the control group (4.5% per year).

### Conclusions

There is much strong, recent evidence to support the indication of bariatric surgery intervention for treatment of severe class II and III (BMI >35) obese, diabetic patients and for prevention of diabetes in class III (>40 ) obese, prediabetic individuals without other comorbidities. The long-term benefit is documented in several studies for up to 10 years postoperatively. Major improvement of diabetes control was observed in more than 80% of treated patients. Complete resolution of diabetes was seen in more than 70% of treated patients after 2 years and remained significantly high at 10 years. A significant part of this improvement was observed within a short time after surgery, most probably in relation to initial visceral fat reduction. The best results were generally noticed in patients with shorter diabetes duration. The benefits of bariatric surgery in diabetic patients varied based on the procedure used. Although mortality rate in relation to bariatric surgery was relatively low, it was not specifically studied in diabetic patients. However, the overall mortality was shown to be lower in severely obese, diabetic patients treated by bariatric surgery compared with those who chose to continue with combined severe obesity and diabetes.

**Suggested reading**


1. Flegal KM, Carroll MD, Ogden CL, Johnson CL. Prevalence and trends in obesity among US adults, 1999-2000. *JAMA*. 2002;288(14):1723-7.
2. Mokdad AH, Serdula MK, Dietz WH, Bowman BA, Marks JS, Koplan JP. The spread of the obesity epidemic in the United States, 1991-1998. *JAMA*. 1999;282(16):1519-22.
3. Mokdad AH, Bowman BA, Ford ES, Vinicor F, Marks JS, Koplan JP. The continuing epidemics of obesity and diabetes in the United States. *JAMA*. 2001;286(10):1195-200.
4. Mokdad AH, Ford ES, Bowman BA, Dietz WH, Vinicor F, Bales VS, Marks JS. Prevalence of obesity, diabetes, and obesity-related health risk factors, 2001. *JAMA*. 2003;289(1):76-9.
5. Kopelman PG. Obesity as a medical problem. *Nature*. 2000;404(6778):635-43.
6. Mokdad AH, Ford ES, Bowman BA, Nelson DE, Engelgau MM, Vinicor F, Marks JS. Diabetes trends in the US: 1990-1998. *Diabetes Care*. 2000;23(9):1278-83.
7. Manson JE, Stampfer MJ, Hennekens CH, Willett WC. Body weight and longevity: A reassessment. *JAMA*. 1987;257(3):353-8.
8. Breeze E, Clarke R, Shipley MJ, Marmot MG, Fletcher AE. Cause-specific mortality in old age in relation to body mass index in middle age and in old age: follow-up of the Whitehall cohort of male civil servants. *Int J Epidemiol*. 2065; 35(1): 169-78.
9. Fontaine KR, Redden DT, Wang C, Westfall AO, Allison DB. Years of life lost due to obesity. *JAMA*. 2003;289(2):187-93.
10. Hoffmans MD, Kromhout D, de Lezenne Coulander C. The impact of body mass index of 78,612 18-year-old Dutch men on 32-year mortality from all causes. *J Clin Epidemiol*. 1988;41(8):749-56.
11. NIH conference. Gastrointestinal surgery for severe obesity. Consensus Development Conference Panel. *Ann Intern Med*. 1991;115(12):956-61.
12. Knowler WC, Barrett-Connor E, Fowler SE, et al. Reduction in the incidence of type 2 diabetes with lifestyle intervention or metformin. *N Engl J Med*. 2002;346(6):393-403.
13. Tuomilehto J, Lindstrom J, Eriksson JG, et al. Prevention of type 2 diabetes mellitus by changes in lifestyle among subjects with impaired glucose tolerance. *N Engl J Med*. 2001;344(18):1343-50.
14. Pan XR, Li GW, Hu YH, et al. Effects of diet and exercise in preventing NIDDM in people with impaired glucose tolerance. The Da Qing IGT and Diabetes Study. *Diabetes Care*. 1997;20(4):537-44.
15. Hamdy O, Ledbury S, Mullooly C, Jarema C, Porter S,. Lifestyle modification improves endothelial function in obese subjects with the insulin resistance syndrome. *Diabetes Care*. 2003;26(7):2119-25.
16. Torgerson JS, Arlinger K, Käppi M, Sjöström L. Principles for enhanced recruitment of subjects in a large clinical trial. The XENDOS (XENical in the prevention of Diabetes in Obese Subjects) study experience. *Control Clin Trials*. 2001;22(5):515-25.
17. Safer DJ. Diet, behavior modification, and exercise: a review of obesity treatments from a long-term perspective. *South Med J*. 1991;84(12):1470-4.
18. Steinbrook R. Surgery for severe obesity. *N Engl J Med*. 2004;350(11):1075-9.
19. Sjöström L, Lindroos AK, Peltonen M, et al. Lifestyle, diabetes, and cardiovascular risk factors 10 years after bariatric surgery. *N Engl J Med*. 2004;351(26):2683-93.

20. Buchwald H, Avidor Y, Braunwald E, et al. Bariatric surgery: a systematic review and meta-analysis. *JAMA*. 2004;292(14):1724-37.

21. Schauer PR, Burguera B, Ikramuddin S, et al. Effect of laparoscopic Roux-en-Y gastric bypass on type 2 diabetes mellitus. *Ann Surg*. 2003;238(4):467-84; discussion 484-5.

22. Sugerman HJ, Wolfe LG, Sica DA, Clore JN. Diabetes and hypertension in severe obesity and effects of gastric-bypass-induced weight loss. *Ann Surg*. 2003;237(6):751-6; discussion 757-8.

23. Pories WJ, Swanson MS, MacDonald KG, et al. Who would have thought it? An operation proves to be the most effective therapy for adult-onset diabetes mellitus. *Ann Surg*. 1995;222(3):339-50; discussion 350-2.

24. Long SD, O'Brien K, MacDonald KG Jr, et al. Weight loss in severely obese subjects prevents the progression of impaired glucose tolerance to type II diabetes: a longitudinal interventional study. *Diabetes Care*. 1994;17(5):372-5.

25. Dixon JB, O'Brien PE. Health outcomes of severely obese type 2 diabetic subjects 1 year after laparoscopic adjustable gastric banding. *Diabetes Care*. 2002;25(2):358-63.

26. Pignone M, Phillips C, Mulrow C. Use of lipid lowering drugs for primary prevention of coronary heart disease: meta-analysis of randomised trials. *BMJ*. 2000;321(7267):983-6.

27. MacDonald KG Jr., Long SD, Swanson MS, et al. The gastric bypass operation reduces the progression and mortality of non-insulin-dependent diabetes mellitus. *J Gastrointest Surg*. 1997;1(3):213-20.

# Counseling on Exercise

Daniel Rooks, PhD

Habitual exercise and physical activity are essential components of long-term weight management. The additional health benefits of exercise and increased physical activity are many and affect every body system. One of the greatest challenges healthcare providers face with weight loss surgery patients is how to facilitate the adoption and long-term maintenance of exercise and increased activity patterns.

The terms *exercise* and *physical activity* are different, yet are commonly used interchangeably. Physical activity is any bodily movement produced by the contraction of skeletal muscle that increases energy expenditure above resting level. This means that any movement, whether purposeful, like walking to your car or carrying groceries, or unconscious, like fidgeting, can be classified as physical activity. Exercise is physical activity that is planned, organized, repetitive, and performed for the purpose of improving or maintaining one or more components of physical fitness.(1) Exercise is at one end of the physical activity continuum and requires some form of guidance or instruction. Using these definitions, everyone is capable of increasing the amount of physical activity performed daily.

Increasing physical activity should be the first step to getting severely obese individuals moving more and increasing their energy expenditure. To help ensure long-term weight loss maintenance, a program of regular exercise should be included in bariatric surgery programs. Information relating to exercise and physical activity for the weight loss surgery patient is still scarce, however. The Betsy Lehman Center for Patient Safety and Medical Error Reduction in Massachusetts convened a panel of experts covering all aspects of weight loss surgery care to assess the state of the field, to make recommendations for evidence-based best practices, and to focus future efforts for advancement on a consensus list of priorities.(2) Recommendations for exercise or specific amounts of physical activity either before or after surgery were not included in the report due to an absence of data. As a result, the recommendations presented in this chapter are based on published guidelines for exercise and physical activity for general health promotion and disease prevention from international scientific organizations and federal committees, scientific articles, and our clinical experience.(1,3-16) The format generally used to quantify the dose of exercise in published guidelines is summarized by the acronym FITT, for frequency, intensity, type, and (duration of) time.(14)

Among the published recommendations for physical activity and exercise over the past 30 years, four documents have great relevance to the severely obese individual. In 1995, the Centers for Disease Control (CDC) in collaboration with the American College of Sports Medicine published a document in the *JAMA* aimed at improving overall health and well-being of Americans.(5)

### American College of Sports Medicine
*Guidelines for Graded Exercise Testing and Exercise Prescription*

| | Frequency | Intensity | Time |
|---|---|---|---|
| 1975 | 3-5 days | 70-90% HRR | 20-45 min |
| 1980 & 1986 | 3-5 days | 50-85% HRR | 15-60 min |
| 1991 | 3-5 days | 40-85% HRR | 15-60 min |
| 1995 | 3-5 days | 40-85% HRR | 20-60 min |
| 2000 | 7 days | 40-85% HRR | ≥20 min |

The report introduced the strategy of performing "moderate level" activities for a total of 30 minutes on most days of the week. These recommendations were underscored with the release of *Physical Activity and Health: A Report of the Surgeon General* in 1996.(1) In addition, the Surgeon General's report acknowledged the popularity of walking and gardening as the main sources of physical activity in the United States and validated the use of moderate activities to promote health and well-being. In 2002, the Institute of Medicine report formally connected the relationship of physical activity for maintaining body weight with promoting health. This association was accompanied by an increase in recommended daily activity from 30 to 60 minutes. In 2005, the US Dietary Guidelines revised the recommendation to include regular physical activity and reduce sedentary activities to promote health, psychological well-being, and a healthy body weight.(17) The Dietary Guidelines divided its physical activity recommendation into three levels based on desired outcome. The first was to reduce the risk of chronic disease and suggested "at least 30 minutes" of moderate activity on most days of the week. For managing body weight and preventing gradual weight gain, the recommendation was to include 60 minutes of "moderate to vigorous" activity on most days of the week. Finally, the recommendation to "sustain weight loss in adulthood" included daily activity of moderate-to-vigorous intensity for 60 to 90 minutes. This transition from recommendations for general health to specifically address the issues of weight loss and long-term weight management respond to the rising epidemic of obesity.

There are many challenges with counseling the severely obese individual to increase energy expenditure. The remaining portion of this paper provides topics to include in conversations with obese patients about introducing regular exercise as part of the lifestyle change that should accompany weight loss surgery. These topics include details of the components of an exercise program for the individual having weight loss surgery.

An exercise program should be individualized and developed around each patient's preferences and functional limitations. No one program fits everyone. The program must be built around each individual's interests, likes, and dislikes. Ask patients what exercise activities they enjoy and build the program around those activities. In addition to activity preference, physical limitation must be considered when choosing exercise activities. Severely obese individuals with symptomatic knee or hip osteoarthritis might resist a recommendation to increase walking due to pain and the associated fear of injury. In this case, recommending an activity that minimizes joint stress can convince a patient to be more active. Activities performed from a seated position or that are water-based are two effective approaches to adapt to lower extremity joint pain. Common activities include recumbent steppers (i.e., NuStep, Ann Arbor, Michigan) and bicycles, swimming, and water-based group exercise for people with arthritis offered by Arthritis Foundation-trained instructors.

## Components of a Complete Exercise Program

- Warm-up
- Exercise training activities
  - Cardiovascular (endurance)
  - Strength (weight/resistance training)
  - Flexibility (stretching)
- Cool down

A total-fitness program is best for the severely obese individual. No single fitness activity alone is sufficient to maximize caloric expenditure and promote physical and emotional well-being. A total of 60 to 90 minutes of exercise on most days of the week is the recommendation for optimal weight management. An exercise program has 5 parts that should be performed in the following order: warm-up, aerobic fitness, strength training, flexibility, and cool down. The warm-up period involves 2 to 5 minutes of slow, rhythmic movements that involve the large muscles of the body. Performing the aerobic fitness activity (i.e., walking) at a slower pace will accomplish this goal. The warm-up activity gradually prepares the person physically to perform the exercise activities. It is especially important for individuals with arthritis and other musculoskeletal issues that require sustained, slow, gentle movement before moving freely. For the most deconditioned patients, the warm-up may be all they can physically do.

## Cardiovascular Training

- Time
  - Start where the individual can and gradually increase (30-60 s/w)
  - Establish short- and long-term goal with the patient
- Type
  - Low to moderate impact (walking, dancing, water exercise, cycling, chair marching)

Aerobic fitness is a cornerstone of a total-fitness program for the severely obese individual. When performed regularly, aerobic fitness can have a myriad of health benefits. The long-term goal for this portion of the exercise program is to be physically moving for an extended amount of time. It is important to begin with an amount of time that a person can do comfortably. In many cases, 5 to 10 minutes is a good place to begin. Most people can walk for 5 minutes, even if they have to stop once or twice to rest. Encouraging patients to walk for 10 minutes a day during the first week can reduce their apprehension and thus align appropriate expectations, as well as prevent over-doing it so that they avoid excessive muscle soreness. The 10 minutes can be divided into two 5-minute walks if the person chooses. After 2 weeks of exercising, 1 minute can be added to every walking session per week (i.e., weeks 1-2: 10 minutes per weekly session; week 3: 11 minutes per session; week 4: 12 minutes per session). Time can be added on a schedule (i.e., weekly) or as the patient chooses, to fit his or her lifestyle. Therefore, if a person begins with 10 minutes a day, it would take an additional 20 weeks to reach 30 minutes (10 minutes + [1 minute per week x 20 weeks])

There is no need to set a specific, objectively measured level of intensity such as heart rate. For some patients on certain medications (i.e., beta-blockers), heart rate does not provide an accurate measure of effort. Instructing people to walk "briskly" or "with a purpose" can be enough to result in substantial health improvements.(18) For individuals who want to assess their effort, the "talk test" provides an easy approach. People who can talk comfortably while walking purposefully are moving at an appropriate pace while the person who cannot complete a sentence without taking a breath needs to slow down a step. This self-regulation of walking effort is important to patients becoming independent with their exercise program.

Most people have clear preferences about the activity to perform, so ask the patient what activities he/she prefers. Walking is the most common form of aerobic exercise, offering the benefits of easy access and no cost and is an integral part of physical independence. The only required piece of equipment is a sturdy pair of walking shoes that offer good support. But the activity does not have to be walking. Any form of gentle, rhythmic, light-to-moderate intensity, total-body activity—such as dancing—works well. Activities that increase stress on joints and bones, (i.e., running) can increase the risk of musculoskeletal injury within the first 10 months after weight loss surgery.

## Strength Training

Recommendations

- Begin with a very low level of resistance
- Use multijoint, functional movements
- Must learn good technique
  - Machine vs nonmachine
  - Book, video, trainer
- Breathing—count out loud
- Movements smooth and controlled through full range of motion

Strength training, also known as resistance training or weight training has become a popular part of a total-fitness program, with its many health and function-related benefits. Strength-training movements should be performed 2 to 3 times a week with at least 1 day of rest between exercise sessions. The 48 hours of rest ensures that the body recovers from the exercise session and minimizes delayed-onset muscle soreness. The intensity of effort performing an exercise should be comfortable and never cause straining or breath-holding. Strength-training exercises can be performed with a variety of equipment, including hand weights, machines, cans of food, household items, resistance bands or cords and a person's body weight. Patients can choose to join a group exercise class, use a video, or perform exercises alone. Community centers, local hospitals, and fitness centers often offer group classes. Having a group exercise instructor who is certified to teach a class promotes a sense of confidence in the obese individual that he/she will be instructed properly. To encourage those patients who are worried about their health, the American College of Sports Medicine (ACSM) is the gold standard for fitness certification for working with people with chronic illness, and they have a Web site with information at www.acsm.org.

Patients should be advised that, when exercising, all movements should be performed smoothly with light resistance and with control maintained throughout the exercise movement. Exercise movements that mimic functional activities, like rising from a chair, are preferred to single-joint movements (i.e., knee flexion). While resistance training is a safe activity, learning and performing proper technique is critical to safe, successful exercise that will result in maximal health benefits. For individuals who are new to strength training, an instructional video or book with clear pictures or drawings and clearly worded descriptions of the exercise movements is essential.(19) Again, instruction from a reliable fitness professional or physical therapist can be extremely valuable to learning proper exercise technique.

## Flexibility Training

- Type
  - Static vs. ballistic stretching
  - Active vs. passive stretching
  - Best performed after warm-up and exercise
  - Alternatives (yoga, tai chi)
- Location
  - Anywhere

Flexibility or comfortable range of joint motion is the third part of a total-fitness program. Also known as *stretching*, these body movements can improve the comfort range of musculoskeletal joint motion and translate to better everyday functional movements, including bathing and dressing, getting in and out of a car and standing for extended periods of time. Stretching exercises can be performed daily and should be done with gentle, smooth movements. The person moves into a particular position until a slight stretch is felt in the body area and held for 15 to 30 seconds. Stretching is performed after aerobic and strength-training exercises to ensure that the muscles and joints are warmed up and pliable to maximize improvement and minimize the risk of injury. Stretching can be performed anywhere and requires a good-quality video or book that describes the exercise movements clearly.

Group activities that involve stretching include yoga, tai chi, and some forms of dance. It is best to begin with whatever form of stretching interests the patient.

## Cool Down

- 5-10 minutes
- Large muscle, slow, rhythmic movements (i.e., walking, cycling, swimming, chair march)
- Breathing exercises
- Relaxation
- Gentle stretching

The final step in the fitness program is the cool down. A cool down is similar to a warm-up, being approximately 5 to 10 minutes in length and involving slow body movements of large muscles. The purpose of the cool-down is to gradually lower the body's systems activity to resting levels. This portion of the exercise program can include listening to relaxing music, meditation, or relaxation and breathing exercises.

A conversation regarding exercise with a weight loss surgery patient is important and should be part of optimal patient care. Currently, no guidelines exist specifically for these patients; however, sound advice will allow the safe adoption of exercise into a new, healthy lifestyle.

## Keys to Exercise Adherence

- Physician reinforcement
- Group/social support
- Safety
- Comfortable environment
- Sufficient challenge
- Fun

The patient should have a short-term exercise plan that includes preferences for aerobic, muscle strengthening, and flexibility activities and a realistic schedule that fits his or her lifestyle. The program should begin with 20 to 30 minutes of activities daily and gradually increase to 60 to 90 minutes per day of physical activity and exercise. The total amount of minutes can be divided into smaller units. Safety is paramount, so it is important to start exercising slowly to reduce the risk of injury and excessive soreness. Like any lifestyle behavior change, it is helped by the clinician's interest and consistent reinforcement, which can contribute greatly to a patient's short- and long-term adherence. Therefore, the entire weight loss surgery team should reinforce adherence to the physical activities the patient values. Success is defined by the patient's increased level of physical activity and habitual participation in appropriate exercise.

**Exercise Counseling Guidelines**

- Identify the patient's interests
- Establish short- and long-term goals that are realistic
- Focus on the first step
- Create the program around the patient's interests and functional limitations

**Patient Resources**

**Books of exercise descriptions**

1. Laliberte R, Byers Kraus V, Rooks D. *The Everyday Arthritis Solution: Food, Movement, and Lifestyle Secrets to Ease the Pain and Feel Your Best!* Pleasantville, NY: Reader's Digest, Inc; 2004. (Paperback. This book contains user-friendly pictures and text describing more than 140 exercises for improving muscle strength and flexibility. It is designed for the person with musculoskeletal issues of various levels of fitness and is very appropriate for the severely obese patient. -DR)
2. Moffat M. *American Physical Therapy Association Book of Body Repair and Maintenance: Hundreds of Stretches and Exercises for Every Part of the Human Body.* New York, NY: Henry Holt & Company, Inc.;1999.
3. The Arthritis Foundation. *Guide to Good Living with Osteoarthritis*. Atlanta, Georgia: The Arthritis Foundation; 2000.

**Web Sites**

Center for Disease Control and Prevention—Physical Activity
http://www.cdc.gov/nccdphp/dnpa/physical/

American Diabetes Association
http://www.diabetes.org/weightloss-and-exercise/exercise/overview.jsp

American Heart Association
http://www.americanheart.org/presenter.jhtml?identifier=1200013

American Academy of Family Physicians
http://familydoctor.org/059.xml

Arthritis Foundation
http://www.arthritis.org/conditions/exercise/default.asp

National Institutes of Health (for older adults)
http://nihseniorhealth.gov/exercise/toc.html

**References**


1. US Department of Health and Human Services. Physical Activity and Health: A Report of the Surgeon General. Atlanta, GA: US Department of Health and Human Services, Centers for Disease Control and Prevention, National Center for Chronic Disease Prevention and Health Promotion; 1996.
2. Commonwealth of Massachusetts Betsy Lehman Center for Patient Safety and Medical Error Reduction expert panel on weight loss surgery: executive report. *Obes Res*. 2005;13(2):205-305.
3. Whaley MH, Brubaker PH, Otto RM, Armstrong L, eds. *ACSM's Guidelines for Exercise Testing and Prescription*. 7th ed. Baltimore, MD: Lippincott Williams & Wilkins; 2006.
4. American College of Sports Medicine Position Stand. The recommended quantity and quality of exercise for developing and maintaining cardiorespiratory and muscular fitness in healthy adults. *Med Sci Sports Exerc*. 1990;22(2):265-74.
5. From the Centers for Disease Control and Prevention. Prevalence of recommended levels of physical activity among women—Behavioral Risk Factor Surveillance System, 1992. *JAMA*. 1995;273(13):986-7.
6. Ashworth NL, Chad KE, Harrison EL, Reeder BA, Marshall SC. Home versus center-based physical activity programs in older adults. *Cochrane Database Syst Rev*. 2005(1):CD004017.
7. Annesi JJ, Otto LM. Relationship between number of exercise counseling sessions attended and adherence to a new exercise program. *Psychol Rep*. 2004;94(3 Pt 1):907-8.
8. Berg AO. US Preventive services task force. Behavioral counseling in primary care to promote physical activity: recommendation and rationale. *Am J Nurs*. 2003;103(4):101-7.
9. Braith RW, Stewart KJ. Resistance Exercise Training: its role in the prevention of cardiovascular disease. *Circulation*. 2006;113(22):2642-50.
10. Bassuk SS, Manson JE. Epidemiological evidence for the role of physical activity in reducing risk of type 2 diabetes and cardiovascular disease. *J Appl Physiol*. 2005;99(3):1193-1204.
11. Chan CB, Ryan DA, Tudor-Locke C. Health benefits of a pedometer-based physical activity intervention in sedentary workers. *Prev Med*. 2004;39(6):1215-22.
12. Giannuzzi P, Mezzani A, Saner H, et al. Physical activity for primary and secondary prevention. Position paper of the Working Group on Cardiac Rehabilitation and Exercise Physiology of the European Society of Cardiology. *Eur J Cardiovasc Prev Rehabil*. 2003;10(5):319-27.

13. Hu FB, Stampfer MJ, Solomon C, et al. Physical activity and risk for cardiovascular events in diabetic women. *Ann Intern Med*. 2001;134(2):96-105.

14. Jakicic JM, Clark K, Coleman E, et al. American College of Sports Medicine position stand. Appropriate intervention strategies for weight loss and prevention of weight regain for adults. *Med Sci Sports Exerc*. 2001;33(12):2145-56.

15. Tanasescu M, Leitzmann MF, Rimm EB, Willett WC, Stampfer MJ, Hu FB. Exercise type and intensity in relation to coronary heart disease in men. *JAMA*. 2002;288(16):1994-2000.

16. Tudor-Locke C, Bassett DR, Jr. How many steps/day are enough? Preliminary pedometer indices for public health. *Sports Med*. 2004;34(1):1-8.

17. Dietary Guidelines for Americans. Agriculture Department; Human Nutrition Information Service and Health and Human Services Department. 2005.

18. Rooks DS, Kiel DP, Parsons C, Hayes WC. Self-paced resistance training and walking exercise in community-dwelling older adults: effects on neuromotor performance. *J Gerontol A Biol Sci Med Sci*. 1997;52(3):M161-8.

19. Laliberte R, Byers Kraus V, Rooks D. *The Everyday Arthritis Solution: Food, Movement, and Lifestyle Secrets to Ease the Pain and Feel Your Best!* Pleasantville, NY: Reader's Digest, Inc.; 2004. [Paperback]

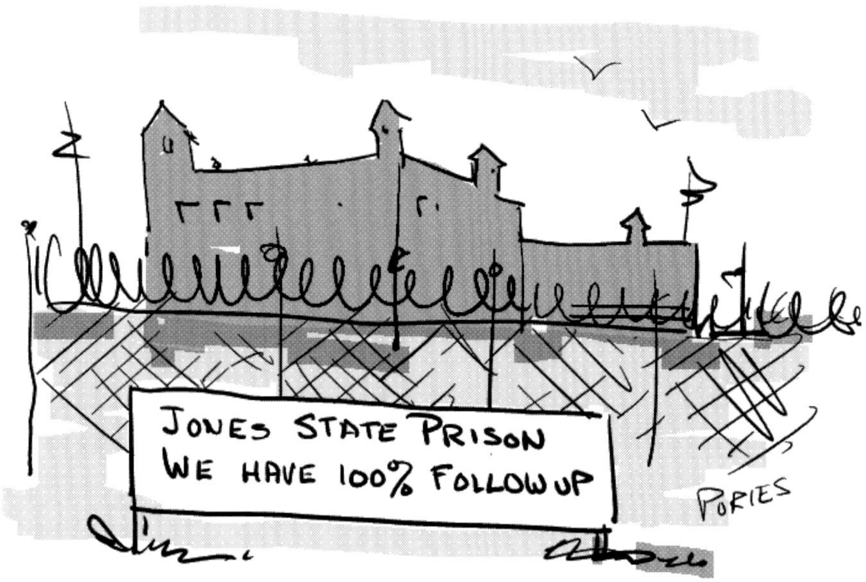
JONES STATE PRISON
WE HAVE 100% FOLLOW UP
PORIES

# Lifelong Medical Follow-up

Edward Hatchigian, MD, MS

All weight loss surgery (WLS) patients are seen preoperatively for their initial medical screening. Several points are emphasized with all candidates, but foremost is that WLS is a lifetime commitment to healthy eating habits and to exercise. The the National Institutes of Health (NIH) guidelines indicate that lifelong medical surveillance after surgical therapy is a necessity and that patients who opt for surgical intervention should be followed by a multidisciplinary team (1). At large centers for the treatment and management of obesity, the team is comprised of surgeons, internists, bariatricians, endocrinologists, nurses, registered dieticians, social workers, psychologists, and exercise physiologists. A very important part of the multidisciplinary team is group support. In smaller programs, such as many of those associated with a community hospital, the team may be comprised of a surgeon with a physician's assistant, nurse practitioner, dietician, and a psychologist. An important part of the lifelong follow-up is the primary care provider, who would be the patient's internist or family physician. It may be even a pediatrician or nurse practitioner. In the long run, WLS patients will have to be seen by their primary care providers. Thus, it is imperative to make the primary care provider aware of the issues that are associated with WLS. There may be many primary care providers who are unfamiliar with the concepts surrounding the treatment and management of morbid obesity. Some providers may tell their patients that WLS is too drastic and that they should be seen by a nutritionist/dietician or enroll in a nonsurgical weight loss program; however, almost all candidates for WLS "have been there, done that." Popular commercial programs such as Weight Watchers and Jenny Craig, popular products such as Slim Fast, diets such as Atkins and South Beach, and prescription medications such as Meridia and Xenical, as well as over-the-counter appetite suppressants and herbal supplements such as Metabolife and Trim-Spa—all of these are examples of the many weight loss efforts that surgical candidates have undertaken. Many have lost weight, be it 5 or 105 lbs. The major obstacle to success is the inability to maintain the weight loss. Primary care providers have to be made aware of the impact that WLS has on the morbidly obese. Based on data from the American Society for Metabolic and Bariatric Surgery (ASMBS), the number of bariatric surgeries performed in 1992 was slightly more than 16,000; by 2004, more than 140,000 surgeries were performed.

The follow-up of patients who have had WLS can be divided into 5 categories: complications, nutritional deficiencies, psychological adjustments, medication management, and weight gain. Complications of WLS associated with the Roux-en-Y gastric bypass procedure may be somewhat different than those associated with the less invasive adjustable LAP-BAND procedure. These are the two most commonly performed surgeries for obesity in this country.

**Table 1**

### Weight Loss Surgery Follow-up

- Complications
- Nutritional deficiencies
- Psychological adjustments
- Medication management
- Weight gain

As Table 1 indicates, the complications following gastric bypass surgery may be medical, surgical, nutritional, or psychological. Examples of these are iron and vitamin $B_{12}$ deficiency, incisional/ventral hernias, cholecystitis, and depression.

From the Roux-en-Y procedure, the two most serious complications that usually occur within the first 4 weeks following surgery are anastomotic leaks (no WLS patient should leave the hospital unless a swallow study is obtained to confirm that everything is intact) and pulmonary embolism. One study indicates that these two complications account for nearly all the deaths following bariatric surgery (2). Patients who are at obvious high risk for thromboembolism should be identified in the preoperative screening process, so that prophylactic measures can be undertaken to minimize the risks. Women who are taking oral contraceptives are advised to discontinue 1 to 2 months prior to surgery and avoid resuming for 1 to 2 months following surgery. These women should be advised to seek other forms of birth control. Morbid obesity, in itself, is a risk for thromboembolism and many morbidly obese patients are immobile from osteoarthritis, or degenerative joint disease with accompanying back and knee pain, and thus may need prophylactic therapy with heparin products. Those deemed at very high risk, such as those having a history of recurrent deep venous thromboses and/or previous pulmonary embolism, should be considered for placement of an IVC (Greenfield) filter as prophylactic measure. The major emphasis, of course, should be on encouraging patients to get up and ambulate as soon as possible after surgery—in other words, no "couch potatoes." With regard to wound infections and the incidence of incisional/ventral hernias, the laparoscopic approach has markedly reduced these complications.

Dehydration is one of the most common complications seen soon after surgery. The restriction provided by the Roux-en-Y gastric bypass and the adjustable gastric LAP-BAND make it difficult for many patients to meet their fluid needs. It is important to encourage postsurgical patients to keep a water bottle with them, whether it is plain water, "Crystal Light," or other brand from which to take frequent sips every 20 to 30 minutes to meet at least 64 ounces of fluids per day. Carbonated beverages (diet or otherwise) should be avoided for their irritating effect on the small pouch and the possibility of gas-bubble formation, which in a small pouch is far more uncomfortable than in the normal stomach. On hot, humid days when dehydration can also occur due to perspiring, sugar-free popsicles should be used as another source of hydration in addition to fluids.

Another common complication following WLS is the nausea/vomiting often due to eating too fast or taking in large portions. The restructuring of the internal anatomy that makes up the malabsorption component of the Roux-en-Y gastric bypass procedure is the dumping syndrome that many, but not all, will experience following gastric bypass surgery. This can last for seconds or for hours after eating foods with high sugar content. Symptoms are often similar to what diabetics experience when blood sugars "bottom out," including dizziness, lightheadedness, headache, facial flushing, shakes, chills, and of course nausea and vomiting. To avoid these unpleasant features associated with gastric bypass surgery, it is emphasized that post-op patients eat very, very slowly, consuming small portions, and chewing their food with extreme care. This may sound simple, but for most post-op patients whose lifetime eating habits have included large portions consumed very fast, this change will take time and much effort to master in order to avoid the dumping syndrome. Vomiting can also be due to psychological issues such as binge-eating—issues that hopefully will be identified in the preoperative screening process and addressed at that time. Vomiting of solid foods and not liquids may occur postoperatively, especially after the patient has gone through the 5 stages of the gastric bypass diet. This is often due to stomal stenosis or stricture. Stomal stenosis is diagnosed by barium study and if confirmed, can be corrected with endoscopy and dilatation. Often this condition is due to eating large portions of food too fast, causing esophageal spasm. Dietary indiscretion can lead to vomiting, which in turn, can cause the restrictive stomach pouch to expand or stretch somewhat. This can eventually lead to cessation of weight loss and then very likely to weight gain.

Morbid obesity is associated with significant comorbidities such as hypertension, type 2 diabetes, obstructive sleep apnea, dyslipidemia, reflux, osteoarthritis/degenerative joint disease, and depression. The significant reduction in weight achieved with surgery has allowed these patients to experience complete resolution or marked improvement in their condition, to the point where they may need to have their medication dosage reduced or stopped completely. In the preoperative evaluation process, those who may have signs and symptoms of a sleep disorder such as snoring, daytime somnolence, and arising in the middle of the night or, in the morning, feeling fatigue and even gasping for air, it is recommended that a sleep study be performed to assess for sleep apnea. Those with a confirmed diagnosis of sleep apnea necessitating wearing a nocturnal continuous positive airway pressure (CPAP) mask may find that with the weight loss achieved, they no longer have to wear the cumbersome device.(4, 5) It is, however, recommended that a repeat sleep study be done at 12 months after surgery before discontinuing treatment for sleep apnea. Many people are on 1, 2 or 3 medications for the control of their hypertension and with the weight loss achieved from surgery, may find that they can have their dosage reduced or medications eliminated; however, there may be some who, although their blood pressure levels are improved, are unable to come off their medications. This may also be true with patients who have had elevated lipid levels controlled by cholesterol-lowering medications (such as Lipitor) prior to surgery. Upon achieving significant weight loss and stopping the medication, they may find their lipid levels rise and thus require them to go back on medication. After all, it is well known that thin people can have hypertension or hyperlipidemia. The association of obesity with type 2 diabetes is well known and to manage a diabetic's blood sugars, physicians and diabetes health educators emphasize limiting the consumption of carbohydrates, reducing weight, and exercising. Several studies have demonstrated rapid improvement in type 2 diabetes with gastric restrictive procedures, and even the resolution of glucose intolerance in many patients (6). Many patients with type 2 diabetes who lose weight with WLS are no longer on medications such as insulin, or are on very low dosages of oral hypoglycemic agents. However, adjustment in medications is different for everyone following WLS. Diabetics must have their blood sugars monitored on a frequent basis perioperatively to ensure good wound healing and postoperatively to avoid complications of hyper- or hypoglycemia.

As patients go through the 5 stages of the gastric bypass diet, their blood sugars will have to be monitored much more regularly, using a glucometer fingerstick, and if necessary, coverage with a sliding-scale regular insulin. The A1C is used preoperatively as an indicator for wound healing ability. Levels under 9% would be acceptable for surgery; those with levels above 9% should achieve better management of their blood sugars prior to undergoing surgery. The A1C level should be followed at intervals postoperatively during "milestone visits," with adjustment in medication or diet made to ensure good control of the diabetes. It should be emphasized to the patient that WLS does not cure diabetes or sleep apnea and that resorting back to practices of dietary indiscretion leading to weight gain, may require the patient to go back on medication or be subjected to use of the CPAP device.

A large percentage of patients who come in for evaluation for WLS are on medication for depression, usually a selective serotonin reuptake inhibitor such as Prozac, Paxil, Celexa, or Effexor. These are often prescribed by the primary care physician for "situational depression" largely related to the patient's obesity. It is interesting to note that many of these psychotropic medications can cause weight gain. However, it is very important that, because of the rapid change in lifestyle and dietary habits, patients with depression remain on medications during their hospitalization and the postsurgery stage to avoid the possibility of decompensation.

With regard to medications following a gastric restrictive procedure, clinicians should avoid prescribing nonsteroidal anti-inflammatory agents (such as ibuprofen) that can increase irritation, leading to the development of marginal ulcers and bleeding. Extended-release drugs also should not be prescribed because of the reduction of transit times. With a gastric bypass procedure, the change in intestinal anatomy can influence the amount of medication that reaches the blood stream. Thus, in the postoperative period, medications that require level checks for therapeutic effectiveness (such as digoxin, dilantin, lithium, synthroid, and anticoagulants) should be monitored closely for any dose adjustments needed to prevent toxicity or subtherapeutic effectiveness.

Nutritional deficiencies can be seen in any procedure that involves restricting oral intake of nutrients, but the Roux-en-Y gastric bypass, because of the restructuring of the internal anatomy that affects absorption, can lead to deficiencies of iron, vitamin $B_{12}$, calcium, and vitamin D. The restructuring of the anatomy raises issues of absorption in the first part of the small bowel (duodenum) and also in the stomach (where the intrinsic factor is produced). Also, the malabsorptive component of the procedure can lead to deficiencies in essential fatty acids, as well as the fat-soluble vitamins A, D, E, and K. Iron deficiency and anemia are common and develop in 20% to 49% of patients who have gastric bypass surgery. Clinical symptoms such as fatigue and lack of energy are common. It is essential to supplement the daily diet with a good multivitamin, preferably in crushed, liquid, or chewable form. Iron supplements can be in the form of iron polysaccharides, ferrous gluconate, or ferrous sulfate and taken with vitamin C (ascorbic acid) to enhance absorption. Ferrous sulfate is one of the more common iron preparations, but is binding and can lead to constipation and black, tarry stools. Ferrous gluconate is a little more tolerable, but the best results are with the iron polysaccharides such as Niferex, which comes in an over-the-counter form, as well as a prescriptive form called Niferex Forte. Severe iron deficiency; however, may warrant intramuscular or intravenous supplementation.

Vitamin $B_{12}$ deficiency following gastric restrictive surgery is common and can be found in 25% to 35% of patients; however, the clinical symptoms are not common. Vitamin $B_{12}$ deficiency is also called combined systems disease, because it is associated with anemia and neurological manifestations. Supplementation of $B_{12}$ can be found in a sublingual, oral, or nasal gel form. Patients who do not respond to oral supplementation will need monthly intramuscular injections of the vitamin. Folate deficiency, which is associated with anemia, does not have neurological manifestations and is not common since a daily multiple vitamin can prevent folic acid deficiency.

As abnormalities in metabolism can occur early after gastric bypass surgery, vitamin D, which is absorbed in the proximal part of the small bowel, can become deficient. Vitamin D deficiency produces secondary hyperparathyroidism, as does hypocalcemia. Calcium absorption is impaired due to the lack of acidity in the gastric pouch and the bypass to the duodenum. Gastric bypass surgery can lead to an increase in bone turnover and decrease in bone mass. Evaluation of bone metabolism and calcium replacement should be undertaken following surgery, and it should be emphasized to the patient that having a bone density exam, which can be arranged by the primary care physician's office, is important. It should be noted that serum calcium measurements are not good indicators of postsurgery calcium deficiency, as levels can be normal at the expense of mobilization of bone. High daily dietary intake of calcium (2 g/d), as well as supplementation of calcium (1.2-1.5 g/d), preferably in the form of calcium citrate, is recommended. For vitamin D, an additional 400 IU daily is recommended. For deficiency states, ergocalciferol (or Drisdol) in a 50,000 IU soft gel can be taken twice weekly for 5 to 10 weeks.

A good multivitamin is to be taken every day, as well as supplements such as vitamin $B_{12}$, vitamin D, and calcium as needed in order to ensure that nutritional recommendations are met. These vitamins can be found in several popular commercial brands (the most common of these taken by patients following gastric bypass is Flintstones Complete Chewables). Again, it is recommended that all medications be taken in a liquid, chewable, or crushed form. Medications that come in large capsules can be opened and sprinkled in yogurt or applesauce, etc.

The psychological changes following WLS are significant. Many patients prior to surgery have pre-existent eating disorder behaviors and require a drastic change in their eating patterns such as fewer meals, less food consumed at each meal, and less eating in response to strong emotions. The positive aspects of rapid weight loss are seen in increase in self-esteem, self-confidence, and assertiveness, thus leading to improvements in social interactions and physical and sexual activity, as well as work performance. However, there are some patients who will find difficulties with coping mechanisms, especially with body-image changes and relationships with intimate partners. These patients would likely benefit from postsurgery follow-up with a psychologist or therapist.

Weight changes following gastric bypass surgery include an average monthly weight loss of 10 to 15 lbs for the first 6 months; therefore, at 6-month follow-up, the average weight loss is 60 to 80 lbs. After 6 months, weight loss may slow to 5 to 7 lbs a month. Weight regain usually begins at 18 to 24 months postoperatively. Often, patients will note a gradual increase in portion size and toleration of the portions eaten. It is not unexpected to see a 7% to 10% regain in weight. The weight regain may be due to physiological factors, anatomical factors such as staple-line disruption, or psychological (inadequate coping) and nutritional (dietary indiscretion) factors.

Most of these issues with WLS are associated with the "gold standard" Roux-en-Y gastric bypass procedure. The less invasive, adjustable gastric LAP-BAND procedure, considered a relatively safe procedure, may have complications such as band infection, band slippage, and band erosion leading to gastric perforation and reservoir leakage.

It should be noted that, with the LAP-BAND being a truly restrictive procedure, there is no restructuring of the internal anatomy and no malabsorptive component, thus weight loss is much slower compared with the gastric bypass procedure, and there is no dumping syndrome. Because there is no malabsorption, nutritional deficiencies are not as common with the LAP-BAND, although it is strongly recommended that a good multivitamin and any required supplements be taken daily.

In conclusion, WLS has become a safe and acceptable treatment for morbid obesity when other measures that have been tried have been unsuccessful. However, the WLS patient should understand that there are postsurgical issues such as complications, nutritional deficiencies, medication monitoring, and psychological adjustments. Early emphasis is placed on adequate hydration, protein intake, multivitamin, iron, calcium, vitamin $B_{12}$, and vitamin D supplementation, with periodic assessment for metabolic bone disease, especially for those with malabsorptive procedures and increased risk for metabolic bone disease (7). Careful long-term follow-up for the patient who has undergone surgery is essential and nearly all of the follow-up care will come from the patient's primary care physician. Physicians and patients will need to be aware of the issues that follow WLS so that measures to identify, treat, and manage these issues can be taken to prevent complications. Weight loss surgery is a tool and successful WLS means a lifetime commitment to healthy eating habits, taking necessary supplements, and to exercise.

**References**

1. National Institutes of Health. Clinical guidelines on the identification, evaluation, and treatment of overweight and obesity in adults—the evidence report. *Obes Res*. 1998;6 (suppl 2):51S-209S (published correction appears in *Obes Res*. 1998;6:464.)

2. Klein S, Wadden T, Sugarman HJ. AGA technical review on obesity. *Gastroenterology* 2002;123:882-932.

3. Buchwald H, Avidor Y, Braunwald E, et al. Bariatric surgery a systemic review and meta-analysis. *JAMA*. 2002;292:1724-37.

4. Kyzer S, Charuzi I. Obstructive sleep apnea in the obese. *World J. Surg*. 1998;22:998-1001.

5. Dixon JB, Schachter LM, O'Brien PE. Sleep disturbance and obesity: changes following Surgically-induced weight loss. *Arch Intern Med*. 2001;161:102-6.

6. Poires WJ, Swanson MS, MacDonald KG et al. Who would have thought it? An operation proves to be the most effective therapy for adult-onset diabetes mellitus. *Ann Surg*. 1995; 222:339-50.

7. Saltzman E, Anderson W, Apovian CM, et al. Criteria for patient selection and multidisciplinary evaluation and treatment of the weight loss surgery patient. Boston, MA: Betsy Lehman Center for Public Safety and Medical Error Reduction. Massachusetts Department of Public Health 2004. *Obes Res*. 2005;13:234-43.

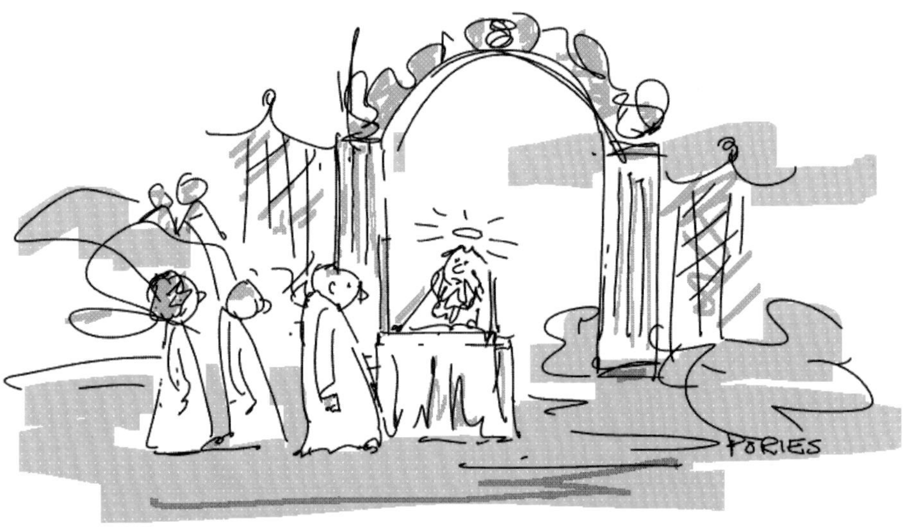


"Ah, yes, you're Doctor Franz, the famous scientist.
You'll be going back to earth as a white rat..."

# Medical Journalism

Colleen M. Hutchinson, MA

Obesity has become a worldwide epidemic, and never before has information on this subject been more needed. Obesity research has garnered a major focus of attention in the medical community by necessity. Medical journalism serves to answer the need for timely and informative research and advancement on the topics of obesity and obesity surgery.

Obesity surgery and care of the bariatric patient encompass several multidisciplinary areas of medicine. One cannot over-emphasize the importance of the healthcare professional's comprehensive approach to best-practices implementation and improvement in these areas. Beyond acquiring knowledge for the sake of clinical advancement, improved standards, and best practices, a comprehensive and thorough approach to a multidisciplinary understanding of obesity is also an inherent component of patient safety. Patient safety outcomes in bariatrics are directly affected by the caregiver's spectrum of knowledge and the resulting methods and level of care provided by that caregiver.

Within the field of obesity surgery, patient behavior plays a uniquely vital role in the outcome of treatment and, therefore, also in the future of a bariatric practice. In a field where increasing emphasis is being placed on accreditation (one of the parameters of which is patient outcomes), the future of bariatric practices will be highly dependent upon the patients' immediate and long-term compliance and success. Regardless of how informed a surgeon is of current research in obesity treatment, if he/she does not continually stay up-to-date and then impart the necessary knowledge to his/her obesity-surgery patient—who has inherited a *permanent* lifestyle-modification regimen—he/she is adhering neither to best practices concerning the patient's safety and success nor the success of the patient outcomes and medical practice.

Reporting of research can now occur first in the *nonmedical* media before being published in medical journals.(1) Keeping current primarily through medical journals is paramount—but it is simply not enough. The average patient today is very informed by the nonmedical media, and if healthcare professionals are not prepared to address and vet that patient knowledge-base, the patient's knowledge scale could prove flawed. Faulty patient education can be detrimental to long-term success because of both consequent problems with compliance and development of unrealistic expectations, which decrease self-efficacy in the obese patient.(2)

At a time when information on obesity is highly sought after and much needed from a variety of perspectives, medical journalism plays an essential role in both establishing and expanding the bariatric healthcare professional's comprehensive knowledge base. As is well-known, the patient does not often see the complete multidisciplinary staff at each visit; yet this does not mean that when patients meet with their surgeon, their questions regarding disciplines other than that of the surgeon are abandoned. For quality-assurance purposes and in an effort to best serve the patient, the surgeon should be as educated as possible on the various multidisciplinary aspects of bariatric care.

Medical journalism meets media's current role as patient educator head-on in an attempt to effectively and accurately address the needs of this growing patient population. Medical journalism's function as healthcare educator in the field of obesity surgery must include surgical, clinical, and allied health disciplines in its scope. Bariatric healthcare professionals must proactively arm themselves with the full armamentarium of knowledge to meet the needs of comprehensive bariatric patient care. Accordingly, it is important to understand the various aspects of medical journalism's role in bariatric patient care and how those aspects affect the surgery practice, the patient, and the care of the bariatric patient.

**The Information-sharing Puzzle: Media, the Informed Patient Population, and Medical Journals**

Patients continually look to news headlines, the Internet, books, and television (news, health specials, reality-show entertainment) as valuable resources for correct medical information. As a result, many now present with not just a general health complaint, but questions and information on symptoms, new related research, possible self-diagnosed conditions, etc. Consequently, the health professional may frequently play the role of clarifier, denouncer, and myth buster. The surgeon must be knowledgeable about what the media is dispensing in terms of new and existing technologies and treatments in bariatrics, not only so he/she can better serve the patient's multidisciplinary needs, but also to counter a sometimes flawed patient knowledge base resulting from misleading, unsubstantiated, or one-sided, media-dispelled information.

As patients become more active in their research, and as the media role in these efforts grows stronger, we must recognize that the need to keep abreast of media coverage in medicine is especially true within the world of weight loss and obesity surgery. While the topic of weight loss is *not* a new one, the growing number of overweight and obese people is, and so is obesity surgery as a first-line treatment. Because this growing trend has an effect on the broader spectrum of society (i.e., national health care, global economics,(3) government policy, adolescent health, etc.), obesity is justifiably and necessarily a topic that must and will continue to be addressed within the media.

One only needs to consider the patients' self-education efforts and the resources available to them to comprehend the value of medical journalism's contribution to bariatric patient care. Obesity surgery specifically is a highly researched topic by past, current, and future obesity surgery patients, especially via the Internet. The Pew Internet & American Life Project determined that 52 million Americans (or 55% of Americans with Internet access) go online to obtain medical information.(4) Typing *obesity* into a Google search turns up over 40 million hits, and *obesity surgery* close to 3 million. Search *obesity chatroom* and view around 1 million links. Chat rooms serve as forums for bariatric patients to share advice, recommend (or discredit) surgeons and centers, meet fellow surgery patients, and provide a support group base for questions and concerns. Unfortunately, some of these "rooms" are virtually unmonitored by bariatric healthcare professionals and often lack essential relevant information.(5) Likewise, news features and mainstream media articles are occasionally misleading, unsubstantiated, or alarmist in nature. You may have already experienced patients asking you about the new "miracle drug" they heard about on the news the night before. Hence the importance of peer-reviewed, validated medical journal content.

By the same token, it is important for the public to become educated on health issues from *knowledgeable* sources—if even from a standpoint of deterrence alone. For example, issues regarding obesity and cardiovascular disease, cancer, bone health, diabetes, sleep apnea, and nutrition may serve to educate the public on the risk of becoming obese and/or leading a sedentary lifestyle. Public education is a significant tool in the fight against obesity and whatever patients can learn stands to improve the state of our overall public health. It will also improve the general knowledge base of those seeking treatment for morbid obesity. The damage done at the above-mentioned venues of misinformation can be undone through the right channels. Bariatric healthcare professionals play a large role in this; as patients come with questions and concerns, the surgeon should be well prepared to discuss different aspects of their care, and also point them in the right direction for legitimate information sources. While the surgeon need not have infinite knowledge of each multidisciplinary area involved in bariatric care, keeping current on accurate, supported research and trends in these areas through medical journal articles is essential. This also underscores the importance of the multidisciplinary approach to medical journalism, discussed later.

Improving patient knowledge will ultimately improve the chances for success in their obesity surgery, as they will be better equipped to handle nutritional, psychological, and physical aspects of care. Beyond the surgery itself, a multidisciplinary approach to treatment and the patient's postoperative compliance effort are paramount factors of surgery success.(6) The more informed patients are from an expectations standpoint regarding postoperative goals and adjustments, the better their self-efficacy and subsequent adherence, and the better the patient outcomes will ultimately be.(7) Patient education offered by staff is also an important element of the informed-consent process.(8)

In addition, educating the obesity surgery patient will improve patient safety, as the patient will be better able to cope with related health issues and conditions, as well as recognize warning signs of complications. The more preoperative and postoperative education and guidance the patient has, the more they (and in turn, bariatric centers) are protected.

### The Importance of Medical Journals in Obesity Care

Keeping abreast of current bariatric care methods and findings in medical journals dedicated to the field is one of the most effective ways of providing the best kind of patient care. One of modern medicine's primary tasks is to communicate and exchange medical information in the quest to improve overall care; our current healthcare system relies on this process of professionals participating in and improving upon the care of patients through such information sharing.(9,10) The dissemination of pertinent medical research and information enables patient care to evolve and improve.(11,12) Peer-reviewed medical journals have developed into an essential vehicle for the dissemination of current research; new concepts, techniques, and technologies; literature reviews; clinical outcomes and findings; best practice recommendations; and reports of individual cases that serve to inform the field.(13) Medical journals enhance best practices as such sharing of information not only educates the healthcare professional, but also advances integration of research and practice, resulting in implementation of new and/or improved strategies in the clinical, practice management, patient management, and multidisciplinary components of health care. Thus, the sharing of informed, validated processes and techniques aids improvement in patient safety, overall prevention of adverse outcomes, and advancement of best practices.

**Multidisciplinary Focus.**

Several components of medical journal publishing introduce inherent value to the final information product. Understanding the general elements of medical publishing that ensure validity, reliability, and relevancy in a particular field is key. Obesity treatment is a distinct medical discipline because of its unique patient population, and bariatric surgical patient care must entail a unique and multidisciplinary approach to care.(13)

With the "paradigm shift" of evidenced-based medicine, scientific and technological advances disseminated via medical journalism for incorporation into patient care,(12) the multidisciplinary approach taken by bariatric medical journals is essential. This learning approach, with focuses that include behavior modification, nutrition, and surgery, will improve clinical treatment and patient safety—both of which are critical components of quality of care.(11)

Multidisciplinary bariatric medical journals aid allied health teams in their coordination of effort and expertise to achieve optimal patient education, selection, consent, care, and short- and long-term management. While multidisciplinary patient involvement is typically well-defined and implemented in an accredited bariatric practice, patients will still want to discuss overlapping disciplines with different staff, and will want to receive guidance in different areas of care. Therefore, one must be aware of all related components of care. In addition, the relationships between these multidisciplinary staff, which determine quality of communications and coordination of patient care, play a significant role in the effort to improve patient safety.(14)

**Surgical Focus**

The surgeon must constantly refresh his/her well of knowledge regarding the various related disciplines, as well as draw from medical journal publications specific to surgery in order to stay informed about relevant surgical research, clinical updates, and new techniques. This is especially the case because obesity surgery, now a recognized subspecialty, continues to define itself through research, surgical advances, and clinical innovations as the science of obesity and its surgical treatment continues to evolve, be built upon, and be disseminated in medical journals.(8) In addition, when many obesity surgeons studied surgery in medical school, obesity surgery was not yet an area in which they could specialize, and multidisciplinary curricula were also nonexistent. While the surgeons' goals did not include overarching coordination of various disciplines and long-term follow-up of chronic conditions and postoperative care, these functions have become a part of their job description by necessity, as evidenced by the American Cancer Society's Statement on Principles Underlying Perioperative Responsibility. The Statement details the surgeon's duty to oversee the patient's overall condition and coordination of treatment.(15)

To effectively arm the bariatric care professional with the tools necessary to provide the highest quality of care, the bariatric medical journal must publish various multidisciplinary perspectives, methodologies, and practices that reliably inform and guide excellent medical decision making. These perspectives include, but are not limited to, surgery, behavior management, nutrition counseling, bariatric-specific nursing, exercise physiology, endocrinology, cardiology, psychology, risk management, and patient-management components of care.(6)

**Patient Safety Focus**

One of the most difficult aspects of improving patient safety is educating healthcare professionals on current, successful techniques and skills, as well as on the skills required for relating this information to patients and fellow staff. Adding to the difficulty is the fact that there is no current universal uniformity to patient-safety best practices or standards, and what is established can be hard to access.(14) All of this underscores the need for findings in patient safety research and evidence-based guidelines for best practices to be disseminated in medical journals.

Further complicating things is the fact that patient-safety education can be challenging because of the difficulty in learning from single instances, where possible improvements can retrospectively be identified (as focus tends to be on individuals involved, rather than the environment).(16) In our present highly litigious, malpractice-bound climate, hospitals are establishing committees and designating staff strictly to oversee patient safety protocols. These hospitals recognize that keeping abreast of successful patient safety methodologies and practices is of paramount importance. In fact, the quest for improvement in patient safety and healthcare quality has led to healthcare institutions training their staff on, and implementing, core innovations that have served to improve the safety record of the airline industry.(17) These innovations focus on improved teamwork objectives, coordination of care, response time, and patient empowerment, and they have helped patient safety protocol development and improvement in the institutions where they have been implemented. Currently these innovations are being utilized in some bariatric centers as well.

Bariatrics is a particularly challenging field of medicine from a patient-safety perspective. The bariatric patient requires different equipment, furniture, products, medical devices, processes (movement, positioning, examination, surgical techniques), and codes of behavior, and therefore requires different standards of care. Timely communication of proactive and successful methods and solutions in patient safety via medical journals is critical to the field of bariatrics, where new challenges are encountered by staff every day. Consequently, patient safety is a necessary focus of journals related to care of the obese patient. It is important to remember that these improvements in methods and protocols that can be shared and learned in bariatric journals serve to improve issues in caregiver injury as well.(18)

**Submissions**

Potential authors of medical journal submissions must exercise skill in recognizing essential research elements, planning and executing the research, assembling the data in an organized fashion, and coherently reporting data in useful, accessible and recognizable ways. Development of writing skills in postgraduate and residency programs would greatly benefit communities that depend on research (i.e., surgical and medical communities).(19)

The submissions process for a particular journal should be well defined in the journal's author information guidelines, and the journal should publish a purpose statement that defines the scope of its content and audience. For a peer-reviewed journal, the submission will undergo peer review by multiple reviewers who are chosen by the editor, based on their expertise in the specific field of the submission's topic. After compiling reviewer comments and recommendations, the editor will decide to accept, reject, or send the paper back to the author for revision. In the bariatric field, a review board should include individuals from the different disciplines involved in bariatric care, so that editorial content in the different areas can be reviewed and improved with validity, as is the objective of this process.

An example of a purpose statement that defines the scope of editorial content and also emphasizes a multidisciplinary focus is the following:

> *Bariatric Times* is designed to provide the most comprehensive readership of surgeons and allied health professionals in bariatric care with timely, relevant news and commentary on developments in obesity treatment. *Bariatric Times* provides a single, concise venue for communications that provide new and detailed information regarding the most updated bariatric total patient care, new clinical findings and industry developments, and all relevant multidisciplinary topics and insights that can be applied to the bariatric allied health professionals' working lives.
>
> Manuscripts that meet our editorial purpose include, but are not limited to, concise articles on surgical technique, reports of preclinical and clinical research that expand existing knowledge, case reports and studies, letters to the editor, and in-depth reviews and reports on treatment, management, prevention, education, ethics, legal issues, and other relevant topics in bariatrics—inclusive of all related allied health disciplines.(20)

**Peer Review and Editorial Board**

According to the American Medical Association, the essence of peer review is to gain expert feedback regarding a paper's importance and/or possibility for improvement.(21) Bias and conflict of interest, as well as the inability to really judge the validity of some research when not a direct witness to it, are deficiencies within the process, underscoring the need for a dedicated, reliable, and varied board of reviewers. A medical journal's editorial board can be independent of a review board, or a journal may have one board that serves both functions. An editorial board's responsibilities can include authoring manuscripts and helping guide the editorial direction of the journal with respect to each member's background. In the case of bariatric medical journals, a varied board of members from the different disciplines related to obesity care is ideal. Editorial board members are expected to help guide editorial direction by suggesting topics, reviewing past content, and helping to make acquisitions of papers on current topics from influential authors in the field. They may advise on advances in the field, as well as on the needs of patients and professionals, and they may provide regular feedback on specific articles and the journal as a whole.

**Columns and Supplements**

Regularly appearing columns within a journal can serve as valuable instruments for disseminating information on obesity surgery specifically because of the multidisciplinary focus, unique patient role in treatment and outcomes, and—historically speaking—relatively new recognized presence in medicine of this medical specialty. Columns can fill certain voids in bariatric editorial content and provide a sense of editorial dependability, as different multidisciplinary sects of the bariatric audience come to regularly rely on them for current information and interesting perspectives within their discipline. Certain columns need not be peer reviewed depending on content, and can be brief and less formal in tone than research-based articles. An example is the *Bariatric Times* Patient Perspective column, in which patients share a unique aspect of their surgical journey (i.e., insurance approval; unrelated, coexisting medical conditions; nutritional observations; age-related surgery issues) so that if and when readers encounter the same or a similar case, they are better prepared to handle it. Obesity surgery is a discipline that, while established in some medical institutions, is just being introduced in others. One example of a journal column that assists new and existing bariatric centers with invaluable guidance is the Bariatric Center Spotlight in *Bariatric Times*, which interviews established, accredited obesity surgery centers and covers everything from staffing information and workflow processes to HIPAA-related solutions to utilization of new bariatric products and techniques. This column fills a void and promotes best practices in providing information-sharing between newer centers looking for guidance and established, successful centers that offer important insights into their decisions and developed processes.

Supplements, which are editorially separate from the regular, peer-reviewed journal articles, but can physically accompany or appear within an issue, are often not funded by the publisher, but by other sources, which necessitates adherence to certain guidelines or set principles regarding content.(1) These supplements provide valuable research information, access to focused content, collaboration between research and industry, and medical education enhancement. Supplements should undergo review by the editor (and, in some cases, additional reviewers), be distinguishable from the other peer-reviewed journal pages, and include citation of funding sources.(1) The same goes for theme issues and special series that can appear in the journal.

**Electronic Media**

In today's technologically advanced society, information can be accessed in multiple formats, and people prefer to receive information by all different means. The greatest advancement has been in the quest to make the information-sharing process faster and more portable. This has had a major impact on modern medicine and its practice. The limitations of time and space in sharing research and other relevant healthcare information are circumvented by computers and their varied offerings of communication methods.(9) Electronic medical media is no exception. It provides healthcare professionals with quick accessibility and the ability to link and share information.(12) Researchers access online sources for reference materials, links to similar works, and verification of accuracy, thoroughness, and timeliness. Practitioners are now able to find sources for more updated and expansive research and findings online than they once could via hard-copy subscriptions, which have become expensive(22) and cumbersome to store. With more than 5,000 journals included in its MEDLINE index, PubMed (www.pubmed.gov), created by the National Library of Medicine, is the most frequently used, free, online database of biomedical journal citations and abstracts.(23) In addition, many journal publishers now offer online journal archives to subscribers, featuring their full-print journal articles, which in some cases are enhanced online with additional commentary or other related editorial information.

Valuable electronic media besides online journal indices and article archives also exist in medical journalism. Continuing medical education (CME), which has traditionally been offered at live events, now trends toward Web-based programs in various formats.(10) Often industry-supported, an educational Webcast is an extremely valuable and innovative tool for bariatric professionals. Providing readers with access to this educational content (which, if archived, is able to be viewed when convenient and also can be shared between colleagues) enhances learning and promotes sharing of information.

Thus, medical journalism plays an indispensable role in the promotion of best practices, patient safety, and enhancement of bariatric patient care. By providing continued multidisciplinary direction and content, sharing new advances in the constantly evolving subspecialty of obesity surgery, and disseminating patient safety innovations and best practice information to the universe of bariatric care professionals, medical journals are an essential part of educating the field of obesity surgery and its patients.

**References**

1. International Committee of Medical Journal Editors. Uniform requirements for manuscripts submitted to biomedical journals: Writing and Editing for Biomedical Publication. Available at: http://www.icmje.org. Updated February 2006.
2. Foster GD, Wadden TA, Phelan S, et al. Obese patients' perceptions of treatment outcomes and the factors that influence them. *Arch Intern Med*. 2001;161:2133-9.
3. Martin L. Economic implications of obesity. In: Buchwald H, Cowan G, Pories W, eds. *Surgical Management of Obesity*. Philadelphia, PA: WB Saunders; 2007:58.
4. Chyna JT. The top 20 healthcare websites: How your patients are using them. *Healthcare Executive*. 2001;16(5);20-5.
5. Madan AK, Frantzides CT, Pesce CE. The quality of information about laparoscopic bariatric surgery on the Internet. *Surg Endosc*. 2003;17(5):685-7.
6. Sarr M, Kendrick M, Clark M, Colazzo-Clavell M, et al. Multidisciplinary team in a bariatric surgery program. In: Buchwald H, Cowan G, Pories W, eds. *Surgical Management of Obesity*. Philadelphia, PA: WB Saunders; 2007:425-431.
7. Gonder-Frederick L, Bauchowitz A, Schirmer B, et al. Patient knowledge in bariatric surgery: Assessment and implications. *Bariatric Times*. 2004;(1)2:10-2.
8. Kaufman D, Kral JG. Academic training of bariatric surgeons. In: Buchwald H, Cowan G, Pories W, eds. *Surgical Management of Obesity*. Philadelphia, PA: WB Saunders; 2007:398.
9. Orthner HF, Scherrer JR, Dahlen R. Sharing and communicating healthcare information: summary and recommendations. *Int J Biomed Comput*.1994;34(1-4):303-18.
10. Iskowitz M. Getting to grips with grants. *Med Marketing & Media*. 2006;41(8):48.
11. Gallagher S. Writing for Publication. In: *The Challenges of Caring for the Obese Patient*. Edgemont, PA: Matrix Medical Communications; 2005:158.
12. Coomarasamy A, Gee H, Publicover M, Khan KS. Medical journals and effective dissemination of health research. *Health Info Libr J*. 2001;18(4):183-91.
13. National Institutes of Health Consensus Development Conference Panel. Gastrointestinal surgery for severe obesity. *Ann Int Med*. 1991;(115):956-61.

14. VanGeest J, Cummins D. An educational needs assessment for improving patient safety: results of a national study of physicians and nurses (National Patient Safety Foundation), page 1. Available at: http://www.npsf.org/download/EdNeedsAssess.pdf. Accessed: January 20, 2007.

15. American College of Surgeons. Statement on principles underlying perioperative responsibility. *Bull Am Coll Surg.* 1996;81(9):39-40.

16. American Association of Clinical Endocrinologists. Patient Safety and Medical System Errors in Diabetes and Endocrinology Consensus Conference, January 11, 2005: Washington, DC. Available at: http://www.aace.com/meetings/consensus/pscc. Accessed January 13, 2007.

17. Olsen K. Rethinking patient safety. *HealthLeaders.* 2006;9:41-42.

18. Gallagher S. Issues of caregiver injury. *Bariatric Times*. 2005;(2)1:16-19.

19. Anaya-Prado R, Toledo AH, Toledo-Pereyra LH. The surgeon as a scientific writer. *J Invest Surg*. 2006;19(6):335-339.

20. Information for Authors: Bariatric Times. Matrix Medical Communications 2005: Edgemont, PA.

21. American Medical Association. Manual of Style, 9th Edition: A Guide for Authors & Editors. Chicago, Ill: Lippincott Williams & Wilkins; 1998:175.

22. Kean G. 18th annual study of journal prices for scientific and medical society journals. JP 2005;3:8. Available at: http://www.allenpress.com/static/newsletters/pdf/JP-2005-03.pdf. Accessed May 26, 2008.

23. National Library of Medicine and National Institute of Health. PubMed. Available at: http://www.ncbi.nlm.nih.gov/entrez/query.fcgi?db=PubMed. Accessed May 26, 2008.

# Media Relations

Jerry Berger

Check out a database catalog of media stories using the words "gastric bypass surgery" or "weight loss surgery" and you will be overwhelmed. Googling the term "gastric bypass surgery" generates 2.7 million hits; "weight loss surgery" returns 5.9 million hits.

Use the LexisNexis database, which captures "serious" news stories from traditional media outlets, and the results are similarly impressive—going back to the first stories in 1983. *The Boston Globe* first covered the procedure in 1988.

Narrow the search by adding the word "death" and the numbers are still startling—more than 250 in the past year. In fact, that 1988 *Boston Globe* story examines the death of a prominent Boston police officer ("Risks of surgery vs. obesity stir medical debate," December 26, 1988.).

But does quality follow quantity? A random examination of many of these stories says the answer, sadly, is no. Overwhelmingly, the stories fall into two broad categories: "Doesn't he/she look great?" or, "What a sad story!" With few exceptions, journalists have not taken the time to look at these procedures with any depth of interest, whether it is to examine the reasons people opt for surgery, to portray the risks inherent in acting or not acting on the condition of obesity, or to highlight what other things people need to do before turning to this tool in the arsenal of weight management.

Beth Israel Deaconess Medical Center (BIDMC) found itself in the center of a media maelstrom after the death of a patient from complications as a result of weight loss surgery. Most of the coverage fell into that broad second category ("What a sad story!"), with some television outlets going so far as to accuse BIDMC of a cover-up because federal patient privacy laws prevented comment beyond expressions of condolence. That case followed closely on the heels of a death at Brigham & Women's Hospital that was tied to postsurgical complications.

Part of the problem facing journalists is what Dr. Ninh T. Nguyen has labeled the "exponential" growth in the procedure. Nguyen, chief of the division of gastrointestinal surgery at University of California-Irvine Medical Center, in a study of Nationwide Inpatient Sample data, notes there were 70,256 cases of this surgery in 2002, rising to more than 150,000 the following year, according to a 2005 study.(1)

Clinicians are well aware of the primary reasons patients turn to surgery to deal with weight issues: the comorbidities that accompany excess weight pose extreme danger. They know that the procedure offers a last, but best, chance for patients who have not been able to control their weight through other means. But for the public, the procedure remains exotic—brought to light by "success" stories such as singer Carnie Wilson's experience and that of television personality Al Roker. For many, obesity is still a reflection of a person's absence of willpower rather than a disease process in itself.

The flip side to that celebrity-driven context is a lack of understanding among the public about the risks and benefits (although Roker has done some good reporting, not only about his experiences, but on the broader issues as well). As journalist and former Harvard School of Public Health instructor David Ropeik observes, risk perception is informed by feelings and lifestyle and needs to be better understood by both journalists and clinicians. He considers standard informed consent documents a "lousy" way to make the case for surgery because their use is an attempt to apply rational processes to deal with something that carries with it a great deal of uncertainty and fear. Ropeik, who coauthored "Risk: A Practical Guide for Deciding What's Really Safe and What's Really Dangerous in the World Around You," notes that people perceive risk differently, that it is not simply a matter of looking at facts. The data are filtered through prisms of perception psychology to powerfully inform the choices that patients make in opting for this surgery and that journalists make in reporting on it. And those prisms must work with a torrent of data that include specialty Web sites, as well as print and broadcast media. Web sites such as www.obesityhelp.com offer opportunities for people to learn about weight loss options and to share experiences they have had with hospitals and clinicians.

As www.obesityhelp.com site founder and Chief Executive Officer Eric Klein notes, the online community offers a dynamic media in which patients may interact to gain the proper perspective on the risk-benefit ratio. The focus ("common people afflicted with a common problem") provides a much needed context for patients, as well as a forum to explore options and vent emotions. Another form of alternative communications has gained popularity—blogging. Patients now can share their personal thoughts and observations online through personal Web logs.

As for the mainstream media, the demands of deadlines, space, and time continue to limit what readers and viewers learn. As *Boston Globe* reporter Liz Kowalczyk acknowledged during her lecture at the Patient Safety in Obesity Surgery course in 2005, there must be a better effort made to look at outcomes, success claims, and why procedures fail. And just as importantly, greater attention should be paid to the question, "What are people who don't have surgery dying from?" The business side of the procedure is also in need of review, Kowalczyk said, reflecting on the gulf between the perception of this surgery as a profit center for hospitals and the contention by surgeons that it is a break-even, or even a money-losing proposition.

But therein lays a potential problem, according to Terry L. Schraeder, MD, a one-time medical television journalist and now a clinician at Mt. Auburn Hospital in Cambridge. He notes that trust levels between clinicians and journalists are not good, although it is a situation best described as "one of ignorance rather than conflicting interests or malice."

For example, while Kowalczyk, who has delved into the underlying issues, stated that "doctors need to talk openly about these stories," Schraeder believes many clinicians are wary of such dialogue, because "given today's realities of covering medical news, an important genetic discovery of a lethal disease often needs to be communicated in one-and-a-half minutes or 500 words."(2). Given this ongoing conflict, it is likely clinicians (and their medical centers) are going to rely on new technology, as well as more traditional public relations and marketing tools, to get their messages across.

In early 2007, BIDMC experimented with the latest technology by providing a 10-minute explanation of obesity, weight loss and bariatric surgery through a link on YouTube (http://www.youtube.com/watch?v=c9-0sYgH0qk&eurl), the popular Web site where videos on a dazzling array of topics are posted. That video is linked back to the medical center's Web site for a fuller description of the overall weight loss program.

BIDMC continues to work with traditional print and broadcast journalists to provide information on the latest research, offering clinicians who function as experts in speaking to reporters, and fielding specific informational requests.

The goal for both clinicians and journalists should continue to be a free and full discussion of the risks, benefits, rewards, and drawbacks of a procedure that offers truly life-saving possibilities to morbidly obese people who have run through every other available option.

**References**

1. Kelly J, Tarnoff M, Shikora S, et al. Best practice recommendations for surgical care in weight loss surgery. *Obes Res.* 2005;13(2):227-33.
2. Schraeder TL. A chasm of distrust in medical reporting: a doctor who was a medical journalist tries to understand why journalists don't trust their sources and sources don't trust reporters. *Nieman Reports*. June 2003.

# Ethics: How to Discuss Medical Errors

Kenneth A. Larsen, DMin, PhD

Complications are expensive and mistakes, if they are not handled well, are even more expensive. Therefore, quality communication is central to any ethics process. In writing about medical errors and how to discuss them with patients and their families, various factors seem to come into play. Current thinking about risks vs. benefits of disclosing medical errors in today's healthcare culture has become a hot topic where disagreements are many. It is not an easy subject by any means, but it is important, it seems to me, to be able to differentiate between a blaming culture, which I believe is largely what we have today, and the more progressive culture where errors are viewed as systems problems and are held collectively. On the other hand, it seems crucial that professionals, as individuals who must traverse this life-and-death territory that is their daily arena, be willing to learn why and how to say *I'm sorry*.

**Risks vs. Benefits of Disclosing Medical Errors**

We live in a very interesting time when there seems to be a groundswell shift in society toward an expectation of professional openness, honesty, and timely disclosure of errors. We have seen the public reaction to *Newsweek's* late retraction of its error in recording Koran abuse at Guantanamo Bay, which led directly to widespread protests and riots in the Muslim world during which at least 17 people were killed in ensuing violence. What can we learn from this case? One, this was a system problem within the magazine itself that led to going with a story lacking the usual level of corroboration. Two, for *Newsweek*, the public perception of failure to disclose and to apologize led to a moral outcry. The one thing you don't want to do is become a portrait on the front page of a major newspaper or national magazine.

So in discussing the errors or "system problems" that might befall us in the medical setting, my first thought is that it is best to be quite upfront with your patients. According to many bariatric surgeons, bariatric surgery is not necessary for any patient; but for the right patient, it can be successful and can significantly improve health.

One of the keys to keeping mistakes down is to choose the correct patient. This is the challenge with back surgeries in the facility I work in and the trick is to choose the right patient. That solves a lot of problems down the road. From my involvement in ethical adjudications, it's always smart to get a patient's mutual buy-in, not only to the inherent risks, but also to what we call the *informed consent.*

Not every clinician gets the true concept of informed consent, even though we deal with it every day. Informed decision-making involves much more than a traditional consent form. It takes extra time and too often we perceive that we don't have that extra time. But experience teaches us that we would lower our risk and serve our patients better if we take that time to sit down and discuss the risks, giving adequate time and opportunity for the patient's questions, and to tease out their unexpressed concerns. It is their *un*expressed or *un*voiced questions that will come back to bite us when something goes wrong, so this time is necessary and will be well spent.

Two celebrity cases demonstrate what happens when things go well and when they don't, in terms of bariatric surgery. For Carnie Wilson, singer and daughter of Beach Boy Brian Wilson, surgery went well. She lost the weight, achieved the health, life balance, and body she always wanted. Everybody was happy. But in the case of Charlie Weiss, former offensive coordinator for the New England Patriots and coach at Notre Dame, the surgery apparently went horribly wrong, as he almost lost his life in the operating room. Charlie spent most of the 2003 football season in a motorized chair on the sidelines.

These highly publicized examples are two sides of this story. The best advice is to carefully rehearse what can go wrong, rehearse how you will discuss the reality of risks to your patients and rehearse how you will approach your patient who does not do well, or has a catastrophic event during the course of his/her procedure. Especially with obesity surgery, there is a lot at stake psychologically. Full disclosure from the onset will go a long way in helping the patient cope with his/her emotional reaction of fear, anxiety, shame, anger, and disappointment when results of surgery turn out to be less than what was hoped for.

A primary reason why hospitals do not disclose errors is fear of malpractice litigation. That's obvious. What is not so obvious, and may be controversial, is that some recent research suggests that hospitals might lower their overall malpractice exposure and its associated costs by instituting a policy of extreme honesty. Increasingly, experience seems to agree with the trend that error disclosure can actually lower malpractice costs. Dr. John Banja, from the Center for Ethics at Emory University, notes that "patients have a right to know about critical incidents, even if they are not physically harmed by them. This rationale for disclosure, based on the ethical issue of autonomy, goes beyond what the law might require one to do."

But often, according to Dr. Banja, "doctors argue that reporting an error may anguish the patient unnecessarily and may breed suspicion in the patient's mind, and that disclosure may erode the patient's trust in their doctors." I think we have heard that argument. I certainly have. What is beginning to change, however, is recognition that although the presumed concerns are plausible, they tend not to be correct and thus, simply don't apply in some situations. Banja also states, "Ethics, law, and the literature suggest that when doctors make mistakes, they have a moral obligation to disclose their errors to the patient in a timely and open fashion. Sweeping errors under the carpet undermines public trust in medicine, because patients feel that doctors are more interested in protecting themselves and their colleagues than they are in protecting the patient's well-being."

**Blaming vs. Faulty Systems in Ascribing Responsibility for Medical Errors**

Findings from several studies of large numbers of hospitalized patients indicate that each year a million or more people are injured and as many as 100,000 die as a result of errors in their medical care. That's astonishing. This makes medical care one of the leading causes of death, accounting for more lives than automobile accidents, breast cancer, or AIDS. In his address to the United States Senate, Harvard School of Public Health patient safety expert, Dr. Lucian Leape, stated that, "While no physician or nurse wants to hurt patients, and mind you, doctors, nurses, and other healthcare workers are highly trained to be careful and take precautions to prevent mistakes, paradoxically, it is precisely this exclusive focus on the individual's responsibility not to make mistakes, reinforced by punishment, that makes health care so unsafe." He continues, "The reason is that errors are seldom due to carelessness or lack of trying hard enough. More commonly, errors are caused by faulty systems, processes, and conditions that lead people to make mistakes. They can be prevented by designing systems that make it hard for people to do something wrong and easy to do it right. Safe industries, such as aviation, chemical manufacturing, and nuclear power, have learned these lessons long ago. While insisting on training and high standards of performance, they recognize that these are insufficient to ensure safety. They pay attention to factors that affect performance, such as hours, workloads, work conditions, team relationships, and the design of tasks, to make errors difficult to make. They create safety by design. Health care must do likewise." Leape concluded, "Approaches that focus on punishing individuals instead of changing systems provide strong incentives for people to report only those errors they cannot hide. Thus, a punitive approach shuts off the information that is needed to identify faulty systems and create safer ones. In a punitive system, no one learns from their mistakes."

From my own personal experience, there is much more to patient safety than just being careful. It takes a village to support a surgeon and to provide the proper healing environment for the patient. Nurses, adjunctive therapists, chaplains, psychologists, intensivists, or hospitalists—all provide the system with valuable checks and balances. We're the extension of the surgeons' eyes and ears and consciousness on the floors. A culture of cooperation, mutuality, and respect is crucial to keeping the patient safe.

At New England Baptist Hospital, we have developed, over the course of 11 years, a 4-step ethics process that works very well. Through it, anyone from housekeeping staff to top administrators can evoke a gathering of all clinicians involved in a patient's care to a patient-care conference whenever there is a patient-care concern. That's our policy. Whenever that conference convenes, the attending physician is always in charge, with the patient, family, and care team present, taking the time necessary to recognize, respond, and resolve the concerns expressed. It is our experience that this type of active communication not only prevents problems from escalating down the road, but also substantively supports the doctor in navigating the disclosure if something should go wrong.

**The Power of Apology**

So, how do we say—and why do we say—*I'm sorry*? The moral courage required to disclose a medical error is great. Making that disclosure is an enormously caring and even loving act. It is painful to admit one's errors, especially to those who have been harmed by them. And though offering an apology may be counterintuitive in a litigious society, it is ultimately healing for the patient, the patient's family, and the healthcare professional who has made the error.

Colorado and Oregon legislatures passed laws a while ago allowing doctors to make statements of apology, sympathy and condolence with the assurance that these statements would not be used against them later in court. There already were similar laws on the books in California, Massachusetts, and Texas. The major barrier to doctors being honest with their patients is fear of malpractice litigation, but now, fortunately, evidence is accumulating that shows this may be a myth. It appears to be the other way around, in fact. It appears to be when things go wrong, the failure to be straightforward in telling patients what happened and the failure to apologize, increases the risk of being sued. When they are angry, people sue because their doctor withheld information, did not take responsibility, or would not apologize for the mishap. We must change this. We must treat patients the way we would like to be treated ourselves, remembering that, armed with Internet search engines and access to medical records as they are today, patients will keep looking until their questions are answered. If the doors to their physician's office or hospital administrators are closed to them, they will go to the lawyers next.

How, then, does one disclose medical errors? The short answer is, by employing the 3-Rs concept: Recognize, Respond, Resolve. Doctors should take the lead, acknowledging what has happened in an objective and a narrative fashion. However, in my view an attending physician should not have to do this alone. He/she is always a part of a bigger team and to convene that team around a patient and family has tremendous healing potential. Let the family and the patient dictate the pace and scope of the discussion, facilitating the expression of unvoiced concerns that they may have. There can be a transcendent quality that emerges out of such conversation. I have often referred to this as a sort of tribal consciousness, in which anger and fear gives way to restored trust and frank exploration of tough questions. Something archetypal can happen in these meetings and a new relationship can be born. But this takes time, commitment, and patience—often in the face of a very disagreeable patient or family member in the beginning. No one can manage the myriad dynamics alone, and timing is everything.

Apologies can definitely come too late, as they did for *Newsweek*. The right time to act is as soon as possible. Because it is human nature to put off painful experiences, it is also important to have an identified system in place that is part of the fabric of the hospital to ensure access to doctor/patient/family communication around all issues of concern, but especially when there has been an error. Some go as far as to suggest that near misses should also be reported to the patient, with the assurance that steps will be taken to correct them.

Because of my unique role in the hospital as a minister and psychologist, I often get to talk with patients who have been "burned" by the medical establishment (obviously not ours). One thing stands out — these patients are genuinely appreciative when someone steps up to the plate and acknowledges wrongdoing and lays out a plan for correction. There is a correlation between litigation and anger; what we must do is to become more skillful in mitigating the anger before the anger litigates us.

Doctors should rehearse what they plan to say. In describing the *balance beam* approach to disclosure, Dr. Pichert from Vanderbilt University School of Medicine refers to 5 basic strategies, each carrying its own sets of risks and benefits. They are listed below and I leave it to those interested to determine which to use when a medical mistake happens.

1. No disclosure at all
2. Disclosure of just the safe facts
3. Limited disclosure made of established facts, with a promise to disclose more facts as they become known
4. Full disclosure right away
5. Full disclosure with assigning of responsibility and how it will be corrected and who will be responsible

**Suggested Reading**


1. Leape LI. Statement of Lucian Leape, MD concerning patient safety and medical errors before the United States Senate; American Psychological Association Public Policy Office. January 25, 2000.
2. Leape LI. Reporting of adverse events. *N Engl J Med.* 2002;347:1633-8.
3. Robeznieks A. The power of an apology: patients appreciate open communication. *AMNews.* July 28, 2003.
4. Wu AW, Cavanaugh TA, McPhee SJ, Lo B, Micco GP. To tell the truth: ethical and practical issues in disclosing medical mistakes to patients. *J Gen Intern Med.* 1997;12:770-5.
5. Kohn LT, Corrigan JM, Donaldson MS, eds. *To Err is Human: Building a Safer Health System*. Washington, D.C., National Academies Press; 2000.
6. Rosner F, Berger JT, Kark P, et al. Disclosure and prevention of medical errors. Committee on Bioethical Issues of the Medical Society of the State of New York. *Arch Intern Med.* 2000;160:2089-92.
7. Kraman S, Hamm G. Risk management: extreme honesty may be the best policy. *Ann Intern Med.* 1999;131:963-7.
8. Hebert PC, Levin AV, Robertson G. Bioethics for clinicians: 23. Disclosure of medical error. Available at: http://www.cma.ca/cmaj/series/bioethic.htm. Accessed September 5, 2007.

# Risk-Management Foundation

John McCarthy, MBA

Many malpractice claims originate when expectations about outcomes are not met. While bariatric surgery has had quite a lot of hype in the press and some high-profile patients have had excellent outcomes, when patients have poor outcomes they might naturally assume that a mistake was made. Patient education leading to well-informed patients who understand the surgical risks of these procedures is a key element in avoiding lawsuits. Expectations must be tempered with well-documented efforts to inform the patient about the procedure, recovery process, and potential complications. It is equally important to involve the patient's family or partner in the discussions, as they may be in the position of making care decisions and organizing support following discharge.

In reviewing malpractice cases from the Harvard system and from other jurisdictions, some common themes have emerged:

1. Provider training and certification is a critical success factor
2. Postsurgery care must be highly organized with staff attuned to the potential complications and key indicators that something is going wrong
3. The hospital must be equipped to care for obese patients
4. A team approach to care and access to the attending physician postsurgery makes early identification of complications much more likely

Malpractice insurers in many US markets have either begun to restrict coverage for bariatric surgery or are questioning whether or not it is an insurable risk. It is not unusual for a new procedure, especially one so heavily marketed, to have a surge in claims right along with the increased volume.

**Figure 1**

National Trend in Weight Loss Surgery

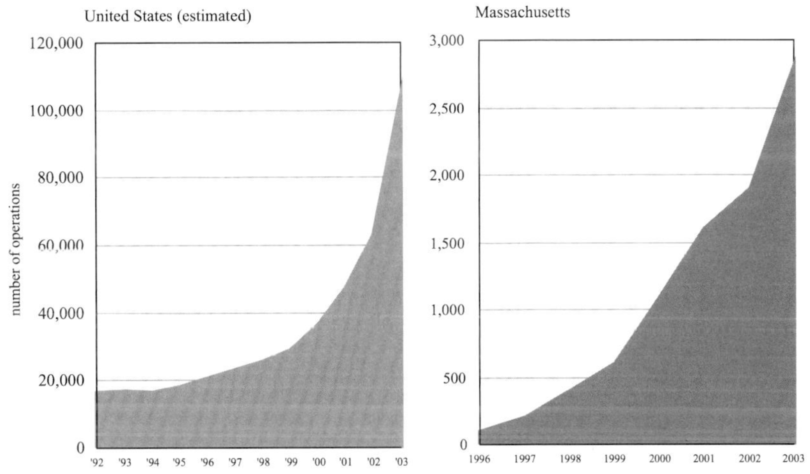


Source: Ridley N. Expert Panel on Weight Loss Surgery—Executive Report. Obesity Research, 2003.

Insurance companies react very badly to situations like the one indicated in Figure 1. When an extremely substantial uptick in instances of a particular surgical procedure occurs, they typically restrict coverage and raise rates hoping that if the climb continues they can moderate their exposure. One prime example of this type of reaction is that of the Medical Liability Mutual Insurance Company (MLMIC), the largest malpractice insurer in New York State. A May 27, 2005, *New York Times* article reported that MLMIC had "notified surgeons that it would end all coverage for bariatric surgery on July 1, unless the state insurance department approved a 50% increase in premiums." As of this writing, MLMIC does provide coverage, but surgeons doing bariatric surgery pay 60.5 % more than other surgeons.

The Harvard teaching hospitals are insured through the Controlled Risk Insurance Company (CRICO), whose program is administered by the Risk Management Foundation. CRICO/RMF is the largest malpractice insurer in Massachusetts. As of the year 2005, it was insuring 10,000 physicians and 18 hospitals. Bariatric claims have exhibited low frequency

**Figure 2**

CRICO Gastric Bypass Cases*

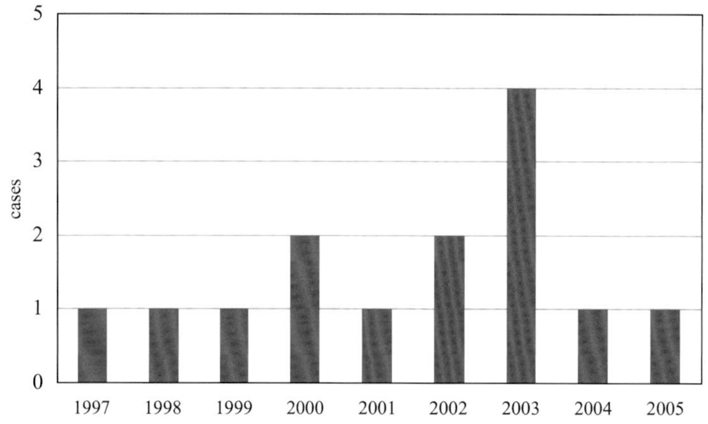


*N=14 cases asserted 1/1/97-6/1/05; surgery done using either an open incision or laparoscopically

While Figure 2 reflects very low frequency for claims, it does not show the number of incidents or adverse events associated with this type of surgery. Claims rates, however, are not at a level that would cause us to institute a higher premium for surgeons doing this type of surgery.

**The "Down Side" of Advertising**

Advertising healthcare services is good for revenue generation, but that same advertising can be used against a provider or hospital organization. One of the byproducts we are seeing in the claims in Massachusetts is a challenge to the law of Regulation of Business Practices for Consumer Protection, and this is based on advertising. In Massachusetts, hospitals have what is called charitable immunity. They can only be sued for up to $20,000 per claim, with the remainder of the liability falling on the physicians involved. But plaintiff lawyers are alleging that since the hospital is marketing these services by advertising, it goes beyond the bounds of charitable immunity and the institution itself should be at more substantial risk. We don't think that's a worthy position, but this new "theory of liability" may be litigated before the question is finally settled.

Our limited claims experience shows that when bariatric surgery cases occur, they tend to be of high severity (64%), with the potential payout at $500,000 or more. When we analyze and code the clinical issues in these cases, technical skills, clinical judgment, and protocol compliance show as significant issues. Communication among providers and appropriate handoffs were also critical to successful management of complications.

It's important to understand the in-depth coding that results from the clinical reviews and depositions. What we found is that most of the challenges in these cases related to inexperience centered around the surgery itself—patient selection, choice of the procedure based on the patient's needs and desires, selection of the right operating technique, technical skill of the surgeon or team, level of postoperative monitoring, and the quality of the long-term follow-up by the surgeon and team after the patient's discharge. What becomes clear is that there is a need to be able to judge which patients are good candidates for this procedure and which are not.

Bariatric patients appear to be much more vulnerable to complications due to obesity-related comorbid conditions. Delays in getting the patient back to the operating room (OR) to explore the problem hamper the defense. If imaging studies are not clear, there should be a documented attempt to redo the study and the patient should be properly informed of the problems being encountered. Coordination of care and postoperative monitoring is imperative. In addition, we found that patients' concerns over complications they are experiencing are not given sufficient attention or credibility.

Preoperatively, patients must be assisted with making genuinely informed decisions about the surgery. Communication of information with regard to high-risk situations is required so that both patient and family fully understand these risks, including the possibility of death. There has been a resurgence in allegations of lack of informed consent in all kinds of clinical settings. Whether it is that the plaintiff bar has done a seminar on how to bring this forward as an issue or that we in the healthcare system are not doing as good a job in informed consent, and documenting the process is not clear; but this seems to be a growing element in the defense of malpractice cases.

From an insurance perspective, the sudden influx of claims is not unusual when new procedures are put into operation. Provider and surgeon reaction was almost immediate as significant patient-management lessons were learned. In particular, it was noted that obese patients require special care, techniques, and equipment, as well as specially trained teams to care for them.

As obesity continues to increase as a public health concern, we believe any efforts expended to stem claims nationwide will be money well spent, because the number of surgeries is only going to continue to grow. As usual, we're scrambling to get out ahead of the issue; however, these issues appear to be receiving more proactive attention than we've seen given to other issues; there remains a need to do more, faster.

We've had a very good experience with simulation training and team training. Several years ago, the anesthesiology chiefs asked if we would provide a premium incentive for attendings to use the anesthesia simulator. A modest incentive was put in place and the program received virtually 100% participation. Ultimately, residents and attending physicians alike completed anesthesia crisis management simulator training. The success of the premium incentive program prompted us to offer obstetricians 1 year of team training, followed by simulation training in the next year, along with online continuing medical education programs. A 10% premium discount is included. The program has proved very promising; early data reflect a drop in both error rates and malpractice claims.

There are excellent training opportunities for minimally invasive surgery as well. Some of the literature suggests it is necessary to do 100 of these surgeries to be proficient, and the idea of doing them on a simulator and not a patient is very appealing to a malpractice insurer. This type of training and credentialing can help us, substantially, to stay ahead of this risk.

The healthcare system presents a great deal of opportunity for variation in complication rates among healthcare institutions, both on a national level and within a given state. In New York, for instance, a state health department study found a 400% variation in cardiac outcomes among high-volume centers. This is a tremendous variation and would be totally unacceptable in industry. The study indicates that these are high-volume centers, which tells us that more volume doesn't necessarily mean higher quality of care.

Thus, there appears to be great opportunity to focus efforts on both credentialing and competency training in order to try to improve quality and reduce some of the claims experience in bariatric surgery.

# Legal and Tort Issues

Luke Sato, MD

Allegations are statements plaintiffs make about what happened and the reasons why they are filing a claim or lawsuit. Allegations are used to take into account what the patient has experienced and to help us aim our efforts in a certain direction.

Experience has taught us when patients traverse through the healthcare system, their unique perspective offers an informative story on how care and services were provided to them and/or how these care and service processes failed within the system. As an illustration of where failures occurred in a given case, a slide is often shown depicting departments of a hospital vertically forming silos and the patient crossing (successfully or otherwise) these silos horizontally.

RMF Patient Safety Process

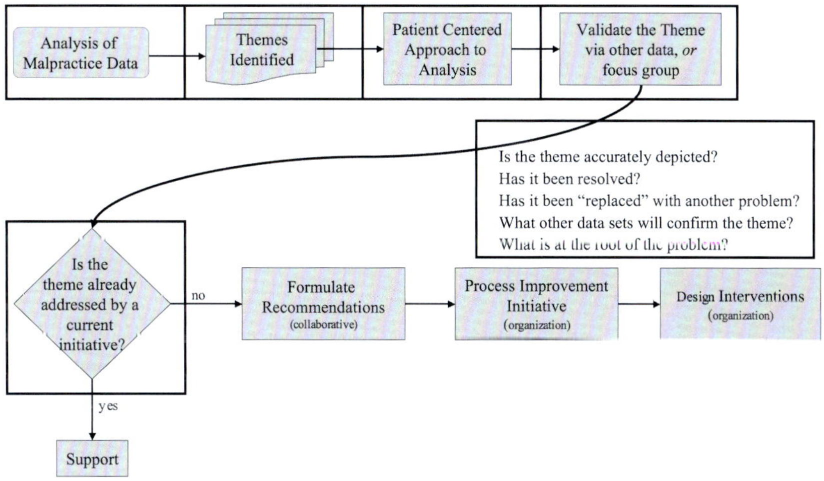


Malpractice claims are thoroughly analyzed in order to determine the factors contributing to an adverse medical event. This is essentially a root-cause analysis. Together with this and the information obtained from plaintiff allegations and depositions, a picture of the event is pieced together using information offered through the investigative process of handling malpractice claims. This methodical approach and the issues that emerge are reconciled and validated with input from the institutions that Controlled Risk Insurance Company (CRICO) serves. The input is collected via a response form asking specific questions:

- Is this risk issue valid?
- Do you recognize it?
- Is it something of concern to you?
- Do you have the same risk issues from your perspective as we do?
- Has it been resolved?
- How do you deal with it and what processes do you see replacing it?
- Do you have any interventions specifically dealing with this risk issue?

If the institution answers yes, CRICO supports the intervention. But if there are no initiatives in place, recommendations, process improvements, and design initiatives are formulated with our institutions in a collaborative manner.

## Underlying Contributing Factors

- No clear indication for surgery—patient selection
- Protracted nature of the postoperative complications
    - Postoperative course extremely complicated and totally unanticipated by the physician, the patient, and the patient's family
- Unexpected death following a low-risk surgical procedure
- Significant delays in diagnosing intra-abdominal pathology
- Residents and fellows failed to notify the attending or a senior surgeon about deteriorating condition
- Patients become emotionally distraught when their surgeon not available (e.g., patients in great pain or require urgent return to OR)
- Failure to listen to patient's problems following discharge—failure to identify the source of patient's symptoms
- Patients felt *"cared for,"* but not *"cared about"*

The figure above outlines issues seen in surgical malpractice claims received by CRICO. One issue often arises during the postoperative period of patient care: complications or unexpected events that occur and are totally unanticipated by the physician, perioperative team, or the patient's family. This places the caregivers in the position of having to become reactive in setting expectations for the family regarding future care of the patient.

A variation on this theme occurs when patients unexpectedly die after a relatively low-risk surgical procedure. How can proper expectations be set with the patient and family if there is a delay in diagnosing conditions such as bowel perforations or nicked arteries—due, of course, to the fact that symptoms of these untoward events manifest for the most part postoperatively and in an insidious manner? The underpinning solution to all of this, of course, is setting the proper expectations for patient and family by having in place a robust, shared, decision-making process.

Another issue to look into involves residents and fellows. We often see these professionals involved in CRICO malpractice cases, although they're not named as defendants quite as often as attending physicians. In such cases, a theme frequently encountered is that the resident or fellow did not involve the attending physicians sooner because of lack of knowledge or experience, or because the environment and culture of the department was not conducive to reporting and following the established chain of command.

Yet another issue arises when patients become extremely anxious and angry if their attending surgeon is not available postoperatively. Residents and fellows are again sent as substitutes for the attending physicians and in these situations, when complications occur or a decision must be made as to whether or not to return to the operating room, significant delays and communication failures can complicate the situation.

Failure to listen to patients' problems belongs on this list of complaints that drive malpractice claims. Patients are at various levels of ability when it comes to communicating their concerns to their caregivers. "I have some issues, some problems, please listen to me," is not always directly stated, allowing for disconnect between the patient and provider. Or perhaps the provider simply doesn't hear what the patient is adamantly trying to say. In fact, there are numerous cases where, sadly, the adage, "The patient often is cared for, but not necessarily cared *about*," can be applied.

## A Care Delivery Model of Layered Processes

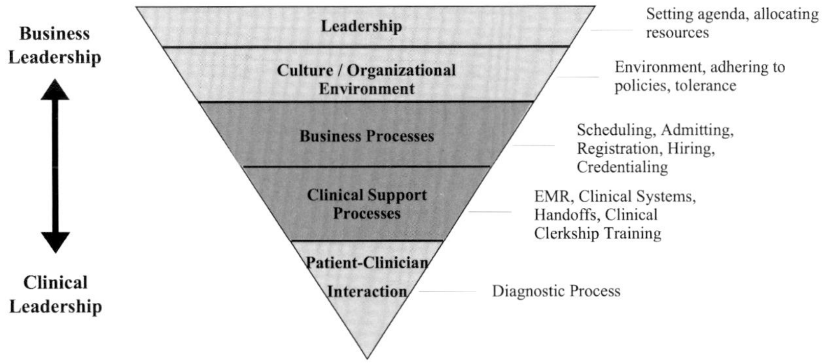


Looking at malpractice cases as a whole, it can be seen that we conceptually describe our observations in a multilayered, care-process model. Each layer consists of processes or functions performed in order to support the bottom of the triangle: the clinical encounter. In the clinical encounter (the "sharp end"), clinicians interface with their patients to directly obtain information such as family history, specific complaints, and findings through the physical examination. This information is fed to the physician's own clinical diagnostic cognitive process, which leads to a preliminary diagnosis. The next layer contains processes that support the clinical encounter. These include systems or clinical processes that, for example, further corroborate the initial diagnosis and add to the information obtained directly from the patient. Clinicians must have access to their patients' medical records to execute the necessary steps based on what information is available to them, along with their clinical judgment. Whether paper-based or electronic, a process and a system must be in place that enables the clinician to properly access all relevant information (clinical notes, medical history, physical examination findings, and laboratory and test results) needed to make the proper diagnosis. In addition, if a clinician should be required to make a referral to another provider, this would also be considered part of the clinical support process.

Next is the business process layer, consisting of processes and functions that are more administrative in nature. These support the running of an office practice, clinic, or hospital. Examples of these functions would include scheduling, admitting, and registration—the type of administrative activities conducted by any organization that deals with patients. Other functions include hiring of staff and credentialing, certifying, and privileging physicians. Each of these may comprise multiple embedded processes.

Finally, in the top two layers, we have culture/organizational environment and leadership.

Although many of the issues we see in medical malpractice claims stem from what happens back down in that "sharp end" of the triangle (where, in other words, something might go wrong between a provider and a patient during a particular clinical encounter and, as a consequence, lead to a claim or suit), we see failures in the other layers as well. The model described is an extremely simplistic construct for health care, but it helps us to understand that systems and process failures account for just as much in terms of medical malpractice claims as does any negligent and non-negligent behavior of individual healthcare providers.

Consider the following: a patient alleges he/she was coerced by the surgeon to have a particular procedure and subsequently experienced an adverse event. The event must be broken down into various subcomponents. From the patient's perspective, the issue is that he/she was being rushed to and through surgery without having the proper time or the appropriate information to make an informed decision as to whether having that procedure was the correct choice. From the healthcare organization's perspective, this patient was thought to be an ideal candidate for the procedure and was taken through a thorough screening process, with all expectations properly communicated and consent obtained.

But did this really happen? If so, the question then becomes, what was the informed-consent process for this procedure? Was there a dialogue between patient and physician, over a period of multiple visits, to appropriately screen him/her as a good candidate for the procedure and set proper expectations? Or was the idea of having such an operation suddenly thrown at the patient?

## Issues/Challenges include …

| "Rush to surgery" perception | vs. | careful patient selection |
|---|---|---|
| Boiler plate informed consent (single visit) | vs. | dialogue with patients (over multiple visits) |
| "Cared for" | vs. | "Cared about" |
| Managing patient expectations (single point in time) | vs. | Managing expectations over time (perhaps a lifetime) |
| Lack of expertise (critical care coverage) | vs. | Dedicated bariatric team 24/7 |

Not only does this relate to the issue of informed consent, but, in a broader context, it also raises the issue of full communication with the patient and his/her family. Are these concerns something we have found with just this particular caregiver or is the environment encouraging this type of rushed informed consent as part of the decision-making process? This also ties into individual inexperience playing a large part in malpractice cases where postoperative complications are missed and problems occur during the bariatric procedure itself. Again, the environment and culture could be playing a role where asking for help is considered "not macho" and, therefore, results in complications going unobserved and treatment being delayed. In terms of interventions that potentially could mitigate these issues, we are currently seeing encouraging results coming from teamwork and communication training. Nevertheless, poor communication, not only between healthcare provider peers, but also between provider and patient, still plays a large part in malpractice claims. The good news, however, is that we have found that good communication is nurtured by having well-designed processes and systems and an environment in which leadership fosters open dialogue between all involved stakeholders delivering care to the patient.

In order to address individual technical competency, we are employing other tools such as surgical simulation centers as potential solutions to these issues. In another chapter, Jack McCarthy, president of CRICO/RMF, has described an incentive premium program where we offer a 10% discount to obstetricians/gynecologists (OB/GYNs) completing simulation/team training and other educationally based requirements. From our perspective, we consider this program to be successful in helping us evaluate a potential reduction in OB/GYN malpractice based on claims over the last several years. We feel that there has been a positive impact made, and an actual return on investment, by giving training that provides an emphasis on communication and team building.

As a malpractice insurance company, we see the risks in obesity surgery to be very similar to those encountered during the introduction of laparoscopic cholecystectomies. We also understand that there are individual human issues, in addition to systems issues, that need to be addressed. For example, training for obesity surgery is challenging and, therefore, we invite tools such as simulation and teamwork training to further educate healthcare professionals. And the idea and benefits of having a cohesive team caring for patients must be impressed upon all stakeholders. For positive surgical outcomes are not only reliant on having excellent physicians; having a team that communicates and the organizational processes that support that team are other components absolutely critical to successful medical outcomes.

# Malpractice/Payers

Robert Hanscom, JD

The Risk Management Foundation, the organization for which I work and which is also known as the Controlled Risk Insurance Company (CRICO), has been the malpractice carrier for the Harvard System for approximately 30 years. As such, we are in a somewhat interesting position with respect to malpractice data. In general, malpractice events are rare. Even in this day and age of lots of press surrounding some of these cases, they are not common occurrences. Thus, as people look at the data that have emerged, many often ask, "Are these data really useful for learning or for gauging performance improvement in our organizations?"

Our answer is an absolute yes. We are convinced that if you analyze the malpractice data correctly, it reveals what specifically needs to be done to start avoiding not only malpractice claims, but also those adverse events in the hospital that may not even become malpractice claims. In other words, you can start to shed light on the themes underlying a much larger geography of healthcare vulnerabilities. We often use an iceberg to illustrate this, with malpractice claims as the tip of the iceberg. They're very visible up there above the surface of the water. A lot of people know about them, but what happens is that people try to link the event to the perceived base of healthcare vulnerabilities beneath the surface of the water. Many times, in the analysis of our malpractice claims, we have seen a very strong thread leading from what's above that surface of the water to what is down beneath.

In general, because our own numerator is so small, we are always looking for what's going on with other malpractice carriers and of course it is not exactly a great arena for sharing information. Organizations tend to hold their information very close. Physician's Insurance Association of America (PIAA) has published a lot of data, but unfortunately we don't have a lot of known denominators in that data, so that can make their information sometimes a bit less valuable to us. COPIC Insurance Company is a malpractice carrier in Colorado. In 2002, COPIC had 5 obesity surgery claims for that particular year. When they looked at the total incurred cost of the 5 claims, it equaled $119,793 per incident and represented 2% of their total claims for that year—again, a very, very small picture. However, similar to what we do, COPIC also looks very hard at what they call their occurrences—what the Risk Management Foundation calls observations. Whenever there are worrisome events that raise the specter of malpractice, we urge our insured population to notify us. In other words, you have either a physician who's worried or a risk manager or a nurse who's worried. Once notified, we can open up a file and be ready for the case; we can start making initial investigations. COPIC does this as well. Covering more than 75% of all the physicians in Colorado, they're a very tightly run organization. We have a lot of respect for them and take the opportunity to share a lot of risk management practices with them.

Instead of looking at those 5 malpractice claims, COPIC shared information on 10 occurrences that took place in 2002. These were made up of 4 deaths and 6 reoperations. Being able to see the breakdown in the system that occurred in that 1-year period was of value to us, as it would be to anyone in this area of healthcare.

Here in the Commonwealth of Massachusetts, we lean heavily toward the defense of individual physicians. The reason for that is that we have a charitable cap in this state set (as of 2005) at the outrageously low level of $20,000 per institution. That means of course, that the plaintiff attorneys rarely ever sue the institution—they sue the individual physician. It's an unfortunate scenario for doctors, but on the other hand, there is an argument that suggests this has kept malpractice awards low in Massachusetts, because juries tend to see these physicians as real human beings, which may mitigate the deep-pocket syndrome. We think there's another downside to all of this, though. Without much of a financial burden to organizations, the institutions haven't been as motivated as we would like them to be to fix systems that should be fixed.

Our own breakdown shows that we had 14 cases over a period of 8½ years, and 44 defendants in those 14 cases.

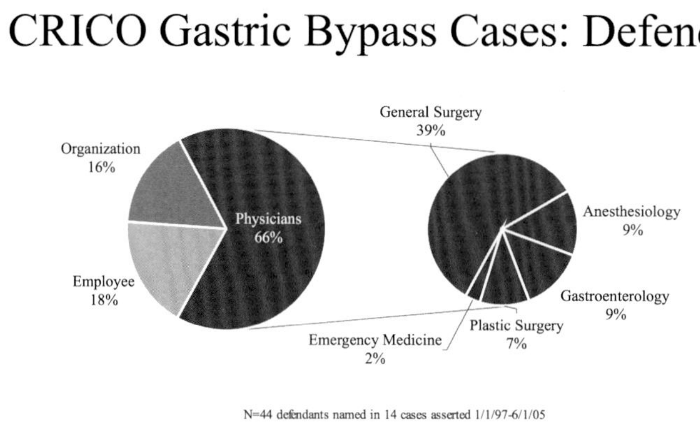


The diagram included here shows the type of defendants. Of them, 66% were physicians. "Employee" means resident, so 18% were residents and the rest were other employees of the organization, such as nurses or anyone else who got pulled into these cases. Of course, each case involves several defendants. Of the physicians, this breakdown shows general surgery as the big player. No surprise there. Then anesthesiology at 9%, gastroenterology at 9%, plastic surgery at 7%, and emergency medicine at 2%.

"Complications" is the name of the game that leads to litigation in these kinds of cases, and our findings came as no surprise.

**Complications leading to litigation included:**

- Anastomotic leaks
- Small bowel obstruction
- Internal hernias
- Hemorrhage
- Anesthesia issues
- Equipment: stapler failures
- Skin injury: decubitus ulcer
- Comorbid conditions
- Death

At the Risk Management Foundation, we believe that there's huge value to capturing the patient's perspective. In our organization, we've taken to reading depositions as though they are stories and they are very rich stories. There is always an element of bias and some of them show a great amount of bias. However, when we read the depositions we begin to understand something more of why the patient actually was compelled to bring a lawsuit.

You know the headline, of course. There's been an adverse outcome for which the patient feels he/she must be compensated. What are eye openers in these depositions are all the other reasons why the patients brought those lawsuits. Many of them relate to communication while others are very reflective of flawed systems within organizations, along with a variety of other matters.

## Top Allegations:
## From the Patient's Perspective

- Alleged inadequate technical skill
- Alleged failures to clearly articulate to the patient and family postoperative risks involved
- Despite disclosures of complications, alleged failures to timely recognize complications and to intervene appropriately
- Alleged failures to appropriately recommend further testing to determine source of pain
- Alleged significant delays to return to OR
- Alleged being left under the care of physicians who were not able to completely care for complication

As a company, we look very carefully at the allegations made in the lawsuits. These are written by the plaintiffs' attorneys, but they are reflective of what the patients believe to be "what went wrong." Here the allegations are presented in descending order, from the most to the least common, with the primary allegation claiming inadequate technical skill. This is the top player in all our surgical cases. Next is alleged failure to clearly articulate to the patient the postoperative risks involved, and then the allegation that despite disclosures of complications, there was a failure to recognize the complication in time and to appropriately intervene. Next is the alleged failure to recommend further testing to determine the source of pain, followed by an allegation around delays in returning to the operating room (OR). Finally, the last allegation is that of being left in the care of physicians unable to completely care for the complication. It seems of interest to note here, too, that (in 2005) the average indemnity in bariatric surgery cases, per the PIAA, was $186,925.

In terms of what we see in our own cases, here are the top concerns:

- Flawed decision making and judgment
- Technical issues
- Communication errors
- Patient issues
- System failures

I should emphasize that we will always be the first to say that malpractice has age to it, and every one of these cases has a unique convergence. In other words, you are unlikely to see a scenario exactly repeated although you will see events that represent very "fluke-like" circumstances. However, with those we apply a methodology to actually create an agenda for process or performance improvement within the organization involved.

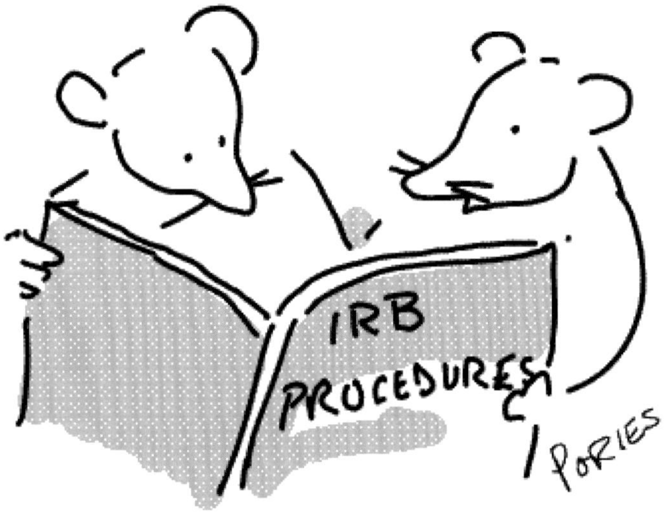


"Hey, hey, hey. I never gave informed consent!"

# Liability in Proctoring

John Kelly, MD

As a surgeon performing minimally invasive and bariatric surgery, I also am currently a proctor—one of a dwindling number in this field. Let me explain why this professional field is diminishing in rank.

We know from a surgeon's perspective what the historical teaching model is. We've taken our training and learned most of our skill set in residency. We may perfect that or put the icing on the cake in fellowship. Then we go out into practice, working to perfect what we've learned even more. In the past, if there's been new technology or things to learn, we picked those up in our journals or in the meetings we attend. We may take courses or site-visit surgeons. Certainly these strategies have worked in the past, allowing us to assimilate new technology and learn new skill sets. Of course, much of the learning is just observational. In addition, in the past, we have had the surgical box (in the form of the abdomen) open and your surgical hands still worked the same way. You could simply emulate what you saw or what you might have observed from another expert surgeon at a course or site visit. Certain procedures or newer technologies might have required an animal or cadaver model, but that was the exception rather than the rule.

The dilemma today is that, compared with the recent past when "new" was likely just an extension, an adaptation, or shift of an existing knowledge or skill set learned in residency, "new" today can often define a technology disruptive to an existing surgical practice or procedure. It truly is a whole new surgical world out there, and the minimally invasive concept is here to stay.

So, how do we work to transfer a new surgical technique that involves minimally invasive surgery and new technology? How do we overcome what I think is the most dangerous thing for patients: the surgical *learning curve*?

Many factors drive this industry, including our patients. If it is really best practice for minimally invasive surgery to enter into many areas of medicine, we have to find a way to transfer this technology and these skill sets to surgeons who are already out there in the field. I find it's important for us to be able to teach today's practicing surgeons and not wait 30 years for a full-turnover cycle of surgeons.

Historically, I think we've done a poor job of this. I believe the training of laparoscopic cholecystectomy is but one example—that if such a procedure were put under the current modern light of scrutiny that gastric bypass is experiencing, we would have had a significant hold on that procedure. The transference of education associated with the gastric bypass is far more significant and, therefore, more dangerous than the laparoscopic cholecystectomy.

What we have available to most surgeons now is in the form of courses and possibly mini-fellowships. More formal fellowships, though perhaps only for a select few, are coming into practice. Preceptorships and the concept of proctorship are also important discussion items. It may be useful for me to offer some quick definitions here. To be a preceptor in a preceptorship is to be a teacher and instructor. When a surgeon comes to me or to my facility for additional training, the preceptorship might be observational only and frequently that's not enough. The best training and what most surgeons would want is a scrubbed-in experience. For that, the surgeon will have to get a temporary state license if he/she is from out of state, and will be required to receive temporary hospital privileges. He/she basically functions as a house officer in the operating room, with no clinical responsibility, and takes orders or directives from me.

As a proctor, many of these definitions seem somewhat humorous and sometimes I feel a bit like an "appointed beggar" or a "member of the clergy" as the definition would suggest. I pray a lot during some of these procedures. But this last definition offers an entirely appropriate meaning when I, as a proctor, leave my facility and supervise an examination, a very high-stakes examination, which is the surgery itself.

Proctoring is off-site teaching for the surgeon. In other words, I go to them, and to me it's a bit of an extension of the preceptorship. You have to build a relationship, a teaching model at your facility; then you have to see those you have taught in practice at their facility. I will have to get temporary hospital privileges at their hospital and perhaps a temporary out-of-state license. The question is, how many cases will there be? This is what we are dealing with in the area of gastric bypass surgery, and we have numbers of 15, 20, or 25 thrown about. The concept becomes quite daunting, considering what the numbers may be.

Who should be a preceptor or a proctor? In general, it should be someone who has a high case number, multiple years of experience, and superior outcomes. In addition, the individual he/she is teaching, preceptoring, or proctoring should probably share a similar philosophy and approach.

Unfortunately, the most daunting issue appears to be that of risk assessment. It is important to recognize that liability and risk are a huge component of what I and other proctors and preceptors go through. If it's a preceptorship (similar to a mini-fellowship of variable time), the patients are coming to my hospital. The individual I am teaching is operating with me on my patients. This is my hospital billing on the procedure and assuming the risk. Any fee that is paid I do not accept personally. It goes into an educational fund, for I feel that this is an educational process that the surgeon is experiencing, and that it is actually taking away from some of the value for residents and fellows in our program. So, I use that fee to help those residents and fellows in educational ways. When a reasonably skilled surgeon is being taught in my operating room under my watch, I don't feel I am assuming any major additional risk, and the visiting surgeon's abilities are often better than those of our present residents and even our fellows. I feel that my liability is acceptable there, also because I am in complete control and in charge in that environment.

A problem with proctorship is that going to someone else's hospital with another surgeon's patient makes the issues more complicated. There is a substantial fee involved for the proctor service, and liability coverage is extremely precarious in this setting. Your hospital attorney will give you a complex answer to what you think may be a simple question. The truth is that no one in this situation can count on coverage if he/she decides to scrub in at an outside hospital.

The question arises, "How have I tried to keep it safe up to this point?" Well, I've used industry to help me identify quality individuals. By "industry" I mean those salespersons on the front line who have a good sense of what *muster* that surgeon that I am going to proctor has in their operating room. These salespersons have a lot of experience traveling around and seeing different operating theaters, but I do follow-up with an extensive questionnaire in any case, and I do phone interviews to make sure for myself, that they "pass muster." I want to hear that they want to follow guidelines much like the ones we wrote for the Betsy Lehman Center or, before those, the Massachusetts Department of Health guidelines. And there are similar philosophies that I would like to share with the proposed surgeon. I prefer to visit just as a supervisor, in examiner mode, and try not to be an enabler. I try to touch as little as possible and not be the assistant surgeon. In fact, the proctored surgeon should have someone else there who is the assistant surgeon. As the proctor, I believe, "You're just the examiner. You don't cheat, you don't take the examination for him/her and, if the patient needs to go open, the surgeon has to have open privileges and you're not going to bail him/her out of any resulting trouble."

What could improve this system? It would probably be better for the proctor to have some type of potential exemption for Good Samaritan training efforts. Would it require a legislative move in order to have that? Possibly, but if laparoscopic bariatric surgery is as important as I think it is, and if we want to make sure everyone in the state who wants it, has access to it, I believe it deserves legislative effort to ensure that access is preserved by expert training. One could imagine other surgeries that may come along, minimally invasive or otherwise, that would be best served by a similar training exemption for proctors.

As far as liability coverage by industry, I know of one particular company that does this well. They have a set of proctors that they use and they do pay for their liability. They arrange for the proctor to go to an institution, get a temporary license and permission to work on the hospital privileges, and even do some of the paper- and footwork for that proctor. It's a very good concept. Of course, the LAP-BAND procedure is a different beast than gastric bypass and the whole risk profile is different with this surgery. To expect industry, which is more in tune with bypass, to pay similarly for this may be a little bit unexpected.

Besides industry, the hospital at which you are proctoring should be considered as the responsible party for liability coverage. Paying for coverage would confirm their dedication to the prospect of offering bariatric surgery at their facility. As you can see, this is a difficult hurdle to cross with no one wanting to take full responsibility for such an important training effort.

Fixing liability and proctored training is important for credentialing purposes. It is most disappointing to take somebody through an extensive proctorship and not be able to give that individual some type of proficiency or credentialing statement. The best you can say is, "I saw you do 10 cases. Good job. You showed you have sufficient skill." It's difficult to go much further in your stamp of approval, credentialing the individual in any way, because of liability issues.

Another problem presents itself when a surgeon "goes off" to proctor. The loss of revenue to both the practice and the hospital can have considerable impact. The reimbursement to the individual might seem reasonable, but when you consider what is lost to the facility by the surgeon's absence, it could be even more prohibitive than the liability issue. One response might be that all the training should be done at the proctor's hospital, which would alleviate most of the liability and travel issues. But, this gets in the way of training residents and fellows. Back when I began proctoring, I was perhaps a bit naïve regarding these issues and happy for the ignorance. Today, though, they are clearly recognizable as powerful obstacles to training and the main reason why proctoring is, as noted at the beginning of this chapter, a dwindling professional arena for surgeons.

The transfer of knowledge remains of critical importance in the postgraduate setting for surgeons. Even those of us who instruct surgeons will continue to need extra training in new techniques and technology so that the surgical world doesn't pass us by. As we learn to disseminate this knowledge better, we will lower the learning curve and thus keep patients safer. But the risk and liability of the proctoring surgeon is not something we can continue to ignore or we will have no teachers. Ultimately, formal credentialing mechanisms must arise out of efforts to resolve the liability and proctoring dilemma.

# Medical Liability Drives Cost

Bruce M. Wolfe, MD

The basic concept of tort law is that persons who are injured by negligence of another should be compensated. The system for identifying this negligence and determining the compensation is the basis for the legal system determining medical malpractice. The advocates of this system would insist that there's an improvement in safety and quality-of-care results. This perhaps is true for such things as product safety. It is difficult to purchase an unsafe toy for a child because of improvements in safety of products, and one can question the role of liability for product safety if an unsafe product is put on the market, and the manufacturer knowingly did so, which would constitute negligence.

In medicine, it is not so straightforward. An analysis of surgical errors in closed malpractice claims revealed a surgery error in 258 of 444 claims (58%).(1) Seventy-five percent of these occurred in intraoperative care. Systems factors were judged to have contributed to error in 82% of cases. Similarly, a recent analysis of 100 malpractice claims against bariatric surgeons revealed potential negligence in 28% of cases.(2) Among these 28 cases, 82% involved a delay in diagnosis.

It is clear that the threat of possible medical-legal action has not adequately addressed the problem of medical errors, including surgical errors. The present emphasis is systematic reporting of errors or potential errors without an associated threat of reprisal.(3) This new emphasis is intended to facilitate complete reporting of errors so that analysis and corrective actions can be accomplished. Examples include establishment of pathways, protocols, and procedures to minimize errors or complications.

The cost of medical malpractice is substantial. The direct cost of medical malpractice—i.e., insurance premiums—that are paid or allocations of funds made by institutions such as Harvard and the University of California, which are self-insured, can be determined. The consumption of a physician's time and the emotional stress endured to investigate and defend a malpractice action is substantial, but cannot be calculated into these costs. Indirect costs, which occur as the result of the practice of defensive medicine, must also be considered.(4)

We have heard much about the rising healthcare costs and malpractice premiums in recent years. Between 2001 and 2002, particularly in general surgery, there was a rate increase in premiums of 21%.(5) A news piece indicated that in the State of Pennsylvania, liability expenses for hospitals were $636 million, or about $3.5 million per hospital, in 2004. Clearly there is a substantial amount of money being spent in this area.

What are the reasons for rising malpractice premiums at the present time? Insurance companies do not generally divulge their finances, but the explanations that are most commonly given are increased claim severity (greater awards per case), increasing contingency, attorney fees, and reduced investment revenue as a result of stock market changes, which impact an important source of revenue for insurance companies. To maintain profits, these companies have increased premiums.

Two attorneys in Pennsylvania, James Saxton and Maggie Finckelstein, have done considerable research in this area.(6) In a survey of premiums for bariatric surgeons, they reported annual premiums ranging from $30,000 up to $300,000 per year. Tail coverage (which covers subsequent actions against a surgeon after he/she retires or changes a practice) can range from 140% to 300% of the annual premium, up to as much as $575,000. Thus it may cost a surgeon several hundred thousand dollars just to retire. In addition, insurance companies are basically using the neurosurgery scale for charging bariatric surgeons. For example, adding a bariatric program at a midsize community hospital in Michigan would raise that hospital's yearly insurance premium by $240,000.

There remains limited data on the topic. A paper was published based on a survey of the American Society for Metabolic and Bariatric Surgery (ASMBS) members in 1999. Of the 165 members who responded, the rate of claims was 1.6 per 1,000 operations. Eighteen of these claims were settled. There was one verdict for the plaintiff. A total of 20% of these claims resulted in some sort of payment (20% is relatively low) and the mean award was $89,000. Thus, Saxton and Finckelstein concluded that bariatric surgeons are being overcharged for malpractice premiums in relation to other specialists.(6) In reality, the payoffs in bariatric surgery are not nearly so high as to justify using the neurosurgery scale to set the rates.

**Table 1**

## Physicians Insurers Association of America

| Average payout for closed claims, 1985-2000 | |
|---|---|
| Neurosurgery | $267,000 |
| OB/GYN | 235,000 |
| Pediatrics | 232,000 |
| Cardiovascular | 199,000 |
| Bariatric surgery | 162,000-189,000 |
| Internal medicine | 169,000 |
| ENT | 168,000 |
| General surgery | 152,000 |

Saxton and Finkelstein, 2005.

The Physicians Insurers Association of America has collected data on all closed claims in the United States. Over a period of about 10 years, there were a total of 192,000 closed cases. Bariatric surgery represented just 0.2% of these claims, demonstrating that this type of surgery is not the predominant cause for malpractice payments. The average payout per closed claim for bariatric surgery is in the middle range: $160,000 to $190,000 (Table 1). Neurosurgical, obstetrics/gynecology (OB/GYN) and pediatric payments, on average, are all substantially higher. Two possible reasons given for why bariatric surgery has a lesser damage potential compared with neurosurgery, pediatrics, and OB/GYN, is that infants and young children are not involved, and central nervous system (CNS) damage is infrequent (Table 2, 3). The damage that ensues as a result of a CNS injury to a baby is calculated over the expected lifetime of the child, producing large direct-cost damages. These situations are where the highest payments occur. In bariatric surgical patients, there is also less damage potential as a result of existing disease and disability and diminished life expectancy. Namely, if the patient dies, it is more difficult to show that they lost many years of expected survival. Finally, among bariatric surgeons and patients, there is presumably a diminished sympathy factor, which is impossible to measure and varies from one jury to another.

Because bariatric surgery is elective, the malpractice risk is diminished. There are accepted eligibility criteria for surgery. As long as these straightforward criteria are followed, it is difficult to claim that the indications for surgery were not present. Patients should, and usually do, undergo extensive preparation and education, and thus claims of having been inadequately informed are infrequent. There are improved outcomes at specialized high-volume centers. The outcomes, complication rates, and safety of bariatric surgery in 2005 are considerably better than they were several years ago.(7) All actions begin with some type of adverse outcome, so if the incidence of complications is reduced, the liability risk is diminished.

Situations in which juries will not be sympathetic to defendant surgeons and hospitals are instances in which poor communication or inadequate informed consent has occurred and when a significant service lapse arises.(8) The usual scenario suggests a complication or problem is present and the response of the healthcare providers, the surgeon in particular, is judged to be inadequate. For example, the surgeon is not available when a problem arises and the covering surgeon does not know what to do. Or a problem arises during off-hours and no one responds. There may be a case of inadequate provider preparation. This is hard to confirm because of the still-evolving criteria governing who should be credentialed to do bariatric surgery; but the claim can certainly be made, particularly as guidelines from the ASMBS and others are evolving. Finally, in any area of medicine, when a complication occurs and is followed by an effort to cover-up, provide misinformation, or not tell the patient the whole story, this becomes problematic, particularly when the patient learns the facts.

There are very little published data on the topic of defensive medicine. A study was done by Studdert et al of attitudes about defensive medicine and the following definition for the term "defensive medicine" is taken from that paper: "A deviation from sound medical practice induced by the threat of liability that may supplement or replace care."(9) Studdert et al surveyed 824 physicians and found that 92% indicated that they may conduct what they termed in this paper "assurance behavior," or some alteration of their practice pattern, in response to the threat of medical legal liability. Unnecessary imaging is the most frequent at 43%, but other unnecessary studies or practice changes are also reported. Secondly, 42% of the respondents indicated that they restrict their practice to eliminate risky or difficult procedures or they avoid complex patients, because they perceive the risk of a complication to be high. An editorial by Budetti states that this approach does not necessarily work.(10) In a *JAMA* article, he indicates that physicians who deviate from sound medical practice statistically are not necessarily the ones at highest risk of medical-legal action. Thus, unfounded deviations from standard care may occur from fear and are in some cases not necessary. Budetti, an attorney, notes that there are situations in which ordering extra studies, such as for cancer detection,(10) may actually be a good thing and that it is obviously positive if physicians who aren't confident avoid accepting complex cases. However, defensive medicine may actually increase the risk of liability, particularly if the patient is injured undergoing an unnecessary procedure.

Why would 92% of physicians who were queried admit they change their practice in order to avoid being sued? This finding was astounding to Budetti, who concluded the antipathy toward the whole malpractice situation is so severe that it outweighs other concerns in a physician's mind at the decisive moment. It is not just malpractice premiums; also involved is the threat of action, a process that is exceedingly painful in terms of the above considerations, consumption of time, and having to relive the experience of the adverse outcome.

Tort reform to date has not led to innovative legal approaches tying liability law to evidence-based changes in medical practice and patient safety. As of this writing, there continues to be a clear disconnect between the medical-legal system and the patient-safety movement, and hopefully revisions can be devised that will lead to a resolution of this serious situation.

**Table 2**

## Bariatric Surgery
## Lesser Damage Potential

- No infants, young children
- Infrequent CNS injury
- Existing disease, disability
- Diminished life expectancy
- Diminished sympathy factor

Saxton and Finkelstein, 2005.

**Table 3**

## Bariatric Surgery Liability Risk Reduced by

- Elective surgery
- Accepted eligibility criteria
- Extensive preparation/education
- Improved outcomes at specialized, high-volume centers
- Lesser potential damage

Saxton and Finkelstein, 2005.

**References**

1. Rogers SO Jr, Gawande AA, Kwaan M, et al. Analysis of surgical errors in closed malpractice claims at 4 liability insurers. *Surgery*. 2006;140:25-33.
2. Cottam D, Lord J, Dallal RM, et al. Medicolegal analysis of 100 malpractice claims against bariatric surgeons. *Surg Obes Relat Dis*. 2007;3:60-6.
3. Gostin L. A public health approach to reducing error: medical malpractice as a barrier. *JAMA*. 2000;283:1742-3.
4. Palmisano DJ. Thomas B. Ferguson lecture: The hidden cost of medical liability litigation. *Ann Thorac Surg*. 2004;78:9-13.
5. Thorpe KE. The medical malpractice 'crisis': recent trends and the impact of state tort reforms. *Health Aff*. 2004;Jan-Jun; Suppl Web Exclusives: W4-20-30.
6. Saxton JW, Finkelstein MM. Bariatric surgery: a comprehensive bariatric program can act to reduce liability risks and to promote patient safety. Stevens & Lee. 2005: Unpublished data.
7. Zhao Y, Encinosa W. Agency for Healthcare Research and Quality (AHRQ). Bariatric surgery utilization and outcomes in 1998 and 2004. Statistical Brief #23. January 2007.
8. Paul NF. Professional Liability Committee, American College of Surgeons. *Professional Liability/Risk Management: a Manual for Surgeons*. 2nd ed. 1997.
9. Studdert DM, Mello MM, Sage WM, et al. Defensive medicine among high-risk specialist physicians in a volatile malpractice environment. *JAMA*. 2005;293(21):2609-17.
10. Budetti PP. Tort reform and the patient-safety movement: seeking common ground. *JAMA*. 2005;293(21):2660-2.

# Tort Reform

Alan Harvey, MD, MBA

Although I am director of Quality Assurance/Quality Improvement and Patient Safety at the Department of Anesthesiology, Perioperative and Pain Medicine at Brigham and Womens' Hospital, as well as chair of the Betsy Lehman Center Task Force on Weight Loss Surgery, I have been fortunate to also fulfill another role as president of the Massachusetts Medical Society (MMS)/*New England Journal of Medicine*. Having had formal training in health law as part of my MBA, with a concentration in health systems management, I am active nationally in medicolegal issues as a delegate to the American Medical Association (AMA). As such, I would like to share with you a national and state perspective on tort reform and discuss how bariatric surgery has been affected by this medicolegal environment. In addition, I will offer a view over the horizon and around the corner of what's to come in terms of fundamental reforms of the tort system.

Let me start by bringing you on a quick tour of recent local news pages and courtrooms of America. The former assistant coach of the New England Patriots gets front-page headlines by suing his physicians 2 years after his gastric bypass surgery. As the story goes on to indicate, "Mr. Weis was in a coma for 2 weeks following his surgery … given last rites by a priest. He recovered completely from his surgery." Another headline, this one from the *Fresno Bee*, reads, "Dying to Lose Weight." It heads one article in an ongoing series on obesity surgery. This particular story was about a man who died following his surgery in 2002.

As you know, these types of reports are frequently in the news. Catchy phrases like "dying to lose weight" grab the reader's attention. Cases such as these come forward in the media and are dealt with through a somewhat unilateral process. Physicians' names are hung out to dry, though retractions may come a few days, months, or years later after the case is settled. However, in the media it seems you're guilty until proven innocent. And, of course, a story has more impact if it comes out on a Monday rather than a Friday when it may disappear over the weekend. In multipart news reports like the one mentioned above, the fact that it goes on day after day gives the story more creditability. This kind of activity operates against the physician and/or the hospital. It becomes part of the legal strategy to coach the patient and inject into the press impressions that influence the public's perception of the case—which in turn forces parties to settle simply because of the unrelenting press coverage day after day.

Lest you think it's only the media that is to blame for this situation, consider the New York law firm whose Web address is www.gastricbypassmalpractice.com. "Are you a victim of gastric bypass malpractice?," the site asks its visitors. To prompt reporting of possible cases, the legal profession even has finder's fees. Nurses or other medical personnel bring cases to the attention of attorneys who then contact the family or the patient. Members of your own team may even be a source for initiating the process. The Web site www.expertwitness.com lists bariatric surgery experts available for testifying against you. Sadly, this is the environment in which we find ourselves working these days.

Since 2002, there has been a steady drumbeat for medical liability reform at the federal and state levels. Initially driven by instances of trauma centers in Nevada being temporarily closed because of the shortage of neurosurgeons and trauma surgeons, the movement quickly attracted national attention. In the years since this campaign began, this has become an issue of interest to those in bariatric surgery due to the increased legal activity and difficulty for some physicians to obtain malpractice coverage.

First, let's examine the issue at the federal level. The AMA was an early advocate for medical liability reform modeled on the legislative package passed in California in 1976 and known by its acronym, MICRA (Medical Injury Compensation and Recovery Act). MICRA's supporters maintain that this California legislation was instrumental in moderating malpractice premium increases.

In 2003, US House of Representatives member Jim C. Greenwood of Pennsylvania introduced HR 5, known as the HEALTH Act (Help Efficient, Accessible, Low Cost, Timely, Healthcare). This became the centerpiece of the federal reform campaign. Its key goals include

- Requiring full compensation for economic losses
- A $250,000 cap on noneconomic losses
- A sliding scale limiting attorney contingency fees
- Eliminating joint and several liability, thus ensuring that defendants pay damages only in proportion to their degree of fault

In 2003, the House passed the measure 219-196, largely along party lines. Only 16 Democrats and 9 Republicans broke their party ranks. Senate Majority Leader Bill Frist introduced a similar bill in the Senate, and forced a vote in the House. However, it fell 11 votes short of the 60 needed to block a filibuster, so the measure failed.

Twice in 2004, the Senate again tried to pass liability reforms. Early in that year, HR 5 was redrafted to target OB-GYNs, but its supporters fell 12 votes short of breaking a filibuster. Two months later, the Senate tried again, this time also targeting physicians involved in emergency services and childbirth, but that, too, fell 11 votes short of breaking a filibuster.

On a parallel track, there has been a great deal of activity in the state legislatures. The AMA has been tracking the liability climate on a state-by-state level to support both federal and state-level reform efforts. If you take a look at the AMA's latest medical liability crisis map (www.ama-assn.org/ama/noindex/category/11871.html), 17 states are described as being in crisis, including Massachusetts. Rhode Island and Tennessee were the most recent states added to the list. Twenty-five states, plus Washington, DC, show serious problems. Just 8 states are considered "OK," meaning that premiums and litigation activity are not having a negative effect on the practice environment.

Texas is a unique case. A few years ago, when Texas was labeled a "crisis" state, voters narrowly approved a constitutional amendment authorizing the state legislature to impose caps on noneconomic damages. The legislation capped noneconomic damages at $250,000, and implemented a number of other MICRA reforms—most notably, the tightening of both the standard of proof and guidelines for expert witnesses. Since that vote, premiums moderated and several insurers have returned to do business in Texas, and Texas is now regarded as a "stable" state.

The drama in Texas has been played out almost identically in every other state. The physician community, allied with the business community and Republican lawmakers, have promoted MICRA reforms. They have been opposed strongly by the trial bar and Democratic lawmakers.

MICRA legislation has generally passed in states where Republicans control the legislature and the governor's office. In Massachusetts, the MMS helped introduce comprehensive MICRA-style reforms in late 2002, just before the beginning of the 2-year session. Despite strong evidence that our healthcare system was suffering, only limited legislative success was secured in the form of a sharp reduction of the interest that accrues on cases while they are working their way through the legal system. This was not a trivial success, but it was far less than what we were hoping for and what we had a realistic chance of securing.

To a large degree, the reform efforts suffered under the dynamics of presidential politics as so much was filtered through the red-state/blue-state paradigm, regardless of a strong, empirical case that consistently made for fundamental liability reform.

**The Key Themes**

MICRA still has a great deal of attraction. Several states have been able to break the doctor-lawyer stalemate and have passed or tightened caps on noneconomic damages. However, some areas still experience stalemates, where MICRA-based legislation hasn't gotten a hearing. Some advocates and legislators are beginning to look at non-MICRA alternatives. We've seen apology and minimum expert witness qualifications legislation enacted, as well as growing interest in programs that have been piloted in other states.

The ballot initiative was a closely watched battle in Florida, where physicians and lawyers put competing, contradictory questions on the state ballot—and both won! Physicians succeeded in capping attorneys' fees at 10% of damages, regardless of the size of the award. However, lawyers one-upped the doctors by successfully pushing for a measure that would end peer-review protections for the investigation of adverse medical events, and they invoked a "3 strikes and you're out" rule for physicians found liable of malpractice in three cases, either by judgment or consent decree (settlements did not count as a "strike"). As everyone predicted, all measures were appealed to the state courts, and things ground to a standstill. In Nevada, however, voters agreed with physicians who wanted to remove two exceptions to its $350,000 cap on noneconomic damages, and they turned away every lawyer-led initiative.

In Oregon, an attempt to re-establish a $500,000 cap on noneconomic damages was defeated and Wyoming experienced mixed results. Voters approved a pretrial screening process, but did not approve a constitutional amendment authorizing caps. The trial bar has challenged caps in the states' highest courts 22 times since 1985, and the results have been mixed. Caps have been upheld in 13 cases, and overturned in 9. In essence, the reform campaign has been a zero-sum game.

**The Joint Commission's Involvement**

Given the real strengths of the physician, business and lawyers' lobbies, this guarantees a virtual stalemate for the foreseeable future—as long as the battle is fought over caps, attorney fees, and other MICRA-based solutions. But what if the campaign to reform the liability system were to be taken to a different playing field? What would happen then? That's the thinking behind the growing effort to bring about non-MICRA reforms—reforms that are *outside* the tort system.

There are many efforts in this vein, but one of the most impressive was a two-year-long roundtable convened by The Joint Commission. The result was a white paper released in February 2005, called *Health Care at the Crossroads*. (Readers may find this paper at www.jcaho.org/news+room/press+kits/tort+reform/medical_liability.pdf.) The roundtable argued that the tort system is beyond repair and toxic to patient-safety improvement. The advisory team included leading figures in patient safety and medical liability reform, including Dr. Lucian Leape, Dr. Troy Brennan, and Philip Howard, the leader of the legal reform advocacy group Common Good. The white paper included 19 recommendations, based on four key concepts:

1. Establish a baseline culture of safety at every healthcare enterprise. This includes the protection of open communication, promotion of teamwork training, and near-miss reporting
2. When avoidable error occurs, full disclosure and appropriate apology must be made to the injured patient, followed by a root-cause analysis and systems improvement to avoid recurrence
3. Injury compensation: early tender/offer to support the patient should be made
4. Alternative dispute resolution techniques such as mediation, arbitration, and medical or administrative courts must be employed. These approaches are designed to avoid the costly overhead and destructive adversarial nature of the current tort system

**Medical Courts**

In 2005, the Robert Wood Johnson Foundation issued a $1.5 million grant to the Harvard School of Public Health and Common Good to pursue a demonstration project on medical courts. In May of 2005, the leaders of the project held a symposium at The Brookings Institution, where input and feedback on how best to structure these courts was collected from advocates in both the medical and legal fields. The goal was to fairly and promptly compensate patients for avoidable injuries, as well as work in concert with patient safety efforts (rather than undermine them). The tort system's shortcomings, as defined by Harvard health researcher, Professor Michelle Mello, are noted as follows:

- The arbitrary and capricious nature of patient compensation
- The very poor job the system does in deterring future adverse events (only 5% of avoidable injuries result in a claim, fewer than 10% of claims go to trial, and most settlements are confidential)
- That it promotes defensive medicine
- That it is grossly inefficient, with 60% of its costs consumed by court overhead and attorney fees

In short, the case for medical liability reform is unimpeachable as the current system is inefficient, arbitrary, and toxic to patient-safety improvements. Indeed, in this current system, even those who win are dissatisfied. There has to be a better way.

**How Do We Reduce Our Medicolegal Risks for Weight Loss Surgery?**

We can standardize our preoperative education, information to the patient and his or her family on the risks and benefits of surgery, and informed consent forms. Further, we can create and follow the best practices from literature such as the Betsy

Lehman Center task force report. We can develop safer systems of care, including raising standards for postoperative monitoring and rapid-response teams. In partnership with physicians, hospitals, and insurers, we can work for alternatives to the current tort system and develop specialized medical courts and higher standards for expert witnesses.

It is up to us to cross the usual boundaries and reach out to coordinate for excellence. We have accomplished this with the Lehman Center process, with the goal of including all weight loss surgery programs in our state. We applaud the American College of Surgeons and the American Society for Metabolic and Bariatric Surgery for setting national practice guidelines in weight loss surgery in order to coordinate for excellence across all states, and create safer systems of care for weight loss surgery patients.

**Other Solutions for the Medical Liability Crisis**

Texas recently established standards for expert witness testimony. If a witness is to testify on a medical issue at a trial in Texas, it is regarded as the practice of medicine. For a nonresident medical witness (who is unlicensed in the state) to fly into the state and testify, a temporary medical license must be issued. The testimony will be submitted to the state's chapter of the national medical specialty society for veracity and, if found to be false, misleading, or not based on the standard of care, the witness could lose the temporary medical license. The advantage is that the incident is reported nationally. This impacts the witness' record, potentially compromising his or her veracity and desirability as a future medical witness in any state. In Massachusetts, this program is under review by the Board of Registration in Medicine, so that in the future, anyone coming into Massachusetts to testify as a medical witness will be held to the national medical specialty society's standard for care, requiring a temporary medical license. This process is just one of the nonlegislative things we can do to promote a solution to the problem of medical liability.

We've looked at ballot initiatives in Massachusetts and find that it can cost \$6 million to \$10 million to put a cleanly worded initiative on the ballot. In addition, our unique state law provides that the legislature can simply take the vote "under advisement," regardless of its outcome. The legislature does not have to act on it, whereas in California, where ballot initiatives are almost an art form, when an initiative is passed, it must be implemented. In Massachusetts, it seemed an unwise use of physicians' business funds, to try to get a ballot initiative that would prove to be advisory only.

Ultimately, the political process can be polarizing. Looking the country over in a general sense, improvement in state legislation for tort reform seems less than promising at this time.

**The Joint Commission Roadmap to Reform**

What, then, are the nonlegislative strategies we can use? Again, as noted, The Joint Commission was effective with its review of our broken liability system. The group's key document, *Health Care at the Crossroads*, which is available at The Joint Commission's Web site, outlines what can be done to support patients who have been genuinely injured (very few actually get compensated) and how the current liability picture is devastating to physicians and practitioners who go to work every day doing their best.

The Joint commission roadmap seems to offer the most reasonable approach in looking at tort reform. It suggests that a baseline culture of safety is necessary, meaning that patient safety and tort reform must be linked. Full disclosure, apology, and a root-cause analysis of the incident are required. Patients want to know what happened. They want to have some apology; either "I'm sorry this happened to you," or, if there was direct physician error, they want to know it. A root-cause analysis on the system issues involved should be initiated to determine what happened and how to prevent it in the future. For injury compensation, early-tender offer for economic damages must be made so that people don't have out-of-pocket expenses. This model, as far as the economic damages component is concerned, is a very good model, supporting patients with economic funds to help them through the medical care needed due to the injury.

Add to this the process of alternative dispute resolution: mediation and/or binding arbitration. The concept of medical courts is supported by Troy Brennan, at the Harvard School of Public Health and Brigham and Women's Hospital, who notes that a specialized court system, where informed judges make decisions on the standard of care, diminishes the need to try to educate a lay jury on these standards and to what care the physician should have given.

## Conclusion

The tort system is broken and is counter to patient interests, patient safety, and full disclosure. Both inefficient and arbitrary, the tort system as a whole has become toxic to our patients' welfare and I am convinced that there is a better way.

The field of bariatric surgery is now a participant in the effort to secure safety and fairness in the tort system. How, as bariatric physicians, do we reduce our medical/legal risks? In addition to proposals already set forth by others, here are some additional thoughts:

- Standardize preoperative education, clarifying the risk/benefits of surgery, and standardize the informed consent forms on either a state or national level. We started this with the Betsy Lehman Center, when we sent out surveys across the state and obtained suggestions on the pre-op education materials and consent forms. This process can yield educated, informed patients who make their decisions for surgery in partnership with their educated and informed physicians
- Recognize that, although the insurance companies pay for procedures, their role is not to stand between patient and physician
- Create and follow the "best practices" set forth in the Lehman Center Report
- Develop safe systems of care. Consider what can happen to the bariatric surgery patient in our hospitals. A safe system of care at night, for instance, can alert nurses or a rapid response team prepared with all the appropriate equipment to take the best care of the bariatric patient. Can there be better monitoring systems? Do we have cordless pulse oximetry? If not, how do we get the technology to create telemetry pulse oximetry as a safety net, with central monitoring? What about respiratory monitors of other types?
- Work with physicians and hospital insurers on expert witness standards for specialized medical courts
- Finally, look at the media component because there is an inherent unfairness in one group being able to get the public to put pressure on a healthcare team. And, when a case is in court process, there must be some control on the media's ability to support one side or the other

Bariatric centers are working together, which means we're stronger. This was part of the Betsy Lehman process that led to a social network that enabled us to benchmark. Working together, we have set a standard of care in Massachusetts that can be fairly and constructively used in court. Let us promote this standard of care using the Betsy Lehman Center recommendations toward the goal of earning support and merit in the national medical/legal system. Keeping in mind that we want to amplify and implement these best practices across the country, let us applaud the American College of Surgeons and American Society for Metabolic and Bariatric Surgery for working with the surgical specialty societies to set a national standard for all bariatric centers. After all, at the end of the day, our collective goal is to create safer systems of care for all bariatric surgery patients.

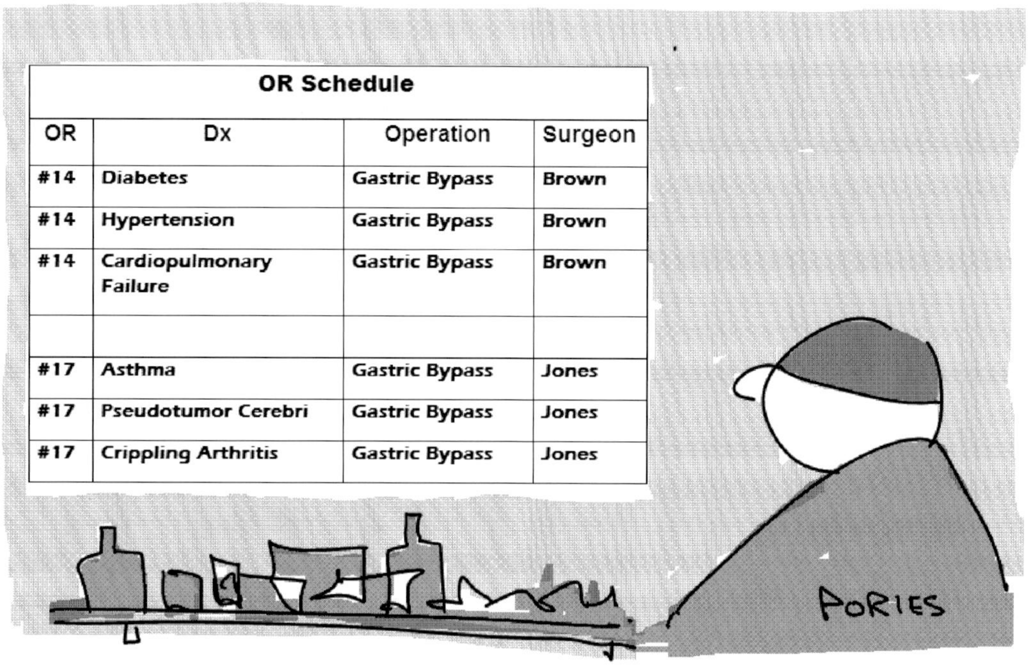
OR Schedule
OR | Dx | Operation | Surgeon
#14 | Diabetes | Gastric Bypass | Brown
#14 | Hypertension | Gastric Bypass | Brown
#14 | Cardiopulmonary Failure | Gastric Bypass | Brown
#17 | Asthma | Gastric Bypass | Jones
#17 | Pseudotumor Cerebri | Gastric Bypass | Jones
#17 | Crippling Arthritis | Gastric Bypass | Jones
PORIES

# Determining Best Practices and Implementing Solutions

Stephanie B. Jones, MD
Daniel B. Jones, MD, MS

*Obesity Surgery: Patient Safety and Best Practices* initiates a real dialogue between our physicians, scientists, healthcare administrators, insurance companies, medical and surgical societies, lawyers, and the media. It shares insights from experts at Harvard Business School and the Harvard School of Public Health. More importantly, the book keeps the focus centered squarely on the patient. Patients share their most intimate fears, concerns, and experiences as they embark on their weight loss surgery journey after years of yo-yo diets, ridicule, and defeat.

The reports of the Betsy Lehman Center for Patient Safety and Medical Error Reduction Expert Panel on Weight Loss Surgery, the American Society for Metabolic and Bariatric Surgery's Centers of Excellence program, and the American College of Surgeons' Bariatric Network have clearly established what we think to be current best practices in 2008. All of these organizations have rallied around the patient—patient safety and best practices. None of these regulatory bodies have tried to expedite training, maximize physician or hospital payment, or lower standards to include all providers. To the contrary, best practices may have the unintended consequence of increasing cost of services, limiting access to the best facilities, and extending training requirements. Patient outcomes, if improved, will determine whether the true objectives are achieved.

Since the first Patient Safety in Obesity Surgery conference in 2005, the American College of Surgeons and American Society for Metabolic and Bariatric Surgery have accredited bariatric programs throughout the United States. The Risk Management Foundation declared intent to partner with the Massachusetts Medical Society to produce uniform consent forms throughout Massachusetts. The malpractice carrier, CRICO/RMF, recognized the need for a Web-based examination for patients prior to surgery as something that would benefit all providers and patients and in so doing decrease malpractice exposure and claims. Surgeons appealed to industry with new ideas for instruments. Journalists gained a better appreciation into some of the restraints of HIPAA, and physicians have become more aware of the need for transparent outcome measures. Several insurance companies—Blue Cross Blue Shield, CIGNA, TRICARE—embraced the concept of establishing Centers of Excellence programs and working with the American College of Surgeons and the American Society for Metabolic and Bariatric Surgery in this process to improve the quality of care. Physicians have been invited by the insurance companies to participate on their advisory boards as they try to establish these policies. Investigators networked with speakers to improve access to research grants, which will help expand our knowledge of the risks and benefits of bariatric surgery. Numerous scientific journals have summarized the science of obesity and explicitly stated needs for future investigation, which may make these operations even better and safer and better understood by the public and payers.

If you don't know where you're going, it's unlikely you'll get there. *Obesity Surgery: Patient Safety and Best Practices* defines the issues and examines the perspective from all angles. Health care policy setters, administrators, and healthcare providers should have a better idea of where we need to go after reading this book, and I'm hopeful that we will get there together as we confront the leading national epidemic obesity.

# Appendix 1

Commonwealth of Massachusetts
Betsy Lehman Center for Patient Safety and Medical Error Reduction
Expert Panel on Weight Loss Surgery

Executive Report
December 12, 2007

PREPUBLICATION COPY/Reprinted with permission from Betsy Lehman Center.
Full report published in Obesity Research, Jan. 2008.

## Table of Contents

**Special Report**

**Commonwealth of Massachusetts**

**Betsy Lehman Center for Patient Safety and Medical Error Reduction**

**Expert Panel on Weight Loss Surgery**

**Executive Report – Update 2007**

**Lehman Center Weight Loss Surgery Expert Panel**

George L. Blackburn, MD, PhD, Chair
Beth Israel Deaconess Medical Center

Matthew M. Hutter, MD, MPH, Vice Chair
Massachusetts General Hospital

Alan M. Harvey, MD, MBA
Immediate Past Chair
Brigham and Women's Hospital

Caroline M. Apovian, MD
Boston Medical Center

Hannah Boulton, RN, MSN
South Shore Hospital

Susan Cummings, MS, RD, LDN
Massachusetts General Hospital

John A. Fallon, MD, MBA, FACP
Blue Cross Blue Shield of Massachusetts

Isaac Greenberg, PhD
Tufts-New England Medical Center

Michael E. Jiser, MD
Saints Memorial Medical Center

Daniel B. Jones, MD, MS
Beth Israel Deaconess Medical Center

Stephanie B. Jones, MD
Beth Israel Deaconess Medical Center

Lee Kaplan, MD, PhD
Massachusetts General Hospital

Marjorie Kaplan, EdD
University of Massachusetts Memorial Medical Center

John Kelly, MD
University of Massachusetts Memorial Medical Center

Rayford S. Kruger, MD, FACS
Tobey Hospital

David B. Lautz, MD
Brigham and Women's Hospital

Carine M. Lenders, MD, MS
Boston Medical Center

Robert LoNigro, MD
Tufts Health Plan

Helen Luce, JD
Consumer Representative

Anne McNamara, RN
Beth Israel Deaconess Medical Center

Ann Mulligan, RN
Newton-Wellesley Hospital

Michael Paasche-Orlow, MD, MPH
Boston University School of Medicine

Frank Perna, PhD
Boston University School of Medicine

Janey S.A. Pratt, MD
Massachusetts General Hospital

Stancel Riley, Jr., MD
Board of Registration in Medicine

Malcolm Robinson, MD
Brigham and Women's Hospital

John Romanelli, MD, FACS
Baystate Medical Center

Edward Saltzman, MD
Tufts-New England Medical Center

Roman Schumann, MD
Tufts-New England Medical Center

Scott A. Shikora, MD, FACS
Tufts-New England Medical Center

Roger L. Snow, MD, MPH
University of Massachusetts Medical School and MassHealth

Stephanie Sogg, PhD
Massachusetts General Hospital

Mary Anna Sullivan, MD
Lahey Clinic and Massachusetts Coalition for the Prevention of Medical Errors

Michael Tarnoff, MD
Tufts-New England Medical Center

Christopher Thompson, MD, MHES
Brigham and Women's Hospital

Christina Wee, MD, MPH
Beth Israel Deaconess Medical Center

Lehman Center
Nancy Ridley, MS, Director
John Auerbach, MBA, Chair, Lehman Board
Frank Hu, MD, PhD, Consulting Clinical Epidemiologist
Leslie Kirle, MPH, Project Manager
Rita Buckley, MBA, Medical Librarian and Medical Editor
Catherine L. Annas, JD, Director of Patient Safety

# Foreword

Sharp increases in the prevalence of severe obesity (BMI > 40 and BMI > 50) have continued to fuel demand for WLS. In 2004, the Betsy Lehman Center for Patient Safety and Medical Error Reduction (Lehman Center) formed an Expert Panel to assess WLS procedures, identify issues related to patient safety, and develop evidence-based best practice recommendations to address those issues.

The resulting document, published as a supplement in Obesity in 2005, set the standard for WLS across the state and well beyond it. The Agency for Healthcare Research and Quality (AHRQ) abstracted the report for broad use, and the American College of Surgeons (ACS) adopted it as the blueprint for its Bariatric Surgery Network Center Accreditation Program. Its recommendations influenced healthcare policy and medical practice at home and abroad.

Since 2004, the literature on WLS has expanded rapidly. New data have been published; new procedures have been developed; and new issues have been brought to our attention. In Massachusetts, weight loss operations increased from over 2,700 in Fiscal Year 2003 to nearly 3,500 in Fiscal Year 2006. We saw a shift from open to laparoscopic operations, and changes in reimbursement policies.

The safety of WLS continues to be of concern. In response, the Lehman Center reconvened the Expert Panel to update the literature review and evidence-based recommendations developed in 2004. Several new members joined the 2007 Expert Panel as well its task groups. All told, there were two additional task groups, bringing the total from 9 to 11. We separated the Psychology Task Group from Multidisciplinary Evaluation and Treatment, and formed a new group, Endoscopic Interventions, to develop best practice guidelines for that emerging technology. In addition, we changed the name of the Coding and Reimbursement Task Group to Policy and Access to better reflect its focus.

The charge to the 2007 Expert Panel was to update the evidence-based best practice recommendations for WLS developed three years ago. Toward that end, its members reviewed weight loss surgical procedures; analyzed the medical literature published since 2004; recommended specific steps to reduce medical errors and improve patient safety; developed credentialing and training standards; identified best practices; and established clinical guidelines and directions for future research.

What follows is a comprehensive evidence-based update to the original best practice recommendations. As with the first report, we hope that these guidelines will have far-reaching effects on clinical practice and healthcare policy, not only in the Commonwealth, but also nationwide. We hope that they will equalize access and reduce variability in performance and outcomes. Ultimately, our objective is to improve the safety of WLS in the state of Massachusetts and protect the well-being of patients who undergo it.

More than 100 individuals created this report. I want to express my deepest appreciation to the Expert Panel and task group members for the monumental work that went into this project. I especially want to thank Dr. George Blackburn, Chair, Dr. Matt Hutter, Vice Chair, Dr. Frank Hu, our clinical epidemiologist, and Rita Buckley, our librarian and medical editor, for their continued leadership and commitment to this project. Last but not least, I want to thank the Department of Public Health and Betsy Lehman Center staff, especially our project manager, Leslie Kirle, and Katie Annas for their diligent efforts in coordinating and facilitating the work of this project.

Nancy Ridley, MS, Director

Betsy Lehman Center for Patient Safety and Medical Error Reduction

**Figure 1**

(A) Estimated number of weight loss procedures performed in the United States, 1992 to 2006 (20, 25, 36).

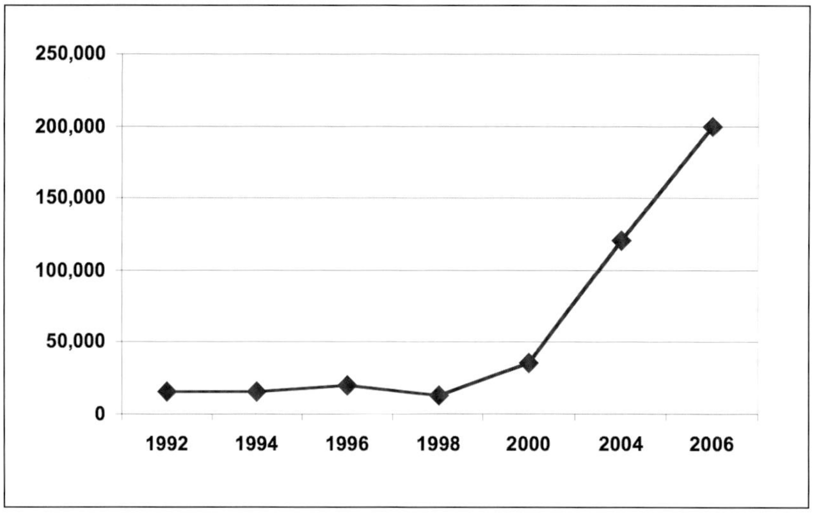


**Figure 2**

(B) The number of weight loss operations performed in Massachusetts, 1996 to 2006 (Dept. of Public Health).

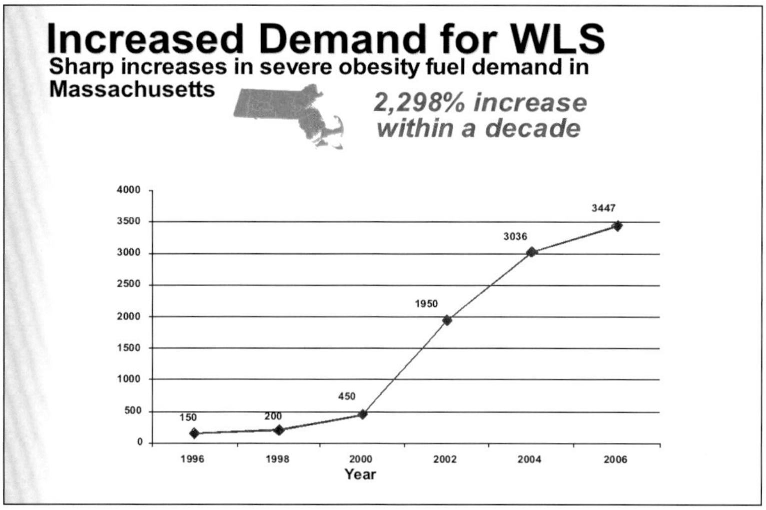

# Preface

Overwhelming data demonstrate reductions in known disease risk factors and improvements in health after weight loss surgery (WLS) (1-3). Recent studies also indicate that WLS confers a survival advantage on patients who undergo it compared with community controls (1, 2). Landmark findings from the Swedish Obese Subjects (SOS) study show an estimated 28% reduction in the adjusted overall mortality rate in the surgical groups compared with conventionally-treated controls (4).

Similar outcomes have been cited in other reports. A collaborative research project in Utah compared 7,925 gastric bypass patients with the same number of age-, gender-, and BMI-matched controls. Data showed that the rate of death from all diseases was 52% lower in the surgery group than in the control group ($P < 0.001$) (5). In a case study that compared 821 obese patients who received laparoscopic adjustable gastric banding (LAGB) with 821 controls treated with medical therapy, Favretti et al. (6) found a statistically significant survival difference in favor of the surgically-treated group.

Perry and colleagues (7) compared a cohort of extremely obese Medicare beneficiaries who underwent WLS to a similar cohort of extremely obese Medicare beneficiaries who did not. At the two-year follow-up, younger (<65 years old) and older patients (≥65) in the surgical group had significantly reduced mortality compared with those in the nonsurgical group. Similarly, Sowemimo et al. (8) reported 50% to 85% mortality reductions with surgical intervention.

Decreased total mortality in the the SOS study (4) surgical groups was primarily due to fewer deaths from cardiovascular disease (especially myocardial infarction) and cancer. In the Utah study (5), significant reductions in mortality were linked to fewer deaths from coronary artery disease, diabetes, and cancer. These results, which show substantial and consistent evidence of a survival advantage for severely obese patients who undergo WLS, are in line with those of earlier reports by Christou et al. (9) and Flum and Dellinger (10). They also confirm previous case series and epidemiologic observations on mortality after weight loss operations in more diverse populations (1,11).

But despite reductions in disease-related mortality after WLS, death rates from other causes, such as accidents and suicides, exceed those of non-surgery patients. In Adams et al. (5), rates of death not caused by disease were 58% higher in the surgery group than in the control group. Reports reveal that a substantial number of severely obese persons have unrecognized presurgical mood disorders or post-traumatic stress disorder, or have been victims of childhood sexual abuse (12).

Data on the association between presurgical psychological status and postsurgical outcomes are limited (13). Although research shows an improved quality of life after gastric bypass surgery (14-17), certain unrecognized presurgical conditions may reappear after surgery (18). Some WLS centers recommend that all patients undergo psychological evaluation, and, if necessary, treatment before surgery and psychologically-related surveillance postoperatively (12, 13, 19). Adams et al. (5) note the need for further research on the optimal approach to evaluating candidates for WLS, including possible presurgical assessment, psychiatric treatment, and diligent postoperative follow-up.

We know from a substantial body of literature that WLS achieves significant and durable weight loss with minimal mortality or complications. We know that laparoscopy shortens length of stay and makes for a faster, easier recovery (20). Now reliable evidence is starting to accumulate on the survival advantage conferred by WLS on those who undergo it. The field is dynamic (21), with surgical approaches being developed and refined at a rapid pace. Yet technical performance of the operations, critical though it may be, is only one of many challenges.

WLS deals with a uniquely vulnerable population in need of specialized resources and ongoing multidisciplinary care. Timely best practice updates are critical to identify new risks, develop strategies to address them, and optimize treatment of WLS patients. As before (22), members of this panel have come together to protect patient safety and prevent medical errors with evidence-based standards of care. This update of best practice guidelines is part of our continued efforts to improve the efficacy and safety of WLS procedures.

George L. Blackburn, MD, PhD, Chair
Matthew M. Hutter, MD, MPH, Vice Chair

### Background

More than 33% of U.S. adults are classified as obese based on objectively measured weight (23), and one-third of American children are either obese or at risk of becoming so (24). Between 2000 and 2005, the proportion of Americans with a BMI ? 40 increased by 50%, while those with a BMI ≥50 increased by 75% (25). Severe obesity has been growing at the fastest rate for the past 20 years (23, 25).

Obesity, particularly abdominal obesity, is associated with increased risk of hypertension, diabetes, hyperlipidemia, sleep apnea, coronary heart disease, and strokes (26, 27). In 1998, medical costs attributable to overweight and obesity accounted for 9.1% of total U.S. medical expenditures, and may have reached as high as $78.5 billion ($92.6 billion in 2002 dollars) (28, 29). In 2000, there were approximately 360,000 deaths associated with obesity (30). It has been suggested that in the 21st century, increasing rates of obesity may lead to a decline in overall life expectancy in the United States (31).

### Update on Common WLS Procedures

Overview. WLS reduces caloric intake by modifying the anatomy of the gastrointestinal tract via restriction, malabsorption, or a combination of the two techniques. Ensuing changes in the gut-brain axis alter peptides that may regulate appetite and satiety (32) (e.g., ghrelin, glucagon-like peptide [GLP-1], and pancreatic polypeptide [PP]). Among the several competing approaches for the management of severe obesity, the general trend is toward combined restrictive-malabsorptive procedures (33). Over the past few decades, the number of weight loss surgeries performed in the U.S. has increased significantly (34, 35). Between 1998 and 2004, weight loss operations rose by 900% to 121,055 (36). In 2006, the estimated total climbed to 200,000 (20,25).

Laparoscopic Roux-en-Y gastric bypass (LRYGB) is considered the gold standard operation for long-term weight control in U.S. (35, 37). Rates of RYGB per 100,000 adults rose significantly from 1998 to 2002, from 7.0 to 38.6. This increase may be attributed, in part, to improved surgical techniques, better patient outcomes, and growing popularity of the procedure (38). Laparoscopic adjustable gastric band (LAGB) is the second most commonly performed operation in the U.S. Despite rapid growth in LRYGB and other weight loss procedures, only an estimated 1% of patients who are eligible for WLS receive it in any given year (39).

### Common WLS Procedures

Laparoscopic Roux-en-Y Gastric Bypass (LRYGB). Gastric bypass involves the creation of a small (20-30 mL) gastric pouch and a Roux limb (typically 75- to 105 cm) (34) that reroutes a portion of the alimentary tract to bypass the distal stomach and proximal small bowel. Following LRYGB, a pleiotropic endocrine response may contribute to improved glycemic control, appetite reduction, and long-term changes in body weight (40). LYRGB also has a profoundly positive impact on obesity-related comorbidities and quality of life (QOL) (41). Other advantages include established long-term effectiveness for sustained weight loss, reduction of comorbidities, minimal risk for long-term nutritional sequelae, and effective relief of gastroesophageal reflux disease (GERD) (21). LRYGB is not without risks. Common causes of death include pulmonary embolism and anastomatic leaks. Nonfatal perioperative complications include venous thromboembolism, wound infections, small bowel obstruction, and bleeding. Postoperative gastrointestinal complications include nausea and vomiting, micronutrient deficiencies, (35) and possible weight regain (22).

**Figure 3**

Roux-en-Y Gastric Bypass (RYGB)

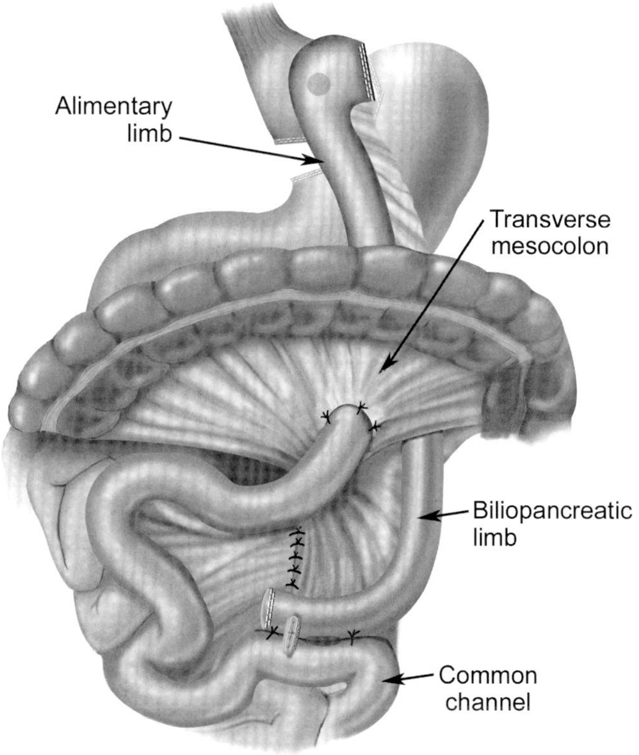


RYGB involves the creation of a small (< 30 mL) gastric pouch and a Roux limb (typically 75- to 105 cm) that reroutes a portion of the alimentary tract to bypass the distal stomach and proximal small bowel. Illustration reprinted with permission from Atlas of Metabolic and Weight Loss Surgery, Jones et al. Cine-Med, 2008. Copyright of the book and illustrations are retained by Cine-Med.

Laparoscopic Adjustable Gastric Band (LAGB). LAGB involves the placement of a band or collar around the upper stomach 1-2 cm below the gastroesophageal junction, thereby creating an approximate 30 mL upper gastric pouch. Degree of stomach constriction can be adjusted by modifying the amount of saline injected into a subcutaneous port, which is linked to a balloon within the band (34). Parikh et al. (42) found that LAGB had fewer and less severe complications compared with LRYGB or laparoscopic malabsorptive procedures. But other data link LAGB with intermediate and long-term complications (e.g., band erosion or slippage, failure to achieve or maintain weight loss) that require reoperation in up to 20% of patients (43, 44).

**Figure 4**

Adjustable Gastric Band (LAGB)

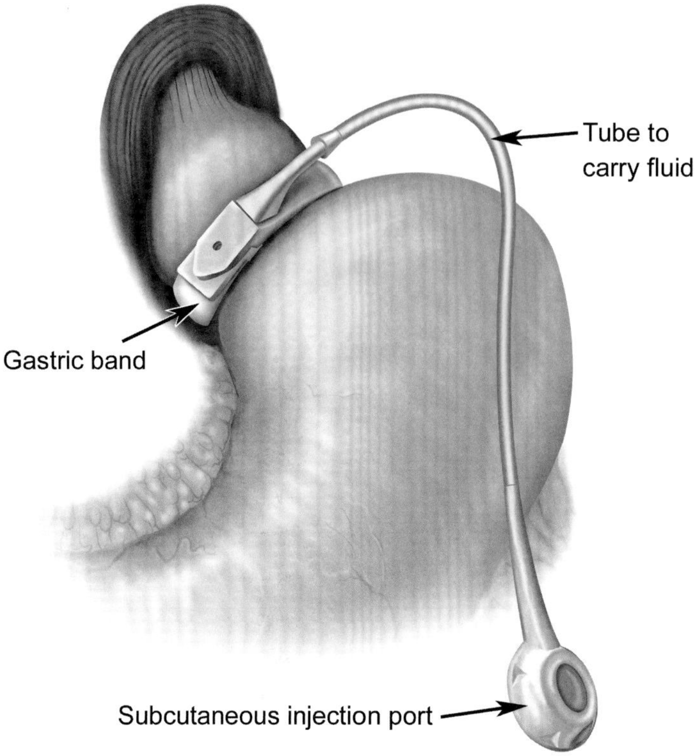


LAGB involves the placement of a band or collar around the upper stomach 1-2 cm below the gastroesophageal junction, thereby creating an approximate 30 mL upper gastric pouch. The band is imbricated to prevent slippage of the stomach in a retrograde manner through the band. Degree of stomach constriction can be adjusted by modifying the amount of saline injected into a subcutaneous port, which is linked to a balloon within the band. Illustration reprinted with permission from Atlas of Metabolic and Weight Loss Surgery, Jones et al, Cine-Med, 2008. Copyright of the book and illustrations are retained by Cine-Med.

Biliopancreatic diversion (BPD). BPD creates malabsorption by maintaining a flow of bile and pancreatic juice through the biliopancreatic limb (45). The procedure is commonly performed with a duodenal switch in which a distal, common channel length of small intestine severely limits caloric absorption (35). The extent of malabsorption is thought to be a function of the length of the common channel (34). The procedure is combined with a sleeve gastrectomy in which the greater curvature of the stomach is resected, creating a tubular section along the lesser curvature of the stomach (34). The BPD described by Scoparino (45) is capable of producing substantial and sustained weight loss, perhaps associated with markedly suppressed ghrelin levels (46). However, increased incidence of stomal ulceration, severe protein-energy malnutrition, diarrhea, and dumping has limited its broad acceptance (21).

**Figure 5**

Biliopancreatic Diversion with Duodenal Switch (BPD)

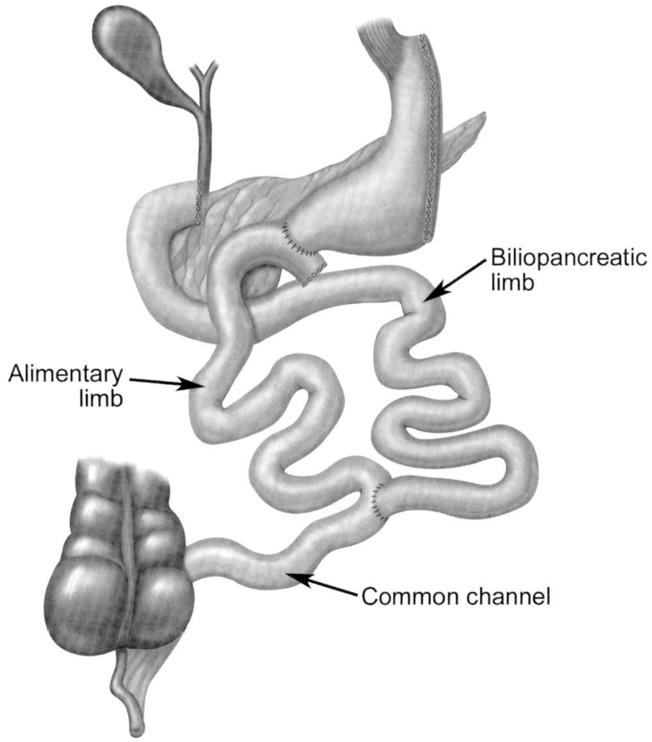


BPD creates malabsorption by maintaining a flow of bile and pancreatic juice through the biliopancreatic limb. The procedure is commonly performed with a duodenal switch in which a distal, common-channel length of small intestine severely limits caloric absorption. The extent of malabsorption is thought to be a function of the length of the common channel. Illustration reprinted with permission from Atlas of Metabolic and Weight Loss Surgery, Jones et al, Cine-Med, 2008. Copyright of the book and illustrations are retained by Cine-Med.

Laparoscopic sleeve gastrectomy (LSG). LSG is a new purely restrictive treatment for severe obesity. The technique consists of the restrictive component of the duodenal switch (DS), a resection of the greater curvature of the stomach over a 45- to 50-F bougie positioned along the lesser curvature. The pylorus and part of the antrum are preserved, resulting in a lesser curvature-based "restrictive" gastric sleeve (21). Early reports of sleeve gastrectomy have shown it to be safe and effective (47, 48), with marked weight loss and significant reduction of major obesity-related comorbidities (49, 50). LSG can be performed as a stand-alone operation or as a bridge to more complex WLS. Following the operation, the stomach empties its contents rapidly into the small intestine, but with little or no vomiting (characteristic of restrictive procedures) (51). There is also a significant reduction in ghrelin associated with resection of the gastric fundus, the predominant area of human ghrelin production (46, 52).

**Figure 6**

Sleeve gastrectomy (SG)

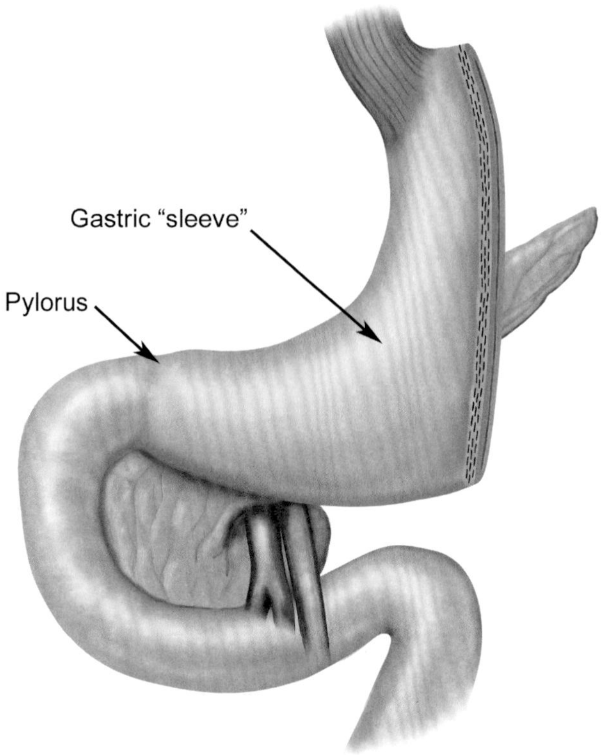


SG consists of the restrictive component of the duodenal switch (DS), a vertical resection of the greater curvature of the stomach creating a long tubular stomach along the lesser curvature. The pylorus and part of the antrum are preserved. Illustration reprinted with permission from Atlas of Metabolic and Weight Loss Surgery, Jones et al. Cine-Med, 2008. Copyright of the book and illustrations are retained by Cine-Med.

**Framework for Evidence-Based Recommendations**

We divided the 35-member Expert Panel into 11 task groups:

- Surgical Care (53)
- Multidisciplinary Evaluation and Treatment (54)
- Behavior and Psychological Care (55)
- Pediatric/Adolescent (56)
- Anesthetic Perioperative Care and Pain Management (57)
- Nursing Perioperative Care (58)
- Informed Consent and Patient Education (59)
- Policy and Access (Coding and Reimbursement) (60)
- Specialized Facilities and Resources (61)
- Data Collection (Registries)/Future Considerations (62)
- Endoscopic Interventions (63)

Panel members joined one or two task groups, each with an assigned coordinator. Participants were asked to update recommendations from the first Lehman Center report (22) based on the best available evidence, including randomized controlled trials (RCTs), observational studies, and expert opinion. A medical librarian performed systematic literature reviews for each group. Searches were limited to English-language studies published between April 2004 and May 2007 in MEDLINE, EMBASE, and the Cochrane Library. Some groups also searched other databases (e.g., CINHAL). The process used to extract data, assess the literature, and grade evidence has been previously described (22).

Each task group prepared a critical summary of its literature review and developed updated best practice recommendations (individual studies are published in this issue of Obesity) based on the most current available evidence. Their reports were reviewed and approved by the Expert Panel. This Executive Report, a summary of key recommendations from all the task groups, was approved by the Expert Panel at its final meeting on July 19, 2007.

**Summary of Evidence-Based Recommendations**

**I. Surgical Care**

The Surgical Care Task Group identified more than 135 papers; the 65 most relevant were reviewed in detail (53). These included randomized control trials, prospective and retrospective cohort studies, meta-analyses, case reports, prior systematic reviews, and expert opinion.

**A. Overview**

Roux-en-Y gastric bypass (RYGB) remains the predominant, gold standard WLS in the U.S., accounting for 93% of all such operations in 2000 (64). Laparoscopic adjustable gastric banding (LAGB) is the second most commonly performed procedure (65, 66). RYGB is known to safely improve or reverse obesity-related comorbidities and produce significant long-term weight loss (21). Long-term data on weight loss after LAGB vary (42, 67, 68).

**B. Types of Weight Loss Surgery**

**Combination Procedures**

Combination procedures join a restrictive component (e.g., gastric stapling) with some form of duodenal bypass. They include RYGB, biliopancreatic diversion (BPD), and duodenal switch. (DS)

*RYGB (Open and Laparoscopic)*

Most gastric bypass operations are now done laparoscopically. LRYGB reduces pulmonary, wound, hernia-related complications, and postoperative pain (Category B), but may have higher internal hernia rates than RYGB (Category C). Weight loss is similar with both approaches (Category B).

*RYGB modifications*

Long-limb RYGB (LL-RYGB) and very very long-limb RYGB (VVLL-RYGB) extend the length of the Roux limb to enhance weight loss. The procedures may increase risk of protein and micronutrient deficiencies (Category C); it has yet to be determined if they produce superior weight loss (Category C).

Banded RYGB may be subject to long-term complications related to reintervention, reoperation, and quality of life (Categories C and D). There is insufficient evidence to make a recommendation (Category D). Long-term drawbacks of mini-gastric bypass might include bile reflux and the need for revisional surgery (Category C). As with banded RYGB, more data are needed to develop recommendations.

*BPD and DS*

BPD and DS produce effective weight loss (Category B). In patients with a BMI > 50, it may be superior to that achieved with RYGB (Category C). However, the procedures may increase severe complications (e.g., protein and micronutrient deficiencies) (Category B). They also require diligent lifelong patient follow-up (Category D).

**Restrictive Procedures**

Restrictive WLS (e.g., LAGB) has no malabsorptive or maldigestive components.

*LAGB*

Short-term data show promising outcomes with LAGB, but long-term studies raise questions on durability and reoperative rates (Category B). We recommend monitoring of long-term data and continuation of current practice patterns, with yearly follow-up of patients (Category D).

LAGB should be performed in accredited, multidisciplinary settings by experienced surgeons. They should have advanced laparoscopic skills, including those needed to revise LAGB to an alternate procedure. Barring that, WLS programs should be able to provide appropriate referrals to facilities that can provide that level of care (Category D). It is safe for obesity medicine specialists, nurse practitioners, physician assistants, residents, and bariatric nurse specialists to adjust bands under the supervision of a weight loss surgeon (Category D).

*Laparoscopic Sleeve Gastrectomy (LSG)*

Several short-term studies suggest safe and effective weight loss with LSG (Categories B and C), but long-term data on safety and efficacy are needed to recommend the approach as anything other than investigational (Category D). If other WLS options are ruled out for reasons of preference or safety, LSG may be considered (Category D).

*Vertical Banded Gastroplasty (VBG)*

VBG is associated with increased peri- and postoperative complications compared with LAGB. Evidence suggests that it should not be used as a primary surgical treatment for obesity (Categories A and B). However, it can be considered when alternative weight loss surgeries are not safe or possible (Category D).

*C. Revision of WLS*

Revisional WLS can address unsatisfactory weight loss or complications after primary WLS. It may also enhance weight loss and further improve comorbidities (Category B). Complications, length of stay, and mortality are higher for revisional WLS (Category B), but it can be safe and effective when performed by experienced weight loss surgeons (Category D).

**D. Intraoperative Techniques**

We recommend the following as standard practice:

- Testing of gastrojejunal anastomosis for leaks intraoperatively or within 48 hours (Category C)
- Strong consideration of whether to close mesenteric defects to avoid internal hernia (Category C)

**E. Patient Selection**

Emerging issues in patient selection include treatment of those with a BMI > 50 and individuals > age 60. Although procedure-specific recommendations for extremely obese patients have yet to be determined (Category C), the literature suggests that combination procedures (e.g., RYGB, BPD, DS) lead to greater excess weight loss (EWL) and resolution of comorbidities than restrictive procedures (e.g., LAGB) (Category D).

Age may remain an independent risk factor following WLS (Category C), but evidence suggests that WLS can be safe and effective in patients > 60 (Categories B and C). We recommend that older patients not be denied improvements in health and quality of life associated with WLS (Category D).

**F. Facility and Surgeon Credentialing Standards**

The following are best practice updates to guidelines in our prior report (69). These recommendations are all based on Category D evidence, unless otherwise noted.

**Facilities**

- All WLS centers should have, or be in the process of obtaining, accreditation by external review
- They should meet WLS volume standards specified by credentialing bodies
- Centers with lower volume should be endorsed if risk-adjusted outcomes fall within benchmarks determined by credentialing body data

**Surgeon – Credentialing**

*General Requirements*

All surgeons seeking WLS credentials for the first time should:

- Complete an accredited general surgery program and be board-certified, board-eligible, or the equivalent
- Have documented training in the fundamentals of WLS, including pre-, peri-, and postoperative care of the WLS patient

*Open Privileges*

Most weight loss surgeries are performed laparoscopically. Those who want only open privileges should complete the general credentialing requirements above, and:

- Be proctored by an experienced weight loss surgeon until proficient
- Have their first 10 cases reviewed by the chief of service and an experienced weight loss surgeon
- Count fellowship cases toward individual surgeon volume requirements

*Full Privileges (Open and Laparoscopic)*

It is no longer practical to require specific and mandatory experience in open WLS prior to applying for laparoscopic privileges. Those seeking full laparoscopic privileges should complete the general requirements and a laparoscopic fellowship of 50 WLS procedures. As an alternative, they can be proctored for a minimum of 25 cases by an experienced (70) (> 200 laparoscopic cases) weight loss surgeon with full privileges. In addition, surgeons should:

- Have their first 10 cases reviewed by the chief of staff and an experienced weight loss surgeon
- Count fellowship cases toward individual surgeon volume requirements

Fundamentals of Laparoscopic Surgery (FLS) certification is also highly recommended for newly trained laparoscopic surgeons.

**Surgeon – Recredentialing**

- Institutions should develop in-house standards for recredentialing based on procedure-specific and risk adjusted outcomes (benchmarks) rather than volume alone
- An annual volume of 25 cases may be sufficient if outcomes are within accepted standards, reported to a central database, and performed at an accredited institution
- Weight loss surgeons should complete at least 12 CME credits related to WLS or obesity every 2 years

**Procedure-specific Credentialing**

Rapid changes in technologies and techniques warrant disclosure of procedure- specific information to patients, and selection of those with lower risk profiles for the first 25 cases. As part of the educational process, surgeons should disclose:

- The type and approximate number of procedures they perform (Category D)
- Alternative WLS options available (Category D)
- Risks, potential benefits, and program outcomes (Category D)

## II. Multidisciplinary Evaluation and Treatment

The Multidisciplinary Care Task Group identified over 150 abstracts related to WLS in general, and to medical, nutritional, and multidisciplinary care in particular; 112 of these studies were reviewed in detail (54).

### A. Multidisciplinary Care

The American Society for Metabolic and Bariatric Surgery (ASMBS) recently changed its name to the American Society for Metabolic and Bariatric Surgery (ASMBS), reflecting growing knowledge that WLS has benefits beyond the treatment of severe obesity. This change expands the scope of multidisciplinary expertise required to provide optimal care for WLS patients. As the nature of multidisciplinary care changes, we recommend:

- Development of uniform minimum standards of multidisciplinary care for WLS patients (Category D)
- Further research on the effectiveness of general medical, surgical, anesthetic, nutritional, and psychological aspects of multidisciplinary treatment (Category D)

### B. Preoperative Education and Patient Selection

Preoperative education allows for more appropriate matching of patients and procedures. It can dispel misperceptions and unrealistic expectations, and help clarify issues related to resolution of comorbid conditions, differences between surgical procedures, and required lifestyle changes after WLS (Category D).

**C. Operative Risk**

Higher BMI and medical comorbidities (e.g., obstructive sleep apnea and coronary heart disease risk factors) increase operative risk and postoperative complications. We recommend assessment of risk factors (71) in each patient (Category C).

*Preoperative Weight Loss*

Preoperative weight loss of 5% to 10% of initial body weight can decrease operation time and may reduce surgical risk. Patients, especially those with a BMI ≥50, should be encouraged to achieve weight loss of 5% to 10% of initial body weight prior to surgery (Category C). Prospective randomized controlled trials are needed to determine optimal preoperative weight loss and improve supervision of preoperative weight reduction (Category C).

*Medical Evaluation*

Specific consideration should be given to WLS patients with a history of CAD or DVT/PE, those who are current smokers, and those with known or suspected abnormal liver function. *H. Pylori* testing and treatment may also be useful, but more evidence is needed to determine its importance. Other risk factors include postprandial hypoglycemia, chronic renal disease, and HIV.

**Coronary Artery Disease (CAD)**

Patients with a history of CAD should receive preoperative assessment of cardiovascular conditions as indicated (Category C). Those with stable or suspected CAD should receive perioperative beta blockade unless contraindicated (Category C).

**Abnormal Liver function**

Patients with known or suspected liver disease should be evaluated to assess severity of cirrhosis and/or portal hypertension (Category B). Intraoperative liver biopsy at the time of surgery may be useful for diagnosis and assessment of liver disease (Category C). WLS is not recommended in patients with Child's Class C cirrhosis (Category B).

**DVT/PE**

We recommend perioperative use of anticoagulants and sequential compression devices to reduce the risk of DVT/PE unless clinically contraindicated (Category B). In patients with increased risk of DVT/PE extended prophylaxis should also be considered (Category D).

**Smokers**

Smokers should be strongly encouraged to stop smoking prior to WLS (Category B). Smoking cessation advice and treatment should be available at the institution or through the WLS program (Category D).

**Hypoglycemia**

Patients with known or suspected hypoglycemia should be assessed by an endocrinologist prior to WLS. In that gastric bypass surgery is already being used to treat diabetes (72), purely restrictive procedures should be considered for WLS patients with a documented history of hypoglycemia (Category D).

**Chronic Renal Disease**

Pre-and postoperative monitoring of renal function is recommended in patients with diabetes and hypertension (Categories A and B). Patients with significant renal disease should be evaluated by a nephrologist prior to WLS (Category D). Special consideration should be given to pre- and postoperative monitoring of fluid and intravascular volume status (Category A).

**HIV Infection**

Patients with HIV should be evaluated by an infectious disease specialist prior to WLS (Category D). Special consideration should be given to preoperative assessment of viral loads, CD4 counts (Category D), and weight gain from antiretroviral medications (Category D).

**D. Nutrition**

**Preoperative and postoperative micronutrients**

WLS, especially malabsorptive procedures, can cause multiple micronutrient deficiencies. Patients should be monitored pre- and postoperatively for deficiencies in vitamin D, thiamine, calcium, iron, vitamin $B_{12}$, and folic acid, with repletion as indicated (Categories A, B, and C).

**E. Exercise and Physical Activity**

WLS patients should be encouraged to increase pre- and postoperative physical activity (Category D) and low-to-moderate intensity exercise (Category A). Guidance and periodic monitoring should be used to help WLS patients remain physically active (Category D).

**F. Pregnancy**

WLS should not be performed in patients who are known to be pregnant; we strongly recommend preoperative testing for women of childbearing age (Category C). Patients should be strongly counseled to not get pregnant for at least 18 months after surgery (Category C).

**G. Post-WLS Body Contouring**

Post-WLS body contouring is an emerging field. The task group identified and reviewed in detail 80 relevant articles, ranging from case reports and expert opinion to prospective randomized trials.

Body contouring can be considered after a patient has achieved a stable weight, generally 18 months (or more) after WLS. Facilities should be accredited, with ready access to intensive care personnel and equipment (Category D).

*Surgeon Criteria*

Body contouring should only be performed by board-eligible or board-certified surgeons with training and experience in the relevant procedures (Category D).

**III. Behavioral and Psychological Care**

The Behavioral and Psychological Care Task Group identified 17 papers; the 13 most relevant were reviewed in detail (55). These included randomized controlled trials, prospective and retrospective cohort studies, meta-analyses, case reports, and prior systematic reviews.

**A. Patient Selection and Preoperative Evaluation**

WLS patients are an emotionally vulnerable population. All candidates for WLS should undergo psychosocial evaluation by a credentialed expert in psychology and behavior change (Category C). Evaluations should be carried out by a social worker, psychologist, or psychiatrist with a strong background in the current literature on obesity and WLS, and some experience in the pre- and postoperative assessment and care of WLS patients (Category D). Though not essential, it is preferable that the evaluator be on staff or affiliated with the WLS center to facilitate communication, maintain the support network, and provide continuity of care (Category D).

To address long-term complications, mental health resources should be made available to patients beyond the standard postoperative period of 6 months (Category D). This recommendation can be met in a variety of ways (e.g., staff mental health professional, referral network).

Mental illness, including eating pathology, should not necessarily be a contraindication to WLS. Evaluations should determine the degree to which mental illness, including eating pathology, may jeopardize the safety or efficacy of WLS (Category C). They should be used to identify patients in need of preoperative psychosocial intervention, and develop recommendations on if, how, and when to best address significant psychosocial risk factors (Category C).

Psychological assessment and support have become essential components of multidisciplinary care in WLS. We recommend that organizations that provide education on obesity and WLS (e.g., The North American Association for the Study of Obesity) offer continuing education units (CEUs) to mental health providers. This will facilitate the development of continuing education standards for mental health specialists in the fields of obesity and WLS (Category D).

**B. Binge Eating Disorder (BED)**

BED in patients seeking WLS is clinically important, especially in the long-term. It should be taken into account in the development of treatment plans. Assessment should be done in a standardized, empirically validated way (e.g., screening with

EDE-Q and follow-up with a brief, standardized interview based on DSM-IV-TR criteria) (Category C). The disorder should not be considered a contraindication for WLS, but rather, a potential complication that may need to be addressed before or after surgery to ensure optimal outcome (Category C).

Patients should know that eating pathology can recur after WLS, and that they may need professional help to deal with recurring patterns of binge eating. BED should be included in the informed consent process and as part of the WLS program's standard educational component (Category C).

**C. Night Eating Syndrome (NES)**

In that there is no clear evidence that NES has any impact on surgical outcome, the condition should not be considered a contraindication for WLS. Rather, it should be seen as a potentially complicating factor that may need to be addressed before or after surgery to ensure optimal outcome (Category D).

**D. Emotional Eating**

Data are insufficient to make recommendations on the assessment and treatment of emotional eating. As with NES, the issue should be considered a potentially complicating factor that may need to be addressed before or after WLS to assure optimal outcome (Category D).

**E. Substance Abuse**

Findings on the prevalence of substance abuse among those seeking WLS are conflicting, and there are few studies on the subject. Evidence is insufficient to conclude that the problem is a frequent one after WLS. Further research is needed to establish the prevalence of substance abuse after WLS as well as its predictors, its relation to surgical outcome, and effective treatment approaches (Category D).

**F. Psychotropic Medications**

Data indicate significantly higher use of psychotropic medications in WLS patients compared with the general population. Further research is needed to determine the relation between various psychotropic medications and their impact on postoperative weight loss and psychosocial adjustment (Category D).

The effects of WLS on the dissolution, absorption, and clinical response to psychotropic drugs are not well understood. For this reason, we recommend close postoperative monitoring of WLS patients, especially after gastric bypass (Category D).

**G. Future Research Needs**

- Adequately powered and controlled prospective trials that examine the relation between psychosocial factors and surgical outcomes
- Randomized controlled trials on the effectiveness of treatments to reduce the impact of psychosocial risk factors on outcomes

**IV. Pediatric/Adolescent**

The pediatric/adolescent WLS Task Group identified more than 1,085 papers; 186 of the most relevant were reviewed in detail (56).

**A. Types of Surgery**

RYGB is considered a safe and effective option for extremely obese adolescents as long as appropriate long-term follow-up is provided (Category B). The adjustable gastric band (AGB) has not been approved by the FDA for use in adolescents, and therefore, should be considered investigational. Off-label use can be considered, if done in an IRB-approved study (Category C).

BPD and DS procedures cannot be recommended in adolescents. Current data suggest substantial risks of protein malnutrition, bone loss, and micronutrient deficiencies. These nutritional risks are of particular concern during pregnancy. In addition, several late maternal deaths have been reported (Category C).

Sleeve gastrectomy should be considered investigational; existing data are not sufficient to recommend widespread and general use in adolescents (Category D).

**B. Comorbidities**

Strong indications for WLS in adolescents include established type 2 diabetes (Category B), moderate to severe OSA with AHI ≥15 (Category C), severe and/or progressive NASH (Category C), and pseudotumor cerebri (Category C). Other indications for WLS in adolescents include mild OSA, mild NASH, hypertension, dyslipidemia, and significantly impaired quality of life (Categories C and D).

All adolescents with obesity should be formally assessed for depression. If found to be depressed, they should be treated prior to WLS (Category B). The presence of eating disturbances is not an exclusion criterion for WLS, but adolescents with such disorders should be treated prior to surgery (Category B).

**C. Patient Selection**

When combination procedures are used in adolescents, physical maturity (completion of 95% of adult stature based on radiographic study) should be documented. In most cases, this criterion will limit surgery to children over age 12 (Category D). Psychological maturity—demonstrated by understanding of the surgery, mature motivations for the operation, and compliance with preoperative therapy—should be assessed prior to WLS (Category D).

BMI cutpoints in children and adolescents who meet other criteria should be ≥35 with major comorbidities (i.e., type 2 diabetes mellitus, moderate to severe sleep apnea [AHI>15], pseudotumor cerebri, or severe NASH) and ≥40 with other comorbidities (e.g., hypertension, insulin resistance, glucose intolerance, substantially impaired quality of life or activities of daily living, dyslipidemia, sleep apnea with AHI > 5) (Categories B and C).

There are no data available to suggest that prolonged preoperative weight management programs are of benefit to adolescents who undergo WLS. However, children and adolescents should demonstrate the ability to comply with treatment regimens and medical monitoring before WLS. In many cases, consistent attendance in a prolonged weight management program will provide important assurance of postoperative compliance (Category D).

Individuals with mental retardation vary in their capacity to demonstrate knowledge, motivation, and compliance; they should, therefore, be evaluated for WLS on a case-by-case basis. For these children, we suggest including an ethicist on the multidisciplinary evaluation team (Category D).

Others who should be screened on a case-by-case basis include: patients with syndromic obesity, endocrine disorders, obesity that appears to be related to the use of weight-promoting medications, and those in whom obesity cannot be controlled through medical interventions and/or carefully designed environmental and behavioral management. Very limited information is available about the outcomes of WLS for such patients (Category D). Patients with uncontrolled psychosis (presence of hallucinations and delusions), bipolar disorder (extreme mood lability), or substance use disorders can be considered for WLS on a case-by-case basis after they have been in remission for one year (Category C).

**D. Team Member Qualifications**

Although few hospitals have sufficient volume for a stand-alone pediatric surgical center, the ideal WLS team should include a minimum of 4 or 5 professionals who are colocated and have at least one preoperative face-to-face meeting to prepare a treatment plan for each patient (Category D). Staff should include:

- Surgeon – experienced adult bariatric surgeon or pediatric surgeon with bariatric fellowship or the equivalent experience
- Pediatric specialist – internist or pediatrician with adolescent and obesity training and experience
- Registered dietician – with weight management certificate and experience in treating obesity and working with children and families
- Mental health professional – with specialty training in child, adolescent, and family treatment, and experience treating eating disorders and obesity
- Coordinator - RN, social worker, or one of the other team members who has the responsibility of coordinating each child or adolescent's care and assuring compliance and follow-up

The ideal setting would be in an adult/pediatric hospital, with a pediatric program partnered with an adult program that has full access to pediatric specialists (Category D). A comprehensive family-based evaluation should be provided to parents seeking surgery for their adolescent children (Category D).

**E. Risks and Outcomes**

Early WLS may reduce obesity-related mortality and morbidity. However, early timing must be weighed against the patient's possible psychological immaturity and the risk of decreased compliance and long-term follow-up (Category C). All adolescents undergoing WLS should be included in prospective longitudinal data collection to improve the evidence base for evaluating the risks and benefits of WLS in this age group (Category D).

Emphasis on compliance strategies, careful monitoring of vitamin and mineral intake, and periodic laboratory surveillance to detect deficiencies is crucial (Category D). Adolescent girls are particularly vulnerable to nutritional deficiencies; this group is at substantial risk of developing iron deficiency anemia and vitamin B deficiencies during menstruation and pregnancy (Category C), and should receive special attention.

Risk of pregnancy increases after WLS. All female adolescents should be informed about increased fertility following weight loss, and possible risks associated with pregnancy during the first 18 months after surgery. They should be counseled to avoid pregnancy during this period, and offered contraception (Category D). In addition to risks for deficiencies of iron, calcium, and vitamin $B_{12}$ after WLS, adolescents may also be at particular risk for osteopenia and thiamine deficiency (Category C).

**F. Informed Consent**

Informed assent by the adolescent should be obtained separately from the parents to avoid coercion (as in other pediatric chronic illnesses that require surgical intervention) (Category D). The patient's knowledge of the risks and benefits of the procedure and the importance of postoperative follow-up should be formally evaluated to ensure true informed assent (Category C). The parental permission process should include discussion of the risks of adult obesity (Category C), available medical treatments (Category B), surgical alternatives, and the specific risks and outcomes of the proposed WLS in the proposed institution.

**V. Anesthetic Perioperative Care and Pain Management**

The Anesthetic Perioperative Care and Pain Management Task Group's literature search yielded 1,788 abstracts, with 162 potentially relevant titles. Following full-text evaluation of the latter, 45 articles were reviewed in detail. Best practice recommendations integrate the latest research on obesity and collaborative multidisciplinary care (57).

**A. Preoperative Evaluation and Preparation**

Mandatory polysomnography (PSG) for WLS patients has been proposed (Category C). However, we recommend that it be used in selected patients as indicated (Category D). When uncertain of the indication for such testing, clinical assessment should be supplemented to include gender, waist-to-hip ratio, and neck circumference (Category B). Preoperative CPAP treatment should be strongly considered for patients with a PSG diagnosis of moderate to severe OSA (Category C). We recommend smoking cessation at least 6 weeks prior to surgery (Category C); the WLS program should provide active support to help patients achieve and sustain compliance (Category D).

**B. Intraoperative Management**

**Induction and emergence**

The ≥30 degree reverse Trendelenburg position prolongs the ability of severely obese patients to tolerate apnea during induction of (Category A), and emergence from (Category D) anesthesia. CPAP of approximately 10 cmH2O may be considered during preoxygenation to prolong non-hypoxic apnea (Category A). Intubating laryngeal mask airway devices provide an alternative mechanical approach to securing the airway (Categories A and B), and may also improve success when attempting ventilation prior to securing the airway (Category D). Intubating laryngeal mask airway devices should be included among the alternative airway management devices immediately available in the operating room (Categories A and B).

**Maintenance of anesthesia**

Preoperative oral administration of clonidine (an alpha-2 agonist) to obese patients with OSA is associated with reduced anesthetic requirements as well as reduced intra- and postoperative opioid requirements. Its use may be considered unless medically or surgically contraindicated (Categories A and C).

**Intraoperative oxygenation**

Several methods to improve intraoperative oxygenation during WLS have been evaluated. We recommend initial treatment of intraoperative hypoxemia with recruitment maneuvers and positive end-expiratory pressure (PEEP) while monitoring their potential hemodynamic effects (Categories A and B).

**Other interventions**

Postoperative nausea and vomiting (PONV) in laparoscopic WLS patients is related to the volume and rate of intraoperative fluid replacement. To reduce PONV, we recommend maintenance of euvolemia (Category C).

**Intraoperative drug dosing**

Pharmacodynamic studies in severely obese patients have suggested optimal dosing requirements for different neuromuscular blocking agents. Cisatracurium and rocuronium should be dosed according to ideal body weight during standard induction of general anesthesia (Category A). The muscle relaxant succinylcholine should be dosed at 1 mg/kg total body weight (Category A). For target controlled infusion (not yet approved in the U.S.), propofol dose should be calculated to more closely reflect total body weight (Category C).

**C. Postanesthesia Care**

Positive outcomes have been reported with early treatment of postoperative hypoxemia employing noninvasive positive pressure ventilatory support (NIV) in nonobese, non-OSA patients at high risk of respiratory failure (Categories A, B, and C). A joint decision between the surgeon, anesthesiologist, respiratory therapist, and nurse should determine NIV use on selected WLS patients (Category D). LRYGB and LAGB have been performed safely as 23-hour stay and outpatient procedures (Category C). However, patients with OSA should not be considered candidates for outpatient WLS (Category D); we recommend adherence to the American Society of Anesthesiologists Practice Guidelines for the Perioperative Management of Patients with OSA (Category D).

**Postoperative pain management**

Based on new evidence of efficacy and safety specific to WLS patients, we recommend use of opioid sparing multimodal analgesic strategies, including local anesthetic wound infiltration and nonsteroidal anti-inflammatory medications, unless contraindicated (Categories A and C). Solutions for thoracic epidural pain management in OSA patients should be opioid-free to reduce the risk of respiratory depression (Category C).

**D. Credentialing**

No evidence indicates that specific credentialing of anesthesia personnel for WLS will improve patient safety or outcomes. We recommend the selection of a board-certified anesthesiologist to coordinate intradepartmental staff education and proctoring to establish proficiency. This individual will also serve as an interdepartmental liaison to WLS programs and the multidisciplinary WLS care team (Category D).

**E. Medical Error Reduction and Systems Improvement**

Optimal outcomes require unimpaired intra- and perioperative multidisciplinary communication among WLS caregivers (Category D). Development of perioperative care pathways for patients with OSA is at an early stage (Category D) and needs further refinement for WLS patients.

**F. Future Research Needs**

Research is needed in the following areas:

- The role and parameters of preoperative OSA treatment for perioperative safety outcomes in WLS
- Intra- and perioperative drug dosing, including prophylactic antibiotic tissue pharmacokinetic assessment
- Appropriate use of alpha-2 agonists in the perioperative care of WLS patients
- Strategies for intra- and postoperative glycemic management

- Impact of advanced monitoring of anesthetic effects on outcomes
- Evidence-based postoperative care guidelines for WLS patients with OSA
- Optimal anesthetic care for WLS patients with increased BMI, age, and quantity and severity of comorbidities
- Impact of an organized multidisciplinary care team on WLS safety outcomes
- Effect of surgical and overall care team pathways to decrease and/or treat perioperative anesthetic and surgical complications

## VI. Nursing Perioperative Care

A systematic review of MEDLINE, nursing journals, and the CINHAL database for nursing and allied health literature identified more than 54 papers; the most relevant were reviewed in detail. Recommendations are based on published evidence and the consensus of the Task Group members (58).

### A. Planning and Communication

Effective communication between all members of the health care team is paramount in the delivery of quality care. It requires sufficient time for the collection of information from patients, site verification in the operating room, timely and concise reporting of symptoms, and the "repeating back" of information exchanged between team members. To optimize communication, we recommend:

- Continued development of clinical pathways (Category D)
- An Advanced Practice Nurse or Clinical Bariatric Nurse Specialist on staff in WLS programs (Category D)
- Development and fostering of good communication skills between patients and practitioners and between members of the health care team (Category D)
- Promotion of collaboration between nurses, physical therapists, discharge planners, social workers, nutritionists, and facilitators of support groups (Category D)

### B. Perioperative Management

Unit-specific triage based on individual comorbidities can promote patient safety (Category D). We also recommend use of the Association of Perioperative Registered Nurses (AORN) Bariatric Surgery Guideline (Category D) and the American Society of Anesthesiologists Practice Guidelines for the Perioperative Management of Patients with Obstructive Sleep Apnea (Category C). Preferably, a dedicated operative team of nurses and surgical technicians should regularly assist in WLS procedures (Category D).

#### Preventing Complications

Risk of venous thromboembolic events (VTE) after gastric bypass is significant. Other postoperative complications include those associated with monitoring of fluid balance, hypoxemia, anastomatic leak, tachycardia, peripheral nerve injury, and risk of skin irritation, infection, ulceration in skinfolds, and decubitus ulcers. We recommend ambulation on the day of surgery, and deep breathing/coughing (Category D); careful positioning to decrease risk of peripheral nerve injury (Categories C and D); and education of emergency department staff on early and late complications in WLS patients (Category D).

#### Perianesthesia

Obese patients present with distinct respiratory care considerations. They should be closely monitored for rapid oxyhemoglobin desaturation and respiratory depression after extubation. Facilities should reference the AORN Bariatric Surgery Guideline (Category D) and educate staff on pulmonary pathophysiology in obese patients (Category D).

#### Postoperative analgesia

The goal of postoperative pain management is to promote participation in activity, ambulation, incentive spirometry, deep breathing, and coughing. Nursing staff should consult with a pharmacist on equianalgesic agents and dosing (Category D), and use multimodal, opioid-sparing strategies to keep patients comfortable (Category D).

### C. Patient and Staff Safety

WLS patients move through many areas of hospitals for tests and procedures. Facilities should review each area and its equipment to make certain they can accommodate extremely obese patients. The weight capacity of tables, beds, stretchers, and wheelchairs should be clearly marked (Categories C and D). A comprehensive ergonomics program, including lifting and transferring equipment, should be used to prevent patient handling injuries (Category B). A designated nurse or back injury resource nurse (BIRN) should coordinate equipment selection, maintenance, staff training, and reporting (Category D).

**D. Outpatient Postoperative Nursing Follow-up**

Dehydration, pulmonary embolisms, and anastomatic leaks are the serious conditions most likely to occur in the early discharge phase. Later complications can include hyperinsulinemic hypoglycemia, metabolic bone disease, problems with redundant skin, nutritional deficiencies, suboptimal weight loss, issues with psychosocial adjustment, and pregnancy.

Medications and vitamin supplements should be reviewed at each postoperative outpatient visit (Categories C and D). Nurses should be knowledgeable about possible late complications, know how to support patients, and be prepared to make referrals to appropriate caregivers (Category D). WLS patients should be encouraged to continue treatment through ongoing WLS support groups and networks (Categories A and D).

**E. Credentialing**

The American Society for Metabolic and Bariatric Surgery (ASMBS) has developed national certification criteria for Clinical Bariatric Nurse Specialists (CBN). We recommend certification (Category D).

**F. Future Research Needs**

Studies are needed in the following areas:

- Clinical pathways for WLS, including emergency departments
- Comprehensive ergonomics programs
- Teach-to-goal educational methods for pre- and postoperative education
- Program retention tools and outcome measures
- Nursing research and involvement in pediatric WLS programs

**VII. Informed Consent and Patient Education**

This Task Group's literature search identified 120 papers, 38 of which were reviewed in detail. No articles were specific to informed consent and WLS. Recommendations are extrapolated from, and supported by, existing data (59).

**A. Content**

**Risks/Complications**

Informed consent should include realistic risk estimates that take into account patient factors (Category C) and relevant institutional and health provider characteristics that might affect risk (e.g., experience and outcomes for specific WLS procedures) (Category B). Short- and long-term risks and complications, and the potential for unknown or unforeseeable long-term risks, should be discussed (Category D).

**Benefits/Effectiveness**

Patients should receive realistic estimates of short- and long-term weight loss, including the potential for weight regain and modest benefits (Category B). They should also be informed if long-term data ( > 5 years) are unavailable (Category D).

They should be advised of the long-term health benefits of weight loss produced by WLS (Category B), but also be made aware that not all pre-existing medical and psychosocial consequences of obesity (including eating disorders) will improve with WLS (Category C). Candidates for WLS should be given realistic estimates for health outcomes if they decline surgical treatment (Categories B and C), and be advised of known factors and interventions that might optimize benefits (Category D). Informed consent and education should consider patient expectations, the value placed on different outcomes, and the risks each candidate is willing to accept. It should also address unrealistic expectations or other misconceptions patients might have (Category C).

**Consequences**

Patients should be advised of required behavioral and dietary changes and other reasonable and foreseeable consequences of WLS that could affect health or quality of life in a substantive way, e.g., gastrointestinal symptoms, cosmetic effects, nutritional restrictions (Category D).

**B. Alternative treatments**

Patients should be advised about alternative WLS procedures and nonsurgical treatment options (e.g., medical and behavioral) (Category C). They should be informed about them even if they are not available through the consenting health provider or institution (Category C).

**C. Patient Comprehension**

Each patient should have their comprehension of the risks, benefits, consequences, and alternatives to WLS evaluated (Category C). Confirmation of comprehension should be included as a protection for patients engaged in the informed consent process (Category C).

**D. Future Research Needs**

Future research is needed to better identify factors that affect short- and long-term outcomes so that patients can be cited appropriate and individualized outcome information. Research should focus on important gaps in knowledge on outcomes and consequences of WLS, and the different approaches that facilitate patient understanding of, and decision-making about, WLS.

**VIII. Policy and Access (Coding and Reimbursement)**

The Policy and Access group identified 51 publications in its literature search; the 20 most relevant were examined in detail (60). These included reviews, cost-benefit analyses, and trend and cost studies from administrative databases.

**A. Policy and Access**

**Access disparities** (All Category D)

Public health policy should be aligned with long-term goals for the treatment of severe obesity. Barriers to WLS in populations with high prevalence of severe obesity should be identified and eliminated, and there should be uniform standards of coverage for all WLS candidates. We recommend advocacy for increased access to WLS for underserved regions and population groups; support for community-based efforts to fight health disparities; and public education about the obesity epidemic and the risks/benefits of WLS.

**Childhood obesity (Categories C and D)**

Sharp increases in childhood obesity lend urgency to the need to address the problem (Category C). Policy initiatives to identify pediatric and adolescent populations most likely to benefit from surgical treatment of obesity are needed. Surgical treatment should be considered a potentially effective option for appropriately selected individuals, and there should be uniform standards of coverage for adolescent patients. We need to educate legislators, community leaders, and other stakeholders on the costs and benefits of WLS for extremely obese adolescents, and leverage opportunities for collaboration between teachers, parents, and community leaders (Category D).

**Insurance policies ( Category A, B, C, and D)**

Controversial issues include required documentation of prior weight loss attempts through more conservative means; access to WLS for those with a BMI of 35 to 40 and obesity-related comorbidities; and proof of extreme obesity for at least 5 years. We recommend:

- Routine examination of weight loss histories during behavioral evaluation to determine whether additional attempts at nonsurgical weight loss are advisable
- Coverage of WLS for those with a BMI of 35 to 40 and comorbid conditions that require ongoing treatment (e.g., CPAP, medication)
- Research to characterize weight loss histories of surgical candidates, and explore the relation between dieting history and postoperative outcomes
- Ongoing collection and dissemination of data on WLS costs, risks, and benefits
- Collaborative efforts between government, industry, and other stakeholders to promote safe and effective delivery of

WLS

**Cost-effectiveness issues**

Obesity is linked to higher health care costs than smoking or drinking, and plays a major role in disability (Category B). Accurate short- and long-term cost savings (and risk/benefits) for employers and insurance companies need to be collected and disseminated. Clinical pathways that reduce unnecessary costs to providers should also be developed (Category D).

**Innovation, evidence-based medicine, and cost containment**

The application of standard cost-containment policies to surgical innovations may stifle new developments. We recommend the use of evidence-based medicine to both guide clinical decisions and show reasonable trends for health care cost containment (Category C).

**Legislation**

We need to keep legislators apprised of the personal and economic costs of obesity in the communities they serve. Dissemination of evidence-based information on the risks, benefits, and cost-effectiveness of WLS can bring these issues to their attention (Categories C and D).

**Stigma (All Category D)**

The highest BMI groups are the fastest growing and the most stigmatized. To address this problem, we recommend targeted education campaigns; community-level public information/education; and sensitivity training for hospital personnel. Hospitals should also acquire obese-appropriate products (e.g., gowns, chairs, commodes).

**B. Coding and Reimbursement**

**Centers for Medicare and Medicaid Services (CMS)**

CMS allows national coverage for Roux-en-Y gastric bypass (open and laparoscopic), laparoscopic adjustable gastric banding (LAGB), and biliopancreatic diversion with duodenal switch (BPD) (open and laparoscopic). Nationally covered procedures and new 2006 CPT codes are available.

**C. Potential Pathways to New Codes**

**Category III and S Codes**

CPT Category III Codes are a temporary set of tracking codes used to identify new and emerging technologies. CPT Category III codes (T codes) support data collection on new services and procedures. CPT Category III codes may be converted to CPT Category I codes if the FDA and CPT Editorial Panel approve the clinical efficacy of the particular service or procedure. Blue Cross/Blue Shield and other commercial payers have developed the category of S codes, which were added to HCPCS Level II to report drugs, services, and supplies. S codes are typically used in conjunction with a non- specific CPT code.

Medicare does not recognize or reimburse for services reported under S codes and may or may not reimburse for CPT Category III codes depending on the service or procedure. Individual commercial insurers may or may not reimburse for S codes or CPT Category III codes as medical policies and reimbursement polices are specific to each insurer.

**D. Issues and Recommendations**

**Alignment of reimbursement policies with clinical objectives**

Reimbursement policies should reflect the importance of comprehensive, multidisciplinary care. There should be full coverage for medical, nutritional, and psychological preoperative evaluation as well as pre-, peri-, and postoperative care required by insurers (Category D).

**CPT codes for WLS and related clinical services (All Category D)**

CPT codes for WLS should be updated to reflect current practice. New CPT Category I codes should be requested and approved as evidence accumulates in favor of new procedures (e.g., vertical sleeve gastrectomy, endoscopic interventions). T codes should be considered for evolving technologies, and procedures. The use of T codes may create a pathway for reimbursement by supporting consistent data collection and development of evidence. Evidence indicating that a promising technology or new procedure leads to improved health outcomes could support conversion of Category III codes to Category I codes. There should be support for the development of appropriate CPT codes for each component of multidisciplinary care (e.g., exercise therapy, pre- and postoperative support groups).

**Data collection, tracking, and reporting systems**

There are several national data collection, tracking, and reporting databases (see Data Collection) (62) as well as proprietary systems. We recommend standardized collection, tracking, and reporting of tiered and risk-adjusted data (Category D).

## IX. Specialized Facilities and Resources

The Specialized Facilities and Resources Task Group identified 1,647 papers in its literature search; the 46 most relevant were reviewed in detail (61). The literature in the area was very sparse. There were no randomized control trials or prospective or retrospective cohort studies. Most of the available literature was in the form of retrospective reviews, prior systematic reviews, and expert or consensus opinion.

### A. Personnel

All medical and support staff must be adequately trained and credentialed as specified in the following task group reports: Surgical Care (53), Anesthesia Perioperative Care and Pain Management (57), Behavioral and Psychological Care (55), and Nursing Care (58). A team of dedicated medical specialists—fully aware of the problems and sensitivities of patients with severe obesity—should be readily available, and all personnel (including ancillary and nonclinical staff) should have obesity-specific education focused on sensitivity training.

### B. Equipment

All facilities performing WLS, including pediatric WLS centers, require the same equipment. We strongly recommend that WLS centers have well-defined plans for the evaluation and treatment of post-WLS surgery patients with potential complications who cannot fit into available diagnostic equipment. Recommended equipment includes:

Ancillary

- Wide wheelchairs, stretchers, and walkers
- Wide BP cuffs
- Biphasic defibrillators
- Size-appropriate sequential compression devices
- Emergency airway equipment
- Wide examination tables bolted to the floor
- Scales of appropriate size and capacity

**Operating Room**

Specially-equipped operating room and ancillary equipment should be available to support patients with severe obesity, including:

- An automated extra-wide operating table with appropriate weight capacity
- Extra-long abdominal instrument sets
- Appropriately sized retractor
- 43- to 46-cm laparoscopes

**Radiology Equipment**

Special diagnostic and interventional equipment is required to support and accommodate WLS patients. Such equipment should include:

- CT scanners with 400 lb weight capacity
- MRI magnet with 400 lb weight capacity
- Fluoroscopic equipment with 300 lb capacity that can study patients in a standing position with high beam voltages
- Interventional facilities available 24 hours a day, 7 days a week

### C. Physical Plant

Size-appropriate facilities should be available in both post-anesthesia and intensive care units (ICUs); postoperatively, dedicated inpatient floors with specially trained personnel should be available. Patient rooms and elevators must have sufficiently wide entrances. Floor-mounted commodes are recommended, but support systems can be used as an alternative. Design of new facilities that will accommodate the WLS patient must comply with the American Institute of Architects Planning and Design Guidelines for Bariatric Healthcare Facilities (73).

### D. Extent of Facility Changes

WLS patients travel throughout hospitals for tests and procedures; there should be size-appropriate accommodations in all inpatient and outpatient points of service. These should include chairs and bathroom facilities, transferring equipment (stretchers and wheelchairs), and monitoring equipment.

### E. Investment

Specialized resources for WLS patients require a significant investment, the size of which depends on everything from geography to patient population. Capital investments are preferred for renovations to existing facilities, and strongly recommended for new construction. WLS centers with lower volume or storage space problems should consider renting equipment.

### F. Staff Injury Reduction

Health care consistently ranks among the top fields for back injuries. Well-established, agreed-upon, and well-known plans for transferring severely obese patients at all points of care can help reduce injuries. We also recommend that proper equipment, as well as training on how to use it, should be immediately available for the transfer of WLS patients. Staff should be well-educated in the use, location, and operation of available lift equipment. Portable equipment is more useful than ceiling lifts, but requires more room clearance. Trained and available on call "lift team" alternatives to equipment (as appropriate) should be considered.

### G. Medical Error Reduction

We recommend dedicated facilities and staff to reduce risk of medical errors, including a dedicated hospital administrator to provide consistent support and oversight. All medical staff should be adequately trained and credentialed in best practice care of WLS patients (53, 57, 58). A team of designated medical subspecialists, fully aware of the problems and sensitivities of extremely obese patients, should be readily available, and all personnel who interact with WLS patients should attend obesity-specific education programs focused on sensitivity training.

### H. Medication Error Reduction

Medication guidelines released by the Joint Commission on Healthcare Organizations (JCAHO) in 2004 (74) emphasize safety. We recommend that facilities follow these recommendations, as well as those specified in our prior report (61). We also recommend an Institutional Pharmacy and Therapeutics Committee to oversee WLS medical dosing regimens, and further research on medication use in the WLS patient.

### I. Systems Improvements

Clinical pathways are required by WLS accreditation programs, such as the American College of Surgeons Bariatric Surgery Center Network Accreditation Program (75) and American Society of Metabolic and Bariatric Surgery's Surgical Review Corporation (76). Clinical pathways specific to WLS patients should be established. These should be procedure-specific, updated frequently, and consistent with order sets. Regular meetings by the WLS team to review patient outcomes and address possible systems changes are essential, as is investment in a WLS database. The database should track patient outcomes and be compatible with the needs of the credentialing body that certifies the center. We recommend risk-adjusted outcomes to adequately evaluate performance.

## X. Data Collection (Registries)/Future Considerations

This Task Group identified 212 papers and reviewed the 63 most relevant in detail. Recommendations are based on available evidence as well as consensus of opinions from Task Group and Expert Panel members (62, 77).

### A. Administrative and Non-administrative Databases

Administrative databases have inherent problems, including unreliable coding and lack of WLS-specific data points. Clinical databases that are not WLS-specific have other shortcomings (e.g., short-term follow-up, sampling of WLS procedures), and single-institution, WLS-specific databases lack standardized definitions and appropriate quality benchmarks. Rather, we recommend collection of WLS-specific data (Categories B and D) on 100% of weight loss surgeries performed (Category D).

### B. New Developments

Longitudinal Assessment of Bariatric Surgery (LABS)

The NIH-funded Longitudinal Assessment of Bariatric Surgery (LABS) consortium has developed a database of standardized information on WLS patients at 6 clinical centers. Data are being collected on patient characteristics, surgical procedures, medical and psychosocial outcomes, and economic factors.

#### Accreditation programs

The Centers for Medicare and Medicaid Services (CMS) made a national decision to cover WLS surgery, but only if performed by institutions and surgeons that are accredited by either the American College of Surgeons (ACS) Bariatric Surgery Center Network or the American Society for Metabolic and Bariatric Surgery/Surgical Review Corporation (ASMBS/SRC) Centers of Excellence program. WLS-specific, longitudinal data collection systems are a major part of each of these accreditation programs. The optimal data collection system should gather information on all WLS procedures using a longitudinal, universal database system. It should be prospective, risk-adjusted, and benchmarked, with WLS-specific data points that track clinical effectiveness and complications following WLS (Categories B and D).

The ACS Bariatric Surgery Network Data Collection System, the Society of American Gastrointestinal Endoscopic Surgeons (SAGES) Bariatric Data Collection System, and the ASMBS/SRC system should meet these criteria. If these systems are not compatible (i.e., cannot agree on the same definitions), an interface should be developed that makes them so (Category D).

### C. Areas That Need More Data

#### Risk adjustment

Risk adjustment helps control for differences in patient risk factors and case mix. Appropriate risk adjustment models should be developed and refined over time to account for these variables (Categories C and D).

#### Determining the best data collector

Data entered into the system must be of the highest quality to ensure accurate analyses on quality of care. To avoid bias, data should be collected by audited, trained data collectors not directly involved in patient care (Categories B and C). That data, in turn, should be analyzed to see if information collected by audited, trained non-nurse reviewers is as valid as that collected by nurse reviewers (Category D).

#### Defining data points

High inter-rater reliability requires data points that are clinically relevant, objective, and easy to identify. Data points, definitions, and systems training programs should be developed that optimize clinical relevance and minimize subjectivity, and in so doing, maximize inter-rater reliability (Categories C and D).

#### Quality indicators and benchmarking capabilities

Definitions of quality and benchmark indicators of progress can be difficult to develop. To advance patient safety, quality indicators and metrics should be appropriate and actionable (Category D).

#### Outliers

Accurate determination of what constitutes an outlier, or bad performer, can have a direct effect on patient safety and access to WLS. Responsible analysis of data and careful definition of outliers is essential to improve quality of care. The means to regularly report that data to stakeholders should be determined (Categories C and D). Poor performers, or high outliers, should be identified, and a mechanism for corrective action developed (Category D).

**Novel therapies**

Safe introduction of novel technologies and assessment of the appropriateness of those procedures in new patient populations are critical for patient safety. Novel and experimental therapies, new patient populations, and expanded indications for WLS should be carefully studied through comprehensive data collection and analysis (Category D). Experimental therapies should be performed with IRB approval, and data collected and audited by a data monitoring board to assess clinical effectiveness and patient safety (Category D).

**Cost-effectiveness and utility analyses**

There is a critical need for well-designed prospective studies that evaluate the cost-effectiveness, cost utility, return on investment, and economic impact of WLS. Cost utility studies should be carried out to guide decision making on the appropriate allocation of resources (Category D).

**State coalition**

We propose the development of a statewide coalition to collectively gather and share data, and determine quality indicators and processes of care that could lead to best practices in WLS (Categories C and D).

## XI. Endoscopic Interventions

This Task Group's literature search identified 18 related articles, all of which were reviewed in detail. All of our recommendations are based on expert opinion (63).

### A. Overview

Endoscopic interventions may provide valuable approaches to the management of WLS complications, and should be a high priority for development and investigation. Similarly, endoscopic interventions, endoscopically-placed devices, and other minimally-invasive, image-guided techniques may also provide valuable approaches to the primary management of obesity; they too should be a high priority for development and investigation (Category D).

### B. Experimental Status

Until formally approved by appropriate regulatory bodies, novel endoscopic interventions and endoscopically-placed devices should only be used in the setting of IRB-approved clinical trials (Category D).

### C. Credentials

Treatment with endoscopic and other image-guided interventions should be performed only by clinicians with specialized training and expertise in their effective and appropriate use (Category D).

### D. Clinical Application

As is the standard for other medical and surgical therapies for obesity, endoscopic interventions should be studied and used only in the context of comprehensive patient evaluation and treatment that reflects the complex medical, nutritional, and behavioral contributors to obesity.

### E. Risks and Benefits

As new technologies become available, choice among therapeutic options for obesity should be determined by the comparative risk-benefit profiles of each modality. These considerations should be matched to the specific clinical characteristics, needs, and treatment goals of each patient (Category D).

### F. Data Collection

To facilitate tracking of utilization, adverse events, and comparative outcomes, all patients who undergo endoscopic and other minimally-invasive interventions for obesity and its complications should be entered into a standard registry. Methods of tracking should be compatible with those used for patients undergoing WLS (Category D).

### G. Coding and Reimbursement

As new devices and minimally-invasive surgical therapies for obesity and its complications are approved for clinical use, a new category of provisional billing codes should be established for these interventions. Reimbursement for novel therapies for obesity should be determined on the basis of scientific evidence of their safety and efficacy (Category D).

**H. Future Research**

Randomized, blinded, sham-controlled clinical trials should be the standard for investigation of the safety and efficacy of endoscopic interventions for the treatment of obesity and its complications (Category D).

**Bibliography**


1. Bray G. The missing link — lose weight, live longer. N Engl J Med 2007;357:818-820.
2. Dixon J. Survival advantage with bariatric surgery: Report from the 10th International Congress on Obesity. Surg Obes Relat Dis 2006;2:585-6.
3. Maggard MA, McGory ML, Shekelle PG, Ko CY. Quality indicators in bariatric surgery: improving quality of care. Surg Obes Relat Dis 2006;2:423-9.
4. Sjöström L, Narbro K, Sjöström D, et al. Effects of bariatric surgery on mortality in Swedish obese subjects. N Engl J Med 2007;357:741-52.
5. Adams TD, Gress RE, Smith SC, et al. Long-term mortality after gastric bypass surgery. N Engl J Med 2007;357:753-61.
6. Favretti F, Segato G, Ashton D, et al. Laparoscopic adjustable gastric banding in 1,791 consecutive obese patients: 12-year results. Obes Surg 2007;17:168-75.
7. Perry CD, Hutter MM, Smith DB, Newhouse JP, McNeil BJ. Survival and changes in comorbidities following bariatric surgery. Ann Surg 2007:in press.
8. Sowemimo OA, Yood SM, Courtney J, et al. Natural history of morbid obesity without surgical intervention. Surg Obes Relat Dis 2007;3:73-77.
9. Christou NV, Sampalis JS, Liberman M, et al. Surgery decreases long-term mortality, morbidity, and health care use in morbidly obese patients. Ann Surg 2004;240:416-23.
10. Flum DR, Dellinger EP. Impact of gastric bypass operation on survival: a population-based analysis. J Am Coll Surg 2004;199:543-51.
11. Kral JG. Studies show reduction in mortality after bariatric surgery. Surg Obes Relat Dis 2006;2:564.
12. McMahon MM, Sarr MG, Clark MM, et al. Clinical management after bariatric surgery: value of a multidisciplinary approach. Mayo Clin Proc 2006;81(10 Suppl):S34-45.
13. Clark MM, Balsiger BM, Sletten CD, et al. Psychosocial factors and 2-year outcome following bariatric surgery for weight loss. Obes Surg 2003;13:739-45.
14. Sarwer DB, Wadden TA, Fabricatore AN. Psychosocial and behavioral aspects of bariatric surgery. Obes Res 2005;13:639-648.
15. Herpertz S, Kielmann R, Wolf AM, Langkafel M, Senf W, Hebebrand J. Does obesity surgery improve psychosocial functioning? A systematic review. Int J Obes Relat Metab Disord 2003;27:1300-14.
16. Arcila D, Velázquez D, Gamino R, et al. Quality of life in bariatric surgery. Obes Surg 2002;12:661-5.
17. Kolotkin RL, Crosby RD, Pendleton R, Strong M, Gress RE, Adams T. Health-related quality of life in patients seeking gastric bypass surgery vs non-treatment-seeking controls. Obes Surg 2003;13:371-7.
18. Elkins G, Whitfield P, Marcus J, Symmonds R, Rodriguez J, Cook T. Noncompliance with behavioral recommendations following bariatric surgery. Obes Surg 2005;15:546-51.
19. Collazo-Clavell ML, Clark MM, McAlpine DE, Jensen MD. Assessment and preparation of patients for bariatric surgery. Mayo Clin Proc 2006 81(10 Suppl):S11-7.
20. Belle SH, Berk PD, Courcoulas AP, et al. Safety and efficacy of bariatric surgery: Longitudinal Assessment of Bariatric Surgery. Surg Obes Relat Dis 2007;3:116-26.

21. Kendrick ML, Dakin GF. Surgical approaches to obesity. Mayo Clin Proc 2006;81(10 Suppl):S18-24.

22. Lehman Center Weight Loss Surgery Expert Panel. Commonwealth of Massachusetts. Betsy Lehman Center for Patient Safety and Medical Error Reduction. Expert Panel on Weight Loss Surgery: Executive Report. Obes Res 2005;13:206-26.

23. Rand Corporation. Research Briefs. Obesity and Disability: The Shape of Things to Come. http://www.rand.org/pubs/research_briefs/RB9043-1/. 2007. Accessed June 9, 2007.

24. Desjardins E, Schwartz AL. Collaborating to combat childhood obesity. Health Aff (Millwood) 2007;26:567-71.

25. Sturm R. Increases in morbid obesity in the USA: 2000-2005. Public Health 2007;121:492-6.

26. Haslam DW, James WP. Obesity. Lancet 2005;366:1197-209.

27. Li Z, Bowerman S, Heber D. Health ramifications of the obesity epidemic. Surg Clin North Am 2005;85:681-701.

28. Finkelstein EA, Fiebelkorn IC, Wang G. National medical spending attributable to overweight and obesity: how much, and who's paying? Health Aff (Millwood) 2003;W3:219-226.

29. Economic Consequences. Centers for Disease Control and Prevention. http://www.cdc.gov/nccdphp/dnpa/obesity/economic_consequences.htm 2007. Accessed June 9, 2007.

30. Mokdad AH, Marks JS, Stroup DF, Gerberding JL. Actual causes of death in the United States, 2000. JAMA 2004;29:1238-45. [Erratum in: JAMA. 2005 293:293-4. JAMA. 2005 293:298].

31. Olshansky SJ, Passaro DJ, Hershow RC, et al. A potential decline in life expectancy in the United States in the 21st century. N Engl J Med 2005;352:1138-45.

32. de Fatima Haueisen Sander Diniz M, de Azeredo Passos VM, Diniz MT. Gut-brain communication: how does it stand after bariatric surgery? Curr Opin Clin Nutr Metab Care 2006;9:629-36.

33. Samuel I, Mason EE, Renquist KE, Huang YH, Zimmerman MB, Jamal M. Bariatric surgery trends: an 18-year report from the International Bariatric Surgery Registry. Am J Surg 2006;192:657-62.

34. Elder KA, Wolfe BM. Bariatric surgery: a review of procedures and outcomes. Gastroenterology. 2007 32:2253-71.

35. DeMaria EJ. Bariatric surgery for morbid obesity. N Engl J Med 2007;356:2176-83.

36. Zhao Y, Encinosa W. Bariatric Surgery Utilization and Outcomes in 1998 and 2004. Statistical Brief #23. Rockville, MD: Agency for Healthcare Research and Quality, January 2007.

37. Kim TH, Daud A, Ude AO, et al. Early U.S. outcomes of laparoscopic gastric bypass versus laparoscopic adjustable silicone gastric banding for morbid obesity. Surg Endosc 2006;20:202-9.

38. Smoot TM, Xu P, Hilsenrath P, Kuppersmith NC, Singh KP. Gastric bypass surgery in the United States, 1998-2002. Am J Public Health 2006;96:1187-9.

39. Wolfe BM, Morton JM. Weighing in on bariatric surgery: procedure use, readmission rates, and mortality. JAMA 2005;294:1960-3.

40. le Roux CW, Aylwin SJ, Batterham RL, et al. Gut hormone profiles following bariatric surgery favor an anorectic state, facilitate weight loss, and improve metabolic parameters. Ann Surg 2006;243:108-14.

41. Peluso L, Vanek VW. Efficacy of gastric bypass in the treatment of obesity-related comorbidities. Nutr Clin Pract 2007;22:22-8.

42. Parikh MS, Laker S, Weiner M, Hajiseyedjavadi O, Ren CJ. Objective comparison of complications resulting from laparoscopic bariatric procedures. J Am Coll Surg 2006;202:252-61.

43. Chapman AE, Kiroff G, Game P, et al. Laparoscopic adjustable gastric banding in the treatment of obesity: a systematic literature review. Surgery 2004;135:326-51.

44. Olbers T, Fagevik-Olsen M, Maleckas A, Lonroth H. Randomized clinical trial of laparoscopic Roux-en-Y gastric bypass versus laparoscopic vertical banded gastroplasty for obesity. Br J Surg 2005;92:557-62.

45. Scopinaro N, Gianetta E, Civalleri D, Bonalumi U, Bachi V. Bilio-pancreatic bypass for obesity: II. Initial experience in man. Br J Surg 1979;66:618-20.

46. Kotidis EV, Koliakos G, Papavramidis TS, Papavramidis ST. The effect of biliopancreatic diversion with pylorus-preserving sleeve gastrectomy and duodenal switch on fasting serum ghrelin, leptin and adiponectin levels: is there a hormonal contribution to the weight-reducing effect of this procedure? Obes Surg 2006;16:554-9.

47. Cottam D, Qureshi FG, Mattar SG, et al. Laparoscopic sleeve gastrectomy as an initial weight loss procedure for high-risk patients with morbid obesity. Surg Endosc 2006;20:859-63.

48. Roa PE, Kaidar-Person O, Pinto D, Cho M, Szomstein S, Rosenthal RJ. Laparoscopic sleeve gastrectomy as treatment for morbid obesity: technique and short-term outcome. Obes Surg 2006;16:1323-6.

49. Silecchia G, Boru C, Pecchia A, et al. Effectiveness of laparoscopic sleeve gastrectomy (first stage of biliopancreatic diversion with duodenal switch) on co-morbidities in super-obese high-risk patients. Obes Surg 2006;16:1138-44.

50. Mognol P, Chosidow D, Marmuse JP. Laparoscopic sleeve gastrectomy (LSG): review of a new bariatric procedure and initial results. Surg Technol Int 2006;15:47-52.

51. Melissas J, Koukouraki S, Askoxylakis J, et al. Sleeve gastrectomy: a restrictive procedure? Obes Surg. 2007;17:57-62.

52. Langer FB, Reza H, M.A., Bohdjalian A, et al. Sleeve gastrectomy and gastric banding: effects on plasma ghrelin levels. Obes Surg 2005;15:1024-9.

53. Kelly J, Shikora S, Jones DB, et al. Best practice updates for surgical care in weight loss surgery. Obes 2007:in press.

54. Apovian CM, Cummings S, Anderson W, et al. Best practice updates for multidisciplinary care in weight loss surgery. Obes 2007:in press.

55. Greenberg I, Sogg S, Perna F. Behavioral and psychological care in weight loss surgery -- best practice update. Obes 2007:in press.

56. Pratt J, Lenders CM, Dionne E, et al. Best practice updates for pediatric/adolescent weight loss surgery. Obes 2007:in press.

57. Schumann R, Jones SB, Cooper B, et al. Update on best practice recommendations for anesthetic preioperative care and pain management in weight loss surgery, 2004 - 2007. Obes 2007:in press.

58. Mulligan A, McNamara A, Boulton H, Trainor L, Raiano C, Mullen A. Best practice updates for nursing care in weight loss surgery. Obes 2007:in press.

59. Wee CC, Pratt J, Fanelli R, Samour P, Trainor L, Paasche-Orlow M. Best practice updates for informed consent and patient education in weight loss surgery. Obes 2007:in press.

60. Shikora SA, Kuger RS, Jr., Blackburn GL, et al. Best practices in policy and access for weight loss surgery. Obes 2007:in press.

61. Lautz DB, Jiser ME, Kelly J, et al. An update on best practice guidelines for specialized facilities and resources necessary for bariatric surgical programs. Obes 2007:in press.

62. Hutter MM, Jones DB, Riley S, et al. Best practice updates for weight loss surgery data collection. Obes 2007:in press.

63. Kaplan LM, Thompson CC, Brugge WR, et al. Best practices in endoscopic intervention for weight loss surgery. Obes 2007:in press.

64. Trus TL, Pope GD, Finlayson SR. National trends in utilization and outcomes of bariatric surgery. Surg Endosc 2005;19:616-20.

65. Galvani C, Gorodner M, Moser F, et al. Laparoscopic adjustable gastric band versus laparoscopic Roux-en-Y gastric bypass: ends justify the means? Surg Endosc 2006;20:934-41.

66. DeMaria EJ, Jamal MK. Laparoscopic adjustable gastric banding: evolving clinical experience. Surg Clin North Am 2005;85:773-87.

67. Suter M, Giusti V, Worreth M, Heraief E, Calmes JM. Laparoscopic gastric banding: a prospective, randomized study comparing the Lapband and the SAGB: early results. Ann Surg 2005;241:55-62.

68. Suter M, Calmes JM, Paroz A, Giusti V. A 10-year experience with laparoscopic gastric banding for morbid obesity: high long-term complication and failure rates. Obes Surg 2006;16:829-35.

69. Kelly J, Tarnoff M, Shikora S, et al. Best practice recommendations for surgical care in weight loss surgery. Obes Res 2005;13:227-33.

70. Schirmer BD, Schauer PR, Flum DR, Ellsmere J, Jones DB. Bariatric surgery training: getting your ticket punched. J Gastrointest Surg 2007;11:807-12.

71. Lautz DB, Jackson TD, Clancy KA, et al. Bariatric operations in Veterans Affairs and selected university medical centers: results of the patient safety in surgery study. J Am Coll Surg 2007;204:1261-72.

72. American Society for Metabolic and Bariatric Surgery. 2007. http://www.asbs.org/. Accessed August 23, 2007.

73. Andrade SD. Planning and Design Guidelines for Bariatric Healthcare Facilities. American Institute of Architects. AIA Academy Journal. 2006. http://www.aia.org/journal_aah.cfm?pagename=aah_jrnl_20061018_award_winner&dspl=1&article=article. Accessed August 6, 2007.

74. Rich DS. New JCAHO medication standards for 2004. Am J Health-Syst Pharm 2004;61:1349-1358.

75. ACS Division of Research and Optimal Patient Care. American College of Surgeons Bariatric Surgery Center Network (BSCN) Accreditation Program Manual. American College of Surgeons. http://facs.org/index.html. Accessed August 23, 2007.

76. Pratt GM, McLees B, Pories WJ. The ASMBS Bariatric Surgery Centers of Excellence program: a blueprint for quality improvement. Surg Obes Relat Dis. 2006 Sep-Oct;2(5):497-503; discussion 503.

77. Lehman Center Weight Loss Surgery Expert Panel. Commonwealth of Massachusetts. Betsy Lehman Center for Patient Safety and Medical Error Reduction. Expert Panel on Weight Loss Surgery: Executive Report. Obes 2007:in press.

# Appendix 2

## The American College of Surgeons **Bariatric Surgery Center Network:** Establishing standards

by **Bruce Schirmer, MD, FACS,** Charlottesville, VA;
and **Daniel B. Jones, MD, FACS,** Boston, MA

Patient demand for bariatric surgical services has been exponential, but meeting that demand has not kept pace with the epidemic of obesity (see Figure 1, page 22).[1] Obesity is defined as a body mass index (BMI) greater than 30 kg/m$^2$, and weight loss surgery is reserved for patients with comorbid conditions and a BMI greater than 35 or a BMI of 40 alone. Severe obesity is defined as having a BMI ≥ 40. In 2003, more than 110,000 bariatric operations were performed in the U.S.[2] With estimates of 11.5 million patients meeting medical necessity for weight-loss surgery, millions of potential patients may not have access to care.[3] Without weight-loss surgery, severe obesity treated by diet and exercise carries its own high mortality.[4-6]

In response to the epidemic of obesity, many surgeons are adding weight-loss surgery (see Figures 2 and 3, page 23) to their practices and bariatric centers are emerging to meet the demand for this operation, for which there are long waiting lists. Societies, licensing boards, and governmental agencies have published guidelines to standardize care and encourage hospital investment in its infrastructure for their patients of size. The Betsy Lehman Center for Patient Safety and Medical Error Reduction convened an expert panel in Massachusetts to establish best practices for weight loss surgery (*www.mass.gov/dph/betsylehman/panel_summary.htm*).[2] The American Society for Bariatric Surgery (ASBS) recognized the importance of establishing "centers of excellence" and established a program for accreditation of surgeons and facilities based on volumes, personnel, and infrastructure.[7] The ASBS endorsed a not-for-profit corporation with a board representing surgeons, industry, and insurance providers to oversee the new corporation. Site visits are conducted by nurses. The best programs would be recognized based on initial criteria of hospital volume and surgeon experience. Lower-volume hospitals could not meet the centers of excellence criteria.

The American College of Surgeons had already recognized the importance of surgeons accrediting surgeons. The ACS had established the Hospital Standards Committee, which became the Joint Commission on Accreditation of Healthcare Organizations (now called The Joint Commission) in 1951. Later the ACS established the accreditation of trauma centers and cancer centers. The ACS established a Bariatric Surgery Center Network (BSCN) Advisory Committee in 2003 to set criteria for accreditation of bariatric surgery centers using the already existing programs for trauma and cancer centers as suggested templates. Key concepts were that surgeons alone, and not industry or nonsurgeons, needed to have oversight of the accreditation process; the professional society—not a separate corporation—should oversee the process; and although institutions, facilities, and programs needed rigorous accreditation, surgeon expertise would be better assessed by local hospital credentialing systems already in existence. The goal was to be inclusive and to use best-practice guidelines to improve patient safety across programs. Central to the goal of the ACS was a database that could be verified, to ensure patient outcomes did not deviate from risk-adjusted benchmarks. Maintenance of accreditation would be based on meeting these benchmarks.

The American College of Surgeons Board of Regents formally approved the BSCN to accredit hospitals in 2005. The standards established for the American College of Surgeons BSCN Accreditation Program delineate four levels for accreditation of inpatient facilities—identified as levels 1a, 1b, 2a, and 2b—and outpatient surgical care facilities, identified as "outpatient."

High-quality surgical care requires documentation of reliable outcome measurements. Level 1a and 2a centers will use the ACS National Surgical Quality Improvement Program (ACS NSQIP) adapted for bariatric surgery, requiring a trained surgical clinical nurse reviewer to collect and submit the required ACS NSQIP data. These centers will have access to benchmark reports containing national aggregate data and individual facility data to assess patterns of care and outcomes relative to national norms. Level 1b, 2b, 2-new, outpatient facilities, and outpatient-new will report outcomes data to the ACS bariatric surgery database for accreditation purposes only. A designated and trained nonsurgeon of the bariatric surgery team will enter the data using the ACS' established protocol. All centers must capture 100 percent of bariatric cases in their data collection.

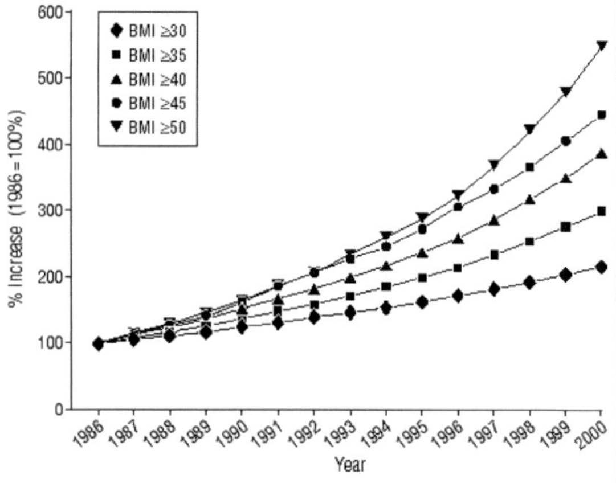


Figure 1. Prevalence of morbid obesity in the U.S. by body mass index.[1]

### *Level 1a and 1b centers*

Level 1 centers will provide complete care, with resources devoted to bariatric surgery. These hospitals can manage the most challenging and complex patients with optimal opportunity for safe and effective outcomes. These centers will engage all levels of obesity and standards of care for weight loss operations, ages, comorbid conditions, and reoperations. They will have high-volume practices of 125 or more weight-loss operations annually, with at least two credentialed and experienced bariatric surgeons, each performing a minimum of 100 weight-loss operations in the previous 24 months. These centers may apply for level 1 accreditation after providing bariatric surgery services for more than one year.

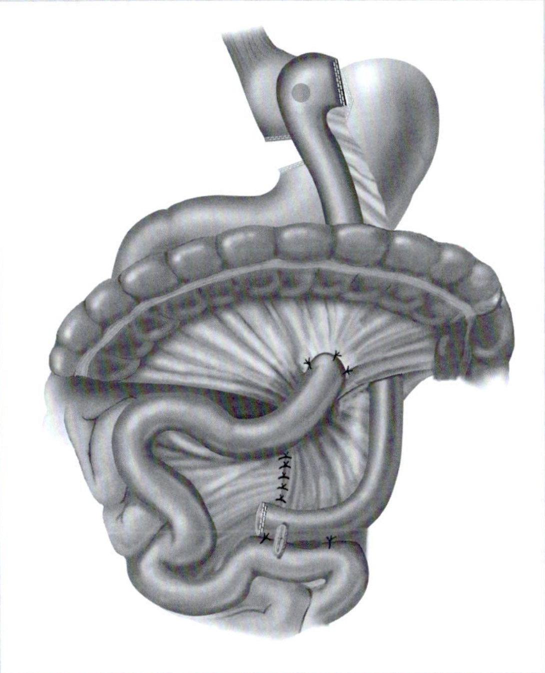

Figure 2. Laparoscopic gastric bypass.

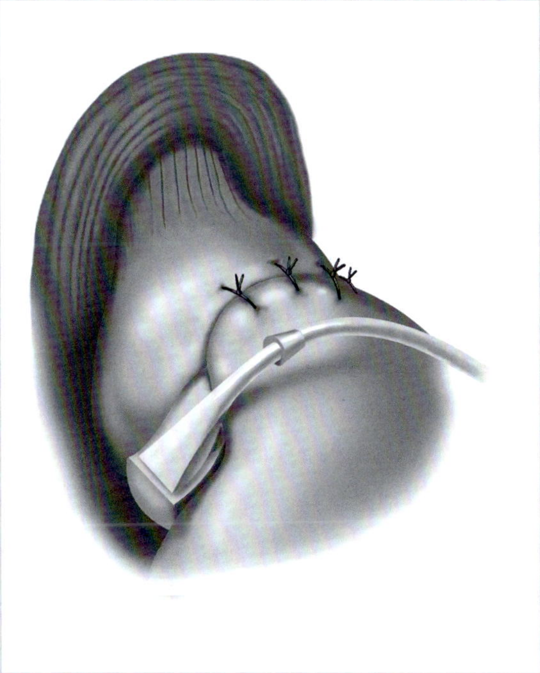

Figure 3. Laparoscopic adjustable gastric band.

Source: Jones DB, Maithel SK, Schneider BE. *Atlas of Minimally Invasive Surgery.* Woodbury, CT: Ciné-Med, Inc.; 2006. Used with permission.

***Level 2a and 2b centers***

Recognizing that high-quality surgical care occurs in centers that don't have a high volume of cases, the ACS will designate certain facilities as level 2 centers. These centers will provide high-quality care to a lower volume of patients—25 or more weight-loss operations annually, with one or more credentialed and experienced bariatric surgeon performing a minimum of 50 weight-loss operations in the previous 24 months. Level 2 bariatric surgery centers are not approved for operations on high-risk patients, such as men with a BMI of 55 or higher, women with a BMI of 60 or greater, or any nonambulatory patients or elective revisional operations. These centers may apply for level 2 accreditation after providing bariatric surgery services for more than one year.

In February 2006, the Centers for Medicare & Medicaid Services (CMS) tied reimbursement for bariatric surgery to already-existing patient-qualification criteria in addition to the requirement that the center be approved as a level 1 ACS center or ASBS-accredited program. In Massachusetts, Blue Cross Blue Shield broadened reimbursement to include ACS level 2a centers reporting excellent patient outcomes. It is hoped that CMS will eventually amend its decision and provide reimbursement for level 2 centers as well.

***Outpatient centers***

Outpatient centers will provide the application and adjustment of laparoscopic gastric bands. These centers will perform 50 or more weight-loss operations annually, with at least one

*continued on page 26*

# ACS-accredited bariatric centers

## Level 1 centers

**Alabama**
University of Alabama at Birmingham Hospital, Birmingham, AL (Level 1a)
Effective 12/7/06–12/7/09

**California**
Community Medical Center–Clovis, Clovis (Level 1b)
Effective 6/26/06–6/26/09

Cedars-Sinai Medical Center, Los Angeles (Level 1a)
Effective 6/20/06–6/20/09

**Connecticut**
Danbury Hospital, Danbury (Level 1a)
Effective 5/5/06–5/5/09

**Florida**
Cleveland Clinic Florida, Weston (Level 1a)
Effective 10/19/06–10/19/09

**Illinois**
Evanston Northwestern Hospital, Evanston (Level 1b)
Effective 1/26/06–1/26/09

**Iowa**
Grinnell Regional Medical Center, Grinnell (Level 1a)
Effective 10/19/06–10/19/09

**Michigan**
Hurley Medical Center, Flint (Level 1b)
Effective 4/14/06–4/14/09

**Minnesota**
Mayo Clinic–St. Mary's Hospital, Rochester (Level 1a)
Effective 10/23/06–10/23/09

**Massachusetts**
Beth Israel Deaconess Medical Center, Boston (Level 1a)
Effective 2/17/06–2/17/09

Brigham and Women's Hospital, Boston (Level 1a)
Effective 8/14/06–8/14/09

Boston Medical Center, Boston (Level 1b)
Effective 12/19/06–12/19/09

Massachusetts General Hospital, Boston (Level 1a)
Effective 10/23/06–10/23/09

Newton-Wellesley Hospital, Newton (Level 1a)
Effective 10/26/06–10/26/09

UMass Memorial Medical Center–Memorial Campus, Worcester (Level 1b)
Effective 7/27/06–7/27/09

**New Jersey**
Hackensack University Medical Center, Hackensack (Level 1a)
Effective 12/8/06–12/8/09

Morristown Memorial Hospital, Morristown (Level 1a)
Effective 1/25/07–1/25/10

**New York**
Albany Medical Center, Albany (Level 1b)
Effective 6/2/06–6/2/09

Lutheran Medical Center, Brooklyn (Level 1b)
Effective 11/8/05–11/8/08

New York-Presbyterian Hospital/Columbia University Medical Center, New York (Level 1a)
Effective 6/14/06–6/14/09

New York-Presbyterian Hospital/Weill Cornell Medical Center, New York (Level 1a)
Effective 8/4/06–8/4/09

St. Luke's-Roosevelt Hospital Center, New York (Level 1b)
Effective 10/11/06–10/11/09

Highland Hospital, Rochester (Level 1b)
Effective 8/30/06–8/30/09

**Ohio**
Cleveland Clinic, Cleveland (Level 1a)
Effective 12/1/06–12/1/09

**Oklahoma**
Saint Francis Hospital, Tulsa (Level 1b)
Effective 10/23/06–10/23/09

**Oregon**
Oregon Health & Science University, Portland (Level 1a)
Effective 6/27/06–6/27/09

**Pennsylvania**
Geisinger Medical Center, Danville (Level 1a)
Effective 1/26/07–1/26/10

Western Pennsylvania Hospital, Pittsburgh (Level 1b)
Effective 10/16/06–10/16/09

**Vermont**
Fletcher Allen Health Care, Burlington (Level 1b)
Effective 6/9/06–6/9/09

**Virginia**
University of Virginia Health System, Charlottesville (Level 1a)
Effective 7/12/06–7/12/09

Sentara Norfolk General Hospital, Norfolk (Level 1a)
Effective 9/29/06–9/29/09

**Washington**
University of Washington Medical Center, Seattle (Level 1a)
Effective 12/5/06–12/5/09

**Wisconsin**
Theda Clark Medical Center, Neenah (Level 1b)
Effective 1/27/06–1/27/09

## Level 2 centers

**Maryland**
Harford Memorial Hospital, Havre de Grace (Level 2b)
Effective 12/21/06–12/21/09

## Outpatient centers

**Texas**
Surgery Center of Richardson, Richardson
Effective 6/21/06–6/21/09

## ACS Bariatric Surgery Center Network Advisory Committee

CHAIR: Bruce Schirmer, MD, FACS, *Charlottesville, VA*
John Alverdy, MD, FACS, *Chicago, IL*
J. Kenneth Champion, MD, FACS, *Marietta, GA*
Edward Felix, MD, FACS, *Fresno, CA*
David Flum, MD, MPH, FACS, *Seattle, WA*
Matthew Hutter, MD, MPH, FACS, *Boston, MA*
Daniel B. Jones, MD, FACS, *Boston, MA*
David Lautz, MD, FACS, *Boston, MA*
Edward Mason, MD, FACS, *Iowa City, IA*
Ninh Nguyen, MD, FACS, *Orange, CA*
J. Patrick O'Leary, MD, FACS, *New Orleans, LA*
C. Daniel Smith, MD, FACS, *Jacksonville, FL*

STAFF:
R. Scott Jones, MD, FACS, *Charlottesville, VA*
Clifford Y. Ko, MD, MPH, FACS, *Los Angeles, CA*
Karen Richards, Administrative Director, *Chicago, IL*
Bianca D. Reyes, BSCN Program Coordinator, *Chicago, IL*
Jane Han, Accreditation Program Coordinator, *Chicago, IL*

credentialed and experienced bariatric surgeon performing a minimum of 50 primary weight-loss operations annually. These facilities must provide bariatric surgery services for more than one year before applying for outpatient accreditation.

***Level 2-new centers***

At an ACS BSCN Advisory Committee meeting in November 2006, committee members approved an additional level of accreditation, level 2-new, for more recently established centers. New programs can apply for accreditation as a level 2-new center without having to provide bariatric services for more than one year, but 25 weight-loss operations within the last 24 months are required. New centers submit outcomes quarterly and can apply for level 1 status after one year with adequate facility and surgeon volumes and all other level 1 standards having been met.

***Outpatient-new centers***

At its meeting in April 2007, the committee approved an additional level of accreditation for newly established outpatient facilities. An outpatient-new center may apply for accreditation after performing a minimum of 25 laparoscopic gastric bands. The program must meet all standards for outpatient facilities with the exception of time and volume requirements. After one year of accreditation, these centers may convert to outpatient center status.

***Grandfather clause***

The ACS BSCN program understands that established bariatric surgeons will relocate, and as such, surgeons with 300 lifetime cases will be considered bariatric surgeons for accreditation purposes. Moreover, fellows completing a formal minimally invasive surgery/bariatric fellowship should be credited for cases performed during fellowship training upon entering practice. However, such cases are not applicable to an institution other than the training center. Certification in fundamentals of laparoscopic surgery is recommended for newly trained laparoscopic surgeons.

***The ACS bariatric surgery database***

Level 1b, level 2b, and outpatient bariatric surgery centers will report their outcomes data to the ACS bariatric surgery database using a Web-based data-entry system. A designated trained nurse or other nonsurgeon of the bariatric surgery service will enter the data using the established protocol. The entered data will be subjected to quality control. The data will be entered into the database encrypted and deidentified to protect the confidentiality of the patients, the hospital, the outpatient facility, and the surgeons. When the hospital or outpatient facility receives the data reports, staff can identify the patients and surgeons. The hospitals and outpatient facilities will receive annual data reports. Center verification visits will include audits of the data, which include chart reviews. These data do not have the same rigor as ACS NSQIP and are not risk adjusted; furthermore, they will not be used to make comparisons or for research because of the lack of rigor. These data will only provide a center's outcomes to the ACS for accreditation.

***Data monitoring***

- *Level 1a and 2a centers*

Level 1a and 2a centers, which are ACS NSQIP participants, can monitor their data on a 24/7/365 basis using the ACS NSQIP Web site. They can compare their data with the average of the other centers in the program. These centers will receive a semi-annual report of their risk-adjusted outcomes in confidential ranking with other center programs. These data will also undergo confidential review by the ACS NSQIP Advisory Committee and the ACS BSCN Advisory Committee. If these reviews reveal trends or variances of concern, the concerns will be communicated to the hospital chief executive officer (CEO), the surgeon director, and the program coordinator. Each ACS NSQIP Center will have interrater reliability visits from a trained, experienced surgical clinical nurse reviewer. This process involves a medical record review to assess the reliability of the submitted data and the variability of data collection and submission.

- *Level 1b, 2b, and outpatient facilities*

Level 1b, 2b, and outpatient facilities are participants in the ACS BSCN database. The hospital CEO, the bariatric surgery director, and the bariatric surgery coordinator will receive a report of their non-risk-adjusted outcome data annually. The ACS BSCN Advisory Committee will review each hospital's deidentified data annually. If these reviews reveal trends or variances of concern, the concerns will be communicated in a special report to the hospital CEO, the bariatric surgery director, and the bariatric surgery coordinator.

### *Finding out more*

To learn more about the necessary physical resources, human resources, clinical standards, surgeon standards, data-reporting standards, and verification/approvals processes required for the designation of American College of Surgeons bariatric surgery centers, log on to the ACS Web site, *www.facs.org,* and click on the link to the program in the left-hand column of the home page. Applications can be downloaded. At the time of application submission, established centers that have been in operation for more than two years will be asked to provide data for the previous two years. Facilities that have been in operation for less than two years will be asked to provide all their data. The applying center's outcomes data are to be reported at 30 days postoperatively or in-house acute care. After successful review of an application, a site visit is scheduled. The committee reviews findings and accreditation is posted. For further inquires, contact the ACS BSCN directly at BSCN@facs.org.

Recognition as an accredited member of the ACS BSCN demonstrates a program's commitment to the highest standards of care by the bariatric surgeons, allied health team, and hospital. Obesity remains a major health problem, and society needs to do more to prevent and treat the disease. The ACS BSCN establishes guidelines to ensure an infrastructure, multidisciplinary program, and patient preparation process to promote best practices and patient safety. Ω

### *References*


1. Sturm R. Increases in clinically severe obestity in the United States, 1988-2000. *Arch Intern Med.* 2003;163(18):2146-2148.
2. Kelly J, Tarnoff M, Shikora S, et al. Best care recommendations for surgical care in weight loss surgery. *Obes Res.* 2005;13:227-233.
3. Encinosa W, Bernard D, Steiner C, Chen C. Use and costs of bariatric surgery and prescription weight loss medications. *Health Aff.* 2005;24(4)1039-1046.
4. Buchwald H, Avidor Y, Braunwald E, et al. Bariatric surgery: A systematic review and meta-analysis. *JAMA.* 2004;292:1724-1737.
5. Flum D, Dellinger E. Impact of gastric bypass operation on survival: A population based analysis. *J Am Coll Surg.* 2004;199:543-551.
6. Christou N, Sampalis J, Liberman M, et al. Surgery decreases long-term mortality, morbidity, and health care use in morbidly obese patients. *Ann Surg.* 2004;240:3,416-424.
7. Gandsas A, Schweitzer M. Bariatric centers of excellence as another pay-for-performance program. *Laparosc Today.* 2006;5(2):5-10.



***Dr. Schirmer** is Chair of the ACS Bariatric Surgery Center Network. He is professor of surgery, department of surgery, division of general surgery, Duke University, Charlottesville, VA.*

***Dr. Jones** is associate professor, Harvard Medical School, as well as chief, section of minimally invasive surgery, and director, bariatric program, division of general surgery, Beth Israel Deaconess Medical Center, Boston, MA.*

# Appendix 3

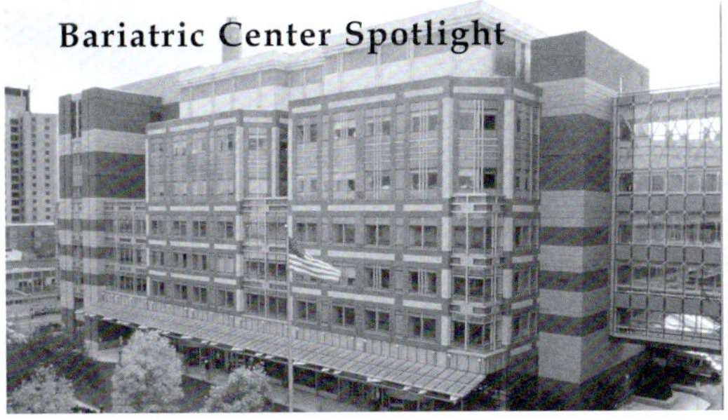


## Beth Israel Deaconess Medical Center (BIDMC)

### Program for Obesity and Weight Loss Surgery

**TELL US ABOUT THE ROLES AND RESPONSIBILITIES OF THE LEAD STAFF AT YOUR FACILITY.**

Over 30 years ago, Dr. George Blackburn laid the groundwork for bariatric surgery in New England and the development of our comprehensive, team-oriented program at Beth Israel Deaconess Medical Center (BIDMC). Currently, he continues his efforts as our senior surgical advisor. Dr. Daniel Jones, Bariatric Program Director, and Dr. Edward Hatchigian, Bariatric Medical Director, work in concert in the care and treatment of people undergoing weight loss surgery.

Dr. Hatchigian began his weight management career with Dr. Blackburn through the Center for the Study of Nutrition Medicine at BIDMC. Now he uses his vast nutrition and medical knowledge to evaluate and oversee patients entering our preoperative screening system and to assist with postoperative medical follow-up.

Dr. Jones was an early champion of laparoscopic gastric bypass and laparoscopic adjustable band in the US, and he has contributed to establishing best practices, training, and accreditation guidelines through the American College of Surgeons Bariatric Committee, American Society for Bariatric Surgery Training Committee, Society of American Gastrointestinal and Endoscopic Surgeons Bariatric Task Force, and locally with the hospital's Patients of Size Committee.

**WHAT IS THE SIZE OF YOUR FACILITY? WHAT DOES IT PHYSICALLY ENCOMPASS?**

A licensed, 585-bed teaching hospital of Harvard Medical School, Beth Israel Deaconess Medical Center is renowned for excellence in patient care, biomedical research, teaching, and community service. Located in the heart of Boston's medical community, it hosts nearly three quarters of a million patient visits annually. BIDMC has a full range of emergency services, including a Level 1 trauma center and roof-top heliport, and the Beth Israel Deaconess Learning Center, which offers patients and families up-to-date health information and online access to research on a wide range of medical conditions.

At BIDMC we have a stand-alone bariatric clinic with offices for bariatrician, nurse, and dietitian visits, and three exam rooms with appropriately sized exam tables and scales. The cabinets are stocked with band fill kits as many of our band adjustments can be done in the office. Conveniently located next to radiology suites, more difficult fills are guided by fluoroscopy.

**PLEASE TELL US ABOUT YOUR STAFF.**

The Obesity Management and Weight Loss Surgery Program has three full-time surgeons who hold academic appointments to Harvard Medical School: Dr. Daniel Jones (Associate Professor), Dr. Benjamin Schneider (Instructor in Surgery), and Dr. Vivian Sanchez (Instructor in Surgery), and medical director Dr. Edward Hatchigian. We also have a senior surgical advisor, Dr. George Blackburn, and a support surgeon, Dr. Jonathan Critchlow, two MIS/Bariatric fellows, and a dedicated multidisciplinary team.

The core team members include three nurses: Angi Walsh, RN, MA, CNOR (Lap Band program coordinator and MIS nurse educator), Michelle Sheppard, RN, BSN, and Anne McNamara, RN, BSN (nursing assessment and preoperative screening coordination); psychotherapist Ronna Casper MEd, LICSW; and two specialized dietitians, Kelly Boyer and June Skoropowski.

Furthermore, we work with the Joslin Clinic for advanced care of diabetic patients; the BeWell Exercise Center for Exercise Physiology; Dan Rooks, PhD, for exercise research; Dr. Loren Borud for plastic surgery and body contouring; and Dr. Stephanie Jones for advancement of specialized anesthesia support. We are fortunate to also have two of our nursing colleagues who have expanded their bariatric expertise as hospital liaisons—Linda DiCenzo, RN,(Practice Manager, Plastic Surgery) and Linda Veglia, RN, RD (Surgical step-down unit and

**Drs. Schneider, Blackburn, Sanchez, Hatchigan, and Jones**

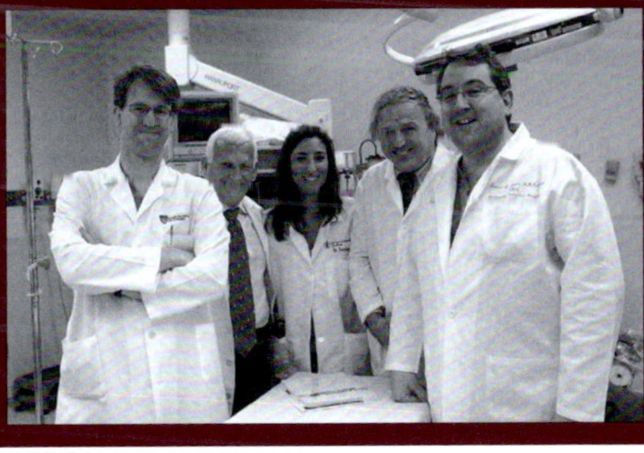

bariatric unit float).

The team at BIDMC has published approximately 600 manuscripts and chapters on nutrition, advances in gastric bypass, laparoscopic adjustable gastric banding, gut physiology, bariatric training, patient safety, and best practices.

**WHAT IS THE NUMBER OF PATIENTS TREATED ON AN ANNUAL BASIS AT YOUR FACILITY?**

In the year 2006–2007, we will evaluate and treat approximately 250 patients. Our surgeons have experience with patients as young as 16 years of age. As an adult hospital we generally see patients 18 to 65 years of age. Patients older than 65 years are considered on a case-by-case basis. Our patients come from the surrounding New England area to be treated by our multidisciplinary team. When we have patients from a great distance, we try to consolidate preoperative appointments and education seminars. We also offer a translated information seminar (presented by Dr. Sanchez) to accommodate our Spanish-speaking patients, a daytime seminar presented by the nurse educator, and discussions, written materials, and videotaped seminars are available for patients of distance.

**HOW IS YOUR FACILITY MANAGED AND BY WHOM?**

Christine Lynch (Bariatric Surgery Division Manager), Eileen Rose, RN (Administrative Manager), and Gina Reidy, RN (Director of Practice Operations), oversee the daily functions of our unit, new staff hiring, and budgets. Staff participates in policy and procedure review, quality improvement, sensitivity training, and patient relations.

**DOES YOUR CENTER HAVE ONE PARTICULAR AREA OF EXPERTISE?**

While we pride ourselves with personalized care for each patient, as a Harvard teaching hospital, BIDMC has been a leader in patient safety and in research advances.

Last summer we hosted an international conference, Patient Safety in Obesity Surgery. This program covered topics in legislation, anesthestic practices, nutritional guidelines, diabetes, media, insurance, risk management, bariatric training for nurses, facilities, and program management. Available as a DVD, the content is currently being updated as a textbook.

George Blackburn spearheaded the Betsy Lehman Center for Risk Reduction, which resulted in best practice guidelines. This report has contributed to American College of Surgeons accreditation criteria, Blue Cross Blue Shield requirements for reimbursement, and Department of Public Health standards in Massachusetts.

BIDMC was the first hospital in he United States to be fully accredited as a level 1-A Bariatric Center by the American College of Surgeons. Dr. Jones serves as a senior ACS site reviewer of bariatric centers.

**PLEASE GIVE A GENERAL SYNOPSIS OF HOW YOUR PATIENTS ARE TREATED WHILE UNDER THE CARE OF YOUR CENTER.**

Our patients are required to attend two general information sessions prior to coming into the program. This gives the potential patient and family a chance to decide if surgical weight management is best for them. Patients are given packets of information or can log onto our website to download an application. Once submitted, Michelle Sheppard, RN, and Anne McNamara, RN, conduct a telephone interview, personalize each patient preoperative assessment, and coordinate studies. Patients are then scheduled to see one of the RNs for a general health history, previous supervised weight loss review, BMI, height/weight, vital signs, EKG, and bioimpedence testing.

**As an adult hospital, BIDMC generally sees patients 18 to 65 years of age.**

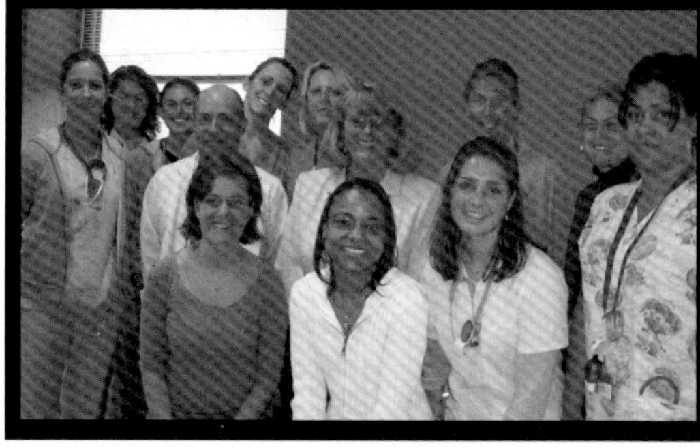

The bariatrician, Edward Hatchigian, MD, conducts a thorough medical evaluation, review of medications, labwork, abdominal ultrasound, cardiac and pulmonary studies, and patient education regarding medical versus surgical weight loss management options. After completing pre-screening appointments with the psychologist and dietitian, the multidisciplinary team discusses each patient's readiness for surgery.

The patient is then scheduled to see the nurse educator, Angi Walsh, RN, the MIS fellow, and the surgeon for preoperative education, short-term goal setting, and the patient contract, which stresses the importance of post-op compliance and follow-up, review of systems and consent. The patient also meets with the administration personnel to schedule preoperative testing and a surgical date and is invited to attend the postoperative support group to be introduced as a peer to other postoperative weight loss surgery patients.

Weight loss surgery is performed in one of two bariatric Endosuites, staffed by a specially trained anesthesia and operating room team. Patients are admitted to our bariatric unit, a dedicated wing of the general surgery floor. Lap-band and bypass patients are discharged on Stage III (full liquid/high-protein/low-sugar) diet for three weeks, then slowly advanced to soft and then full diet during the next 5 to 6 weeks.

Postoperative visits are scheduled with the team at three and eight weeks for advancement of diet; four months; six months; and one year for Roux-en-Y (RNY) patients, or every 2 to 3 months for Lap-band patients. Labwork is repeated at regular intervals during the first year, and annually thereafter.

Communication is maintained with the PCP, diabetologist, and/or other special care provider throughout the process.

**BIDMC was the first hospital in the United States to be fully accredited as a level 1-A Bariatric Center by the American College of Surgeons.**

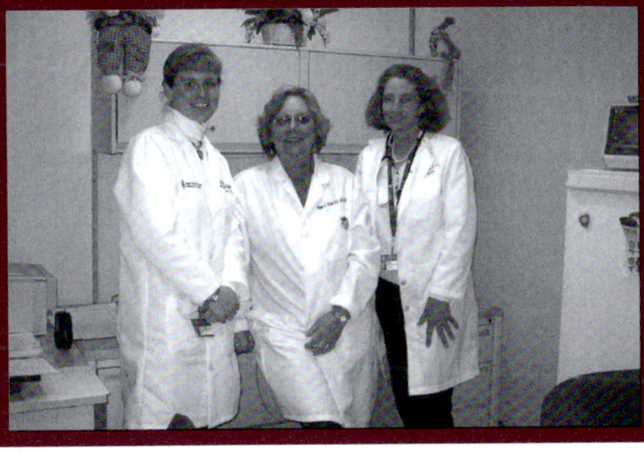

**WHAT ARE SOME OF THE NEW EQUIPMENT, DEVICES, AND PRODUCTS YOU USE?**

We have two state-of-the-art Endosuites for our bariatric procedures. Dr. Jones has developed a series of laparoscopic gastric banding and laparoscopic gastric bypass instruments, including the anvil grasper, band pusher, and hooker.

**WHO HANDLES YOUR PROCEDURE SCHEDULING?**

Our administrative staff schedules our patients through the surgical scheduling office. Nursing and administrative staff schedule any additional appointments. Surgeons have block operating and clinic days. The nurses and dietitians triage patient calls and schedule emergency appointments as needed. We use software that is common to all caregroup locations so that we are able to access off-site lab work, x-rays, and online medical records.

**HOW IS INVENTORY MANAGED IN YOUR FACILITY?**

Supplies are ordered as needed and everyone helps with this task. The banding nurse orders all band supplies as well as requests for special equipment through the OR supplies management team.

**HAVE YOU WITNESSED A SPIKE IN ANY SPECIFIC ELEMENT OF BARIATRIC PATIENTS?**

We have seen a real explosion in the percentage of our patients seeking laparoscopic gastric banding from 4 to 40 percent in the last two years. Whether banding or bypass, almost all of our patients seek the laparoscopic approach.

**HOW HAS MANAGED CARE AFFECTED YOUR FACILITY AND THE CARE THAT IT PROVIDES PATIENTS?**

Managed care means more paperwork and hurdles to providing access to care. In general, it also results in lower reimbursement for physicians and institutions. We just do what is right for the patient. The hospital understands that different patients will have different needs, consume different resources, and have variable hospital stays. We comply with best practice guidelines.

**DOES YOUR FACILITY HAVE AN OUTPATIENT PROGRAM?**

We have a clinic that is ideally located one block from the main hospital and Harvard Medical School. The bariatric clinic has chairs, scales, gowns, and educational materials. Beth Israel Deaconess Medical Center has two multispecialty regional outpatient centers. At this time we do not perform bariatric procedures on an outpatient basis.

**HOW DOES YOUR FACILITY DEAL WITH THE ISSUE OF PATIENT SAFETY AND STAFF SAFETY?**

The Patients of Size Working Committee was established in 2004 to develop a risk assessment and intervention strategy for patients at increased safety risk due to large size. We use several lift and transfer devices, such as Hover mattresses.

**PLEASE DESCRIBE YOUR PATIENT EDUCATION PROGRAM.**

Patients are required to attend two information seminars prior to surgery, conducted by the nurse educator and surgeons, that focus on the entire weight loss surgery journey from medical management to preoperative evaluation, surgical procedures performed, identification and roles of team members, statistics, and outcome studies. Each patient receives an information packet describing the surgical process, nutrition, exercise, and long-term follow-up information. In addition, each patient has a group and individual appointment with the dietitian for nutritional education, and one with the nurse educator for preoperative education prior to surgery.

**WHAT TYPES OF PATIENT SUPPORT PROGRAMS ARE OFFERED AT YOUR FACILITY?**

Support groups are offered twice monthly for all surgical weight loss patients. Facilitated by one of the nurses/dietitians, the meetings are structured around a topic or theme of the month for discussion. Our surgeons and OR and bariatric unit staff will often attend, and family members and referring physicians are invited. The last half of the meeting consists of a breakout session for patients 0 to 12 months postoperative and

**In the last two years, the percentage of BIDMC patients seeking laparoscopic gastric banding has grown from 4 to 40 percent.**

greater with a patient cofacilitator. Our nurse educator has received certification as a support group and success habits facilitator. We are currently expanding our Boston support group to accommodate our MetroWest, North, and South Shore patients in alternate locations.

We also have a monthly online newsletter to help patients stay connected when they cannot attend meetings, and our website includes patient-oriented activities, such as clothing exchange, buddy system, peer-to-peer support activities (shopping, taste-testing new products), and an annual weight loss surgery reunion.

### WHAT LONG-TERM FOLLOW-UP MEASURES ARE PRACTICED AT YOUR FACILITY?

Annual chart audits, quality improvement projects, postoperative questionnaires, and surveys. Our Lap-band database has tracked postoperative weight loss since 2003.

### DO YOU UTILIZE ANY ALTERNATIVE THERAPIES?

In collaboration with gastroenterologists, we have developed novel endoscopic therapies pending FDA approval.

### WHAT QUALITY CONTROL ASSURANCE MEASURES ARE PRACTICED IN YOUR FACILITY?

BIDMC is Joint Commission on Accreditation of Healthcare Organizations (JACHO)-compliant, and staff is required to complete CPR recertification, sensitivity training, and hospital-based competencies on an annual basis. Our bariatric program is Level 1-A certified as an ACS Center of Excellence.

### WHAT TRENDS DO YOU SEE EMERGING?

A significant trend is the increase in the number of laparoscopic adjustable gastric bands performed as an ambulatory procedure.

**The team at BIDMC has published approximately 600 manuscripts and chapters on nutrition, advances in gastric bypass, laparoscopic adjustable gastric banding, gut physiology, bariatric training, patient safety, and best practices.**

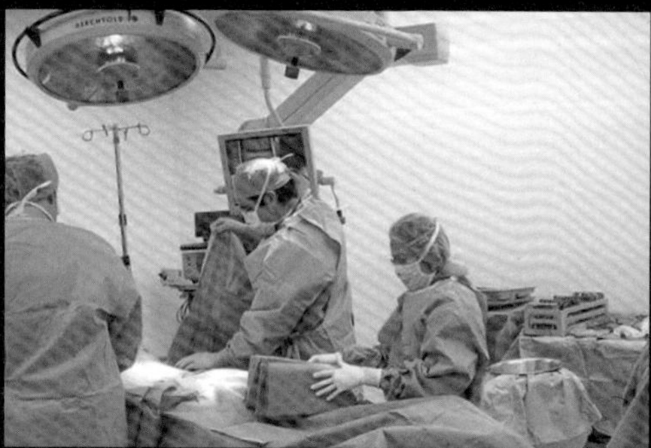

### WHAT TECHNOLOGIES AND EQUIPMENT DO YOU WORK WITH THAT HAVE HELPED YOUR PROGRAM?

We have a state-of-the-art Simulation and Skills Center used by multiple medical/surgical specialties. All medical students, residents, and fellows have mandatory skills checklists and verification of skills prior to advancement. This assures that all healthcare providers are competent. We have also opened our virtual OR and ICU for advanced training of physicians and ICU, ER, anesthesia, and OR staffs.

### WHAT EFFORTS DO YOU MAKE TO MAINTAIN HIPAA COMPLIANCE?

We have web-based HIPAA training and online medical record signoff for employees. Patients are informed of healthcare rights and sign an informed consent. Updated insurance information is done via telephone registration in a separate area of the clinic for confidentiality.

### WHAT MAKES YOUR FACILITY UNIQUE?

Commitment to perioperative education and life long follow-up. We have a strong commitment to staff education, publishing, and research. We are also the official hospital of the Boston Red Sox and have established several community outreach and mentoring programs in partnership with the sports club.

# Index

## C

## H

## N

## Q



## R



## S